Case-Based Lessons in the Management of Complex Hepato-Pancreato-Biliary Surgery

Timothy M. Pawlik · Sharon Weber
T. Clark Gamblin
Editors

Case-Based Lessons in the Management of Complex Hepato-Pancreato-Biliary Surgery

Springer

Editors
Timothy M. Pawlik
The Ohio State Wexner Medical Center
The Ohio State University School of Medicine
Columbus, OH
USA

T. Clark Gamblin
Medical College of Wisconsin
Milwaukee, WI
USA

Sharon Weber
Division of General Surgery
University of Wisconsin-Madison
Madison, WI
USA

ISBN 978-3-319-50867-2 ISBN 978-3-319-50868-9 (eBook)
DOI 10.1007/978-3-319-50868-9

Library of Congress Control Number: 2016959745

Printed on acid-free paper

This Springer imprint is published by Springer Nature
The registered company is Springer International Publishing AG
The registered company address is: Gewerbestrasse 11, 6330 Cham, Switzerland

We dedicate this book to our families and to our patients

Foreword

The only source of knowledge is experience

Albert Einstein (1879–1955)

We learn from our experiences. When faced with unusual and difficult situations in which we have limited experience and are out of our comfort zone, we depend on the experiences of others. This is at the core of training in surgery, where residents and fellows learn from experienced surgeons and mentors. What do you do when you are faced with a patient with a difficult or unusual condition and do not have ready access to a colleague with whom to discuss the case, or even seek assistance with the operation? We depend on the literature.

The editors of this book have assembled in one source an international team of experts in hepato-biliary and pancreatic surgery to share their experiences with the management of difficult Hepato-Pancreato-Biliary (HPB) conditions and new therapeutic alternatives. Collectively, the individual authors have well in excess of 300 years' experience with complex HPB patients. The case study approach is the foundation of this book. It allows the reader to learn from experiences in the management of unique patients and the application of innovative techniques. The case method provides the learner with immediate information concerning pattern recognition of the problem at hand, the pre-operative thinking of the surgeons and, importantly, the intraoperative management and technical approach to the patient. Some of the patients presented are incredibly complex and represent one-of-kind situations, others represent difficult management issues or technical challenges, and still others present controversies in treatment. In addition, the content includes excellent discussions of minimally invasive and robotic approaches.

Whether you are a surgeon in training or an experienced hepato-biliary pancreatic surgeon, I think you will find this text an essential complement to your library.

Columbus, OH

E. Christopher Ellison, MD, FACS
Robert M. Zollinger Professor
Department of Surgery
The Ohio State University College of Medicine

Preface

Hepato-Pancreato-Biliary Surgery is a field filled with unique challenges and requires perspective for rare cases. Such cases commonly demand a set of complex skills. While cases are not routine, the clinical scenarios demand an expertise and insight to offer patients state of the art therapy.

Our goal was to create a case based learning resource based on authorities in the field who share their patients and experience with the reader. Each chapter contains relevant facts and applies expert lessons learned to a particular patient case. Perioperative and intraoperative decisions are discussed in a manner that a colleague would share with a partner, and key points or takeaways are featured in each chapter. The book contains a diverse team of renowned international authorities to guide the reader through challenging HPB topics.

It is our hope that this book will serve as a resource that is often visited by surgeons at all stages of their career. We also hope to stimulate students, residents and fellows regarding the breadth and depth of their knowledge in HPB surgery.

Columbus, OH, USA — Timothy M. Pawlik
Madison, USA — Sharon Weber
Milwaukee, USA — T. Clark Gamblin

Contents

Contributors

Daniel Abbott University of Wisconsin School of Medicine and Public Health, Madison, WI, USA

Victoria Ardiles Department of HPB Surgery, Hospital Italiano de Buenos Aires, Buenos Aires, Argentina

Francesco Ardito UOC Chirurgia Epatobiliare, Fondazione Policlinico Universitario A. Gemelli, Rome, Italy

Jean-Michel Aubin Department of Surgery, Foothills Medical Centre, University of Calgary, Calgary, AB, Canada

Daniel Azoulay Department of HPB Surgery and Liver Transplant Unit, Henri Mondor Hospital, Creteil, France

Chad G. Ball Department of Surgery, Foothills Medical Centre, University of Calgary, Calgary, AB, Canada

Domenico Bassi UOC Chirurgia Epatobiliare e Trapianti Epatici, Università degli Studi di Padova, Padua, Italy

Jennifer Berumen Department of Surgery, University of California, San Diego, La Jolla, CA, USA

Riccardo Boetto UOC Chirurgia Epatobiliare e Trapianti Epatici, Università degli Studi di Padova, Padua, Italy

Christophe Bourdeaux Department of Digestive Diseases, Institut Mutualiste Montsouris, Université Paris Descartes, Paris, France

Richard A. Burkhart Department of Surgery, The Johns Hopkins Hospital, Baltimore, MD, USA

Alex Chang Department of Surgery, University of Cincinnati, Cincinnati, OH, USA

Xiao-ping Chen Tongji Hospital, Tongji Medical College, Huazhong University of Science and Technology, Wuhan, China

John D. Christein Department of Surgery, University of Alabama at Birmingham (UAB), Birmingham, AL, USA

Kathleen K. Christians Department of Surgery, Medical College of Wisconsin/Froedtert Hospital, Milwaukee, WI, USA

Umberto Cillo UOC Chirurgia Epatobiliare e Trapianti Epatici, Università degli Studi di Padova, Padua, Italy

Philippe Compagnon Department of HPB Surgery and Liver Transplant Unit, Henri Mondor Hospital, Creteil, France

Christina L. Costantino Department of Surgery, Massachusetts General Hospital, Boston, MA, USA

Elijah Dixon Foothills Medical Centre, University of Calgary, Calgary, AB, Canada

Michael I. D'Angelica Department of Surgery, Division of Hepatopancreatobiliary Surgery, Memorial Sloan Kettering Cancer Center, New York, NY, USA

Douglas B. Evans Department of Surgery, Medical College of Wisconsin/Froedtert Hospital, Milwaukee, WI, USA

Benjamin D. Ferguson Department of Surgery, University of Chicago, Chicago, IL, USA

Alessandro Ferrero Division of General and Oncologic Surgery, Mauriziano Hospital "Umberto I", Torino, Italy

Cristina R. Ferrone Massachusetts General Hospital, Boston, MA, USA

Douglas L. Fraker Department of Surgery, University of Pennsylvania, Philadelphia, PA, USA

David Fuks Department of Digestive Diseases, Institut Mutualiste Montsouris, Université Paris Descartes, Paris, France

Robert Gandy Department of Hepatobiliary and Upper Gastrointestinal Surgery, Institute of Academic Surgery, Royal Prince Alfred Hospital, Camperdown, NSW, Australia

Brice Gayet Department of Digestive Diseases, Institut Mutualiste Montsouris, Université Paris Descartes, Paris, France

Felice Giuliante UOC Chirurgia Epatobiliare, Fondazione Policlinico Universitario A. Gemelli, Rome, Italy

Concepcion Gomez Gavara Department of HPB Surgery and Liver Transplant Unit, Henri Mondor Hospital, Creteil, France

Bruno A. Gonzalez-Nolasco Department of General Surgery, National Institute of Medical Sciences and Nutrition "Salvador Zubiran", Mexico City, Mexico

Ryan T. Groeschl Department of Surgery, Mayo Clinic, Rochester, MN, USA

Salila S. Hashmi Emory University Hospital School of Medicine, Atlanta, GA, USA

Alan Hemming Department of Surgery, University of California, San Diego, La Jolla, CA, USA

O. Joe Hines Department of Surgery, David Geffen School of Medicine at UCLA, Los Angeles, CA, USA

Melissa E. Hogg Department of Surgery, Division of Surgical Oncology, University of Pittsburgh Medical Center, Pittsburgh, PA, USA

Caroline C. Jadlowiec Division of Transplantation Surgery and Department of Surgery, Mayo Clinic, Rochester, MN, USA

Robert T. Jensen Digestive Diseases Branch, National Institutes of Health, Bethesda, MD, USA

E. John Harris Division of Vascular Surgery, Stanford University Medical Center, Stanford, CA, USA

Gyulnara G. Kasumova Department of Surgery, Beth Israel Deaconess Medical Center, Harvard Medical School, Boston, MA, USA

David A. Kooby Emory University School of Medicine, Atlanta, GA, USA

Eylon Lahat Department of HPB Surgery and Liver Transplant Unit, Henri Mondor Hospital, Creteil, France

William P. Lancaster Department of Surgery, Indiana University, Indianapolis, IN, USA

Russell C. Langan Department of Surgery, Division of Surgical Oncology, Memorial Sloan Kettering Cancer Center, New York, NY, USA

Steven K. Libutti Montefiore Medical Center and Albert Einstein College of Medicine, Bronx, NY, USA

Chetana Lim Department of HPB Surgery and Liver Transplant Unit, Henri Mondor Hospital, Creteil, France

Jeffrey B. Matthews The University of Chicago, Chicago, IL, USA

Michael McCall Department of Surgery, Division of General Surgery, Foothills Medical Centre, University of Calgary, Calgary, AB, Canada

Emmanuel Melloul Mount Sinai Liver Cancer Program, Recanati/Miller Transplantation Institute Icahn School of Medicine at Mount Sinai, New York, NY, USA

Miguel-Angel Mercado Department of General Surgery, National Institute of Medical Sciences and Nutrition "Salvador Zubiran", Mexico City, Mexico

Jennifer L. Miller-Ocuin Department of Surgery, University of Pittsburgh Medical Center, Pittsburgh, PA, USA

Anubhav Mittal Royal North Shore Hospital, St Leonards, NSW, Australia

Katherine A. Morgan Medical University of South Carolina, Charleston, SC, USA

David M. Nagorney Department of Surgery, Mayo Clinic, Rochester, MN, USA

Attila Nakeeb Indiana University School of Medicine, Indianapolis, IN, USA

Jeffrey A. Norton Department of Sugery, Stanford University Medical Center, Stanford, CA, USA

Lee M. Ocuin Division of Surgical Oncology, Department of Surgery, University of Pittsburgh Medical Center, Pittsburgh, PA, USA

Michael Ossesis Department of HPB Surgery and Liver Transplant Unit, Henri Mondor Hospital, Creteil, France

Sanjay Pandanaboyana Department of Hepatobiliary and Pancreatic Surgery, Auckland City Hospital, Auckland, New Zealand

Rowan W. Parks Department of Clinical Surgery, University of Edinburgh, Royal Infirmary of Edinburgh, Edinburgh, UK

Henry A. Pitt Department of Surgery, Temple University Health System, Philadelphia, PA, USA

Dario Ribero Division of Hepatobilio-Pancreatic Surgery, European Institute of Oncology, Milano, Italy

J. Robert O'Neill Department of Clinical Surgery, University of Edinburgh, Royal Infirmary of Edinburgh, Edinburgh, UK

Agostino Maria De Rose UOC Chirurgia Epatobiliare, Fondazione Policlinico Universitario A. Gemelli, Rome, Italy

Charles B. Rosen Division of Transplantation Surgery and Department of Surgery, Mayo Clinic, Rochester, MN, USA

Yoshihiro Sakamoto Hepato-Biliary-Pancreatic Surgery Division, University of Tokyo Hospital, Tokyo, Japan

Chady Salloum Department of HPB Surgery and Liver Transplant Unit, Henri Mondor Hospital, Creteil, France

Charbel Sandroussi Department of Hepatobiliary and Upper Gastrointestinal Surgery, Institute of Academic Surgery, Royal Prince Alfred Hospital, Camperdown, NSW, Australia

Eduardo de Santibañes Department of HPB Surgery, Hospital Italiano de Buenos Aires, Buenos Aires, Argentina

Martin de Santibañes Department of HPB Surgery, Hospital Italiano de Buenos Aires, Buenos Aires, Argentina

Myron E. Schwartz Mount Sinai Liver Cancer Program, Recanati/Miller Transplantation Institute Icahn School of Medicine at Mount Sinai, New York, NY, USA

Matteo Serenari Department of HPB Surgery, Hospital Italiano de Buenos Aires, Buenos Aires, Argentina

Junichi Shindoh Hepatobiliary-Pancreatic Surgery Division, Department of Gastroenterological Surgery, Toranomon Hospital, Tokyo, Japan

Alexander P. Stark Department of Surgery, David Geffen School of Medicine at UCLA, Los Angeles, CA, USA

Parissa Tabrizian Mount Sinai Liver Cancer Program, Recanati/Miller Transplantation Institute Icahn School of Medicine at Mount Sinai, New York, NY, USA

Roberto Lo Tesoriere Division of General and Oncologic Surgery, Mauriziano Hospital "Umberto I", Torino, Italy

Jennifer F. Tseng Department of Surgery, Beth Israel Deaconess Medical Center, Harvard Medical School, Boston, MA, USA

Allan Tsung Division of Hepatobiliary and Pancreatic Surgery, Department of Surgery, University of Pittsburgh Medical Center, Pittsburgh, PA, USA

Mario Vilatoba Department of General Surgery, National Institute of Medical Sciences and Nutrition "Salvador Zubiran", Mexico City, Mexico

Tyler S. Wahl Department of Surgery, University of Alabama at Birmingham (UAB), Birmingham, AL, USA

Go Wakabayashi Ageo Central General Hospital, Ageo, Japan

Matthew J. Weiss Department of Surgery, The Johns Hopkins Hospital, Baltimore, MD, USA

John Albert Windsor HBP/Upper GI Unit, Department of General Surgery, Auckland City Hospital, Auckland, New Zealand

George Younan Department of Surgery, Medical College of Wisconsin/Froedtert Hospital, Milwaukee, WI, USA

Herbert J. Zeh III Department of Surgery, Division of Surgical Oncology, University of Pittsburgh Medical Center, Pittsburgh, PA, USA

Bi-xiang Zhang Tongji Hospital, Tongji Medical College, Huazhong University of Science and Technology, Wuhan, China

Bin-hao Zhang Tongji Hospital, Tongji Medical College, Huazhong University of Science and Technology, Wuhan, China

Amer H. Zureikat Department of Surgery, Division of Surgical Oncology, University of Pittsburgh Medical Center, Pittsburgh, PA, USA

Nicholas J. Zyromski Indiana University School of Medicine, Indianapolis, IN, USA

Abbreviations

AA	Anterior approach
AC	Acute cholecystitis
ADC	Apparent diffusion coefficient
AFP	Alpha-fetoprotein
AGA	American Gastroenterological Association
ALK	Alkaline phosphatase
ALPPS	Associating liver partition and portal vein ligation for staged hepatectomy
ALTPS	Associating liver tourniquet and portal ligation for staged hepatectomy
APBJ	Abnormal pancreatico–biliary junction
ARHA	Accessory of the right hepatic arteries
ASA	American Society of Anesthesiologists
AST, ALT	Serum aspartate and alanine aminotransferases
BCLC	Barcelona clinic liver cancer
BD-IPMN	Branch-duct intraductal papillary mucinous neoplasm
BMI	Body mass index
BW	Body weight
CA 19-9	Carbohydrate antigen 19-9
CA	Carbohydrate antigen
CA	Celiac artery/ies
CABG	Coronary artery bypass graft
CALI	Chemotherapy-induced liver injury
CASH	Chemotherapy-associated steatohepatitis
CBD	Common bile duct
CEA	Carcinoembryonic antigen
CHA	Common hepatic artery/ies
COPD	Chronic obstructive pulmonary disease
CP	Chronic pancreatitis
CRLM	Colorectal liver metastases
CT	Computed tomography
CV	Caudate vein
CVP	Central venous pressure

DCD	Donation after cardiac death
DFS	Disease-free survival
DGE	Delayed gastric emptying
DSS	Disease-specific survival
DVT	Deep vein thrombosis
DW-MRI	Diffusion-weighted MRI
EC	Emphasematous cholecystitis
ED	Emergency department
EGD	Esophagogastroduodenoscopy
ERAS	Enhanced recovery after surgery
ERC	Endoscopic retrograde cholangiography
ERCP	Endoscopic retrograde cholangiopancreatography
EUS	Endoscopic ultrasound
EUS-FNA	Endoscopic ultrasound and fine needle aspiration
FAMMMS	Familial atypical multiple mole melanoma syndrome
FDA	Food and Drug Administration
FFP	Fresh frozen plasma
FISH	Fluorescence in situ hybridization
FLR	Future liver remnant
FNA	Fine-needle aspiration
GC	Gangrenous cholecystitis
GDA	Gastroduodenal artery
Gem/Cis	Gemcitabine and cisplatin
GGT	Gamma glutamyl transferase
HALS	Hand-assisted laparoscopic surgery
HBV	Hepatitis B virus
HC	Hilar cholangiocarcinoma
HCC	Hepatocellular carcinoma
HPB	Hepato-pancreato-biliary
HTK	Histidine-tryptophan-ketoglutarate
IBC	Intrahepatic biliary cystadenoma
IBCC	Intrahepatic biliary cystadenocarcinoma
ICG	Indocyanine green
ICG	International Association of Pancreatology Consensus Guidelines
IDUS	Intraductal ultrasound
IJ	Internal jugular
INR	International normalized ratio
IOUS	Intraoperative ultrasonography
IRHV	Inferior right hepatic vein
ISGPF	International Study Group on Pancreatic Fistula
ISGPS	International Study Group of Pancreatic Surgery
IVC	Inferior vena cava
LCRT	Long-course radiation therapy
LDP	Laparoscopic distal pancreatectomy
LFTs	Liver function test(s)

LHM	Liver hanging manoeuver
LHV	Left hepatic vein
LLR	Laparoscopic liver resection
MARS	Molecular Adsorbents Recirculating System
MDC	Multidisciplinary conference
MDCT	Multidetector computed tomography
MD-IPMN	Main-duct intraductal papillary neoplasm
MHV	Middle hepatic vein
MIS	Minimally invasive surgery/surgical (approaches)
MRCP	Magnetic resonance cholangiopancreatography
MRHV	Middle right hepatic vein
MRI	Magnetic resonance imaging
NCCN	National Comprehensive Cancer Network
NED	No evidence of disease
NET	Neuroendocrine tumors
OLR	Open liver resection
OS	Overall survival
PD	Pancreaticoduodenectomy
PDA	Pancreatic ductal adenocarcinoma
PF	Pancreatic fistula
PNET(s)	Pancreatic neuroendocrine tumor(s)
POD	Postoperative day
PPT	Partial parenchymal transection
PSA	Pseudoaneurysm
PSC	Primary sclerosing cholangitis
PTBD	Percutaneous transhepatic biliary drainage
PTC	Percutaneous transhepatic cholangiography
PTFE	Polytetrafluoroethylene
PTPE	Percutaneous transhepatic portal vein embolization
PVE	Portal vein embolization
PVL	Portal vein ligation
PVO	Portal vein occlusion
RALPP	Radio-frequency-assisted liver partition with portal vein ligation
RAMPS	Radical antegrade modular pancreatosplenectomy
RCC	Renal cell carcinoma
RFA	Radiofrequency ablation
RHV	Right hepatic vein
RPV	Right portal vein
RRHA	Replacement of the right hepatic arteries
SA	Splenic artery
SAPE	Sentinel acute pancreatitis event
SBNET	Small bowel neuroendocrine tumors
SBRT	Stereotactic body radiotherapy
SHV	Short hepatic vein
SIRS	Systemic inflammatory response syndrome

SMA	Superior mesenteric artery
SMPV	Superior mesenteric-portal vein
SMV	Superior mesenteric vein
SMV-PV-SVV	Superior mesenteric vein–portal vein–splenic vein confluence
SV	Splenic vein
SVT	Splenic vein thrombosis
TACE	Transarterial chemoembolization
TG	Tokyo Guidelines
TIGAR-O	Toxic/metabolic, idiopathic, genetic, autoimmune, recurrent pancreatitis, obstructive
TLV	Total liver volume
TNM	Tumor node metastasis
TPIAT	Total pancreatectomy with islet autotransplantation
TPN	Total parenteral nutrition
TSH	Two-stage hepatectomy
TVE	Total vascular exclusion
US	Ultrasound
UW	University of Wisconsin [solution]
VARD	Video-assisted retroperitoneal debridement
WOPN	Walled-off pancreatic necrosis

Part I
Liver

Resection of Large Hepatocellular Carcinoma: Hanging Technique

1

Bin-hao Zhang, Bi-xiang Zhang and Xiao-ping Chen

Introduction

About 70% of the tumors in patients diagnosed with hepatocellular carcinoma (HCC) are categorized as either large (5–10 cm in diameter) or huge (larger than 10 cm in diameter). A prevalent belief in the medical community is that large and huge tumors cannot be removed.

We hypothesized that while the resection of large liver tumors had proved difficult in clinical practice, the procedure was safe in theory. In anatomic resections of equal size, which involve removing liver tissue along functional lines, less tumor-free tissue was resected for larger tumors and more tumor-free tissue was resected for smaller tumors. In the 1980s, intraoperative blood loss from liver resection was reported to be around 2,000 ml and the mortality rate caused by intraoperative massive hemorrhage was about 10%. The liver-hanging maneuver (LHM) is one of the improved techniques to reduce bleeding and mortality. Improved techniques reduced intraoperative blood loss during liver resection for large and huge tumors to around 250 ml and caused the mortality rate to drop below 0.7%.

Conventionally, for right hepatectomy, full mobilization of the right hemi-liver is necessary before liver parenchymal transaction [1, 2]. This approach is not always feasible in patients with huge tumor or diaphragmatic tumor invasion. For large tumors, even when full liver mobilization is technically possible, several increased risks are observed, including tumor rupture from excessive pull, tumor cell dissemination from excessive manipulation, and massive bleeding from tear of short hepatic veins from the inferior vena cava (IVC). More surgeons now use an

B. Zhang · B. Zhang · X. Chen (✉)
Tongji Hospital, Tongji Medical College, Huazhong University of Science and Technology, 430030 Wuhan, China
e-mail: chenxp@medmail.com.cn

T.M. Pawlik et al. (eds.), *Case-Based Lessons in the Management of Complex Hepato-Pancreato-Biliary Surgery*, DOI 10.1007/978-3-319-50868-9_1

anterior approach (AA) for these patients, with parenchymal transection starting from the anterior surface of the liver toward the IVC [1, 2]. This anterior approach has a problem of controlling bleeding from the deeper liver parenchymal tissue because of poor exposure.

To overcome this problem, LHM was proposed by surgeons, allowing surgeons to hang the liver during right hepatectomies without primary liver mobilization.

Belghiti et al. [3] proposed a LHM using a tape to pass through the retrohepatic space between the anterior surface of the IVC and the liver parenchyma. The most important step for this maneuver is the dissection of the anterior plane of the IVC, which is a blind procedure deep in the retrohepatic space. Several short hepatic veins drain directly from the liver into the IVC. These veins vary in size, number, and position. The retrohepatic IVC often becomes compressed or bent in cirrhosis, which increases the risk of injury to the IVC and its branches during the blind dissection. A success rate of 80–92% for blind retrohepatic dissection and a massive bleeding rate caused by injured short hepatic veins of 4–6% have been reported [4–6], which explains why some surgeons are still reluctant to use this technique.

The liver double-hanging maneuver was proposed to develop a retrohepatic tunnel on the right side of the IVC [7]. The tunnel goes through a true avascular space that contains loose connective tissues only. This improved double-hanging maneuver is more safe and easy.

LHM has been reported to have numerous advantages, especially in terms of shortened operative time and reduced blood loss. Moreover, the LHM avoids liver rotation with lower risk for tumor dissemination and higher possibilities of oncologic benefits, helps to reduce remnant liver manipulation with potential improvement in postoperative liver function, and allows better exposure and hemostasis of the deeper section plane with safer IVC protection. Additionally, the tension on the elastic tape would help to obtain a linearly cut surface and would avoid the zigzag manner, thereby contributing to protection of the IVC from surgical injury. Furthermore, the hepatectomies in cases of huge tumors with diaphragm adhesions would be facilitated.

Belghiti-Hanging Maneuver

The liver is exposed through an abdominal incision using either a bilateral subcostal or a J-shaped incision. After performing intraoperative ultrasonography, confirming the absence of tumor contact toward the IVC, a cholecystectomy is performed and the portal pedicle encircled. The upper surface of the liver is exposed up to the anterior surface of the suprahepatic IVC. The space between the right and middle hepatic veins is dissected on 2 cm downward. Without any mobilization of the right liver, the hilum's tape is pulled upward and to the left to allow exposure of the anterior surface of the infrahepatic portion of the IVC. If present, a vein of the caudate process is ligated and divided, and a right inferior hepatic vein is dissected but not ligated.

The most important step of this maneuver is the dissection of the anterior plane of the IVC. The dissection starts with a long vascular clamp posterior to the caudate lobe on the left side of the right inferior hepatic vein, if present, proceeding cranially with great care along the middle plane of the IVC toward the space between the right and middle hepatic veins previously dissected. After 4–6 cm of blind dissection the clamp appears between the right and middle hepatic veins (Fig. 1.1). A tape is seized with the clamp and passed around the hepatic parenchyma. This allows the elevation of the liver away from the anterior surface of the IVC. Before the parenchymal transection, the right pedicle was divided, devascularizing the right liver. The parenchymal transection is conducted from the anterior surface down to the posterior plane in front of the IVC. During parenchymal division, upward traction on the tape-hanging maneuver leads to follow the direct plane and facilitates the exposure and hemostasis of the deeper parenchymal plane in front of the IVC (Fig. 1.1). After completing the exposure of the anterior surface of the IVC, the right side of the IVC is dissected with division and ligation of the inferior hepatic veins and the IVC ligament. Then the trunk of the right hepatic vein is either stapled with a vascular stapler or divided between vascular clamps and oversewn. The coronary and right triangular ligaments are then transected and the specimen removed.

The Belghiti's LHM prerequisite is the existence of a longitudinal avascular plane between the IVC and the liver (Fig. 1.2), which was first anatomically suggested by Couinaud in 1981 [8, 9]. However, 7–15% of this channel passage is not truly avascular but only vascularized by lower density of veins [10].

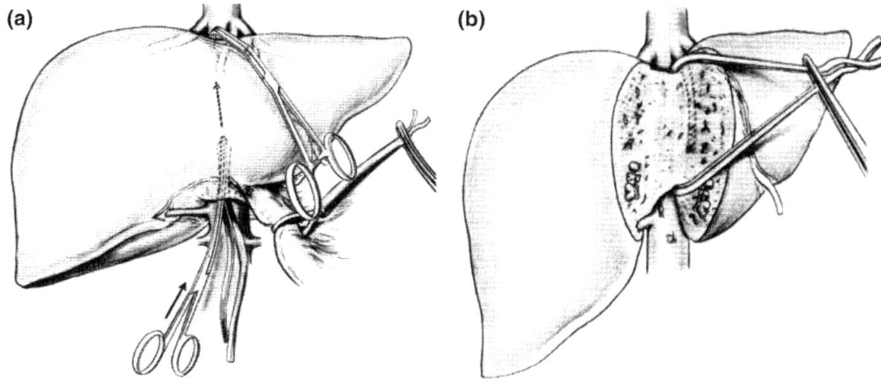

Fig. 1.1 Belghiti's liver-hanging maneuver. **a** The most important dissection time is the blind passage of a long vascular clamp inserted along the midline of the anterior surface of the vena cava and on the left side of the inferior right hepatic vein, if present, **b** proceeding cranially up to the space between the right and the middle hepatic vein trunks. Reprinted from J Am Coll Surg 193; Belghiti J, Guevera OA, Noun R, Saldinger PF, Kianmanesh R. Liver-hanging maneuver: a safe approach to right hepatectomy without liver mobiliztion. p.109–111; copyright © 2001; with permission from Elsevier

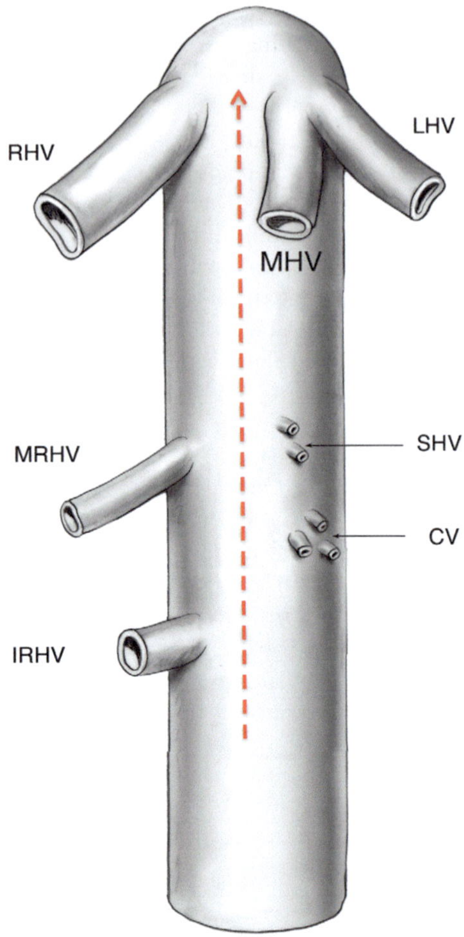

Fig. 1.2 Direction and position for the clamp during Belghiti's liver-hanging maneuver. *RHV* right hepatic vein; *LHV* left hepatic vein; *MHV* middle hepatic vein; *SHV* short hepatic vein; *CV* caudate vein; *MRHV* middle right hepatic vein; *IRHV* inferior right hepatic vein. Reprinted from Am J Surg 193; Gaujoux S, Douard R, Ettorre GM, Delmas V, Chevallier J-M, Cugnenc P-H. Liver-hanging maneuver: an anatomic and a clinical review. p.488–492; copyright © 2007; with permission from Elsevier

Belghiti's LHM uses a tape to pass through the retrohepatic tunnel between the anterior surface of the inferior vena cava (IVC) and the liver parenchyma. This technique has been found useful in selected patients who undergo left or right hepatectomy. The key to this maneuver is the blind dissection of the retrohepatic space anterior to the IVC using a long vascular clamp. After blind dissection starting inferiorly, the clamp appears between the right and the middle hepatic veins. A tape is seized with the clamp and is passed through the retrohepatic tunnel. During parenchymal division, upward traction on this tape around the liver contributes to better exposure and hemostasis of the deeper hepatic parenchyma in front of the IVC. Many surgeons are still reluctant to use this maneuver. Some consider it too complicated and difficult, whereas others are afraid of bleeding from an injured short hepatic vein during retrohepatic dissection, the reported incidence of which is about 4–6% [4–6].

To overcome these difficulties, a modification of this technique—the liver double-hanging maneuver—was devised. This technique has the advantage of being technically simple and safe.

Chen's Double-Hanging Maneuver

The liver is exposed through a right subcostal incision with midline extension, which can be extended to the left side for better exposure if necessary. The ligamentum teres and the falciform ligament are dissected. A tape is placed around the duodenohepatic ligament and the infrahepatic IVC, respectively (Fig. 1.3). These tapes can be used to control hemorrhage if necessary. The peritoneum on the right side of the IVC just inferior to the liver is open to expose the right adrenal gland. The operator then uses his/her right index finger to dissect the space from below upward between the hepatic parenchyma and the anterior and superior edge of the right adrenal gland, and then along the right side of the IVC.

The right coronary ligament is open suprahepatically on the right side of the IVC for 2–3 cm. The operator uses his/her left index finger to dissect the retrohepatic space from above downward along the right side of the IVC. The retrohepatic tunnel is built when the fingers touch each other. A kidney pedicle forceps is used to place two tapes around the liver for liver suspension. One tape is pulled to the right, and the other is pulled to the left. Liver transection is performed along a plane to the right of the middle hepatic vein as determined by intraoperative ultrasound. The liver double-hanging maneuver contributes to better exposure of the operative fields and is easier to manipulate during liver parenchymal transection (Fig. 1.4).

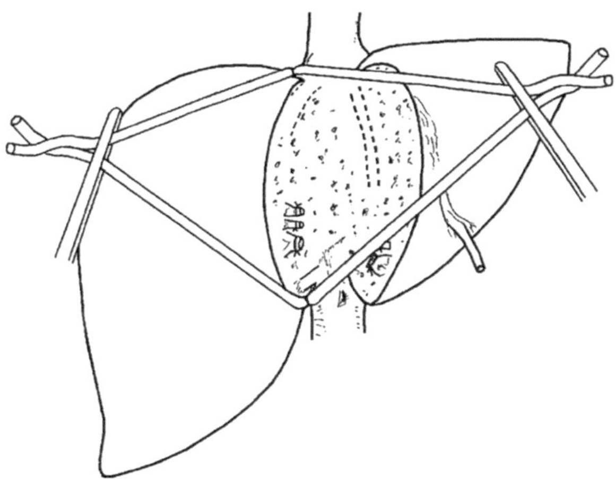

Fig. 1.3 Liver double-hanging maneuver. Reprinted from Surgery 144; from Chen XP, Zhang WG, Lau WY, Qiu FZ. Right hepactectomy using the liver double-hanging maneuver through the retrohepatic avascular tunnel on the right of the inferior vena cava. p. 830–833; copyright © 2008; with permission from Elsevier

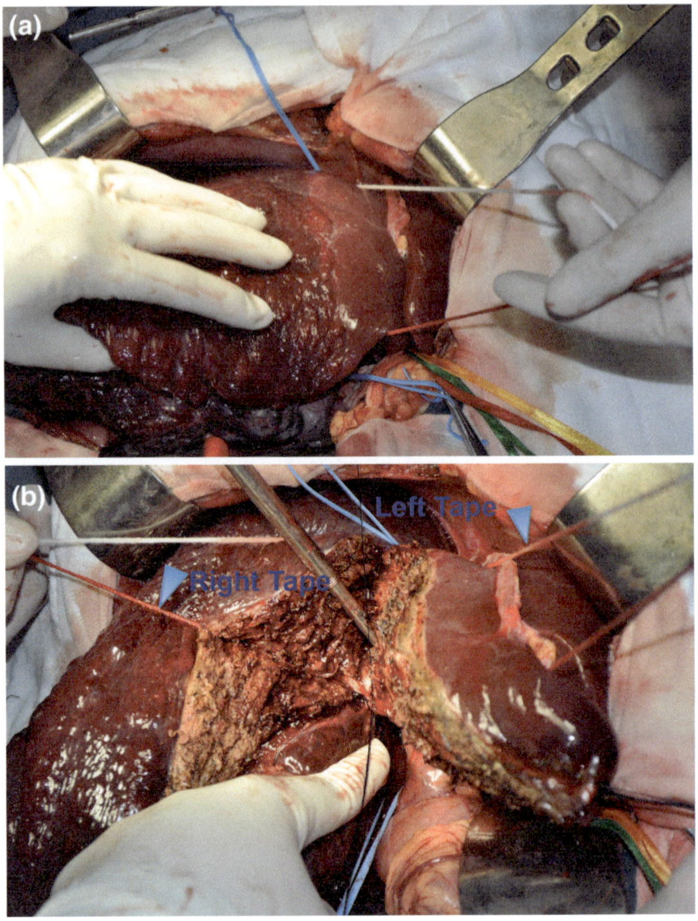

Fig. 1.4 Chen's liver double-hanging maneuver during surgery. The two-hanging tapes were used to guide the transection plane, control bleeding, minimize tumor touch, and protect the IVC. Figure A is reprinted from Surgery 144; Chen XP, Zhang WG, Lau WY, Qiu FZ. Right hepactectomy using the liver double-hanging maneuver through the retrohepatic avascular tunnel on the right of the inferior vena cava. p. 830–833; copyright © 2008; with permission from Elsevier

When the liver parenchymal transection reaches to the right hepatic vein, the origin of the right hepatic vein from the IVC is dissected, doubly ligated, and divided. Liver transection is then carried out along the right border of the IVC, which divides the caudate process and then ligates and divides the short hepatic veins.

In this improved technique, the tunnel goes through a true avascular space that contains loose connective tissues only. The right adrenal grand is an important anatomic structure in this retrohepatic space. If it is not injured, then the risk of bleeding is very low. During the dissection of the retrohepatic tunnel, the operator should keep his or her index finger close to the back of the liver. This maneuver is simple and safe because blind dissection of the space between the right and middle hepatic veins is not needed.

In this technique of right hepatectomy, the entire caudate lobe is left intact, whereas in Belghiti's liver-hanging technique, parts of the paracaval portion and the caudate process are resected. Although the difference in the amount of liver tissue resected between these two techniques is minimal, Chen's technique represents a right hepatectomy, which is more correct anatomically.

In conclusion, the liver double-hanging maneuver for major right hepatectomy has several advantages: First, the operator can feel the retrohepatic tissues with the index fingers, which is safer than blind dissection using forceps. Second, it is not necessary to dissect between the right and the middle hepatic veins. Third, a true avascular space that contains loose connective tissue exists only behind the liver parenchyma on the right side of the IVC. The success rate of tunneling through this retrohepatic space is 100%. Fourth, the leftward and rightward traction on the tapes contributes to better exposure of the deeper parenchymal tissue during liver transection. Tightening the tapes helps to control bleeding from the hepatic transection plane, especially for bleeding coming from branches of the hepatic veins. In conclusion, the liver double-hanging maneuver through the retrohepatic tunnel on the right side of the IVC is a safe and easy procedure.

Modified double-hanging maneuver, namely single-hanging tape on the remnant side, may be applied to guide the transection plane during right hemi-hepatectomy when the liver can be exposed well (Fig. 1.5). When the abdominal cavity has enough space to expose the liver, or when the right liver lobe could be partially mobilized, the right tape is not necessary in some cases. In this condition, the single left tape is used to guide the transection plane and protect the IVC. This single-hanging maneuver through the retrohepatic avascular tunnel on the right of the IVC has also been applied successfully to laparoscopic or robotic-assisted laparoscopic right hemi-hepatectomy in more than 100 cases in our center (Fig. 1.5).

Case Presentation

A 68-year-old woman, who is a hepatitis B virus (HBV) carrier, claimed abdominal distension, without jaundice or fever. No family or genetic history was found. She had hepatitis B virus infection, but had not accepted any therapy before admission. Neither history of cigarette smoking nor alcohol drinking was found. Preoperative computed tomography (CT) revealed huge HCC in the right lobe of the liver, with suspected diaphragm invasion. Neither intrahepatic metastasis nor lymphonode metastasis was shown in CT scanning. It also showed suspected tumor thrombus in the right branch of the portal vein, but tumor pressure of the portal vein could not be excluded (Fig. 1.6). However, ultrasonography did not show portal vein tumor thrombus. Preoperative biochemical examinations revealed AFP: 8760 ng/ml, HBV-DNA 3.43×10^3 copies/ml and Child-Pugh A grade.

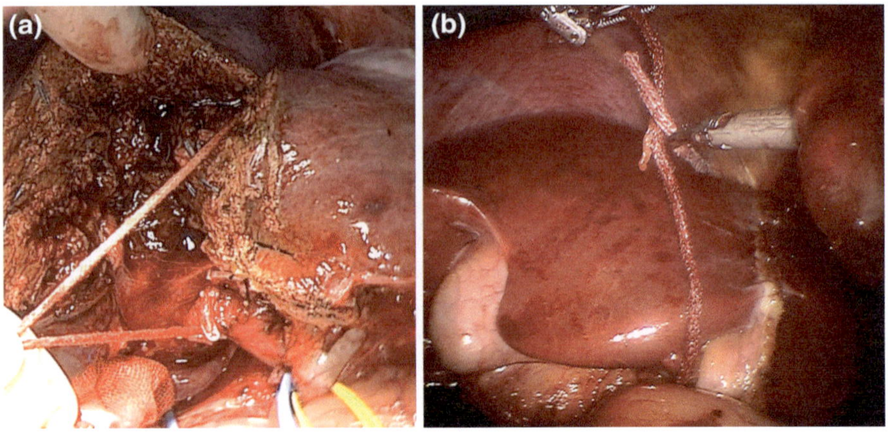

Fig. 1.5 Modified double-hanging maneuver. **a** Single-hanging tape on the remnant side was applied to guide the transection plane and protect the IVC. **b** The single-hanging maneuver through the retrohepatic avascular tunnel on the right of the IVC was applied to robotic-assisted laparoscopic right hemi-hepatectomy

Our Management

1. Evaluation of the Remnant Liver Function
2. Antiviral Therapy with Entecavir
3. Right Hemi-hepatectomy with Chen's Double-Hanging Maneuver

Diagnosis and Assessment

This patient had definite abdominal distention, and more than 10 years HBV history without antiviral treatment. HBV-DNA was positive, and AFP level was extremely high. CT scanning showed specific enhancement of HCC with tumor size of 15 cm. Although portal vein thrombus was suspected with CT scanning, ultrasonography did not show portal vein tumor thrombus. Her physical status scoring is zero, and liver function is Child-Pugh A (score 6). According, HCC (BCLC stage B) was definitely diagnosed.

CT scanning is essential for diagnosis of HCC and evaluating the feasibility of liver resection (Fig. 1.6). The arterial phase showed identical HCC enhancement and suspected diaphragm invasion, but no lymphonode metastasis was presented; the portal vein phase showed suspected tumor pressure or tumor thrombus in the right branch of the portal vein; the delayed phase clearly showed the common branch of middle hepatic vein and left hepatic vein, and indicated that the middle hepatic vein was pressed by the tumor. CT 3-D reconstruction (Fig. 1.7). was performed to evaluate the future liver remnant (FLR).

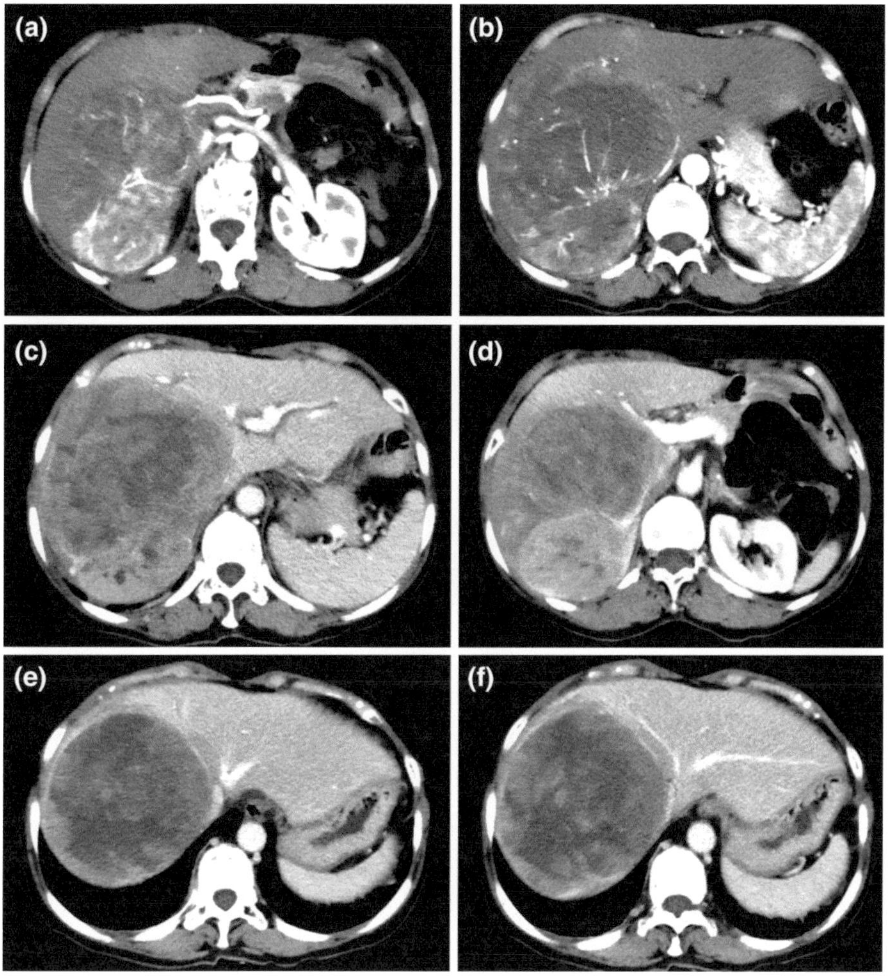

Fig. 1.6 CT scanning for the patient with HCC located in the right lobe. The arterial phase showed identical HCC enhancement (**a**) and suspected diaphragm invasion (**b**), but no lymphonode metastasis was presented; **c**, **d** the portal vein phase showed normal left branch of the portal vein, and suspected tumor pressure or tumor thrombus in the right branch of the portal vein; **e**, **f** the delayed phase showed the common branch of middle hepatic vein and left hepatic vein (**e**), and indicated that the middle hepatic vein was pressed by the tumor (**f**). The right hepatic vein could not be distinguished, probably was circled or pressed by the tumor

FLR/standardized liver volume (SLV) ratio > 20% was considered safe hepatectomy for patients with normal liver function, but >31% with impaired liver function [11–13]. SLV was calculated according to the following formula: $-794.41 + 1267.28 \times$ body surface area (m^2) [14]. For this patient, the FLR/SLV ratio is 46% for right hemi-hepatectomy, indicating safe surgery.

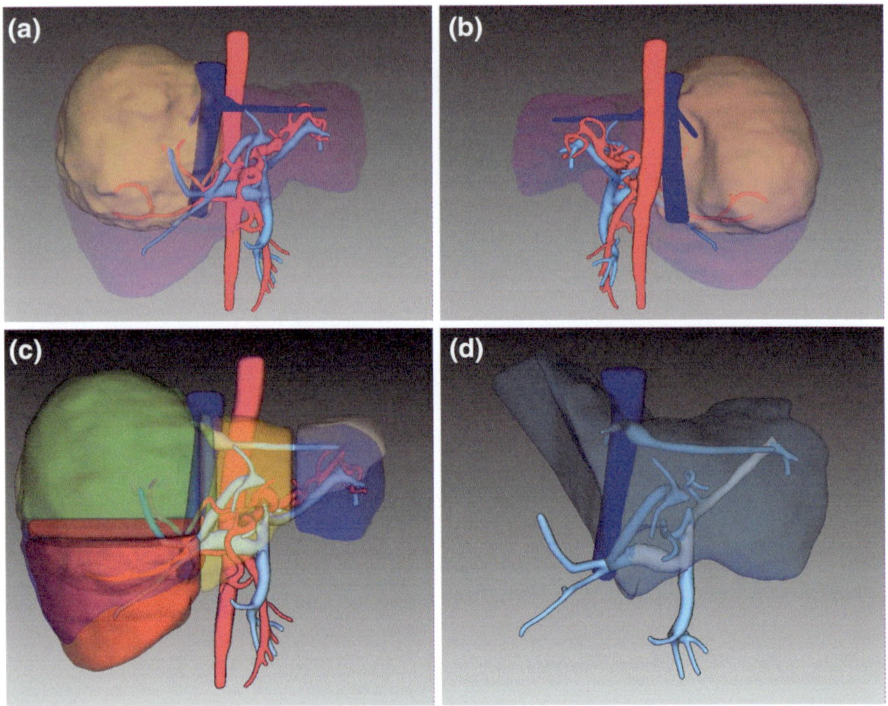

Fig. 1.7 3D CT reconstruction and future liver remnant (FLR) estimation. **a** General view (anterior) of the whole liver. *Red color* for artery; *light blue* for portal vein system; *navy blue* for hepatic vein and IVC; *pine* for normal liver; and *orange* for tumor. **b** Posterior general view of the whole liver. The middle hepatic vein was pressed to left by tumor, and the right hepatic vein was not shown as a result of tumor growing. **c** The tumor is majorly located in segment 7 and 8, partially in segment 5 and 6. **d** Future liver remnant after right hemi-hepatectomy. The middle hepatic vein was protected and kept

In our center, we routinely perform 3-D CT reconstruction and calculate the remnant liver volume (Fig. 1.7). In our experience, FLR/ body weight (BW) ratio > 0.8% is considered safe hepatectomy for patients with no cirrhotic live, but >1% for those with cirrhotic liver. In this case, the total liver volume was 2216.7 cm^3, the tumor volume was 1444.6 cm^3, the ratio of tumor/whole liver 65.2%, FLR (left liver lobe) after right hemi-hepatectomy was 561.2 cm^3, the FLR (left liver lobe)/total liver ratio is 25.3%, the body weight of this patient is 45.6 kg, the FLR (left liver lobe)/BW ratio is 1.2%.

The evaluation of present hepatic function was based on the Child-Pugh scoring system [15]. This system has been widely accepted by clinicians to evaluate liver function, and to predict postoperative recovery. This patient did not show any sign of hepatic encephalopathy or ascites. ALB is 33 umol/L, total bilirubin and PT are normal. Therefore, the liver function of this patient is Child-pugh A (score 6). In addition, indocyanine green retention rate at 15 min (ICGR15) was examined to evaluate the liver functional reserve estimation [16–18]. The ICGR15 for this patient is 4.8%, indicating normal liver functional reservation. Gastroscopy was also performed and did not show obvious esophageal varices, indicating no portal hypertension.

Nutritional assessment was performed at admission according to Subjective Global Assessment (SGA) [19] and Nutrition Risk Index (NRI); 83.5–97.5 was considered as mildly malnourished, while <83.5 was considered as severely malnourished [19–21]. NRI was calculated with the formula: 1.519 $\times$ serum albumin (Alb) (g/L) + 0.417 $\times$ (current weight/usual weight) $\times$ 100. Malnutrition was considered if the patients met at least one of two criteria: [20, 21]: (1) NRI $\leq$ 100, (2) any two of the following: current weight/ideal weight was $\leq$95%; serum Alb $\leq$ 35.0 g/L; or serum prealbumin was $\leq$200 mg/L. This female patient had mild malnutrition, as her serum prealbumin was 156 mg/L and NRI was 96.3%.

Management

Perioperative antiviral treatment was initiated as soon as the DNA level was identified. Entecavir tablet 0.5 mg was orally administered every day without interruption, and was administered via the nasogastric tube at the day of surgery. We highlighted the role of antiviral therapy, as clinical studies has proved that antiviral treatment for HBV relative HCC has the role of reducing postoperative complications and prolonging tumor-free survival [22, 23].

Right hemi-hepatectomy was performed in an open surgery for this patient. Laparoscopic hepatectomy was not considered, owing to the following factors: (1) the tumor is too huge to expose under laparoscopy; (2) diaphragm invasion or adhesion results in difficulty of right liver mobilization; (3) thrombectomy is required in case that thrombus existed in the right branch of the portal vein, which is hard to perform under laparoscopic surgery. Therefore, open surgery was performed through a right subcostal incision with midline extension.

The Chen's double-hanging maneuver was applied to assist liver parenchyma transection (Fig. 1.8). In this case, the two-hanging tapes played the following roles: (1) guide the transection plane; (2) hemorrhage control; (3) protect the middle hepatic vein and IVC; (4) expose the transection tunnel; (5) minimize the pressure of the tumor during operation to reduce tumor spreading. No bleeding presented when we built the retrohepatic tunnel and set up the hanging tapes.

The whole liver parenchyma transection time is less than 30 min, and total intraoperative hemorrhage is 150 ml. The middle hepatic vein and IVC were protected well. No tumor thrombus was observed in the portal vein system, after we dissected the right branch of the portal vein. The remnant liver has light liver cirrhosis, but its volume was more than enough for this thin woman.

We provided omega-3 fatty acid-based parenteral nutrition for the patient for 5 days after surgery, as a lower content of n-6 unsaturated FA in lipid emulsion than in conventional pure soybean oil emulsion was suggested by the European Society of Enteral and Parental Nutrition (ESPEN) for cirrhotic patients [24]. Our

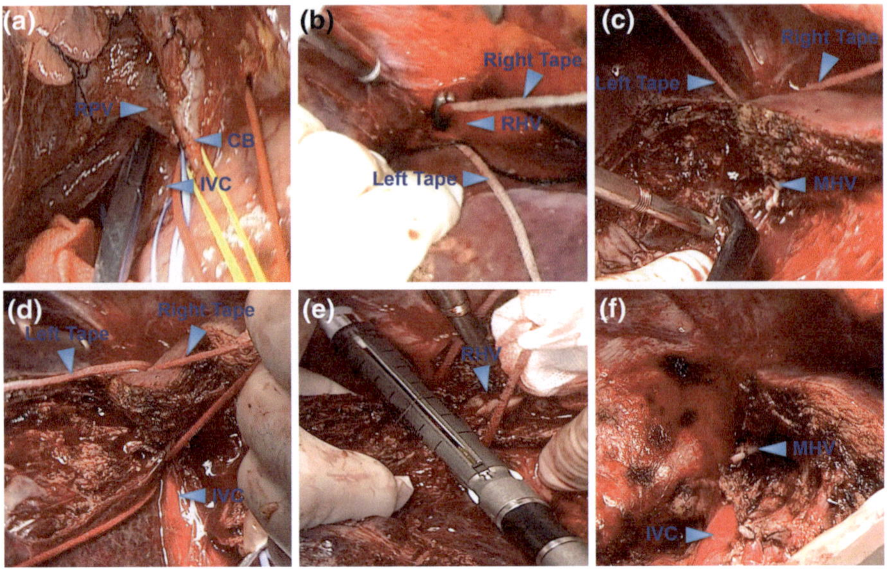

Fig. 1.8 Right hemi-hepatectomy with Chen's double-hanging maneuver. **a** The kidney pedicle forceps was inserted into the retrohepatic tunnel. **b** The tip of the kidney pedicle forceps passed through the retrohepatic space and arrived at the right side of the suprahepatic IVC. Two tapes around the liver are pulled toward the left and the right, respectively. **c** The MHV was exposed in the transection plane of the remnant liver. **d** The tapes guided the transection plane and protect the IVC. **e** The RHV was exposed and transected. **f** Remnant liver with MHV and IVC in the transection plane. *RPV* right branch of portal vein; *CB* common bile duct; *IVC* inferior vena cava; *RHV* right hepatic vein; *MHV* middle hepatic vein

unpublished clinical study provided evidences that this omega-3 fatty acid-based parenteral nutrition improves postoperative recovery for cirrhotic patients with HCC.

Outcome

The removed tumor mass showed adequate liver resection and negative transection margin (Fig. 1.9). The tumor was 15 cm × 10 cm × 10 cm in size and showed clear tumor margin. Histologic examination of the tumor was consistent with HCC of moderate differentiation.

The patient in this case was discharged from the hospital 7 days after surgery. Diet was started the 2 day after the operation, and liver function was recovered to normal 3 days postoperatively. No major complication presented, except minor pleural effusion that did not require any treatment.

AFP and ultrasonography were examined every month, while CT scanning and HBV-DNA were examined every 3 months. After 13 months follow-up, CT scanning did not shown recurrence or metastasis. HBV-DNA was controlled in the normal level (<100 copies/ml). AFP level waved at different follow-up time point, but lower than 500 ng/ml.

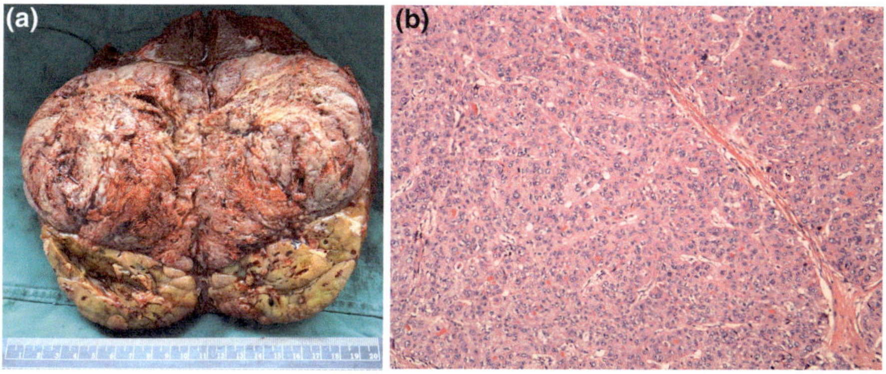

Fig. 1.9 Tumor mass and pathology. **a** Removed tumor mass showed clear tumor margin and en-block tumor resection. **b** Hematoxylin–eosin staining showed hepatocellular carcinoma with moderate differentiation

References

1. Chen XP, Qiu FZ, Wu ZD, Zhang ZW, Huang ZY, Chen YF. Long-term outcome of resection of large hepatocellular carcinoma. Br J Surg. 2006;93:600–6.
2. Lai EC, Fan ST, Lo CM, Chu KM, Liu CL. Anterior approach for difficult major right hepatectomy. World J Surg. 1996;20:314–7; discussion 318.
3. Belghiti J, Guevara OA, Noun R, Saldinger PF, Kianmanesh R. Liver hanging maneuver: a safe approach to right hepatectomy without liver mobilization. J Am Coll Surg. 2001;93:109–11.
4. Kokudo N, Imamura H, Sano K, Zhang K, Hasegawa K, Sugawara Y, et al. Ultrasonically assisted retrohepatic dissection for a liver hanging maneuver. Ann Surg. 2005;242:651–4.
5. Meng WC, Shao CX, Mak KL, Lau PY, Yeung YP, Yip AW. Anatomical justification of Belghiti's 'liver hanging manoeuvre' in right hepatectomy with anterior approach. ANZ J Surg. 2003;73:407–9.
6. Aydin U, Yazici P, Zeytunlu M, Kilic M, Coker A. Bimanual 'bi-finger' liver hanging maneuver: an alternative and safe technique for liver hanging. HPB (Oxford). 2007;9:195–8.
7. Chen XP, Zhang WG, Lau WY, Qiu FZ. Right hepatectomy using the liver double-hanging maneuver through the retrohepatic avascular tunnel on the right of the inferior vena cava. Surgery. 2008;144:830–3.
8. Couinaud C. Controlled hepatectomies and exposure of the intrahepatic bile ducts: anatomical and technical study. Paris: published by author; 1981.
9. Sutherland F, Harris J, Couinaud C. A passion for the liver. Arch Surg. 2002;137:1305–10.
10. Ettorre GM, Douard R, Corazza V, Santoro R, Vennarecci G, Santoro E. Anatomical basis of liver hanging maneuver: a clinical and anatomical in vivo study. Am Surg. 2007;73:1193–6.
11. Kishi Y, Abdalla EK, Chun YS, Zorzi D, Madoff DC, Wallace MJ, et al. Three hundred and one consecutive extended right hepatectomies: evaluation of outcome based on systematic liver volumetry. Ann Surg. 2009;250:540–8.
12. Ferrero A, Vigano L, Polastri R, Muratore A, Eminefendic H, Regge D, Capussotti L. Postoperative liver dysfunction and future remnant liver: where is the limit? Results of a prospective study. World J Surg. 2007;31:1643–51.

13. Vauthey JN, Chaoui A, Do KA, Bilimoria MM, Fenstermacher MJ, Charnsangavej C. et al. Standardized measurement of the future liver remnant prior to extended liver resection: methodology and clinical associations. Surgery. 2000;127: 512–9.
14. Vauthey JN, Abdalla EK, Doherty DA, Gertsch P, Fenstermacher MJ, Loyer EM, et al. Body surface area and body weight predict total liver volume in Western adults. Liver Transpl. 2002;8:233–40.
15. Pugh RN, Murray-Lyon IM, Dawson JL, Pietroni MC, Williams R. Transection of the oesophagus for bleeding oesophageal varices. Br J Surg. 1973;60:646–9.
16. Moody FG, Rikkers LF, Aldrete JS. Estimation of the functional reserve of human liver. Ann Surg. 1974;180:592–8.
17. Kawamura H, Kamiyama T, Nakagawa T, Nakanishi K, Yokoo H, Tahara M, et al. Preoperative evaluation of hepatic functional reserve by converted ICGR15 calculated from Tc-GSA scintigraphy. J Gastroenterol Hepatol. 2008;23:1235–41.
18. Manizate F, Hiotis SP, Labow D, Roayaie S, Schwartz M. Liver functional reserve estimation: state of the art and relevance to local treatments. Oncology. 2010;78(Suppl 1):131–4.
19. Detsky AS, McLaughlin JR, Baker JP, Johnston N, Whittaker S, Mendelson RA, et al. What is subjective global assessment of nutritional status? JPEN. 1987;11:8–13.
20. Buzby GP, Williford WO, Peterson OL, Crosby LO, Page CP, Reinhardt GF, et al. A randomized clinical trial of total parenteral nutrition in malnourished surgical patients: the rationale and impact of previous clinical trials and pilot study on protocol design. Am J Clin Nutr. 1988;47:357–65.
21. Baker JP, Detsky AS, Wesson DE, Wolman SL, Stewart S, Whitewell J, et al. Nutritional assessment: a comparison of clinical judgement and objective measurements. N Engl J Med. 1982;306:969–72.
22. Zhang B, Xu D, Wang R, Zhu P, Mei B, Wei G, et al. Perioperative antiviral therapy improves safety in patients with hepatitis B related HCC following hepatectomy. Int J Surg. 2015;15:1–5.
23. Hosaka T, Suzuki F, Kobayashi M, Seko Y, Kawamura Y, Sezaki H, et al. Long-term entecavir treatment reduces hepatocellular carcinoma incidence in patients with hepatitis B virus infection. Hepatology. 2013;58:98–107.
24. Plauth M, Cabre E, Campillo B, Kondrup J, Marchesini G, Schutz T, et al. ESPEN guidelines on parenteral nutrition: hepatology. Clin Nutr. 2009;28:436–44.

2 Debulking of Extensive Neuroendocrine Liver Metastases

Douglas L. Fraker and Steven K. Libutti

Introduction

The incidence of neuroendocrine tumors (NET) primarily in the mid-gut, but also of the pancreas, has increased significantly over the past two decades. The cause for this increase in incidence is not clear. Patients with mid-gut NET may present with symptoms of diarrhea as well as flushing, but a large number of patients, despite volume disease and elevated secretory products, may be asymptomatic. Similarly, patients with pancreas NET often present as asymptomatic lesions of the liver. These malignancies frequently metastasize to the liver and nowhere else. Patients who die from this malignant disease typically succumb to liver failure.

Patients with NET metastatic to the liver frequency have large numbers of lesions distributed evenly throughout the liver. The approach to these patients surgically is very different from the approach employed in the more well-defined patient population of metastatic colorectal cancer to the liver. Specifically, in treatment of colon cancer metastasis, there are clear guidelines related to numbers of lesions as well as the importance of doing a negative margin resection. For debulking of metastatic neuroendocrine tumors to the liver, there is no limitation in terms of number of lesions, and it is not important to have negative margins. In fact, it is more appropriate to resect lesions right on their capsule. Also, it is felt that

D.L. Fraker
Department of Surgery, University of Pennsylvania, 4 Silverstein, 3400 Spruce Street, Philadelphia, PA 19104, USA
e-mail: frakerd@uphs.upenn.edu

S.K. Libutti (✉)
Montefiore Medical Center and Albert Einstein College of Medicine, 3400 Bainbridge Avenue, 4th Floor, Bronx, NY 10467, USA
e-mail: slibutti@montefiore.org

T.M. Pawlik et al. (eds.), *Case-Based Lessons in the Management of Complex Hepato-Pancreato-Biliary Surgery*, DOI 10.1007/978-3-319-50868-9_2

surgical debulking is beneficial to patients even if up to 30% of the disease is not able to be treated.

Case 1: Mid-Gut Neuroendocrine Tumor Metastatic to the Liver

The patient is a 62-year-old man with a past history of papillary thyroid cancer 6 years earlier, in complete remission, who presented with flushing and a change in bowel habits with going from one bowel movement per day to two to three loose bowel movements per day. He had imaging with CT scan that showed a dominant 6 cm right inferior segment hepatic lesion, additional lesions up to 3 cm in the right hepatic lobe, a 3 cm caudate metastasis, and small lesions in the left liver (Fig. 2.1). The pancreas appeared normal, and the official reading said there was no evidence of any small bowel lymphadenopathy or lesions in the small intestine. A biopsy was performed of the large level 6 lesion and it showed a metastatic neuroendocrine tumor. Twenty-four hour urinary 5HIAA was elevated at 13 mg/24 h (upper limits of normal 7.5). He was treated with Sandostatin, with resolution of his flushing and improvement in his bowel function. No other efforts at treatment and no endoscopic

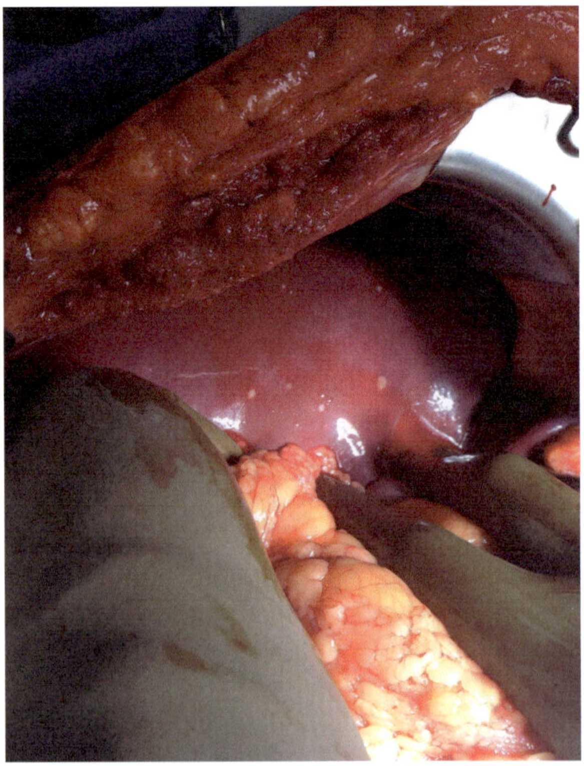

Fig. 2.1 Intraoperative picture of left lobe of liver in patient with metastatic small bowel NET to the liver. Large 8 cm lesion in inferior right lobe with other lesions in right lobe and caudate. Multiple small lesions in left liver make it clear that there is no curative option, and also demonstrates why right hepatectomy is not indicated due to extensive contralateral disease

studies were performed at an outside institution. An initial interval scan at 6 months showed an increase in size of his right segment 6 hepatic metastasis from 6 cm up to 8 cm. The remaining lesions were stable, and no new lesions appeared and there were no other findings. He was referred to our multidisciplinary neuroendocrine tumor group.

An octreoscan was obtained and it showed activity in the hepatic metastasis; no activity in the small bowel mesentery, small bowel, or pancreas. Serum serotonin was elevated at 1,433 ng/mL (normal range 85–220). We performed upper endoscopy and colonoscopy, which showed no lesions. He had a capsule endoscopy which was negative.

He was seen in surgical consultation and was recommended to have an exploration with liver debulking, including intraoperative identification of his mid-gut primary and planned resection. He had been receiving monthly Sandostatin injections, and an intravenous Sandostatin drip was prepared for infusion as needed for carcinoid storm. The approach was right subcostal incision with extension to the left side. The lateral aspects of the subcostal incision was not curved superiorly as is typical for right hepatic lobectomy, but rather went more inferiorly to allow exploration of the abdominal cavity for his primary to facilitate exploration of the abdominal cavity for a primary lesion. The initial part of the operation was to assess the primary. It was found immediately on palpation of the distal small bowel which was in the pelvis. The hepatic flexure of the colon and area of the ileo-cecal valve was completely mobilized with some tethering of the primary lesion and palpable lymph nodes in a loop of distal small bowel mesentery in the pelvis. This distal small bowel was brought up into the subcostal incision and there was careful palpation of the bowel from the ligament of Treitz to the ileocecal valve. The solitary lesion approximately 8 cm proximal to ileocecal valve was the only mass palpated. This had not been visualized by colonoscopy.

For mid-gut NET that are more than 20% proximal to the ileocecal valve, every effort is made to try to preserve the ileocecal valve and do a segmental small bowel resection. At this site and with the location of the lymph node metastasis necessitating resection of the right colic trunk, a right hemicolectomy with resection of segment of small bowel and nodal metastasis was performed with standard anastomosis. Once the bowel resection and anastomsis was completed, the retractors were completely shifted from exposing the lower aspect of the abdomen to exposing the liver. The liver was completely mobilized and assessed by palpation and intraoperative ultrasound. The dominant segment 6 lesion was easily felt, there were four to five additional lesions in the right lobe > 1 cm and a large palpable caudate mass. The left and right liver had multiple small palpable metastases (Fig. 2.2). A cholecystectomy was performed. In this case, it was not necessary to remove the gallbladder to address any of the hepatic nodules, but for patients with NET with a laparoscopic approach, or certainly with an open approach liver metastasis, it is mandatory to remove the gallbladder as long-term use of Sandostatin will lead to formation of gallstones and ability to approach the gallbladder laparoscopically is compromised after such an extensive hepatic debulking procedure. To address the dominant lesion in the right segment 6, the right hepatic lobe

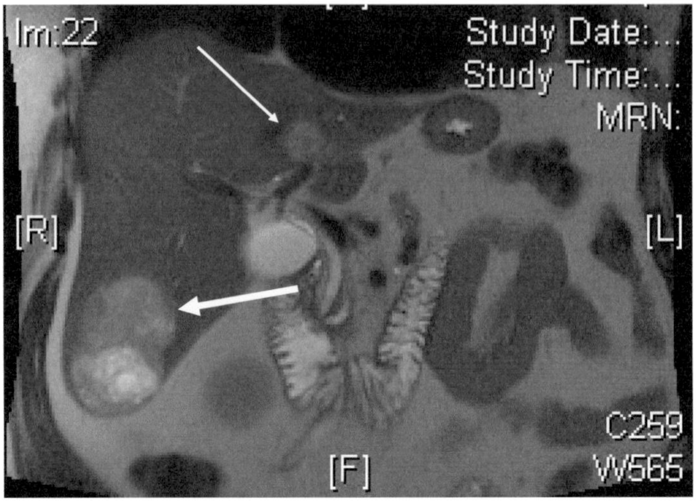

Fig. 2.2 Axial MRI of patient with metastatic NET to liver. Large right segment 6 lesion has grown significantly over 6-month interval (*large arrow*). Caudate lesion is second largest tumor (*small arrow*). At laparotomy, attempts were made to remove this lesion, but concerns over damaging left portal triad resulted in radiofrequency ablation of this tumor

was completely mobilized off the inferior vena cava. The feeding vasculature from the inferior segmental portal triad was assessed by surgeon-directed ultrasound and entered the lesion at the inferior medial border of this mass. The approach was to identify the margin of this large hepatic metastasis in a lateral avascular area. As is typical, it was firm, white, and once we were on the capsule either with blunt dissection with a finger or with a right angle, the surrounding parenchyma was swept away. When bridging vessels were seen, they were controlled with clips or Aquamontys ablation. Intraoperative ultrasound-guided dissection to where the main trunk was plastered over this and a vascular stapler was used to divide the main trunk. This large lesion was removed with very little surrounding parenchyma and very little blood loss (Fig. 2.3a). The cut parenchyma of the base was controlled with argon beam laser. All other small nodules were then addressed. Any nodule larger than 5 mm on the surface was resected with cautery and some exophytic lesions sharply resected with the base treated with cautery. Lesions just under the surface in the range of 1–3 cm had a circular incision made with cautery right over the palpable nodule. Once the white capsule of the nodule was identified, again blunt dissection either with the finger or right angle clamp was used to go around this often resecting 3 cm lesions in under 30 s. Several small 2–4 mm lesions were controlled with Aquamontys ablation on the surface with the typical popping noise (Fig. 2.3b). Ultrasound revealed two lesions, one in the caudate that was medially posterior to the main left segmental portal triad (Fig. 2.1) and a second lesion that was deep anterior to the right portal triad. An attempt was made to enucleate the caudate lesion, but it was too close to the main left portal structures.

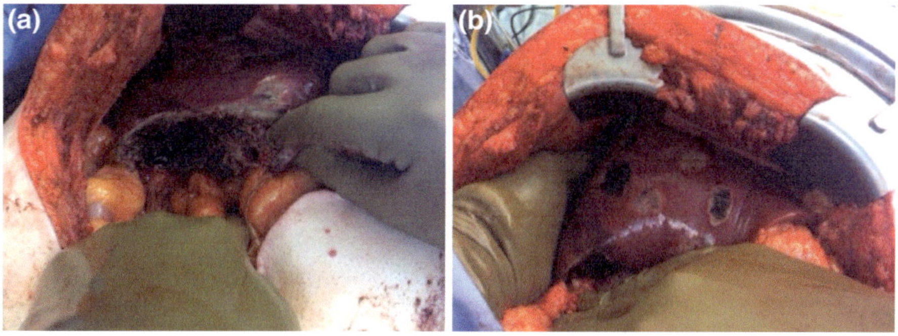

Fig. 2.3 Post-treatment photographs of patient with mid-gut NET. Panel **a** shows resection of 8 cm segment 6 lesion with hepatic parenchymal preservation. Panel **b** shows treatment of smaller lesions by enucleation (dark areas) or surface ablation (light areas)

These were treated with radiofrequency ablation with ultrasound guidance following standard ablation algorithms.

Postoperatively, the patient recovered with no significant change in hepatic functions postoperatively and was discharged on postoperative day 6 without complication. His pathology showed his small bowel lesion was a grade 1, 2.3 cm mass, solitary mid-gut primary with a Ki-67 of <1%. There were 4/22 lymph nodes with metastatic disease. All margins were negative. His large segment 6 lesion which at presentation had been 6 cm, was measured at 8.8 cm and had a Ki-67 of 9.7% with positive tumor margin as expected. There were five left liver nodules between 4 and 6 mm with Ki-67 of zero with no mitoses identified. There were 12 resected right hepatic nodules between 5 and 30 mm and had zero mitoses identified in these lesions.

This patient illustrates several aspects relevant to debulking of neuroendocrine lesions from a mid-gut primary. First, the patient had negative cross-sectional imaging and negative endoscopy in terms of the primary tumor in the terminal ileum and was labeled as an unknown or occult primary with extensive hepatic metastases. He had symptoms related to serotonin production and had an elevated 5HIAA. He had marked elevation of his serum serotonin, essentially confirming a mid-gut primary despite the negative imaging with colonoscopy, capsule endoscopy, and cross-sectional assessment of the bowel. Of note, his postoperative serotonin had dropped to near normal levels at 230 ng/mL. His primary lesion measured 2.3 cm in size despite the negative imaging, negative octreoscan, and negative capsule endoscopy. It was able to be palpated very easily on exposure of the bowel. This is very typical, and extensive efforts sometimes are costly to identify the primary and are not necessary with this clinical scenario. Also patients may sometimes be discouraged from undergoing surgical debulking of the hepatic metastases because of the occult primary and this should not be a hindrance, as again it can virtually always be identified by surgical exploration and treated simultaneously with debulking liver metastases.

The initial strategy employed for this patient was a watch and wait with Sandostatin and although the majority of the lesions in his liver remain stable, he had a solitary lesion increase from 6 to 8 cm that then was 8.8 cm at the time of resection. This is somewhat unusual, but prompted a referral to a tertiary center which led to this successful debulking. The final pathology demonstrated that specific lesion had an intermediate and almost high grade Ki-67 of 9.7%, whereas both the primary lesion and the other liver metastases had Ki-67 of <1%. Clearly a secondary mutation had occurred in this specific lesion, leading to its rapid growth, and also demonstrating the importance of removing that before it became too large or it had metastasized outside the liver. This patient has been followed for over 12 months with no clear new lesions appearing, with complete resolution of the symptoms, and no postoperative complications.

Technical Pearls for Debulking Liver Metastases from Neuroendocrine Tumors

- Utilize cross-sectional imaging CT with contrast or MRI scans to assess for extent of hepatic metastasis. Plan a procedure to do as much hepatic parenchymal preservation with enucleation of lesions instead of anatomic resection even for large metastases.
- Approach neuroendocrine liver metastases with a blunt dissection on the firm white capsule of the lesion with the right angle or sometimes finger dissection. Make no attempt to obtain any hepatic margin. Use the argon beam laser or other energy devices such as cautery at high level or Aquamantys to burn the cut surface of the liver.
- Utilize surgeon-directed intraoperative ultrasound to guide resection of deeper nodules. Frequent use of ultrasound can identify approaches to lesions that are not even palpable in a vascular space, and then employ the blunt dissection technique once the metastasis is visualized to do an extraction.
- Reserve segmental resections for clusters of nodules at the lateral tip of the left lateral segment 2/3 or inferior right liver segment 6. Formal lobectomy is infrequently indicated due to distribution of metastases
- Use ablative techniques for deep lesions next to central portal structures in radiofrequency ablation and microwave ablation. Use energy such as high-level cautery or Aquamantys to burn surface nodules 4 mm or less and expect a popping sound as these are burned.

Case 2: Pancreas NET Metastatic to Liver

The patient is a 52-year-old man who worked at a steel mill and had a back injury. As part of his imaging for this injury he had an abdominal CT, which showed over 25 liver metastases in a bilobar distribution up to 3–4 cm in size and a 4 cm tail of the pancreas mass (Fig. 2.4a). Despite this bulky disease, his liver functions were completely normal. He had absolutely no abdominal or back pain related to his tumor burden. He had a percutaneous biopsy of a liver lesion which showed low-grade NET. He started on monthly long-acting Sandostatin shots and was treated with Everolimus. He had an interval 4-month scan which showed some progression of liver nodules. He underwent sequential bilobar Yttrium-90 embolizations and had a >80% response in his disease.

He sought out our multidisciplinary tumor group as his tertiary center, where he had been receiving treatment who did not recommend surgical debulking. At the time he was seen, it was an interval of 3–4 months after his radio-embolization and a repeat scan showed fairly significant progression back to the levels they were prior to embolization. On physical examination he looked completely healthy and well nourished and had absolutely no symptoms. The disease seemed to be almost too extensive to do a meaningful debulking, so he underwent another set of very closely spaced Yttrium-90 radio-embolizations at his home institution. He had a planned surgery date 3 weeks after the second one and he had a scan just 2 days prior to the surgery with another remarkable response again of >80% decrease in size of his bilobar lesions (Fig. 2.4b). His pancreas lesion has been stable throughout.

He was approached with a bilateral subcostal incision. He had two segmental resections, one of segment 2 in the left lateral area, where there was probably a

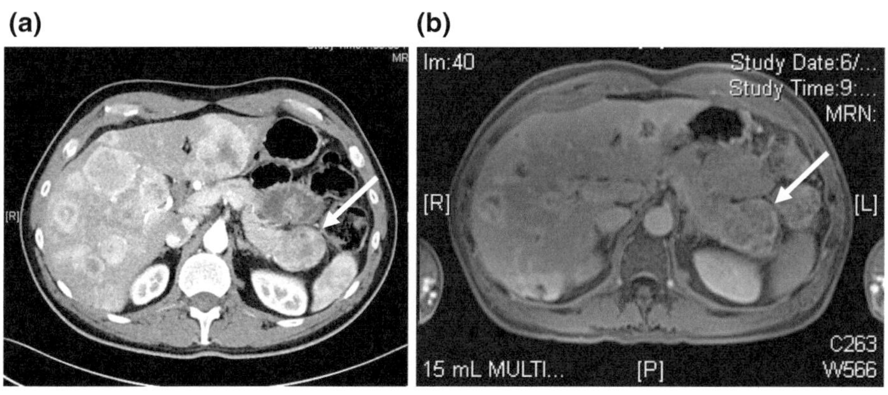

Fig. 2.4 Pretreatment and post-treatment CT and MRI of patient with metastatic pancreatic NET to liver. The patient had 5 cm primary in tail of pancreas (*arrow*) and large bilobar liver metastases (Panel **a**). After Yttrium-90 the liver lesions had an 80% response and appear necrotic (Panel **b**). The patient underwent distal pancreatectomy for the PNET primary and debulking of >95% of hepatic disease with no surgical complications

dozen tumor nodules all clustered, and another one in segment 5/6, with multiple tumor nodules. The other lesions were treated with enucleation on the capsule of the lesion, as well as five lesions treated with radiofrequency ablation by ultrasound guidance. He underwent a distal pancreatectomy with no evidence of extrapancreatic spread from his primary lesion. He did well postoperatively and was discharged on postoperative day 5 and flew across country back to his home institution on postoperative day 7. His pathology showed a well-differentiated intermediate-grade pancreas neuroendocrine tumor, 5.4 cm in size, with a Ki-67 of 5.9%. There was perineural invasion and lymphatic invasion, but there were 0/12 lymph nodes with metastasis. His left lateral partial hepatectomy showed more than 12 nodules between 4 mm and 21 mm, with 25% of the tumor viable. Similarly, his right inferior partial hepatectomy showed over 15 nodules between 4 and 20 mm, somewhat diffuse, with 20% of the tumor viable. He had over 10 left hepatic metastases resected between 4 and 24 mm, and over 15 right hepatic metastases resected between 4 and 25 mm.

This patient had removal of his primary, and probably debulking of greater than 95% of hepatic lesions with zero blood loss and completely normal hepatic functions postoperatively. Although the number of nodules were too great to completely render him disease-free, all of the Ki-67 indices in the liver metastases in the viable components were <2%, and the majority of these had been stable. Removing his intermediate-grade primary lesions to prevent further metastases and debulking of this large number of low-grade slow-growing lesions with an operation that causes minimal morbidity should improve his overall survival.

This case demonstrates the utilization of nonsurgical treatments to address bulky liver metastases, specifically in this case radio-embolization to optimally debulk with appropriate timing between the interventional radiology treatment and the surgical treatment.

These two cases illustrate that for the appropriately prepared patient, significant and sometimes bulky liver disease can be safely resected/ablated with minimal morbidity. If the primary is in place, this too can be safely resected at the time of liver debulking. Multiple lesions can be safely enucleated and segmental or sector resections should be reserved for areas of the liver where maximal debulking can be safely accomplished and the number of lesions exceeds that which can safely be enucleated. With the advent of systemic therapies that have shown activity for established disease, it may be possible to prolong the progression-free survival following maximal debulking of liver metastases.

Alternative Approach/Controversies in Management of Neuroendocrine Liver Metastases

- For extensive liver lesions with pathologically proven low Ki-67 (<2%), a "watch and wait" approach may be appropriate to assess the rate of growth supplemented by long-acting Sandostatin. Asymptomatic patients may be

followed with serial examinations for years with minimal change and good quality of life.
- Utilize interventional radiology techniques prior to surgery to decrease the bulk of disease and facilitation surgical debulking. Specifically, bland embolization, TACE, or intra-arterial injection of radiospheres may lead to significant responses with appropriately timed surgical debulking.
- Utilize interventional radiology techniques such as percutaneous radiofrequency or microwave ablation or alcohol injection for residual or recurrent disease after extensive tumor debulking.

Overall Management of Patients with Extensive Neuroendocrine Hepatic Metasasis

- For patients with numerous bilobar lesions in the liver at presentation, a complete cure is unrealistic. Plan treatment strategies to maximize overall survival and minimize morbidity from the neuroendocrine tumor.
- For incurable patients, hepatic debulking may significantly increase the overall survival and may significantly increase the quality of life due to a decreased amount of secretory products from the neuroendocrine metastasis.
- Patients with extensive neuroendocrine metastases frequency present with unknown primaries. The most common location of the primary is mid-gut NET, and the second most common area is pancreas NET. Occasionally, patients present with chest NET or gastric carcinoids with bulky liver lesions. Work-up should include MRI/EUS for evaluation of pancreas, and a chest CT with the stomach assessed at the time of EUS. If all these studies are negative, virtually all patients have a mid-gut NET that can easily be felt and resected at the time of liver debulking. Assess cross-sectional imaging looking for distortion of the mesentery due to nodal metastases that are much more commonly visible than the primary NET in the small bowel.
- Utilize secretory products to assess for progression of disease as well as to assess the success of debulking treatment. Specifically, serum serotonin is far more reliable than chromogranin A for a marker for mid-gut carcinoid.
- Utilize nuclear medicine imaging including Indium octreoscan, MIBG, and gallium scan if available to look primarily for nonhepatic metastasis frequently occurring in bone or other unusual places.

Conclusion

In conclusion, surgical resection of metastatic neuroendocrine tumors to the liver is a completely different procedure than any other liver resection, and different than almost any resection for abdominal malignancy. Metastatic NET are basically "shucked out" on the margin of the tumor, with no attempt to get negative margins. Patients who would never be considered to be surgical candidates for any other type of malignancy can benefit from surgical debulking. It is imperative that this group of patients have their liver imaging reviewed by surgeons experienced in treatment of neuroendocrine tumors.

Treatment of Neuroendocrine Liver Metastases

1. Assess the volume and number of tumors on cross-sectional imaging.
    a. Volume of metastaic lesions up to 50% of the overall liver volume may be debulked.
    b. The number of lesions is not prohibitive if there is satisfactory residual hepatic parenchyma.
    c. Goal may be to remove at least 70% (for mid-gut NET) and >90% to select pancreas NET.
2. Identify the primary NET and make plans to resect
    a. For mid-gut NET:
        i. Do segmental small bowel resection or right colectomy
        ii. Palpate for multifocal primary lesion (>35%)
        iii. Preserve the ileo-cecal valve if possible
        iv. Remove bulky root of mesentery lymph nodes by resecting off vessels
    b. For pancreas NET:
        i. Distal pancreatectomy/splenectomy for body and tail pancreas PNET
        ii. Assess head/uncertain primary PNET for well-defined margins and enucleate if a reasonable margin from the main pancreatic duct
        iii. Consider pancreatico-duodenectomy for select patients (young, no co-morbidities) with complete excision of liver metastases.

c. Occult primary:

   i. Chest CT to rule out bronchial/thymic carcinoid.
   ii. EGD to rule out gastric and EUS/MRI to evaluate the liver. Carefully examine small bowel mesentery for signs of mid-gut carcinoid.
   iii. If all negative, palpate small bowel for primary mid-gut carcinoid.

3. Resection/Ablation of liver metastases

   a. Incision virtually along bilateral subcostal to allow mobilization of right lobe of liver.
   b. Assess deep lesions with IOUS.
   c. Plan resection ablation to normal hepatic parenchyma.

      i. Enucleate any lesion away from major portal triad structures and major hepatic vein branches.
      ii. Dissect bluntly right on the capsule of the metastasis
      iii. Ablate deep lesions near major vessels

   d. Perform prophylactic cholecystectomy as patients will be on long-acting sandostatin
   e. For mid-gut NET have infusion of sandostatin available to prevent carcinoid crisis

Resection of Centrally Located Cystadenoma/Cystadenocarcinoma

3

Emmanuel Melloul, Parissa Tabrizian and Myron E. Schwartz

Introduction

Intrahepatic biliary cystadenoma (IBC) is a rare biliary cystic tumor, accounting for approximately 5% of all hepatic cysts [1]. IBC arises centrally in segment 4 disproportionately more often than elsewhere in the liver. While benign, malignant transformation to intrahepatic biliary cystadenocarcinoma (IBCC) has been reported in up to 30% of resected cases; IBCC accounts for 0.41% of malignant hepatic epithelial tumors [2, 3]. Patients are most commonly asymptomatic; jaundice may result from tumor invasion or compression of the porta hepatis. Painful intracystic hemorrhage, rupture, fever due to secondary infection, ascites, and retrohepatic vena cava obstruction/thrombosis have also been reported [4, 5].

Nonneoplastic simple biliary cysts are considerably more common than IBC; a solitary, septated cystic mass with solid mural components on imaging should raise suspicion of IBC. A central location further increases the likelihood of this diagnosis. Treatment consists of resection. Benign cystadenomas are readily amenable to enucleation, which could be viewed as a pericystectomy; if there is any

E. Melloul · P. Tabrizian · M.E. Schwartz (✉)
Mount Sinai Liver Cancer Program, Recanati/Miller Transplantation Institute Icahn School of Medicine at Mount Sinai, New York, NY 10029, USA
e-mail: myron.schwartz@mountsinai.org

E. Melloul
e-mail: emmanuelmelloul@hotmail.com

P. Tabrizian
e-mail: parissa.tabrizian@mountsinai.org

T.M. Pawlik et al. (eds.), *Case-Based Lessons in the Management of Complex Hepato-Pancreato-Biliary Surgery*, DOI 10.1007/978-3-319-50868-9_3

indication of malignancy, however, resection through normal tissue planes with negative margins is mandatory [6, 7]. Reported 5-year survival rates after resection of IBCC range from 25 to 100% [8].

Case 1

History

A 59-year-old woman was referred for evaluation after abnormal liver enzymes were noted on routine blood tests, with alkaline phosphatase in the 400s and elevated ALT. She had an unremarkable past medical history and no underlying liver disease; she was first noted to have a centrally located hepatic cyst 8 years prior to presentation on imaging performed for an unrelated issue. Six months prior to presentation she developed appendicitis; an abdominal CT at that time showed the cyst to be unchanged from past imaging, measuring 7 cm and resulting in mild left-sided biliary dilatation. Imaging at presentation showed increased left-sided biliary dilatation as well as occlusion of the left portal vein and new enhancing mural nodules (Fig. 3.1a–e). She remained asymptomatic other than some upper abdominal fullness and dyspepsia.

Procedure

Based on the imaging and, in particular, the recent changes observed, invasive malignancy was strongly suspected; accordingly, extended left and caudate hepatectomy (segments 1, 2, 3, 4, and 8) was performed. The patient's anatomy was such that the segment 5 pedicle arose from the "posterior" right pedicle, facilitating salvage of segment 5. The left hepatic artery and portal vein were dissected and ligated extrahepatically, and the left hepatic duct was transected close to the bifurcation and oversewn. The caudate was elevated off of the cava after dividing short hepatic veins. The left and middle hepatic veins were encircled above the liver and taken flush with the cava using a stapling device. Anteriorly, the parenchymal division began through liver parenchyma away from the cyst, using an electrosurgical device without hilar occlusion, between segments 4 and 5; the dissection subsequently proceeded to the right, following the contour of the tumor, up along the right anterior portal structures in an extra-Glissonian plane, and the segment 8

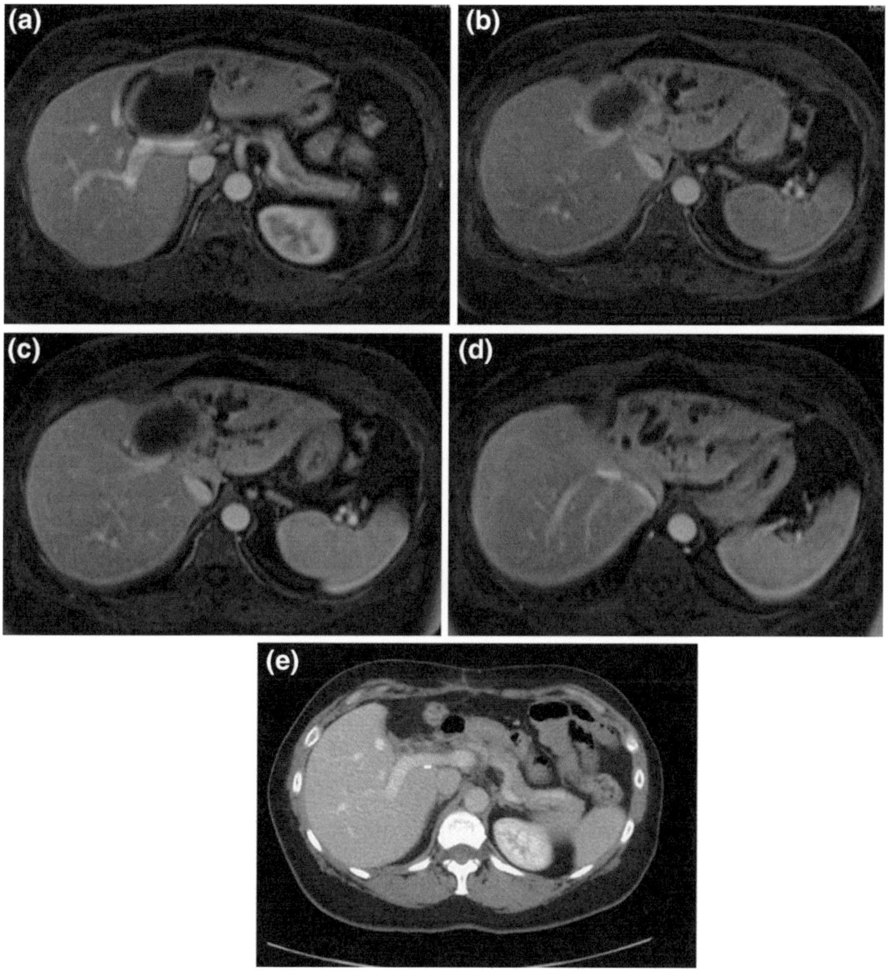

Fig. 3.1 Imaging studies of the first case that exhibit a symptomatic centrally located cystic lesion with enhancing intramural projections. The cystic lesion abuts the left hepatic duct, producing significant left hepatic duct dilation (**a**–**d**). No vascular invasion was apparent. In **e**, the postoperative imaging after extended left hepatectomy. The lesion proved to be an intrahepatic cystadenocarcinoma

pedicle was taken within the parenchyma. Dorsally, the cyst/tumor extended rightward to the right hepatic vein; dissection was carried out in the plane of the vein and the tumor was successfully separated away except for a small point of adherence, whereupon a side-biting vascular clamp was applied onto the vein, a portion of the vein wall was excised, and repair was carried out with 6-0 polypropylene.

Outcome

The postoperative course was uneventful, and the patient was discharged on postoperative day 4. Pathology showed moderately to poorly differentiated IBCC with extensive lymphovascular and perineural invasion arising in an IBC; margins and lymph nodes (0/2) were free of tumor. She received adjuvant gemcitabine for 6 months, and was alive and free of recurrence on followup 3 years after surgery.

Case 2

History

A 52-year-old male with no significant past medical history presented with upper abdominal fullness and abnormal liver tests, with alkaline phosphatase 492, ALT 163, and bilirubin 1.4. CEA and CA19-9 were normal. MR showed a 20 cm multiloculated cyst involving segments 4/5/8 and compressing but not invading the left and right anterior portal structures (Fig. 3.2a–d). There was no evidence of portal hypertension.

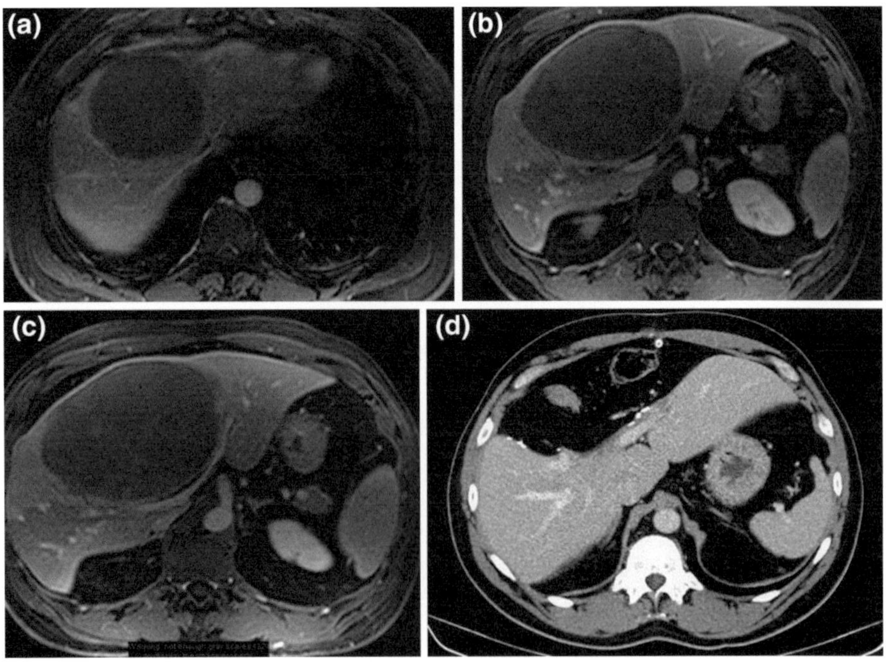

Fig. 3.2 Study imaging of the second case presenting with asymptomatic centrally located cystic lesion (**a**–**c**). There are no intracystic projections and no vascular involvement. The intrahepatic biliary tree is not dilated. The patient underwent a central pericystectomy (**d**). The lesion proved to be an intrahepatic cystadenoma with foci of cystadenocarcinoma

Procedure

Based on the smooth, well-defined border of the cyst with compression but with no evidence of invasion of portal structures, central resection in the enucleation plane of the lesion was undertaken. After taking down the gallbladder, tying and dividing the gallbladder mesentery, and lowering the portal bifurcation in an extra-Glissonian plane, the segment 4 structures were dissected and ligated in the umbilical fissure. The capsule of the liver was scored with electrocautery around the edge of the cyst. The porta hepatis was occluded en masse with a broad vascular clamp for 19 min, during which the cyst was separated from segments 2–3 in the enucleation plane using scissors dissection, clipping vessels, and ducts that traversed the transection plane with a multiclip applier. After a 5-minute period of reperfusion, the porta was once again clamped for 20 min, during which the cyst was similarly enucleated away from segments 5–8. The main trunk of the middle hepatic vein, which was closely applied onto the cyst, was ligated at its junction with the left hepatic vein and removed along with the specimen.

Outcome

The patient had an uneventful recovery and was discharged home on postoperative day 4. Pathology revealed an 18 cm hepatobiliary mucinous cystadenoma with areas of carcinoma; extensive necrosis, cystic degeneration, and limited lymphovascular invasion were noted. No adjuvant therapy was given. The patient was alive and free of recurrence at 2 years after surgery.

Technical Pearls

- Dissection of the portal structures in the extraglissonian plane by lowering the hilar plate is the most expedient and safest approach.
- If complete right anterior resection is planned the right anterior sectoral structures can be encircled and divided using the ultrasonic dissector.
- Dissection and encircling of the middle hepatic vein above the liver can generally be accomplished, and is facilitated by making a short incision into the liver parenchyma overlying the confluence.
- A scissors dissection technique, using the blunt scissors tip to dissect through parenchyma and identify small vascular structures, which can be clipped, can be used for parenchymal transection.

Discussion

The central portion of the liver comprises segments 4, 5, and 8; depending on the nature, size, and location of the pathology to be dealt with, resection of centrally located tumors may require removal of part or all of one or more of these segments (Fig. 3.3). Central resection requires division of the liver twice, with two resultant cut surfaces and the attendant risks. Extended right or left hepatectomy is an alternative that has, over the years, been commonly employed because of its relative technical simplicity; central resection has become more common of late with the recognition of the value of parenchyma-sparing surgery, both for primary liver tumors where there is concern about hepatic functional reserve, and for metastatic tumors where it is desirable to maintain options to treat possible future recurrence [9].

Anatomical Considerations

Segment 4 is commonly described as having two subsegments, 4A and 4B, although there are typically multiple portal branches to segment 4 rather than two discrete pedicles. Be that as it may, the left portal vein runs transversely to the umbilical fissure under segment 4B and then up the umbilical fissure, terminating in the obliterated umbilical vein, often designated as the round ligament. The segment 4 portal branches, along with those from the hepatic artery and hepatic duct, enter segment 4 in the umbilical fissure and course through segment 4 from left to right (see Fig. 3.3). These portal structures are readily clipped or ligated in the umbilical fissure when complete resection of segment 4 or 4B is planned, but the fact that they run from left to right makes it possible to divide through segment 4 at any distance from the umbilical fissure without preliminary dissection while maintaining perfusion and biliary drainage to the portion of segment 4 that is left behind [10]. As they approach the liver, the portal vein, hepatic artery, and bile duct are invested and subsequently distributed through the liver within a common sheath derived from the reflection of Glisson's capsule, and in many circumstances dissection of these structures in the extra-Glissonian plane is both the most expedient and the

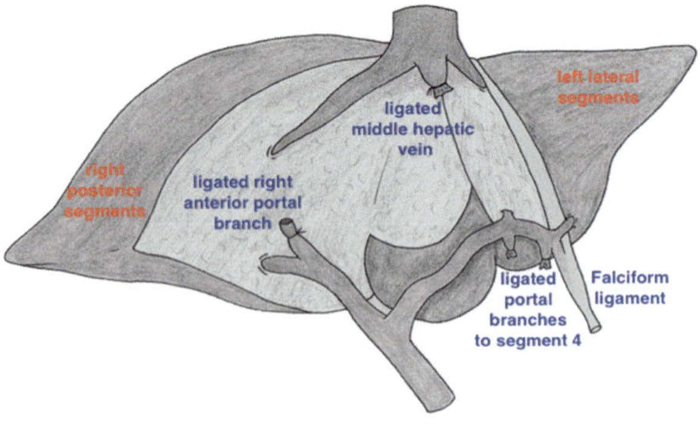

Fig. 3.3 Schematic representation of a central hepatectomy (removal of segments 4, 5, 8)

safest approach [10]. Separating the portal structures away from the parenchyma of segments 4B and 5 is a key maneuver when complete resection of these segments is planned. This so-called lowering of the hilar plate is accomplished by first removing the gallbladder if present, ligating and dividing the tissue at the base of the gallbladder fossa (commonly called the gallbladder mesentery; there are often small structures there that are of no consequence, but that can be troublesome if not ligated), dividing the peritoneum under segments 4B and 5 as it envelopes the portal structures, and separating the portal structures from the liver parenchyma outside of Glisson's sheath. It typically requires the division of a few small portal branches near the portal bifurcation to establish this extra-Glissonian plane. While this process of lowering the hilar plate can be carried out with simple scissors dissection, an ultrasonic dissector, when available, is a useful tool to establish and maintain the correct plane of dissection.

For complete segment 4 resection the extra-Glissonian dissection of the left portal structures is continued out to the umbilical fissure. A substantial segment 4 duct is invariably present near where the left portal vein makes its 90° turn up the umbilical fissure; if, as in most cases, the segment 4 structures in the umbilical fissure have been dissected individually, it is most expedient, unless constrained by the presence of immediately adjacent tumor, to enter the hepatic parenchyma with a fine clamp and encircle, ligate, and divide this duct within the liver. This is a reliable way to avoid injury to the segment 2–3 ducts that may otherwise easily be injured when dissecting in this area. It may be noted that the dissection described herein is identical to that required in performing extended right hepatectomy.

Dissection of the right anterior portal structures can be similarly carried out in the extra-Glissonian plane; again, clean precise dissection is facilitated by the use of an ultrasonic dissector. The right anterior sectoral structures are readily encircled and may be ligated or stapled and divided if complete right anterior resection is planned. Otherwise, with further dissection into the liver it is possible (albeit not without some effort) to encircle the segment 5 or 8 pedicles should complete resection of segment 5 or 8 be planned. It is also possible, when the situation of a tumor dictates, to dissect the right anterior portal structures in a way conceptually like the segment 4 dissection, dividing those pedicles that supply the medial portion of segments 5–8 and leaving those feeding the lateral part of segments 5–8 intact, though this dissection is typically carried out during the course of parenchymal transection rather than as a preliminary step.

Careful review of high-quality imaging that clearly demonstrates the vascular anatomy of the liver is essential in these cases because anatomical variations are common [11]; the right anterior structures, for example, may arise as a common trunk with the left structures, or the first major branch on the right side may supply either more or less of the right liver than is classically considered to be segments 5 and 8.

The left and middle hepatic veins nearly always join to form a common trunk before entering the inferior vena cava. The line between segment 4 and segments 2–3 is defined externally by the falciform ligament; following an imaginary line continuing the line of the falciform to the dorsalmost limit of the liver reliably indicates where the confluence of the middle and left hepatic veins lies. It goes without saying that intraoperative ultrasound, here as in so many situations in liver surgery, is useful to precisely localize intrahepatic structures.

Dissection and encircling of the middle hepatic vein above the liver can generally be accomplished, and is facilitated by making a short incision into the liver parenchyma overlying the confluence; here again, an ultrasonic dissector is useful to define the vein atraumatically. The middle hepatic vein may be viewed conceptually as running between the right and left livers, but practically speaking it follows a diagonal course, originating in segment 5 with tributaries from segment 4B and receiving tributaries from segment 8 as it courses through segment 4A to join with the left hepatic vein.

The right hepatic vein defines the lateral extent of segments 5–8, and serves as the margin of resection when complete resection of the right anterior sector is planned. When the contemplated procedure involves complete resection of segment 4A, the middle hepatic vein is necessarily divided close to its confluence with the left hepatic vein. Bleeding from the hepatic veins, and in the case of central resection from the middle hepatic vein, is usually the greatest source of intraoperative risk in liver surgery; on the other hand, there is enough adaptability of the venous outflow of the liver that division of the middle hepatic vein during hepatic resection while preserving parts of the liver that seemed to be primarily drained by it does not, practically speaking, lead to clinically significant hepatic congestion.

Alternative Approaches

- Extended right or left hepatectomy is an alternative, technically simpler approach and the proper technique in larger tumors with adjacent small liver segments.
- Central resection is a useful parenchyma-sparing surgery, both for primary liver tumors where there is concern about hepatic functional reserve, and for metastatic tumors where it is desirable to maintain options to treat possible future recurrence.
- Total vascular isolation is a useful technique for very large cysts distorting the confluence of the major hepatic veins with the vena cava.

Enucleation Technique

IBCs are readily enucleated from the liver, and if they do not contain invasive cancer, enucleation is a curative procedure [6, 7]. As these tumors grow, the intrahepatic structures are pushed aside; when a central IBC has grown to a substantial size the portal structures are typically splayed around it inferiorly, and the hepatic veins, in particular the middle vein, are stretched around and closely applied onto the tumor. It is important to carry out enucleation in a relatively bloodless field, as visibility is paramount; we routinely employ hilar occlusion. Total vascular isolation is a useful technique for very large cysts distorting the confluence of the major hepatic veins with the vena cava when it can be difficult to avoid entry into large veins; with increasing experience over time on the part of both our surgical team and our anesthesia group, our use of total vascular isolation has gradually diminished. We most commonly employ a scissors dissection technique, using the blunt scissors tip to dissect through parenchyma and identify small structures which are clipped [12]. It is important to get into the correct plane immediately adjacent to the tumor early on and to recognize when major portal or venous structures are closely applied on to the tumor, in which circumstance it is key to establish the dissection plane between the structures and the tumor, rather than dissecting the structures together with the tumor away from the surrounding parenchyma.

Determining the Approach

In planning surgery for central tumors, the surgeon must weigh the value of preserving parenchyma against the greater technical complexity and larger cut liver surface associated with central resection. In cases where segment 4 has been replaced by the tumor and the left lateral segment is small, expediency may warrant performance of left or extended left hepatectomy. In Case 1, discussed earlier, the centrally located IBCC was closing off the left hepatic duct as demonstrated by the significant dilatation of the left hepatic duct on the preoperative imaging. In addition, left portal vein thrombosis was present. These findings led to suspicion of invasive cancer preoperatively, and the decision to perform an extended left lobe resection with caudate with a parenchymal margin rather than to employ an enucleation technique.

In Case 2, discussed earlier, while large, there was no suggestion of invasive cancer, the vessels and ducts were all patent, and the left lateral segment was large, leading us to perform a central resection using an enucleation approach.

Management

- Treatment of cystadenocarcinoma consists of liver resection because of difficult accurate preoperative diagnosis and high recurrence rate.
- Benign cystadenomas can be managed with enucleation if there is no indication of malignancy.
- Careful review of high-quality imaging that clearly demonstrates the vascular anatomy of the liver is essential because of common anatomical variations.

- The use of intraoperative ultrasound is useful to precisely localize intra-hepatic structures.
- In planning surgery, the value of preserving parenchyma must be weighed against the greater technical complexity and larger cut liver surface associated with central resection.

References

1. Del Poggio P, Buonocore M. Cystic tumors of the liver: a practical approach. World J Gastroenterol. 2008;14(23):3616–20.
2. Kubota E, Katsumi K, Iida M, Kishimoto A, Ban Y, Nakata K, et al. Biliary cystadeno-carcinoma followed up as benign cystadenoma for 10 years. J Gastroenterol. 2003;38 (3):278–82.
3. Ammori BJ, Jenkins BL, Lim PC, Prasad KR, Pollard SG, Lodge JP. Surgical strategy for cystic diseases of the liver in a western hepatobiliary center. World J Surg. 2002;26(4):462–9.
4. Dixon E, Sutherland FR, Mitchell P, McKinnon G, Nayak V. Cystadenomas of the liver: a spectrum of disease. Can J Surg. 2001;44(5):371–6.
5. Ramacciato G, Nigri GR, D'Angelo F, Aurello P, Bellagamba R, Colarossi C, et al. Emergency laparotomy for misdiagnosed biliary cystadenoma originating from caudate lobe. World J Surg Oncol. 2006;4:76.
6. Sang X, Sun Y, Mao Y, Yang Z, Lu X, Yang H, et al. Hepatobiliary cystadenomas and cystadenocarcinomas: a report of 33 cases. Liver Int. 2011;31(9):1337–44.
7. Martel G, Alsharif J, Aubin JM, Marginean C, Mimeault R, Fairfull-Smith RJ, et al. The management of hepatobiliary cystadenomas: lessons learned. HPB (Oxford). 2013;15 (8):617–22.
8. Vogt DP, Henderson JM, Chmielewski E. Cystadenoma and cystadenocarcinoma of the liver: a single center experience. J Am Coll Surg. 2005;200(5):727–33.
9. de'Angelis N, Pascal G, Salloum C, Lahat E, Ichai P, Saliba F, et al. Central hepatectomy versus extended hepatectomy for malignant tumors: a propensity score analysis of postoperative complications. World J Surg. 2016 Jun 6. [Epub ahead of print].
10. Liau KH, Blumgart LH, DeMatteo RP. Segment-oriented approach to liver resection. The Surgical clinics of North America. 2004;84(2):543–61.
11. Soler L, Delingette H, Malandain G, Montagnat J, Ayache N, Koehl C, et al. Fully automatic anatomical, pathological, and functional segmentation from CT scans for hepatic surgery. Comput Aided Surg. 2001;6(3):131–42.
12. Schwartz ME, Miller CM, Roayaie S, Gomatos IP, Konstadoulakis MM. Metzenbaum-assisted liver resection: a safe and effective liver resection technique. Dig Surg. 2014;31(4–5):312–7.

4 Management of Patients with Bilateral Multi-focal Colorectal Liver Metastasis: Two-Stage Approach

Dario Ribero, Roberto Lo Tesoriere and Alessandro Ferrero

Introduction

Despite major advances in chemotherapy and local treatments, surgical resection of colorectal liver metastases is still the therapeutic modality offering the best chance for cure, with 5-year overall survival rates reported to approach 60%. Nevertheless, fewer than 25% of patients are considered to have resectable disease. In particular, patients with multiple, bilobar metastases are among those with the highest chance to be deemed unresectable because of the impossibility to completely remove all tumor deposits while preserving an adequate future liver remnant (FLR) volume. If there are currently no morphological limits in terms of number and distribution of liver metastases to define resectability [1] the key point remains the adequacy of the FLR. During the past decades, considerable efforts were directed toward developing innovative approaches to improve resectability in these patients, including conversion chemotherapy followed by rescue surgery, portal vein embolization (PVE), and use of radiofrequency ablation (RFA). Another option, termed "two-stage hepatectomy," has been conceived by Adam et al. [2] who proposed a potentially

D. Ribero (✉)
Division of Hepatobilio-Pancreatic Surgery, European Institute of Oncology,
Via Ripamonti 435, Milano, Italy
e-mail: dario.ribero@ieo.it

R.L. Tesoriere · A. Ferrero
Division of General and Oncologic Surgery, Mauriziano Hospital "Umberto I",
Largo Turati 62, 10128 Torino, Italy
e-mail: rlotesoriere@mauriziano.it

A. Ferrero
e-mail: aferrero@mauriziano.it

T.M. Pawlik et al. (eds.), *Case-Based Lessons in the Management of Complex Hepato-Pancreato-Biliary Surgery*, DOI 10.1007/978-3-319-50868-9_4

curative strategy consisting in planned, sequential liver resections: during the first stage, one hemiliver is cleaned; the initial operation is then followed by a period of time to hallow hypertrophy of the remaining liver; then, a second operation is performed to resect the remaining disease, when adequate parenchymal hypertrophy has reduced the risk of postoperative liver insufficiency. After its seminal proposal, in a few years this approach has been standardized. In patients responding to chemotherapy, attention is first focused on extirpating the low-volume disease in the planned FLR with limited resections; performing the minor hepatectomy first permits to protect the FLR by avoiding repeat dissection and resection in a small, friable, hypertrophic remnant, which would be required if minor resection is performed second. In addition, if disease progresses between stages, the patient who would have not benefitted from an aggressive surgery is spared the morbidity of a major hepatectomy. Conversely, in the absence of tumor progression in the FLR, the hypertrofic response to PVE or portal vein ligation (PVL) permits the selection of candidates with the lowest operative risk to undergo major or extended resections. Finally, targeting at first the "easy side" of the liver, with minor hepatic resection, allows consideration of resecting the primary during the first stage in patients with synchronous metastases [3].

In the following paragraphs, we will present general and technical aspects of the two-stage hepatectomy and we will discuss the short- and long-terms results as well as alternative approaches.

Case Presentation

A healthy 59-year-old woman, complaining of recent changes in her bowel habit with constipation and narrowing of the stool, presented to the emergency department of a community hospital with symptoms of acute bowel obstruction. A CT scan was performed, revealing an obstructing left colon cancer with multiple bilateral liver metastases. A colonic stent was placed, with prompt relief of the symptoms. After 9 days the patient underwent an uneventful left hemicolectomy. Pathology showed a moderately to poorly differentiated adenocarcinoma pT3 pN2a (4/18) with lymphovascular invasion; K-RAS status was tested identifying a mutation in the exone 2 (G12D). Chemotherapy with Folfox plus Bevacizumab was started after restaging of the disease (Fig. 4.1a). Pretreatment CEA was 187 ng/ml. After six cycles of chemotherapy, the CT scan (Fig. 4.1b) showed a partial response, concomitant with a normalization of the serum CEA level (4.6 ng/ml). Therefore, the patient was sent to our department for surgical evaluation and treatment recommendation. An MRI was performed and all radiological images were reviewed by a dedicated liver multidisciplinary team that recommended surgery with a two-stage approach.

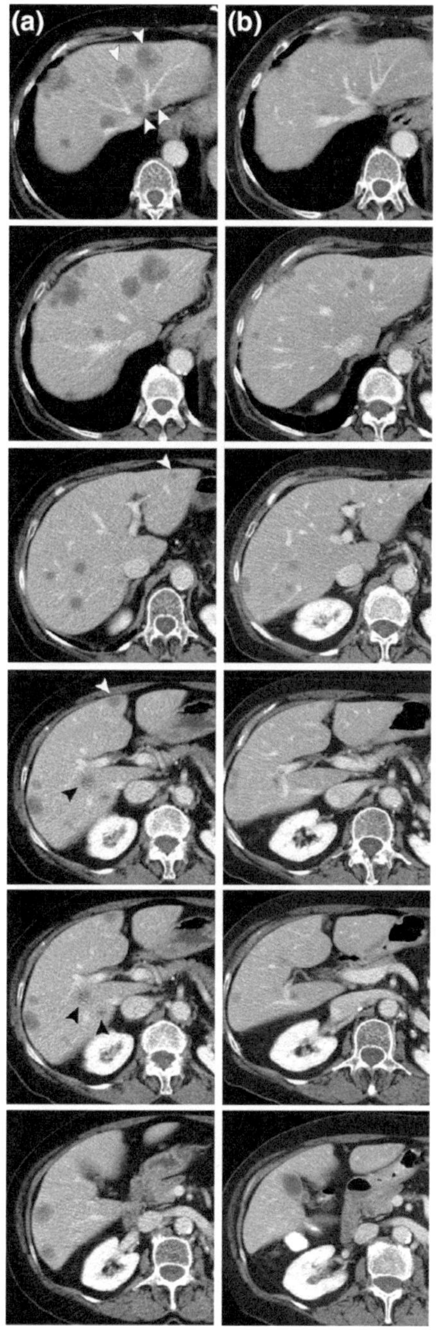

Fig. 4.1 CT scan at diagnosis **a** shows multiple bilobar liver metastases. The entire right hemiliver is involved, with two metastases (*black arrowheads*) located in contact with the second-order right portal bifurcation making unfeasible any resection less than a right hepatectomy. As opposite, the left hemiliver is relatively speared; six lesions (*white arrowheads*) are identified. After six cycles of neoadjuvant chemotherapy, CT scan **b** shows a partial response with reduction in size of all lesions; none of the lesions in the left liver has disappeared

Technical Pearls

- Accurately stage the disease with IOUS since the chance of finding new lesions is high, and use ultrasound to guide the parenchymal spearing clearance of the FLR.
- Prefer wedge resection and detachment of metastases from vessels, especially hepatic veins, to reduce the parenchymal sacrifice of the FLR; in these cases the extraheaptic control of the root of the hepatic veins is desirable.
- When portal vein ligation is performed, 10 ml of absolute alcohol should be injected into the right portal vein to reduce formation of intrahepatic porto-portal venous collaterals and right portal vein recanalization.
- In patients undergoing portal vein ligation, avoid performing cholecystectomy in order to reduce postoperative adhesions and facilitate hepatic pedicle dissection during the second stage. Likewise, during the first stage, reduce to a minimum the right liver mobilization.
- Prefer the use of standardize volumetry to evaluate the FLR hypertrophy and precisely estimate the DH and the KGR to predict the safety of the second-stage resection.

Preoperative Assessment

Since in recent years the concept of resectability has changed toward a technically based definition that considers solely the possibility to radically extirpate all metastatic deposits (i.e., to obtain an R0 resection), accurate detection and precise localization of all liver metastases is essential to select appropriate candidates for surgery and to determine the overall surgical strategy (one- vs. two-stage approach). Computed tomography (CT) remains the mainstay of liver imaging since it accurately assess both the intra- and extra-hepatic extent of disease. Use of multidetector-row CT allows us to obtain high-quality, thin (2.5 mm) slices, which have been shown to improve detection of small metastases as compared to thicker ones (5-, 7.5- or 10-mm) [4]. The liver should be examined with a specific protocol including an unenhanced scan followed by the acquisition of 3 sets of images after intravenous injection of a non-ionic iodine contrast medium (100–150 ml at a flow rate of 3–5 ml/s): late arterial phase (after 25–35 s); portal venous phase (after 55–70 s); and delayed phase (after 180 s). Data indicate that the dual-phase evaluation (late arterial and portal venous) improves the detection and characterization of colorectal liver metastases when compared with portal venous phase imaging alone [5]. In addition, CT data can be used for vascular reconstruction and liver volumetry that is nowadays an essential preoperative evaluation to increase the safety of major hepatectomies. Therefore, we do strongly recommend obtaining high-quality studies before making any clinical decision. However, in the subset of patients with multiple bilateral metastases, CT is often insufficient. In fact, these patients share specific features to be considered. First, almost all patients undergo chemotherapy that significantly reduces the sensitivity of preoperative imaging as compared to that observed in chemotherapy-naïve patients (CT: 65.3% vs. 87.5%; PET 49% vs. 93.3%, respectively) [6]. Second, multiple small lesions are often present at diagnosis or as a consequence of chemotherapy-induced tumor shrinkage. Several studies have reported that the sensitivity of contrast-enhanced magnetic resonance imaging (MRI) is significantly higher than that of CT, with the largest difference observed in the detection of metastatic lesions of less than 1 cm [7]. In addition, use of the liver-specific MRI contrast agent Gd-EOB-DTPA has further increased the detection rate and thus the diagnostic accuracy [8].

Recently, by analyzing a large homogeneous series of patients with colorectal liver metastases who had undergone preoperative chemotherapy, we have shown that the combined assessment of DWI sequences with Gd-EOB-DTPA-enhanced MRI sequences yielded a greater diagnostic accuracy and sensitivity (89.2 and 91%, respectively) compared to those of each individual method [9]. Worthy of note was the observation that assessment of DWI was pivotal in identifying small lesions, which may be missed or misinterpreted as peripheral vasculo-biliary structures or artifacts in contrast-enhanced sequences. Therefore, we strongly recommend to complete the preoperative evaluation with a Gd-EOB-DTPA-enhanced MRI with DWI. The major limitation is that, in many cases, the same study has not been performed before commencing chemotherapy and thus comparable pretreatment images are not available. Thus, we also suggest performing an MRI as a basal evaluation whenever possible in patients with liver-only disease. Due to restricted availability and high cost, in our practice FDG-PET and PET-CT are not prescribed in all patients, but in selected cases in whom diagnosis is not clear following diagnostic conventional modalities.

Surgical Management

Once liver resection has been considered feasible and oncologically appropriate, the patient is scheduled for surgery. A standardized operative technique is used. The patient is placed supine with the right arm tucked in a 15° reverse Trendelenburg position. A chevron incision with or without an upper midline extension up to the xiphysternum or a *J*-shaped incision are used. The type of incision is selected based on patient size, the costal arch morphology, and the presence of abdominal incision from previous surgeries. After a thorough abdominal exploration, the round and falciform ligaments are sectioned. As a general recommendation, the deeper part of the falciform ligament and the coronary ligaments should be preserved to avoid penetration of air at the hepatocaval confluence; air that generates artifacts might mask anatomical details essential for surgical planning. In our patient, two lesions are in contact with the middle and left hepatic veins (Figs. 4.1a and 4.2a), whose relationship are best visualized in the absence of artifacts from dissection. Intra-operative ultrasonography (IOUS) is performed with a 7.5–10 MHz dedicated probe. Our preference is for a microconvex echoprobe (Hitachi-Aloka Medical; Tokyo, Japan) because of the optimal compromise between small size, wide scanning window, and stability along its handling. Aims of IOUS are to stage the disease by confirming preoperative findings and, excluding previously undetected lesions, to visualize the anatomic relationships between vasculo-biliary structures and tumors, to plan the definitive surgical strategy, and to guide resection by delineating proper transection planes and controlling them during the parenchymal dissection. Despite major advances in preoperative imaging, IOUS remains an essential staging tool. In a recent bi-institutional study, data from 515 patients who had undergone liver resection for colorectal liver metastases in the years 2005–2009 were reviewed [10]. All patients had an intensive preoperative workup, with a median of three high-quality imaging modalities per patient, including MRI in half of them; nevertheless, IOUS detected new nodules in 132 patients (25.6%) and its findings prompted a change of the preoperatively planned type of resection in 27.2% of the cases. Interestingly, on multivariate analysis bilobar (OR 1.66) and multiple more than >3 metastases (OR 1.85) were independent predictors of intraoperative detection of new nodules. Therefore, in patients undergoing the first operation of a two-stage hepatectomy, a meticulous IOUS exploration should be performed, since the chance of unexpected findings is high.

Once resectabilty has been definitively confirmed, the first operation focuses on the clearance of the FLR, usually the left liver or segments 2–3. The left liver is thus fully mobilized by dividing the left coronal and triangular ligaments while the mobilization of the right lobe is limited to a minim. In our patient, since two lesions were in contact with the middle and the left hepatic vein, the hepatocaval confluence was widely exposed to permit encircling the common trunk (Fig. 4.2c). To increase the safety of resection we do recommend this maneuver whenever exposure of these vessels is required. Recent evidence from a cohort of 226 consecutive patients indicates that in those undergoing detachment of colorectal metastases from major intrahepatic vessels, defined as "vascular R1" because of an exposed tumor in that specific site, the risk of local recurrence was similar to that of patients having a R0 resection (5.3% vs. 4.3%) [11]. Therefore, whenever signs of infiltration are not evident at IOUS, peeling off the metastases with preservation of the vascular skeleton is advisable.

The parenchymal transection can be performed with different techniques. We systematically use the ultrasonic dissector together with irrigated bipolar forceps and absorbable clips or suture ligature for minor and larger vessels or bile ducts, respectively. The Pringle's maneuver is not systematically performed for several reasons. Almost all patients had undergone preoperative chemotherapy and thus the liver might be more susceptible to the ischemic damage; in addition, during the first stage, removal of the primary, if present, might be associated to liver resection; [3] in such cases, to avoid clamping of hepatic pedicle might prevent intestinal venous

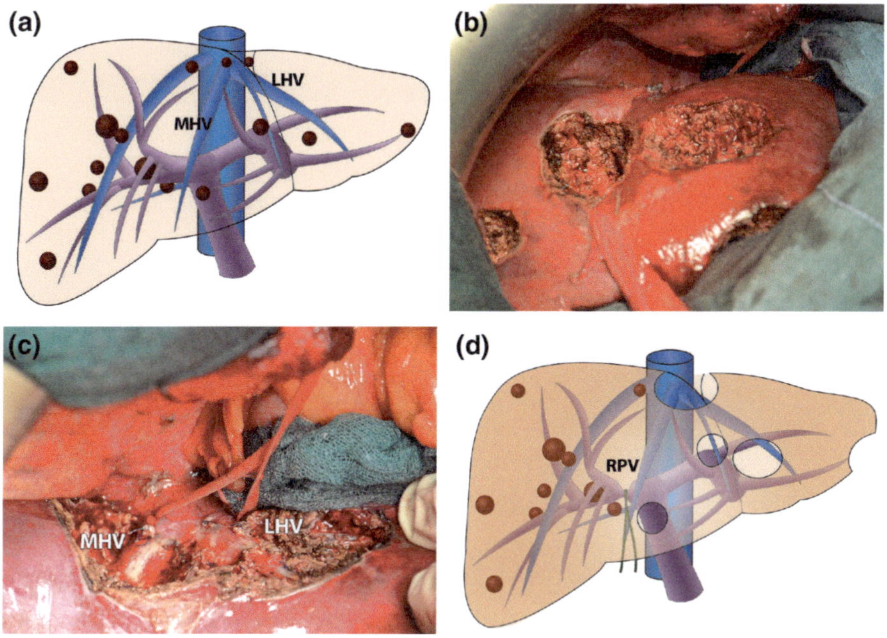

Fig. 4.2 Two-stage hepatectomy, the first step. **a** Schematic representation of the location of all metastatic deposits in our patient. **b** Atypical resections of segments 3 and 4b. **c** Resection of two lesions in S4a with exposure of the left hepatic vein (LHV) and the middle hepatic vein (MHV) on the cut surface; the common trunk has been taped. **d** Schematic representation of the state at the end of the first stage. All left liver lesions have been cleared and the right portal vein (RPV) has been ligated

congestion which, in theory, can jeopardize a prompt anastomotic healing. Therefore, on a routine basis we adopt a "no-clamping policy" with salvage clamping in case of bleeding or persisting oozing [12]. Overall, the clearance of the FLR is performed either through anatomical or atypical resections. Several authors have found no significant difference in oncological outcomes between anatomical and atypical resections for colorectal liver metastases [13–15]. For this reason, IOUS-guided parenchymal-sparing resections should be the preferred option. Figure 4.2a–d depict the surgical approach and the final result of the first operation in our case.

After completing the parenchymal resection, in most patients we do perform a PVL to stimulate the FLR hypertrophy. The efficacy and safety of this technique has been repeatedly proved. A recent metanalysis evaluating the hypertrophic effect of PVL and PVE revealed a statistically comparable increase of the FLR volume, albeit corresponding percentages (27% vs. 39%) pointed to a more pronounced effect of PVE [16]. This difference might be due to a more effective occlusion of distal portal vein branches that prevent shunting between the right and left portal vein. Therefore, before ligating the right portal branches we systematically inject

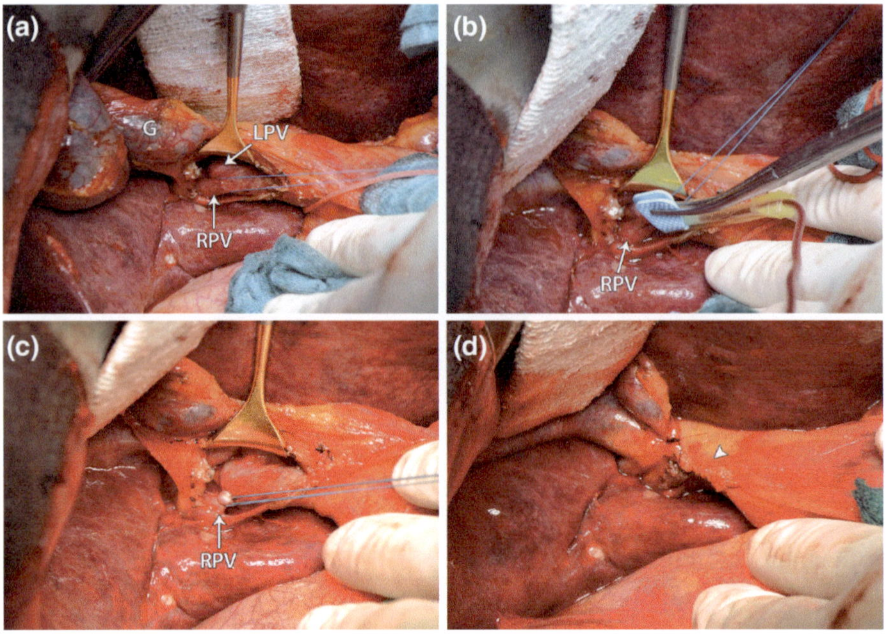

Fig. 4.3 Technique of right portal vein ligation. **a** The right side of hepatic pedicle is dissected and the right (RPV) and left (LPV) portal veins are identified. RPV is controlled on a loop. Gallbladder (G) is not removed whenever possible. **b** 10 cc of alcohol are injected in RPV. Then the injected alcohol is flushed into the right portal system by briefly loosening the loop before its ligation. **c** The RPV is ligated with two nonabsorbable sutures. **d** The peritoneum of the hepatic pedicle is closed in order to reduce adhesions

10 cc of ethanol, which has been successfully used as embolizing material for PVE. The technique of PVL is detailed in Fig. 4.3. In our experience, key points are: (i) it is not necessary to remove the gallbladder; in fact, after opening the peritoneum of the right border of the hepatic pedicle, using a Gil-Vernet retractor positioned under the bile duct permits us to easily dissect the portal vein; keeping the gallbladder in situ reduces the formation of postoperative adhesion and serves as a guidance to the hepatic pedicle during the second operation; (ii) before injecting the alcohol or ligating the right portal vein, the patency of the main and left portal vein should be checked with the color-doppler; (iii) we always inject 10 cc of alcohol which is a cheap, safe, and readily available sclerosing agent that might enhance the hypertrofic response of the FLR. Not all patients, however, undergo PVL during the first stage. In patients with very small FLR volumes, or in those undergoing extensive resection of the FLR, PVE is scheduled 7–10 days after resection to permit recovery of liver function, thus reducing the risk of complications.

It is not clear if the routine use of chemotherapy between the first- and second-stage hepatectomy can lower tumor progression and dropout rates. In fact, multiple evidences indicate a significantly higher rate of tumor growth after portal vein occlusion (PVO), a phenomenon due to changes in cytokines and growth factors, alteration in hepatic blood supply, and enhanced cellular host response promoting local tumor growth [17–22]. While data from international cancer centers showed that administration of chemotherapy between stages could prevent tumor progression [17], in our series of patients selected for a two-stage hepatectomy, interval tumor progression, observed in 53% of the cases, was independent of whether the patient had or had not had chemotherapy [22]. Notably, the administration of chemotherapy did not significantly reduce the dropout rates. Therefore, we do not routinely perform chemotherapy after the first operation.

Four weeks after PVO a CT scan is performed to measure the FLR volume, since after an initial phase of rapid growth, at this time point the kinetic of FLR hypertrophy reaches a plateau [23]. If a volume of at least 30% of the total liver volume (TLV) is documented, and no tumor progression in the liver remnant is observed, the second operation is scheduled. As mentioned above, it is not uncommon to observe an interval tumor growth in the liver to be removed; [17, 19, 20, 22]; in our opinion, this should not be considered per se a formal contraindication to proceed with the second stage, since it appears more a consequence of local factors promoting the growth of the known metastases rather than a true "tumor progression."

Alternative Approaches and Current Controversies

- One-stage approach with ultrasound-guided parenchymal-sparing resections has been proposed as a comparable alternative. However, concerns still remain on whether patients selected for a one-stage strategy are the same to those undergoing a two-stage hepatectomy, and on the oncological outcomes due do the absence of robust long-term data.
- One-stage plus RFA might be an appealing alternative. However, while limited data indicate comparable results, many evidences suggest a real efficacy of RFA only when one lesion of <2 cm is treated. Therefore, while waiting further studies, use of RFA should be limited.
- ALPPS has the potential to reduce the dropout rate, albeit mortality remains high and initial data suggest higher recurrence rate and reduced survival compared to the two-stage approach, a fact that might nullify the benefit of a reduced dropout.

Different methodologies of liver volumetry have been described as being the most popular based on direct measurement of the functional TLV, obtained by subtracting tumors' volume from the measured TLV, or based on the estimation of the TLV (eTLV), obtained with a formula (eTLV [cm^2] = $-794.41 + 1267.28 \times$ BSA) that, using the body surface area, standardizes the liver size to the patients size [24]. The latter method is called standardized volumetry. Although many studies have investigated the critical residual liver volume associated with the development of hepatic insufficiency, few data exist on the implications of the method used to measure liver volumes. In a series of 243 noncirrhotic patients we have directly compared the two methods, demonstrating that the adoption of the standardized volumetry might be clinically relevant since it identifies a subset of patients in whom the measured liver volumetry underestimates the risk of hepatic insufficiency [25]. In addition, in patients with multiple lesions, such as those selected for a two-stage hepatectomy, mathematical errors in measuring tumor volume cumulate because of multiple measurements that, besides, are time consuming. In some patients who have received extensive and complex atypical resections to clean the FLR, the actual volume after resection might not correspond to that obtained by simply subtracting tumors' volume from the FLR volume. Therefore, four to five days after resection it might be useful to perform a CT scan on which to calculate an accurate "basal" FLR volume by delineating the contours of the actual liver remnant. With this basal assessment is also possible to precisely evaluate the kinetic measures of FLR hypertrophy, such as the degree of hypertrophy (DH %, defined as the percentage-point difference between the FLR volume before and after PVO) [23] and the kinetic of growth rate (KGR %/week, calculated as: DH at first post-PVO volume assessment (%) ÷ time elapsed since PVO (weeks) at first post-PVO volume assessment) [26, 27]. Both measures have been shown to predict the safety of major or extended hepatectomies with cutoffs of 5–7.5% and 2%/week, respectively [23, 26]. When directly compared, the accuracy of KGR to predict postoperative morbidity and mortality was superior to that of DH, with KGR values of >2%/week associated with less than 10% risk of hepatic insufficiency and null risk of 90 days' mortality from liver failure [26]. In fact, by standardizing the DH to time, the KGR provides an estimation of individual regeneration curves after PVO that contributes additional prognostic information beyond the FLR volume and the DH.

The second stage of the two-stage hepatectomy entails removal of the residual disease, usually with a right or an extended right hepatectomy. The surgical approach is similar to that of the first stage. After opening the abdomen through the same incision, IOUS is performed to exclude the presence of new undetected metastases in the FLR. Then, the right liver is fully mobilized and cholecystectomy is performed, if the gallbladder is present. We usually dissect the right border of the hepatic pedicle to isolate the right hepatic artery and the right portal vein, which are sectioned between ligatures. As opposite, the right biliary duct is interrupted almost at the end of the parenchymal transection. In some patients, dissection of the pedicle might be very difficult due to the presence of inflammation or dense adhesions from previous PVL plus ethanol injection or PVE. In such circumstances, we suggest an intrahepatic suture-ligation of the right Glissonian pedicles. Alternatively, a "Glissonian approach" might be considered [28]. It consists of performing a small incision of the liver parenchyma in front of the hilum and to bluntly dissect it to disclose the anterior surface of the right glissonean pedicle and its limit. Then, a second incision is made perpendicular to the hepatic hilum on the right border of S1. A large-curved clamp (Mixter clamp) is introduced through the first incision on the left side of the right glissonean sheath with the tip allowed to slide from left to right diagonally at a 30° angle. This maneuver allows us to encircle with a tape the right main sheath, which can be sectioned with a linear stapler after applying a firm countertraction of the tape to avoid the risk of an extended left clamping. Before firing, IUOS with color-Doppler might be used to ascertain the maintenance of a left portal flow.

Figure 4.4a, b show the PVL induced changes of the FLR volume in our patient. Four weeks after PVL a good hypertrophy was observed. A DH of 9.9% and a KGR of 2.47%/week indicate an excellent regeneration curve and a low postoperative risk. Accordingly, the patients recovered uneventfully after a right hepatectomy (Fig. 4.4c) and was discharged from the hospital on postoperative day 5.

Outcome of Two-Stage Hepatectomy and Its Current Role

Table 4.1 summarizes technical aspects and short- and long-term outcomes following two-stage hepatectomy in the largest published cohorts. Despite two-stage hepatectomy is performed in patients with advanced disease at high risk of recurrence, 5-year survival estimates of $\sim 50\%$ have been obtained when both the stages are completed [28]. The main aspect that emerges from all series is that approximately 20–30% of patients cannot proceed to the second-stage resection because of tumor progression, insufficient hypertrophy of the FLR, or complications either related to surgery or PVE [29]. This dropout rate has stimulated surgeons to explore alternative strategies. Associating Liver Partition and Portal Vein Ligation for Staged Hepatectomy (ALPPS) is one of these. With this technique the liver growth seems much faster than after PVO, permitting surgeons to reduce to 7–10 days the delay between the two stages. However, the associated morbidity is high, and mortality rates of approximately 6% in patients undergoing ALPPS for colorectal liver metastases have been reported [30]. In addition, despite the theoretical advantages of reducing the dropout rate, higher recurrence and reduced survival rates have been observed [31], suggesting that two-stage hepatectomy by selecting optimal candidates who do not progress during a long period of time might be oncologically more adequate.

Recently, it has also been reported that offering patients with multiple bilobar liver metastases a one-stage hepatectomy with [32] or without [33] RFA might guarantee comparable long-term outcomes but no dropout that has been advocated as a loss of chance. However, while data regarding two-stage hepatectomy are robust, outcomes of one-stage approaches remain unclear for several reasons. First, since a two-stage hepatectomy should be considered only if a one-stage hepatectomy cannot be performed, a direct comparison of the two strategies remains questionable, as it is possible that patients are different. Second, because of a short follow-up or an intensive use of intraarterial adjuvant chemotherapy, at present, the long-term outcomes cannot be considered equivalent. Finally, despite enthusiasm for RFA, numerous studies suggested a real efficacy only in very selected patients

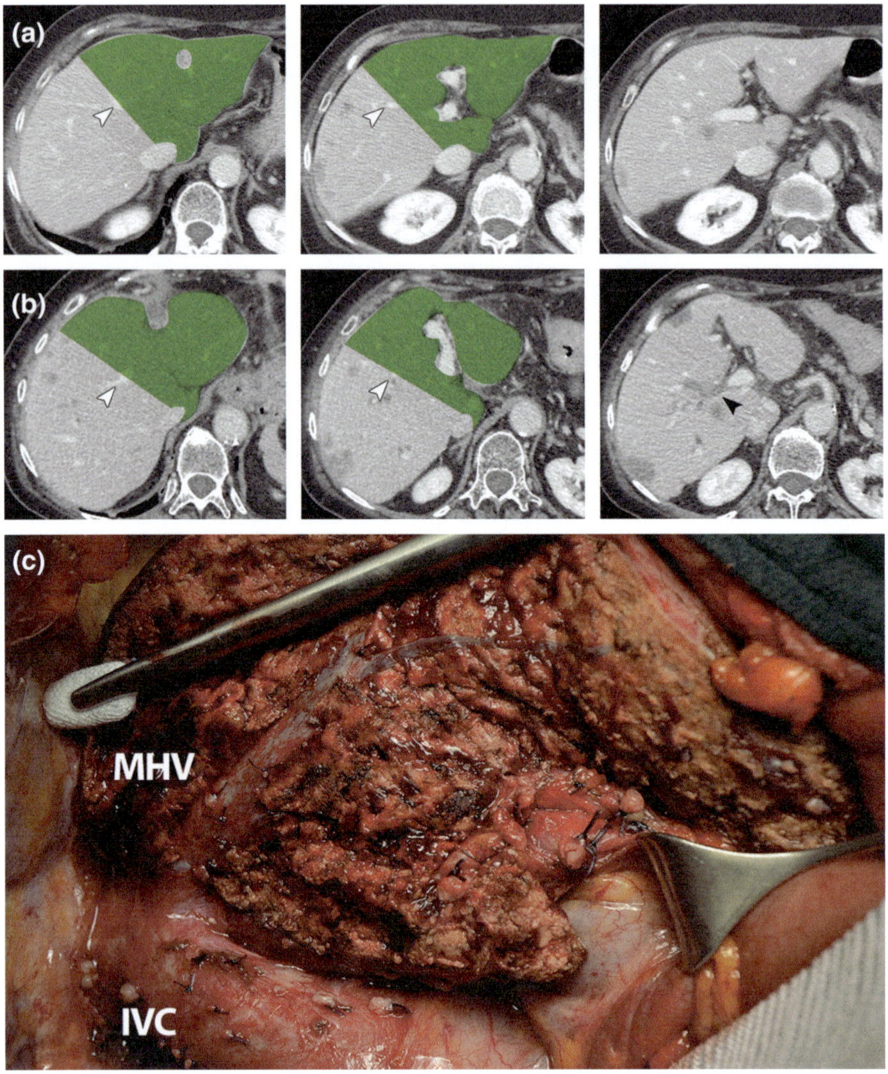

Fig. 4.4 Liver volumetry before and after PVL and the result of the second operation. **a** The FLR volume before PVL is 402.2 cc corresponding to a 26.2% of an estimated TLV of 1546 cc (the patients was 168 cm height with a weight of 72.5 kg [BSA 1.84]). **b** Liver volumetry performed four weeks after PVL shows a good hypertrophy of FLR which measures 538 cc, corresponding to 36.1% of the eTLV; the DH and the KGR are 9.9% and 2.47%/week, respectively. As a consequence of segment 4 hypertrophy, the main portal scissure (white arrowheads) slightly rotated to the right. The *black arrowhead* indicates the right portal vein closed. **c** Second stage completed by performing a right hepatectomy. The middle hepatic vein (MHV) is exposed on the cut surface. Inferior vena cava (IVC) is shown

Table 4.1 Technical aspects, short- and long-term outcomes following two-stage hepatectomy in recent series

Author	Year	*n* of pts	Preop CTx (%)	Simultaneous colorectal resection (%)	Completion rate (%)	PVE/PVL	Interval CTx	Morbidity		Mortality		OS post two-stage#		
								1st stage (%)	2nd stage (%)	1st stage (%)	2nd stage (%)	Median (months)	3-years (%)	5-years (%)
Tanaka [35]	2007	24	64	NR	92	17/0	0	13	23	0	0	NR	33	NR
Wicherts [36]	2008	59	97	20	69	32/0	78	7	29	0	7	42	60	42
Tsai [37]	2010	45	71	50	78	33/2	62	26	26	4	5	36	58	NR
Karoui [3]	2010	33*		100	76	5/17		21	32	0	4		80	48
Muratore [22]	2011	47	79	50	77	27/11	53	19	44	0	0	38	65	NR
Narita [38]	2011	80	82	40	76	3/74	31	14	54	0	0	40	59	32
Tsim [39]	2011	38	97	0	87	0/36	13	11	33	0	0	35	50[a]	NR
Bowers [40] §	2011	39	74	NR	82	0/28	15	23	56	0	4	24 [b]	28[b]	NR
Turrini [41]	2012	48	100	37	71	0/48	29	18	23	0	0	44	59	35
Giuliante [42]	2014	130	87	55	78	55/59	30	17	35	0	3.9	43	NR	32
Jamal [43]	2014	74	100	NR	52	48/0	NR	26	48	0	0	NR	68	75
Passot [29]	2016	109	100	23	82	80/0	44	6	26	0	7	57	68	49

CTx chemotherapy; *PVE* portal vein embolization; *PVL* portal vein ligation; *OS* overall survival (# data reported refer to survival after completion of two-stage hepatectomy); *NR* not reported

[a]In patients with R0 liver resection

[b]Survival in patients with colorectal liver metastases only

*Included only patients with concomitant colorectal resection

§Included patients with liver metastases from colorectal cancer (n = 33) and other tumors (n = 6)

with a single, small lesion (<2 cm) [34]. Therefore, two-stage hepatectomy remains the most reliable and standardized approach for patients with multiple bilateral colorectal liver metastases.

Overall Management of Patients with Bilateral Colorectal Liver Metastases

- Two-stage hepatectomy allows treatment of patients with advanced disease while providing an optimal oncological selection based on response to chemotherapy and absence of rapid progression between stages. A role of RAS as a selection criterion is emerging, albeit robust data are lacking.
- Preoperative and intraoperative staging is pivotal to optimize surgical results. Therefore, high-quality imaging (CT scan with a liver protocol and MRI with hepato-specific contrast medium) should be obtained in these patients.
- All patients who are candidates for a two-stage hepatectomy should undergo preoperative chemotherapy; use of interval chemotherapy is debatable.
- Combination of resection with ablation techniques such as RFA might increase the resectability rate, albeit RFA should be limited to a single lesion less than 2 cm in diameter.
- Monitor response to chemotherapy, absence of progression between stages, tumor biology.
- Adoption of two-stage hepatectomy is supported by several studies and strongest evidences than alternative strategies such as one-stage hepatectomy with or without multiple RFAs or ALPPS.

References

1. Adam R, De Gramont A, Figueras J, Guthrie A, Kokudo N, Kunstlinger F, et al. The oncosurgery approach to managing liver metastases from colorectal cancer: a multidisciplinary international consensus. Oncologist. 2012;17(10):1225–39.
2. Adam R, Laurent A, Azoulay D, Castaing D, Bismuth H. Two-stage hepatectomy: a planned strategy to treat irresectable liver tumors. Ann Surg. 2000;232:777–85.
3. Karoui M, Vigano L, Goyer P, Ferrero A, Luciani A, Aglietta M, et al. Combined first-stage hepatectomy and colorectal resection in a two-stage hepatectomy strategy for bilobar synchronous liver metastases. Br J Surg. 2010;97(9):1354–62.
4. Weg N, Scheer MR, Gabor MP. Liver lesions: improved detection with dual-detector-array CT and routine 2.5-mm thin collimation. Radiology. 1998;209:417–26.
5. Scott DJ, Guthrie JA, Arnold P, Ward J, Atchley J, Wilson D, et al. Dual phase helical CT versus portal venous phase CT for the detection of colorectal liver metastases: correlation with intra-operative sonography, surgical and pathological findings. Clin Radiol. 2001;56 (3):235–42.

6. Lubezky N, Metser U, Geva R, Nakache R, Shmueli E, Klausner JM, et al. The role and limitations of 18-fluoro-2-deoxy-D-glucose positron emission tomography (FDG-PET) scan and computerized tomography (CT) in restaging patients with hepatic colorectal metastases following neoadjuvant chemotherapy: comparison with operative and pathological findings. J Gastrointest Surg. 2007;11:472–8.
7. Regge D, Campanella D, Anselemetti GC, Cirillo S, Gallo TM, Muratore A, et al. Diagnostic accuracy of portal phase CT and MRI with Mangafodipir trisodium in detecting liver metastases from colorectal carcinoma. Clin Radiol. 2006;61:338–47.
8. Koh DM, Brown G, Riddell AM, Scurr E, Collins DJ, Allen SD, et al. Detection of colorectal hepatic metastases using MnDPDP MR imaging and diffusion-weighted imaging (DWI) alone and in combination. Eur Radiol. 2008;18:903–10.
9. Macera A, Lario C, Petracchini M, Gallo T, Regge D, Floriani I, et al. Staging of colorectal liver metastases after preoperative chemotherapy. Diffusion-weighted imaging in combination with Gd-EOB-DTPA MRI sequences increases sensitivity and diagnostic accuracy. Eur Radiol. 2013;23(3):739–47.
10. Ferrero A, Langella S, Giuliante F, Viganò L, Vellone M, Zimmitti G, et al. Intraoperative liver ultrasound still affects surgical strategy for patients with colorectal metastases in the modern era. World J Surg. 2013;37(11):2655–63.
11. Viganò L, Procopio F, Cimino MM, Donadon M, Gatti A, Costa G, et al. Is tumor detachment from vascular structures equivalent to R0 resection in surgery for colorectal liver metastases? An observational cohort. Ann Surg Oncol. 2016;23(4):1352–60.
12. Viganò L, Jaffary SA, Ferrero A, Russolillo N, Langella S, Capussotti L. Liver resection without pedicle clamping: feasibility and need for "salvage clamping". Looking for the right clamping policy. Analysis of 512 consecutive resections. J Gastrointest Surg. 2011;15:1820–8.
13. Kokudo N, Tada K, Seki M, Ohta H, Azekura K, Ueno M, et al. Anatomical major resection versus non anatomical limited resection for liver metastases from colorectal carcinoma. Am J Surg. 2001;181(2):153–9.
14. Gold JS, Are C, Kornprat P, Jarnagin WR, Gönen M, Fong Y, et al. Increased use of parenchymal-sparing surgery for bilateral liver metastases from colorectal cancer is associated with improved mortality without change in oncologic outcome: trends in treatment over time in 440 patients. Ann Surg. 2008;247(1):109–17.
15. Mise Y, Aloia TA, Brudvik KW, Schwarz L, Vauthey JN, Conrad C. Parenchymal-sparing hepatectomy in colorectal liver metastasis improves salvageability and survival. Ann Surg. 2016;263(1):146–52.
16. Pandanaboyana S, Bell R, Hidalgo E, Toogood G, Prasad KR, Bartlett A, et al. A systematic review and meta-analysis of portal vein ligation versus portal vein embolization for elective liver resection. Surgery. 2015;157(4):690–8.
17. Fischer C, Melstrom LG, Arnaoutakis D, Jarnagin W, Brown K, D'Angelica M, et al. Chemotherapy after portal vein embolization to protect against tumor growth during liver hypertrophy before hepatectomy. JAMA Surg. 2013;148(12):1103–8.
18. Hoekstra LT, van Lienden KP, Doets A, Busch ORC, Gouma DJ, van Gulik TM. Tumor progression after preoperative portal vein embolization. Ann Surg. 2012;256(5):812–7.
19. Elias D, De Baere T, Roche A, Mducreux, Leclere J, Lasser P. During liver regeneration following right portal embolization the growth rate of liver metastases is more rapid than that of the liver parenchyma. Br J Surg. 1999;86:784–8.
20. Kokudo N, Tada K, Seki M, Ohta H, Azekura K, Ueno M, et al. Proliferative activity of intrahepatic colorectal metastases after preoperative hemihepatic portal vein embolization. Hepatology. 2001;34:267–72.
21. de Graaf W, van den Esschert JW, van Lienden KP, van Gulik TM. Induction of tumor growth after preoperative portal vein embolization: is it a real problem? Ann Surg Oncol. 2009;16:423–30.

22. Muratore A, Zimmitti G, Ribero D, Mellano A, Viganò L, Capussotti L. Chemotherapy between the first and second stages of a two-stage hepatectomy for colorectal liver metastases: should we routinely recommend it? Ann Surg Oncol. 2012;19(4):1310–5.
23. Ribero D, Abdalla EK, Madoff DC, Donadon M, Loyer EM, Vauthey JN. Portal vein embolization before major hepatectomy and its effects on regeneration, resectability and outcome. Br J Surg. 2007;94(11):1386–94.
24. Vauthey JN, Abdalla EK, Doherty DA, Gertsch P, Fenstermacher MJ, Loyer EM, et al. Body surface area and body weight predict total liver volume in Western adults. Liver Transpl. 2002;8:233–40.
25. Ribero D, Amisano M, Bertuzzo F, Langella S, Lo Tesoriere R, Ferrero A, et al. Measured versus estimated total liver volume to preoperatively assess the adequacy of the future liver remnant: which method should we use? Ann Surg. 2013;258(5):801–6.
26. Shindoh J, Truty MJ, Aloia TA, Curley SA, Zimmitti G, Huang SY, et al. Kinetic Growth Rate after portal vein embolization predicts posthepatectomy outcomes: toward zero liver-related mortality in patients with colorectal liver metastases and small future liver remnant. J Am Coll Surg. 2013;216(2):201–9.
27. Leung U, Simpson AL, Araujo RL, Gönen M, McAuliffe C, Miga MI, et al. Remnant growth rate after portal vein embolization is a good early predictor of post-hepatectomy liver failure. J Am Coll Surg. 2014;219(4):620–30.
28. Takasaki K. How to tape the whole right segmental branch. In: Takasaki K, editor. Glissonean pedicle transection method for hepatic resection. Springer Japan 2007. p. 56–61.
29. Passot G, Chun YS, Kopetz SE, Zorzi D, Brudvik KW, Kim BJ, et al. Predictors of safety and efficacy of 2-stage hepatectomy for bilateral colorectal liver metastases. J Am Coll Surg. 2016;223(1):99–108.
30. Linecker M, Stavrou GA, Oldhafer KJ, Jenner RM, Seifert B, Lurje G, et al. The ALPPS risk score: avoiding futile use of ALPPS. Ann Surg. 2016. [Epub ahead of print].
31. Adam R, Imai K, Castro Benitez C, Allard MA, Vibert E, Sa Cunha A, et al. Outcome after associating liver partition and portal vein ligation for staged hepatectomy and conventional two-stage hepatectomy for colorectal liver metastases. Br J Surg. 2016;103(11):1521–9.
32. Faitot F, Faron M, Adam R, Elias D, Cimino M, Cherqui D, et al. Two-stage hepatectomy versus 1-stage resection combined with radiofrequency for bilobar colorectal metastases: a case-matched analysis of surgical and oncological outcomes. Ann Surg. 2014;260(5):822–7; discussion 27–8.
33. Viganò L, Torzilli G, Cimino M, Imai K, Vibert E, Donadon M, et al. Drop-out between the two liver resections of two-stage hepatectomy. Patient selection or loss of chance? Eur J Surg Oncol. 2016;42(9):1385–93.
34. Lee H, Heo JS, Cho YB, Yun SH, Kim HC, Lee WY, et al. Hepatectomy vs radiofrequency ablation for colorectal liver metastasis: a propensity score analysis. World J Gastroenterol. 2015;21(11):3300–7.
35. Tanaka K, Shimada H, Matsuo K, Ueda M, Endo I, Togo S. Remnant liver regeneration after two-stage hepatectomy for multiple bilobar colorectal metastases. Eur J Surg Oncol. 2007;33 (3):329–35.
36. Wicherts DA, Miller R, de Haas RJ, Bitsakou G, Vibert E, Veilhan LA, et al. Long-term results of two-stage hepatectomy for irresectable colorectal cancer liver metastases. Ann Surg. 2008;248:994–1005.
37. Tsai S, Marques HP, de Jong MC, Mira P, Ribeiro V, Choti MA, et al. Two-stage strategy for patients with extensive bilateral colorectal liver metastases. HPB. 2010;12(4):262–9.
38. Narita M, Oussoultzoglou E, Jaeck D, Fuchschuber P, Rosso E, Pessaux P, et al. Two-stage hepatectomy for multiple bilobar colorectal liver metastases. Br J Surg. 2011;98(10):1463–75.
39. Tsim N, Healey AJ, Frampton AE, Habib NA, Bansi DS, Wasan H, et al. Two-stage resection for bilobar colorectal liver metastases: R0 resection is the key. Ann Surg Oncol. 2011;18 (7):1939–46.

40. Bowers KA, O'Reilly D, Bond-Smith GE, Hutchins RR. Feasibility study of two-stage hepatectomy for bilobar liver metastases. Am J Surg. 2012;203(6):691–7.
41. Turrini O, Ewald J, Viret F, Sarran A, Goncalves A, Delpero J-R. Two-stage hepatectomy: who will not jump over the second hurdle? Eur J Surg Oncol. 2012;38(3):266–73.
42. Giuliante F, Ardito F, Ferrero A, Aldrighetti L, Ercolani G, Grande G, et al. Tumor progression during preoperative chemotherapy predicts failure to complete 2-stage hepatectomy for colorectal liver metastases: results of an Italian multicenter analysis of 130 patients. J Am Coll Surg. 2014;219(2):285–94.
43. Jamal MH, Hassanain M, Chaudhury P, Tran TT, Wong S, Yousef Y, et al. Staged hepatectomy for bilobar colorectal hepatic metastases. HPB. 2012;14(11):782–9.

5 Management of Patients with Bilateral Multifocal Colorectal Liver Metastases: ALPPS

Matteo Serenari, Martin de Santibañes, Victoria Ardiles and Eduardo de Santibañes

Case Presentation

A 44-year-old female patient was referred to our surgical department with symptoms of abdominal pain and obstipation. A computed tomography (CT) demonstrated bilobar hypodense images in the liver and a complete obstruction of the sigmoid colon due to a 40 mm enhanced mass. The presence of extrahepatic disease was excluded by chest and pelvis scans. Carcinoembryonic antigen (CEA) and carbohydrate antigen 19-9 (CA 19-9) levels at the time of diagnosis were 12 ng/ml and 31.7 U/ml, respectively.

The patient underwent a laparoscopic converted to open left hemicolectomy with primary colorectal anastomosis since the mass was close to the parietal wall and to the left ovary, which was resected en-bloc with the sigmoid colon. A biopsy of one superficial lesion situated in the right lobe was performed. The postoperative course was uneventful and the patient was discharged without major complications. The

M. Serenari · M. de Santibañes · V. Ardiles · E. de Santibañes (✉)
Department of HPB Surgery, Hospital Italiano de Buenos Aires,
Juan D. Perón 4190, C1181ACH Buenos Aires, Argentina
e-mail: eduardo.desantibanes@hospitalitaliano.org.ar

M. Serenari
e-mail: matteo.serenari@gmail.com

M. de Santibañes
e-mail: martin.desantibanes@hospitalitaliano.org.ar

V. Ardiles
e-mail: victoria.ardiles@hospitalitaliano.org.ar

T.M. Pawlik et al. (eds.), *Case-Based Lessons in the Management of Complex Hepato-Pancreato-Biliary Surgery*, DOI 10.1007/978-3-319-50868-9_5

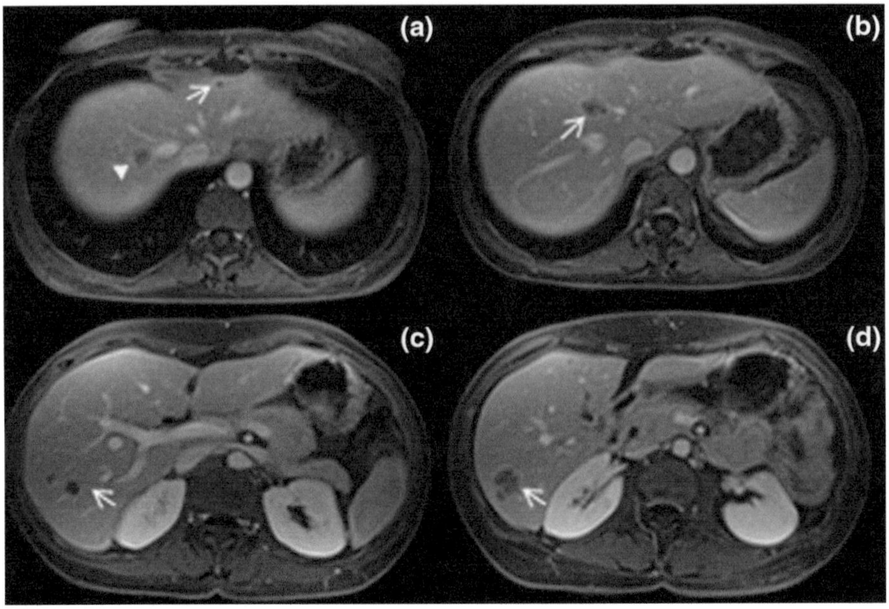

Fig. 5.1 Preoperative magnetic resonance imaging (MRI) after three cycles of preoperative chemotherapy, showing **a** a lesion in segment 7 (*arrowhead*) infiltrating the right hepatic vein and a lesion in segment 2 (*arrow*); **b** other lesions (*arrows*) were found in segment 8 infiltrating the middle hepatic vein; **c** in segments 6/7; and **d** in segment 6

histology revealed an adenocarcinoma of the colon with synchronous liver metastases (T3N0M1).

The patient received three cycles of chemotherapy with FOLFOX and Bevacizumab. Post-chemotherapy magnetic resonance imaging (MRI) showed one small lesion (5 mm) in segment 2 and four lesions in segment 6, 6/7, 7, and 8 respectively. The maximal diameter of the lesions in the right lobe was 25 mm and revealed a slight (<30%) decrease in size (Fig. 5.1) compared with the previous MRI [1].

My Management

1. Two-stage hepatectomy with portal vein occlusion (PVO)
2. ALPPS
3. Mini-ALPPS

Diagnosis and Assessment

Colon cancer is the third malignancy worldwide in terms of incidence [2]. At diagnosis, 15–25% of patients with stage IV have synchronous detected liver metastases [3]. Chest/abdominal/pelvis CT has been already demonstrated as the best option for initial staging [4]. Use of F-18 fluorodeoxyglucose positron emission tomography/computed tomography (18 FDG-PET/CT) has been suggested for detecting distant metastases when suspicious lesions on abdominal CT were seen, but PET-CT compared with CT alone did not result in frequent change in surgical management or better survival among patients with potentially resectable hepatic metastases [5].

MRI combined with liver-specific contrast agents such as gadoxetic acid or gadobutrol, seems to be more sensitive than CT in detecting liver metastases for subcentimetre lesions [6]. Additionally, the apparent diffusion coefficient (ADC), derived from diffusion-weighted MRI (DW-MRI), may provide information on predicting response to chemotherapy [7, 8].

Regardless of which technique is used, the accurate assessment of number and location of hepatic metastases is a crucial issue for adequate treatment planning and successfully therapy [9]. At initial diagnosis, about 25–30% of patients are not resectable due to the extent of hepatic disease or a small future liver remnant (FLR). Computed tomography is routinely used as a method for preoperative calculation of the remnant liver. With a normal parenchyma, FLR should range between 20% and 30% of estimated total liver volume [10], with a minimum cut-off set at 20%, below which risk of liver failure [11], infections, and liver mortality is significantly increased. Whereas, when an underlying liver disease preexists (steatosis, cholestasis, fibrosis, cirrhosis, or chemotherapy), FLR should be greater than 30–40% [12]. Liver toxicity due to chemotherapic agents, namely chemotherapy-induced liver injury (CALI), is common in patients who received prolonged treatment for colorectal liver metastases. In this setting, multimodality treatment for colorectal liver metastases suggested a minimal FLR ratio of at least 40% [13] or higher [14] in patients heavily pretreated with chemotherapy. The two typical histological patterns are represented by the sinusoidal injury (sinusoidal obstruction syndrome) in oxaliplatin-based regimens, and chemotherapy-associated steatohepatitis (CASH) secondary to the use of irinotecan [15]. More than six cycles of oxaliplatin need a longer time interval before major hepatectomy, even though accountability for PHLF still remains a matter of debate [16]. Whereas, use of irinotecan has been demonstrated to be associated with an increased risk of peri-operative mortality [15].

In addition to preoperative liver volume calculation, nuclear imaging techniques (^{99m}Tc-galactosyl serum albumin scintigraphy or ^{99m}Tc-mebrofenin hepatobiliary scintigraphy) have gained wider acceptance and to date are able to measure more precisely both total and future remnant liver function combining SPECT/CT images, and potentially identifying patients at higher risk for post-hepatectomy liver failure [17, 18].

Management

When marginally resectable or unresectable colorectal liver metastases are detected at the time of diagnosis, preoperative chemotherapy is recommended [19] with first-line therapy including doublets (e.g., FOLFOX, FOLFIRI, CAPOX) or triplets (e.g., FOLFOXIRI) combined with targeted therapy (e.g., monoclonal antibodies) [20]. When the primary tumor is represented by a mid-low rectal cancer, short- or long-course radiation is also provided followed by chemotherapy.

Assessment of response to neoadjuvant treatment should be performed every 2 months. Disease progression while undergoing preoperative chemotherapy predicts poor outcome, and a change to a second-line regimen is usually recommended [21]. Whereas, if cross-sectional imaging demonstrates partial response to treatment or stable disease, surgery can be reconsidered. Overall, a total duration of 6 months of preoperative and adjuvant chemotherapy should be administered [22].

A controversial topic is represented by the management of synchronous colorectal cancer and bilateral liver metastases. Roles and timings of resection depend mainly on the tumor status and/or the need for emergency surgery. When the primary tumor is symptomatic (bleeding, obstruction, or perforation), colorectal resection is always preferred before liver surgery (classical approach), otherwise simultaneous resection (combined approach) seems favorable [23]. Simultaneous colorectal resection and minor hepatectomy can be done safely with a comparable risk to both procedures in staged patients [24]. Caution must be exercised when associating major hepatectomy and/or low anterior rectal surgery, due to the reported high rate of postoperative complications [25]. However, at experienced centers and in selected patients, low morbidity and mortality rates can be achieved [26]. Instead, patients with substantial burdens of liver metastases in comparison to a lower risk of the primary tumor to progress or cause complications, may benefit from a liver-first surgery (reverse approach) [23]. Randomized controlled trials are needed to further investigate differences in clinical outcomes of these three different approaches.

When assessing resectability, the proximity of hepatic lesions to the inflow and/or outflow of the liver can be more important for surgical decision than the number or the largest dimension of the tumors, requiring frequently extended resection with an increased risk for post-hepatectomy liver failure. At present, parenchymal-sparing techniques are widely used, thus avoiding unnecessary major hepatectomies and at the same time increasing the chance of salvage resection in case of liver recurrence [27]. However, when size of FLR is regarded to be not sufficient to sustain liver function in the postoperative course, techniques of PVO such as portal vein embolization (PVE) or portal vein ligation (PVL) can be considered to increase the volume of the FLR [28, 29]. Such techniques can be used in the context of a staged hepatectomy for bilobar liver metastases, to enable a faster hepatic regeneration in the interval. PVE is classically performed through a percutaneous transhepatic ipsilateral approach using CT guidance, which provides embolization by means of a variety of substances (histoacryl, lipiodol, gelfoam, and n-butyl cyanoacrylate) of the diseased hemiliver including segment 4 branches when right extended hepatectomy is planned [30]. About 4–8 weeks after PVE, the liver volume is evaluated again to reassess resectability [31].

Portal vein occlusion may also be achieved by ligation of right/left portal branch, during a first-step laparotomy [32]. Hypertrophy after PVL is reported to be inferior to PVE, likely due to incomplete vascular interruption of collaterals between the two hemilivers [33]. Nevertheless, there are no controlled studies clearly showing superiority of PVE versus PVL [34]. Regardless of which technique is used, cleaning the FLR in the first stage is mandatory to avoid tumor growth in the interval.

In the classic TSH, between 12% and 32% of patients do not complete the second stage due to progression of disease or insufficient FLR hypertrophy [35]. Uni- and multivariate analysis showed that age over 70 years, male gender, larger lesions > 5 cm, serum carcinoembryonic antigen level before PVE greater than 200 ng/ml, three or more metastases in the FRL, progression during preoperative chemotherapy, and the presence of extrahepatic disease were significant factors predicting failure to achieve completion of hepatectomy [29, 36]. It is not clear whether the use of chemotherapy between the first and second stage can lower tumor progression and dropout rates [37, 38]. What is more likely is that liver regeneration can be impaired or altered by use of some chemotherapy agents, thus increasing the risk of postoperative liver failure and overall morbidity after completion of stage 2 [15].

In 2012, Schnitzbauer et al. [39] reported an innovative two-stage technique for patients with bilobar colorectal liver metastases. In the first stage, right portal vein ligation and in situ splitting of the liver on the right side of the falciform ligament was performed; in the second stage, after a median time interval of 9 days, extended hepatectomy was completed in 100% of patients with an impressive liver hypertrophy registered between the two stages. Thereafter, the so-called advanced liver partition and PVL for staged hepatectomy, namely ALPPS, has spread to many centers worldwide [40]. An International Registry was created [41] and counted in March 2015 more than 500 patients from 78 centers in 48 countries. High rate of morbidity and 90-day mortality were reported after ALPPS [42] and many concerns were addressed to the safety of such procedure [43]. However, before rejecting ALPPS as unsafe, wide variability in outcomes among different centers has to be taken into account, which can be explained in two ways. First, while many concerns have been raised in patients with biliary tumors [44, 45], ALPPS is a powerful and safer [44] tool for colorectal liver metastases to induce FLR volume increase. Second, many surgical techniques have been described from its inaugural description, confirming the need of a standardization of such a surgical practice: radio-frequency-assisted liver partition with portal vein ligation (RALPP) [46], associating liver tourniquet and portal ligation for staged hepatectomy (ALTPS) [47], partial transection of the liver parenchyma during stage 1 of ALPPS (partial

ALPPS) [48], and more recently, parenchymal transection in stage 1 of ALPPS followed by portal vein embolization (hybrid ALPPS) [49].

Clinical Pearls

- 4–8 weeks are needed to obtain adequate volume hypertrophy in conventional PVO
- 12–32% of patients submitted to conventional two-stage hepatectomy did not proceed to second stage
- parenchymal damage due to prolonged chemotherapy can increase the risk of PHLF

Hybrid ALPPS was first [50] described in two patients affected by gallbladder carcinoma with right portal vein infiltration. PVE, in place of PVL, was performed on postoperative day (POD) 2 after the first stage of ALPPS: the volumetric increase was 113 and 65% after 6 and 14 days, respectively. The patients did well and were discharged without major complications. A similar procedure had been performed by Robles et al. [47] using a tourniquet technique and sequential PVE to achieve liver partition in a patient with perihilar tumor burden.

Our group proposed a paradigm change during the 1st ALPPS International Consensus Meeting at Hamburg in February 2015, and the initial results of this modified ALPPS technique, called "mini-ALPPS," were reported in a recent publication [49].

When approaching a mini-ALPPS right trisectionectomy, in the first stage a supraumbilical midline incision or a J-shaped incision is performed. After exploration of the abdominal cavity to rule out extrahepatic disease, intraoperative ultrasound (IOUS) is performed to confirm numbers and position of the lesions, limiting as minimum as possible liver mobilization to avoid future adhesions and reduce surgical stress. If planned ALPPS is confirmed and bilateral involvement is present, enucleation of liver metastases in the FLR has to be performed. Partial parenchymal transection (PPT) is performed along the falciform ligament, using cavitron ultrasonic surgical aspirator in combination with harmonic scalpel and cautery. Depth of liver transection should not exceed 3–5 cm, to avoid injury of the middle hepatic vein and biliary branches of segment 4. Regardless of tumor localization and/or portal vein infiltration, the hepatic pedicle is not dissected at all and should remain untouched during the entire procedure.

PVE is approached through dissection and cannulation of the inferior mesenteric vein with a 5 Fr introducer. Under real-time fluoroscopic digital subtraction, the right portal vein and segment 4 branches are identified and then selectively embolized by interventional radiologists using a mixture of cyanoacrylate and lipiodol ultra-fluid. Afterwards, a control portogram is performed to demonstrate the patency of the left lateral segment portal vein branches and at the same time to make sure of the devascularisation of collaterals to the right portal vein. At the end of the procedure, the catheter is removed from the inferior mesenteric vein, which can be ligated or repaired whenever possible. As an alternative, the ileocolic vein or any other dilated splanchnic vein could be cannulated for PVE.

Volumetry is usually performed 6 days after the first stage and assessment before completion of stage 2 is performed by calculation of sFLR, in conjunction with ^{99m}Tc-mebrofenin hepatic scintigraphy, which helps to confirm a simultaneous increase of liver function in the remnant liver.

When future liver remnant volume and function as well as patient conditions are considered adequate to proceed to second stage, the second surgery can be scheduled.

In the second stage, fewer adhesions are encountered between the parenchymal resection surfaces and access to hepatic pedicle is facilitated by lesser hilar inflammation adherences. Parenchymal splitting is completed following the previous transection line and the right hepatic vein is dissected and divided by a vascular stapler, finally completing the hepatectomy. At the end of the operation, a hydraulic test is performed through cannulation of the cystic duct to rule out any bile leaks. If there are any doubts on the indemnity of the remnant biliary system, a cholangiography can be performed.

Clinical Pearls

- depth of liver transection should not exceed 3–5 cm, to avoid injury of the middle hepatic vein and biliary branches of segment 4
- the hepatic pedicle is not dissected at all and should remain untouched during the entire procedure
- PVE is approached through dissection and cannulation of the inferior mesenteric vein with a 5 Fr introducer.

Outcome

The patient in this case presented a preoperative non-tumoral volume of the left lateral section (segments 2–3) plus the caudate lobe (segment 1) of 294 cc, representing 26% of the standardized total liver volume. During the first stage, IOUS confirmed the presence of one lesion in segment 7, infiltrating the right hepatic vein, and another one in segment 8, infiltrating the middle hepatic vein. Therefore, a right trisectionectomy by means of ALPPS due to the insufficient FLR was indicated. Partial parenchymal transection along the falciform ligament followed by

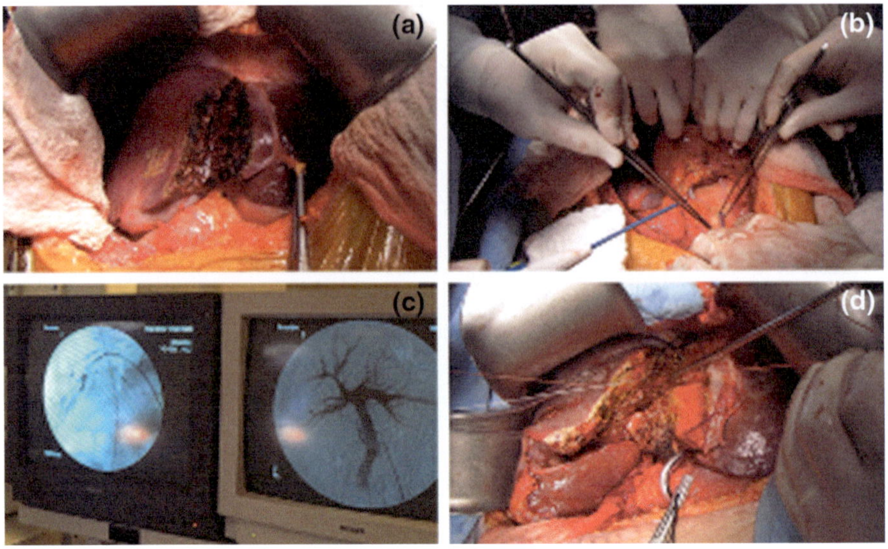

Fig. 5.2 “Mini-ALPPS” approach: **a** partial parenchymal transection during first stage. **b** Isolation of inferior mesenteric vein for its cannulation. **c** Intraoperative portal vein embolization. **d** Completion of hepatectomy during second stage

embolization of the right portal vein including segment 4, was performed (Fig. 5.2). Two other lesions were found in the left lateral section, which were resected to clean the remnant liver. A plastic sheet was left in the abdomen to cover the surfaces of resection. After 7 days, a first CT volumetry was performed and showed a sFLR of 33%. Although the good volumetric hypertrophy, the function of the remnant liver measured by means of ^{99m}Tc-mebrofenin scintigraphy was not considered enough to proceed to stage 2. Thereby, hepatobiliary scintigraphy and CT volumetry were repeated on POD 14, this time showing a 38% of sFLR and a satisfying remnant liver function (Fig. 5.3). No major complications or post-hepatectomy liver failure occurred until this point. Completion of right tri-sectionectomy was finally performed on POD 16 and the patient was discharged 5 days after, without any complications. Histological analysis of the specimen confirmed the preoperative diagnosis and tumor-free (R0) resection margins. The patient received adjuvant chemotherapy with FOLFOX, and 6 months after surgery is still alive and free of disease.

The above-described technique allows adequate hypertrophy as seen in ALPPS but with a less aggressive procedure in the first stage. PPT has already been shown to trigger a similar rate of liver hypertrophy compared to complete transection [51]. Furthermore, risk of bile leak and/or ischemia of segment 4, secondary to incidental transection of small bile duct and arteries, can be avoided. Association of PPT with intraoperative PVE results in a less eventful recovery before the second stage, the

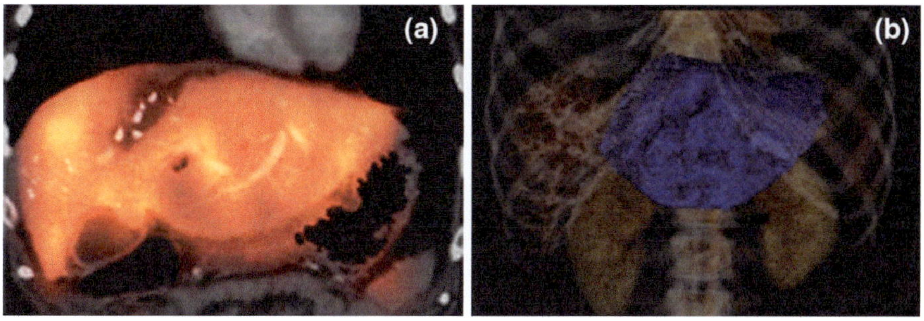

Fig. 5.3 **a** SPECT/CT image fusion with 99mTc-mebrofenin, and **b** three-dimensional CT liver volumetry of segments 1-2-3, representing the 38% of standardized future liver remnant performed on postoperative day 14

latter simplified by avoiding hepatic hilum dissection and liver manipulation in stage 1.

In our experience, 22 patients were submitted to ALPPS surgery between June 2011 and March 2016 for bilateral colorectal liver metastases (Table 5.1). There were 14 males and eight females. Liver metastases were synchronous in 20 of 22 cases (90.9%) and metachronous in two patients (9.1%). In seven patients with synchronous metastases, simultaneous colorectal resection was performed. Major complications (Dindo-Clavien $\geq$ 3a) occurred in 18.2% and no mortality within 90 days was observed. Free of tumor (R0) margins of resection were obtained in 19 of 22 patients (86.4%). When looking at "mini-ALPPS" series for bilateral colorectal liver metastases (four patients), only one wound infection was encountered as a surgical complication. Median liver hypertrophy was 47% (range 26–79%) with a median interval between the first stage and the last volumetric evaluation before the second stage of 11 days (range 6–16 days). Overall survival at 1, 3, and 5 years was 80.4, 70.4, and 43.2%, respectively.

When comparing outcome following ALPPS to other available treatments for bilateral CRLM, it must be kept in mind that patients treated with ALPPS represent a subgroup that cannot be compared to conventional one-stage hepatectomy or patients submitted to preoperative PVE with monolobar disease. These results have to be compared to chemotherapy alone and at best to conventional two-stage hepatectomy (TSH) for bilobar disease with FLR hypertrophy obtained by means of interstage PVO. A case-match analysis of patients submitted to ALPPS (multicenter) versus TSH (single center) demonstrated significantly higher morbidity (41.7%) after stage 2 in the ALPPS group, although complications in the TSH group was fairly lower (17.6%) than in other series [52]. The International Registry [44] reported a major morbidity of 29% for patients submitted to ALPPS for CRLM; that is comparable to TSH, ranging from 20% [36] to 59% [53]. Further-

Table 5.1 Descriptive of all patients submitted to ALPPS for bilateral colorectal liver metastases at Hospital Italiano between 2011 and 2016

Variable	$n = 22$
Age, median (range), years	57 (29–81)
Sex, male/female	14/8
Charlson index, median (range), number	7 (6–10)
BMI, median (range), kg/m^2	24.4 (16.9–31.2)
Preoperative chemotherapy, number (%) Oxaliplatin-based Irinotecan-based Biologic agent	21 (95.5) 18 (81.8) 7 (31.8) 12 (54.5)
Cycles of chemotherapy, median (range), number	7 (2–15)
Synchronous/metachronous, number	20/2
Number of lesions on imaging, median (range), number	5 (2–33)
Maximal diameter of the largest lesion, median (range), mm	57.5 (20–160)
sFLR prior to stage 1, median (range), %	25.4 (6.7–30.6)
FLR/BW prior to stage 1, median (range), %	0.55 (0.14–0.69)
sFLR prior to stage 2, median (range), %	44.4 (25.8–68)
FLR/BW prior to stage 2, median (range), %	0.94 (0.54–1.53)
FLR increase, median (range), %	106 (26–286)
KGR, median (range), %/day	15.1 (0.8–28.3)
Time interval, median (range), days	11 (6–16)
Feasibility of stage 2, number (%)	22 (100)
Simultaneous colorectal resection, number (%) Left hemicolectomy Anterior rectal resection Transverse colectomy	7 (31.8) 4 (57.1) 2 (28.6) 1 (14.3)
Type of liver resection, number (%) Right hepatectomy Right trisectionectomy Left trisectionectomy	8 (36.4) 13 (59.1) 1 (4.5)
Partial parenchymal transection, number (%)	17 (77.3)
PPT + PVE (mini-ALPPS), number (%)	4 (18.2)
Major morbidity after stage 1, number (%)	5 (22.7)
Major morbidity after stage 2, number (%)	4 (18.2)
Hospital stay, median (range), days	19 (9–49)
90-day mortality, number (%)	0
Resection margins, number (%) R0 R1	19 (86.4) 3 (14.6)

sFLR standardized future liver remnant; *BW* body weight; *KGR* kynetic growth rate; *PPT* partial parenchymal transection; *PVE* portal vein embolization; *ALPPS* associated liver partition and portal vein ligation more, a 90-day mortality of 5% after ALPPS seems acceptable when compared to TSH, for which mortality is reported up to 7% [53].

Although only a short-term follow-up is yet available from the last ALPPS registry report [44], the overall survival (OS) of 59 and 41% and the disease-free survival (DFS) of 88 and 74% at 1 and 2 years, respectively, compare favorably with that provided in the few existing international series of two-stage hepatectomies [35]. The most relevant aspect is that survival in ALPPS takes into consideration patients in whom PVE or PVL have failed ("salvage ALPPS") and patients who theoretically would have dropped out between stages due to progression of disease in conventional TSH.

Conclusion

ALPPS is not intended to supplant conventional two-stage hepatectomies, but rather to expand the armamentarium for hepatic resection, and to date, represents the only chance of cure in patients in whom PVO have failed (salvage ALPPS) or with very small FLR. Randomized controlled trials comparing ALPPS versus TSH are currently underway and at present any comparison between these two surgical strategies can only be suggestive, not definitive. Mini-ALPPS represents a further refinement of classic ALPPS technique and may be useful to reduce the clinical impact of stage 1 before completion of stage 2 [45, 54], obtaining a comparable degree of hypertrophy with a lower rate of complications. An additional oncologic advantage, due to avoiding hepatic hilum dissection and liver manipulization, is not to be underestimated. Further studies are needed to validate the findings of this original report.

Overall

- ALPPS represents the only chance of cure in patients in whom PVO have failed (salvage ALPPS) or with very small FLR
- Mini-ALPPS represents a further refinement of classic ALPPS technique to reduce the clinical impact of stage 1 before completion of stage 2
- ALPPS survival includes patients in whom PVE or PVL have failed and patients who theoretically would have dropped out between stages due to progression of disease in conventional TSH
- Randomized controlled trials comparing ALPPS versus TSH for colorectal liver metastases are currently underway.

References

1. Eisenhauer EA, Therasse P, Bogaerts J, Schwartz LH, Sargent D, Ford R, et al. New response evaluation criteria in solid tumours: Revised RECIST guideline (version 1.1). Eur J Cancer. 2009;45(2):228–47.
2. Iarc. IA for R on CWHO. GLOBOCAN 2012: estimated cancer incidence, mortality and prevalence worldwide in 2012. Globocan 2012;1–6.
3. Steele G, Ravikumar TS. Resection of hepatic metastases from colorectal cancer. Biologic perspective. Ann Surg. 1989;210(2):127–38.
4. Dewhurst C, Rosen MP, Blake MA, Baker ME, Cash BD, Fidler JL, et al. ACR appropriateness criteria (R) pretreatment staging of colorectal cancer. J Am Coll Radiol. 2012;9(11):775–81.
5. Moulton C-A, Gu C-S, Law CH, Tandan VR, Hart R, Quan D, et al. Effect of PET before liver resection on surgical management for colorectal adenocarcinoma metastases: a randomized clinical trial. JAMA. 2014;311(18):1863–9.
6. Scharitzer M, Ba-Ssalamah A, Ringl H, Kölblinger C, Grünberger T, Weber M, et al. Preoperative evaluation of colorectal liver metastases: comparison between gadoxetic acid-enhanced 3.0-T MRI and contrast-enhanced MDCT with histopathological correlation. Eur Radiol. 2013;23(8):2187–96.
7. Elias D, Youssef O, Sideris L, Dromain C, Baton O, Boige V, et al. Evolution of missing colorectal liver metastases following inductive chemotherapy and hepatectomy. J Surg Oncol. 2004;86(1):4–9.
8. Donati OF, Fischer MA, Chuck N, Hunziker R, Weishaupt D, Reiner CS. Accuracy and confidence of Gd-EOB-DTPA enhanced MRI and diffusion-weighted imaging alone and in combination for the diagnosis of liver metastases. Eur J Radiol. 2013;82:822–8.
9. Harsha Tirumani S, Won Kim K, Nishino M, Howard SA, Krajewski KM, Jagannathan JP, et al. Update on the role of imaging in management of metastatic colorectal cancer. RadioGraphics. 2014;34(1):1908–28.
10. Vauthey JN, Abdalla EK, Doherty DA, Gertsch P, Fenstermacher MJ, Loyer EM, et al. Body surface area and body weight predict total liver volume in western adults. Liver Transplant. 2002;8(3):233–40.
11. Abdalla EK, Barnett CC, Doherty D, Curley SA, Vauthey J-N. Extended hepatectomy in patients with hepatobiliary malignancies with and without preoperative portal vein embolization. Arch Surg. 2002;137(6):675–80; discussion 680–1.
12. Shoup M, Gonen M, D'Angelica M, Jarnagin WR, DeMatteo RP, Schwartz LH, et al. Volumetric analysis predicts hepatic dysfunction in patients undergoing major liver resection. J Gastrointest Surg. 2003;7(3):325–30.
13. Adam R, Miller R, Pitombo M, Wicherts DA, de Haas RJ, Bitsakou G, et al. Two-stage hepatectomy approach for initially unresectable colorectal hepatic metastases. Surg Oncol Clin N Am. 2007;16(3):525–36, viii.
14. Narita M, Oussoultzoglou E, Fuchshuber P, Pessaux P, Chenard M-P, Rosso E, et al. What is a safe future liver remnant size in patients undergoing major hepatectomy for colorectal liver metastases and treated by intensive preoperative chemotherapy? Ann Surg Oncol. 2012;19 (8):2526–38.
15. Vauthey JN, Pawlik TM, Ribero D, Wu TT, Zorzi D, Hoff PM, et al. Chemotherapy regimen predicts steatohepatitis and an increase in 90-day mortality after surgery for hepatic colorectal metastases. J Clin Oncol. 2006;24(13):2065–72.
16. Nakano H, Oussoultzoglou E, Rosso E, Casnedi S, Chenard-Neu MP, Dufour P, et al. Sinusoidal injury increases morbidity after major hepatectomy in patients with colorectal liver metastases receiving preoperative chemotherapy. Ann Surg. 2008;247(1):118–24.

17. de Graaf W, van Lienden KP, Dinant S, Roelofs JJTH, Busch ORC, Gouma DJ, et al. Assessment of future remnant liver function using hepatobiliary scintigraphy in patients undergoing major liver resection. J Gastrointest Surg. 2010;14(2):369–78.
18. Togashi H, Takahashi K, Onodera Y, Adachi T, Suzuki A, Karasawa T, et al. Separate analysis of asialoglycoprotein receptors in the right and left hepatic lobes using 99mTc-GSA SPECT in patients with acute hepatic damage. Hepatol Res. 2006;36(2):130–8.
19. Mentha G, Majno PE, Andres A, Rubbia-Brandt L, Morel P, Roth AD. Neoadjuvant chemotherapy and resection of advanced synchronous liver metastases before treatment of the colorectal primary. Br J Surg. 2006;93(7):872–8.
20. Loupakis F, Cremolini C, Masi G, Lonardi S, Zagonel V, Salvatore L, et al. Initial therapy with FOLFOXIRI and bevacizumab for metastatic colorectal cancer. N Engl J Med. 2014;371(17):1609–18.
21. Nordlinger B, Sorbye H, Glimelius B, Poston GJ, Schlag PM, Rougier P, et al. Perioperative chemotherapy with FOLFOX4 and surgery versus surgery alone for resectable liver metastases from colorectal cancer (EORTC Intergroup trial 40983): a randomised controlled trial. Lancet. 2008;371(9617):1007–16.
22. Adam R, de Gramont A, Figueras J, Kokudo N, Kunstlinger F, Loyer E, et al. Managing synchronous liver metastases from colorectal cancer: a multidisciplinary international consensus. Cancer Treat Rev. 2015;41(9):729–41.
23. Kelly ME, Spolverato G, Lè GN, Mavros MN, Doyle F, Pawlik TM, et al. Synchronous colorectal liver metastasis: a network meta-analysis review comparing classical, combined, and liver-first surgical strategies. J Surg Oncol. 2015;111(3):341–51.
24. Feng Q, Wei Y, Zhu D, Ye L, Lin Q, Li W, et al. Timing of hepatectomy for resectable synchronous colorectal liver metastases: for whom simultaneous resection is more suitable—a meta-analysis. PLoS One. 2014;9(8).
25. Reddy SK, Pawlik TM, Zorzi D, Gleisner AL, Ribero D, Assumpcao L, et al. Simultaneous resections of colorectal cancer and synchronous liver metastases: a multi-institutional analysis. Ann Surg Oncol. 2007;14(12):3481–91.
26. Capussotti L, Ferrero A, Viganò L, Ribero D, Lo Tesoriere R, Polastri R. Major liver resections synchronous with colorectal surgery. Ann Surg Oncol. 2007;14(1):195–201.
27. Torzilli G, Procopio F, Donadon M, Del Fabbro D, Cimino M, Montorsi M. Safety of intermittent pringle maneuver cumulative time exceeding 120 minutes in liver resection. Ann Surg. 2012;255(2):270–80.
28. Serenari M, Cescon M, Cucchetti A, Pinna AD. Liver function impairment in liver transplantation and after extended hepatectomy. World J Gastroenterol. 2013;19(44):7922–9.
29. Yang C, Rahbari NN, Mees ST, Schaab F, Koch M, Weitz J, et al. Staged resection of bilobar colorectal liver metastases: surgical strategies. Langenbecks Arch Surg. 2015;400(6):633–40.
30. Madoff DC, Abdalla EK, Gupta S, Wu T-TT, Morris JS, Denys A, et al. Transhepatic ipsilateral right portal vein embolization extended to segment IV: improving hypertrophy and resection outcomes with spherical particles and coils. J Vasc Interv Radiol. 2005;16(2 Pt 1):215–25.
31. Abulkhir A, Limongelli P, Healey AJ, Damrah O, Tait P, Jackson J, et al. Preoperative portal vein embolization for major liver resection: a meta-analysis. Ann Surg. 2008;247(1):49–57.
32. Kianmanesh R, Farges O, Abdalla EK, Sauvanet A, Ruszniewski P, Belghiti J. Right portal vein ligation: a new planned two-step all-surgical approach for complete resection of primary gastrointestinal tumors with multiple bilateral liver metastases. J Am Coll Surg. 2003;197(1):164–70.
33. Broering DC, Hillert C, Krupski G, Fischer L, Mueller L, Achilles EG, et al. Portal vein embolization vs. portal vein ligation for induction of hypertrophy of the future liver remnant. J Gastrointest Surg. 2002;6(6):905–13.
34. Aussilhou B, Lesurtel M, Sauvanet A, Farges O, Dokmak S, Goasguen N, et al. Right portal vein ligation is as efficient as portal vein embolization to induce hypertrophy of the left liver remnant. J Gastrointest Surg. 2008;12(2):297–303.

35. Lam VWT, Laurence JM, Johnston E, Hollands MJ, Pleass HCC, Richardson AJ. A systematic review of two-stage hepatectomy in patients with initially unresectable colorectal liver metastases. HPB (Oxford). 2013;15(7):483–91.
36. Giuliante F, Ardito F, Ferrero A, Aldrighetti L, Ercolani G, Grande G, et al. Tumor progression during preoperative chemotherapy predicts failure to complete 2-stage hepatectomy for colorectal liver metastases: results of an italian multicenter analysis of 130 patients. J Am Coll Surg. 2014;219:285–94.
37. Hoekstra LT, van Lienden KP, Doets A, Busch ORC, Gouma DJ, van Gulik TM. Tumor progression after preoperative portal vein embolization. Ann Surg. 2012;256(5):812–8.
38. Fischer C, Melstrom LG, Arnaoutakis D, Jarnagin W, Brown K, D'Angelica M, et al. Chemotherapy after portal vein embolization to protect against tumor growth during liver hypertrophy before hepatectomy. JAMA Surg. 2013;148(12):1103–8.
39. Schnitzbauer AA, Lang SA, Goessmann H, Nadalin S, Baumgart J, Farkas SA, et al. Right portal vein ligation combined with in situ splitting induces rapid left lateral liver lobe hypertrophy enabling 2-staged extended right hepatic resection in small-for-size settings. Ann Surg. 2012;255(3):405–14.
40. Schadde E, Schnitzbauer AA, Tschuor C, Raptis DA, Bechstein WO, Clavien P-A. Systematic review and meta-analysis of feasibility, safety, and efficacy of a novel procedure: associating liver partition and portal vein ligation for staged hepatectomy. Ann Surg Oncol. 2015;22(9):3109–20.
41. de Santibañes E, Clavien P-A. Playing Play-Doh to prevent postoperative liver failure: the ALPPS approach. Ann Surg. 2012;255(3):415–7.
42. Nadalin S, Capobianco I, Li J, Girotti P, Königsrainer I, Königsrainer A. Indications and limits for associating liver partition and portal vein ligation for staged hepatectomy (ALPPS). Lessons Learned from 15 cases at a single centre. Zeitschrift für Gastroenterol. 2014;52(1):35–42.
43. Aloia TA, Vauthey J-N. Associating liver partition and portal vein ligation for staged hepatectomy (ALPPS): what is gained and what is lost? Ann Surg. 2012;256(3):e9; author reply e16–9.
44. Schadde E, Raptis DA, Schnitzbauer AA, Ardiles V, Tschuor C, Lesurtel M, et al. Prediction of mortality after ALPPS stage-1: an analysis of 320 patients from the international ALPPS registry. Ann Surg. 2015;262(5):780–5; discussion 785–6.
45. Serenari M, Zanello M, Schadde E, Toschi E, Ratti F, Gringeri E, et al. Importance of primary indication and liver function between stages: results of a multicenter Italian audit of ALPPS 2012-2014. HPB (Oxford). 2016;18(5):419–27.
46. Gall TMH, Sodergren MH, Frampton AE, Fan R, Spalding DR, Habib NA, et al. Radio-frequency-assisted liver partition with portal vein ligation (RALPP) for liver regeneration. Ann Surg. 2015;261(2):e45–6.
47. Robles R, Parrilla P, López-Conesa A, Brusadin R, de la Peña J, Fuster M, et al. Tourniquet modification of the associating liver partition and portal ligation for staged hepatectomy procedure. Br J Surg. 2014;101(9):1129–34; discussion 1134.
48. Petrowsky H, Györi G, de Oliveira M, Lesurtel M, Clavien P-A. Is partial-ALPPS safer than ALPPS? A single-center experience. Ann Surg. 2015;261(4):e90–2.
49. de Santibañes E, Alvarez FA, Ardiles V, Pekolj J, de Santibañes M. Inverting the ALPPS paradigm by minimizing first stage impact: the Mini-ALPPS technique. Langenbecks Arch Surg. 2016;401(4):557–63.
50. Li J, Kantas A, Ittrich H, Koops A, Achilles EG, Fischer L, et al. Avoid "All-Touch" by hybrid ALPPS to achieve oncological efficacy. Ann Surg. 2016;263(1):e6–7.
51. Alvarez F, Ardiles V, de Santibañes M, Pekolj J, de Santibañes E. Associating liver partition and portal vein ligation for staged hepatectomy offers high oncological feasibility with adequate patient safety: a prospective study at a single center. Ann Surg. 2015;261(4):723–32.

52. Ratti F, Schadde E, Masetti M, Massani M, Zanello M, Serenari M, et al. Strategies to increase the resectability of patients with colorectal liver metastases: a multi-center case-match analysis of ALPPS and conventional two-stage hepatectomy. Ann Surg Oncol. 2015;22(6):1933–42.
53. Wicherts DA, Miller R, de Haas RJ, Bitsakou G, Vibert E, Veilhan L-A, et al. Long-term results of two-stage hepatectomy for irresectable colorectal cancer liver metastases. Ann Surg. 2008;248(6):994–1005.
54. Truant S, Scatton O, Dokmak S, Regimbeau JM, Lucidi V, Laurent A, et al. Associating liver partition and portal vein ligation for staged hepatectomy (ALPPS): impact of the inter-stages course on morbi-mortality and implications for management. Eur J Surg Oncol. 2015;41 (5):674–82.

Management of Low Rectal Cancer with Synchronous Liver Metastases

6

Robert Gandy and Charbel Sandroussi

Introduction

One-quarter of patients with rectal adenocarcinoma have stage IV disease at presentation, and over two-thirds of patients have metastases limited to the liver. Unresectable liver colorectal liver metastases (CRLM) are associated with only 30% 1-year survival, and long-term survival is worse for patients presenting with synchronous disease [1].

Successful completion of treatment to all sites of disease is the only chance of cure and is associated with 5-year survival of 55% [2, 3]. Indeed 5-year survival rates of 67% [4] have been achieved with the addition of neoadjuvant systemic therapy to control micrometastatic disease and select biologically favorable disease [5, 6].

Uncertainty remains regarding the optimal sequencing of therapy, the applicability of synchronous resections and the role of pelvic radiotherapy in stage IV rectal adenocarcinoma [7–11]. The overall goal of treatment is surgical resection of disease and minimizing delay in systemic treatment.

Case Presentation 1

A 65-year-old man with a background of chronic obstructive pulmonary disease and type 2 diabetes presented with diarrhea and 10 g of unwanted weight loss over 2 months. Colonoscopy revealed an obstructing low rectal tumor. MRI of the

R. Gandy · C. Sandroussi (✉)
Department of Hepatobiliary and Upper Gastrointestinal Surgery,
Institute of Academic Surgery, Royal Prince Alfred Hospital,
Missenden Road, Camperdown, NSW 2050, Australia
e-mail: Charbel.Sandroussi@gmail.com

T.M. Pawlik et al. (eds.), *Case-Based Lessons in the Management of Complex Hepato-Pancreato-Biliary Surgery*, DOI 10.1007/978-3-319-50868-9_6

rectum was suggestive of a T3N1 tumor with threatened circumferential resection margin. CT scan revealed a 13 mm hypodense lesion in segment 3 of the liver. CEA was elevated at 3.22 µg/L.

Clinical Pearls

- Pelvic radiation for locally advanced low rectal cancers improves local control and disease-free survival and may facilitate a liver-first approach.
- In the setting of synchronous metastatic disease, neoadjuvant radiotherapy regimes should include oxaloplatin-based chemotherapy.
- Consider performance status prior to synchronous resection. Major hepatic resections, when combined with synchronous rectal resection, are associated with high morbidity.
- For large-volume liver disease, neoadjuvant "sandwich" chemotherapy (+-concurrent pelvic radiotherapy) and a liver-first approach is favored.
- For low-volume liver disease, multimodal treatment of the rectal disease, followed by completion chemotherapy is favored. Hepatic resection may be combined with reversal of ileostomy.

Multidisciplinary Management

Neoadjuvant chemoradiation was undertaken with short-course radiation therapy to the rectum (5 × 5 Gray over two weeks). At the completion of week 2, systemic FOLFOX was delivered for six cycles over 6 weeks. CT imaging was repeated showing no progression of disease but no objective tumor response in the pelvis. Laparoscopic low anterior resection with colo-anal anastamosis and diverting ileostomy was completed. The postoperative course was uneventful and pathological analysis confirmed complete tumor extirpation (T3N1bR0). Eight weeks after rectal resection, synchronous laparoscopic left lateral sectionectomy and reversal of ileostomy was performed. Again, the postoperative recovery was uneventful, both rectal and hepatic resections were complete, and no further systemic therapy was required (Figs. 6.1 and 6.2).

Case Summary

The background of a patient with a symptomatic primary tumor, low volume CRLM, and limited performance status requires careful consideration. Long-course radiation to the pelvis combined with combination chemotherapy was considered too toxic for this patient [12]. Short-course radiotherapy (SCRT) followed by combination chemotherapy only delayed receipt of systemic therapy by2 weeks and

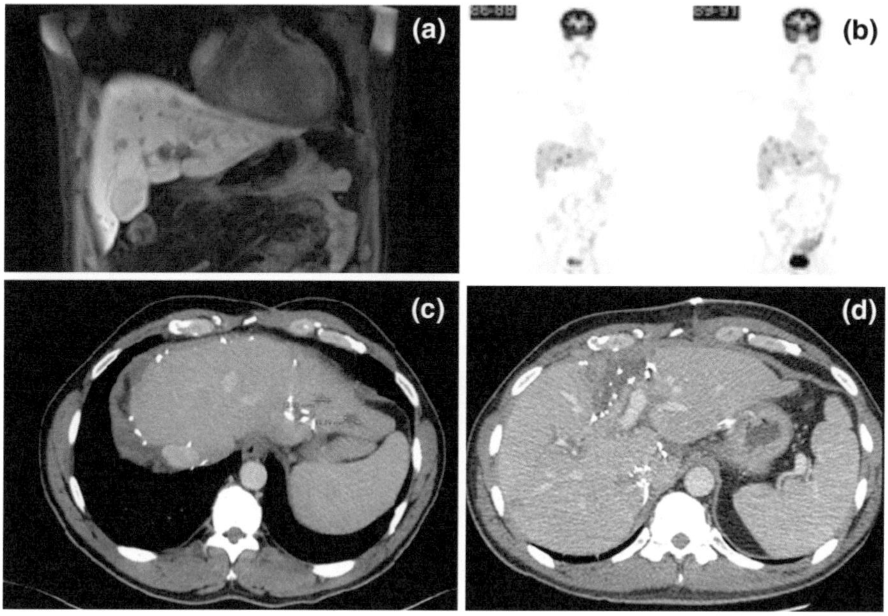

Fig. 6.1 Case 3. **a** Contrast enhanced T1 weighted MRI of the liver showing multiple liver metastases and segment 4 lesion threatening left portal vein margin. **b** FDG-18 Positive emission topography showing multiple liver metastases and primary in pelvis. **c** Computed tomography 6 months after surgery revealing 2 recurrent lesions in the left lobe of the liver which were subsequently resected. **d** Computed tomography scan of the liver following first ALLPPS procedure showing dissection along portal vein margin and ligation of right portal vein

allowed good control of the symptomatic primary disease [13]. Low anterior resection (with diverting ileostomy) and left lateral sectionectomy were both surgically amenable to a combined laparoscopic approach. This was not undertaken due to the higher risk of complications from combined liver and rectal resection, in a comorbid patient [14], as well as the fact that an ileostomy reversal could be combined with laparoscopic left lateral sectionectomy.

Controversies in Management

- Complete extirpation of malignant disease is possible for patients undergoing minor liver resections and left-sided bowel resections, although not always appropriate.
- Patient fitness and performance status is the main determinant of whether this approach is appropriate.

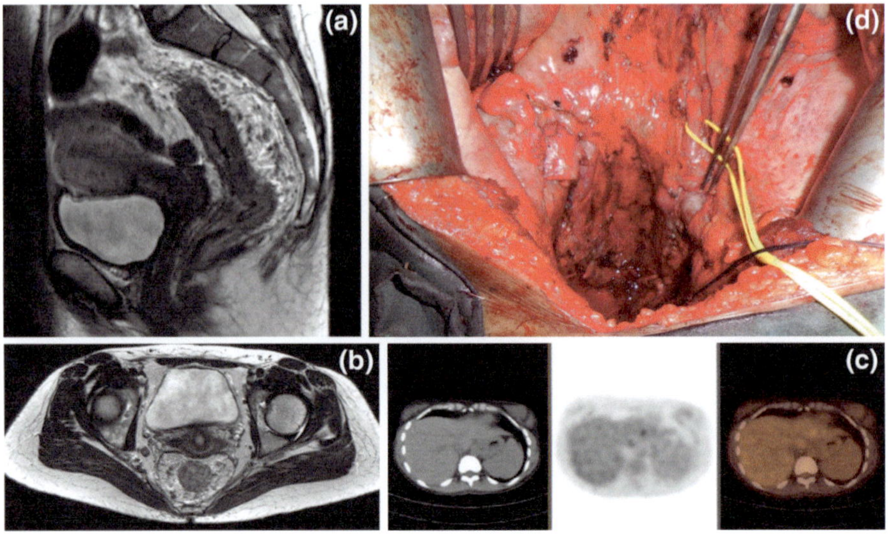

Fig. 6.2 Case 2. **a**, **b** T2 weighted MRI of the pelvis showing extensive low rectal adenocarcinoma with multiple enlarged mesorectal and iliac lymph nodes. **c** FDG-18 PET/CT showing increased uptake in segment 2/3 of the liver, this lesion was not identifiable on imaging following chemotherapy. **d** Operative photograph following partial anterior exenteration and bilateral ileac node dissection

Case Presentation 2

A 35-year-old woman, with no significant past medical history, presented to her general practitioner with lethargy and was found to have iron-deficiency anemia. A history of intermittent rectal bleeding was elucidated. Digital rectal examination revealed a firm anteriorly fixed mass, 6 cm from the anal verge. Colonoscopy confirmed a nonobstructing rectal mass and biopsy proved adenocarcinoma.

Computed tomography of the chest, abdomen, and pelvis, and magnetic resonance imaging of the pelvis was performed for staging. A 2 cm hypodense lesion in segment 2/3 was observed, with no evidence of extrahepatic disease. Pelvic MRI revealed a very large low rectal tumor with invasion to the rectovaginal septum as well as extensive mesorectal and iliac lymphadenopathy (T4b, N2b, M1a). Staging was completed with 18F-FDG PET/CT, which confirmed oligometastatic disease in the left lateral section of the liver. CEA levels were not elevated at 1.2 µg/L.

Multidisciplinary Management

Neoadjuvant long-course chemoradiation was commenced. Fractionated external beam radiation was delivered to the rectum and pelvic side walls for a total of five weeks and 50 Gray. The chemosensitiser 5-FU was delivered in combination with oxaloplatin, irinotecan, leucovorin, and bevacizumab for 7 months.

Repeat MRI of the pelvis and CT of the chest, abdomen, and pelvis showed significant response to neoadjuvant therapy in the pelvis, "ghosting" of the lesion in the left lobe of the liver, and no new metastatic deposits.

Synchronous ultralow anterior resection (incorporating the posterior wall of the vagina), diverting loop ileostomy, bilateral iliac node dissection, and left lateral sectionectomy of the liver was performed. The liver lesion was not detectable on intraoperative high definition ultrasound, and there was minimal iliac nodal tissue and a fibrotic rectovaginal septum.

Pathological analysis revealed a moderate response to neoadjuvant therapy of the primary lesion, extensive necrosis was seen in most lymph nodes sampled, with viable tumor cells in only three of 31 mesorectal nodes. A complete pathological response was observed in the liver lesion, with no viable tumor.

The perioperative course was complicated by severe thrombocytopenia and a return to theater for suspected pelvic bleeding, subsequent abdominal and pelvic collections requiring percutaneous drainage, and intravenous antibiotics. Postoperative chemotherapy was delayed for 4 months due to complications from surgery.

Case Summary

The extensive nature of the pelvic disease, despite limited symptoms, meant that the potential for downstaging with standard radiotherapy was favored [15]. The patient was able to tolerate combination chemotherapy, radiotherapy, and a biological agent with minimal toxicity and excellent response. Synchronous open resection was performed, but due to the extensive nature of the pelvic dissection, multiple complications were observed. Clear surgical margins, minimal lymph node involvement, and complete response to disease in the liver were good prognostic indicators.

Controversies in Management

- Longer durations of chemotherapy prior to surgery increase the risk of perioperative complications.
- Systemic recurrence is the most likely determinant of long-term survival and this may be improved with a longer duration of preoperative chemotherapy.
- Preoperative chemotherapy allows assessment of the biology of the disease.

Case Presentation 3

A 42-year-old man presented to his general practitioner with epigastric pain. He underwent an ultrasound scan of the abdomen, which revealed multiple bilobar solid liver lesions. Subsequent digital rectal examination revealed a mid-to-low rectal mass. Referral to colonoscopy and an examination by a colorectal surgeon confirmed a low rectal adenocarcinoma. MRI of the rectum revealed the tumor to focally extend beyond the muscularis propria, with multiple enlarged lymph nodes confined to the mesorectum. CT imaging of the liver revealed hypodense lesions in all segments of the liver, but no evidence of peritoneal or extrahepatic spread. 18FDG PET/CT confirmed the innumerable FDG-avid lesions in the liver, but with no extrahepatic disease. CEA level was elevated at 9.0 μg/L.

Multidisciplinary Management

Systemic chemotherapy with palliative intent was commenced and, given his excellent performance, two cycles of FOLFOX were delivered. Repeat CT scan revealed a measurable reduction in size of the liver lesions. There was also some objective evidence of shrinkage of the primary lesion. Referral to a specialist liver surgeon prompted primavist MRI of the liver and consideration of staged hepatectomy. The two superficial lesions in segments 2 and 3 of the liver were resectable prior to portal vein embolization, with extended right hemi-hepatectomy as a second-stage procedure. However, a 2 cm segment 4 lesion was close to the left portal inflow, which if enlarged following the first-stage hepatectomy, may have precluded extended right hemi-hepatectomy. Dissection on the plane of the left portal pedicle and the requirement to minimize time without chemotherapy made an ALLPPS procedure ideal. The patient completed five further cycles of FOLFOX chemotherapy, suffering only with fatigue and mild peripheral neuropathy. Repeat imaging was completed before proceeding to surgery three weeks after the seventh cycle of chemotherapy. Six wedge resections of segments 2 and 3 were performed at the first stage along with caudate lobectomy, liver partition along the left portal pedicle, and ligation of the right portal vein. Of the six lesions, only one contained viable adenocarcinoma, with necrosis, inflammation, and fibrosis, indicating a good response to neoadjuvant chemotherapy. Extended right hemi-hepatectomy was performed 11 days later, revealing more than 40 lesions of the liver with a maximum diameter of 25 mm. Pathological analysis revealed no metastasis in portal lymph nodes and no lymphovascular invasion. Postoperatively, chemotherapy was recommenced at 6 weeks with a further six cycles of FOLFOX. MRI of the pelvis at 6 months revealed a complete radiological response in the rectum, and this was confirmed at proctoscopy. Repeat primovist MRI of the liver revealed two new lesions in segment 2 of the liver (in a watershed of a wedge resection). A third hepatectomy was performed to remove segment 2. After a further 3 months with no chemotherapy, a single-stage low anterior resection was performed, and pathological review of the specimen analysis revealed a complete pathological response.

Case Summary

Hepatic metastases defines the prognosis of the patient. The patient was initially deemed unresectable at colorectal MDT and started "palliative" chemotherapy. After a response to initial chemotherapy was observed, referral to a specialist HPB surgeon was performed. The risk of involved margins at hepatectomy favored prolonged systemic therapy and a short interval to aggressive two-stage hepatectomy removing approximately 50 liver lesions. Early low-volume recurrence in the left lateral section has necessitated further chemotherapy and a third liver resection. The primary tumor has undergone near-complete response and can be observed, as further metastatic disease will dictate outcome.

Controversies in Management

- Longer durations of preoperative chemotherapy may improve tumor response at the expense of causing liver injury as a consequence of sinusoidal obstructive syndrome and steatohepatitis.
- Liver-first surgery is appropriate when the burden of disease is high, or the surgery to remove the tumors is complicated.

Discussion: Symptomatic Primary Tumors

The referral pattern of patients diagnosed with primary rectal cancer often dictates sequencing of therapy, with a primary first approach still favored by most centers [8]. Symptomatic disease is often cited as the reason for upfront resection, prior to systemic therapy. Sporadic rectal bleeding and anemia are common symptoms, but bleeding requiring ongoing transfusion is rare. Large bowel obstruction due to a low rectal tumor is also a rare event and should be managed with diverting colostomy followed by neoadjuvant therapy rather than upfront resection. For partially obstructed or endoscopically obstructed rectal adenocarcinoma, colostomy can be avoided in 96% of patients who are able to undergo radiation therapy prior to surgery [16]. This results in less delay to neoadjuvant therapy, and should reassure oncologists that treatment is unlikely to be interrupted.

Neoadjuvant Therapy

In nonmetastatic rectal cancer, short-course radiation therapy (SCRT) followed by surgery and long-course radiation therapy (LCRT) with chemosensitization (5-FU) then surgery, is associated with decreased rates of local recurrence [17]. LCRT has the added benefit of downstaging primary tumors for sphincter-sparing resections, and can increase R0 resection rates and local control [15]. In stage IV disease the use of standard SCRT/LCRT regimes followed by rectal surgery can delay the provision of effective systemic therapy by over 3 months. This delay may be dramatically increased should complications be encountered following rectal resection, which risks disease progression in the liver and subsequent unresectability [5]. Similarly, untreated rectal disease and a systemic therapy/liver-first approach is associated with 26% of rectal tumors being found to be unresectable [18].

The addition of more effective systemic therapy to LCRT (typically oxaloplatin compounds and leucovorin) is an aggressive approach of neoadjuvant treatment to the liver and rectum. It is associated with increased toxicity and may be poorly tolerated in patients with comorbidities [12].

A less toxic approach is short-course radiotherapy with surgery delayed until systemic therapy can be completed. This is associated with radiological response rates in 74% of patients [19] and this allows for modifications in subsequent treatment sequence, i.e., liver-first approach. The sequence of radiation therapy—systemic therapy then repeat imaging—may also be reversed with the advantage of early assessment for disease progression and avoiding radiation therapy in patients with progressive unresectable liver disease [17].

Aggressive systemic therapy may be applied in patients with excellent performance status, and may convert initially stage IV unresectable disease in 15% of patients [20]. Response rates of the primary tumor to standard combination chemotherapy rates are in the order of 55% [20], however, a proportion of patients may progress despite treatment [18]. The addition of biological agents in eligible patients increases response rates. Meta-analysis has revealed that overall response rates are around 64% and conversion to R0 resectability possible in 22.5% [21].

Combination chemotherapy may be complicated by nonalcoholic steatohepatitis, steatosis, and liver cell injury. This may delay or preclude major liver resection, especially in patients with borderline liver function, or necessitate a two-stage procedure. Even successful chemotherapy with a complete or near-complete response may cause radiological "ghosting" of lesions, making resection complex.

Surgical Resection

The classical approach (primary first) to synchronous colorectal cancer and CRLM remains the most widely accepted and commonly practiced approach [7, 22]. This may in part be due to patterns of referral and can allow the full metastatic burden of disease be appreciated. The liver-first approach incorporating neoadjuvant chemotherapy, in which the metastatic disease is prioritized and not delayed by local treatment to the primary tumor, is a newer approach. The requirement and effect of rectal chemoradiation and the higher risk of septic complications with rectal resection, compared to colonic resection make a liver-first approach ideally suited to synchronous rectal adenocarcinoma [23]. Although no benefit has been proven in overall survival, and morbidity and mortality appear to be similar in both groups [7, 8], a higher proportion of patients complete all treatment in a liver-first approach [5]. Meta-analysis has shown that only 19% of patients progress in their liver disease prior to hepatic resection with neoadjuvant chemotherapy [5]. Although 55% response rates are observed in the rectal primary [24], a high proportion of patients (26%) are observed to have progression in the pelvis after completion of all therapy to the liver [18]. The addition of radiotherapy (either short-course immediately followed by systemic therapy, or long-course with effective systemic therapy) may negate the risk of an unresectable primary [12, 13].

Conclusion

A synchronous approach to colorectal resection of all tumor sites at one operation would seem the ideal approach, with similar mortality and morbidity to staged resections, as published by multiple authors [7, 10, 14, 23, 25, 26]. However, these studies are biased by the limited numbers of rectal resections included and the low-volume of metastatic disease (i.e., need for major hepatectomy). One study limited to patients with undergoing synchronous resection in the setting of a rectal primary showed it is safe, but that 5-year survival is lower than other published studies [25]. This study was also limited by less than 1/3 of patients undergoing low anterior resection and only 22% major hepatectomy [25]. Other studies have reported high rates of complications (58%) and lower overall survival (32%) [14]. There is general consensus that in all but the fittest patients, combined low rectal resection and hepatectomy should be avoided.

The decision to perform a primary or liver-first approach should be impacted by the volume of disease at both sites. The likelihood of involved margins or progression preventing resection at each site must be assessed, and treatment prioritized, to avoid positive margins or unresectable disease.

References

1. Manfredi S, Lepage Cm, Hatem C, Coatmeur O, Faivre J, Bouvier A-M. Epidemiology and management of liver metastases from colorectal cancer. Ann Surg. 2006;244(2):254–9.
2. Kopetz S, Chang GJ, Overman MJ, Eng C, Sargent DJ, Larson DW, et al. Improved survival in metastatic colorectal cancer is associated with adoption of hepatic resection and improved chemotherapy. J Clin Oncol. 2009;27(22):3677–83.
3. Adam R. The oncosurgery approach to managing liver metastases from colorectal cancer: a multidisciplinary international consensus. Oncologist. 2012;17(10):1225–39.
4. Verhoef C, van der Pool AEM, Nuyttens JJ, Planting AST, Eggermont AMM, de Wilt JHW. The "liver-first approach" for patients with locally advanced rectal cancer and synchronous liver metastases. Dis Colon Rectum. [Research Support, Non-U.S. Gov't]. 2009;52(1):23–30.

5. Jegatheeswaran S, Mason JM, Hancock HC, Siriwardena AK. The liver-first approach to the management of colorectal cancer with synchronous hepatic metastases: a systematic review. JAMA Surg. [Review]. 148(4):385–91.
6. Vigano L, Karoui M, Ferrero A, Tayar C, Cherqui D, Capussotti L. Locally advanced mid/low rectal cancer with synchronous liver metastases. World J Surg. 35(12):2788–95.
7. Brouquet A, Mortenson MM, Vauthey J-N, Rodriguez-Bigas MA, Overman MJ, Chang GJ, et al. Surgical strategies for synchronous colorectal liver metastases in 156 consecutive patients: classic, combined or reverse strategy? J Am Coll Surg. 210(6):934–41.
8. Mayo SC, Pulitano C, Marques H, Lamelas J, Wolfgang CL, De Saussure W, et al. Surgical management of patients with synchronous colorectal liver metastasis: a multicenter international analysis. J Am Coll Surg. 216(4):707–16.
9. Kelly ME, Spolverato G, Le GN, Mavros MN, Doyle F, Pawlik TM, et al. Synchronous colorectal liver metastasis: a network meta-analysis review comparing classical, combined, and liver-first surgical strategies. J Surg Oncol. [Meta-Analysis Review]. 111(3):341–51.
10. Martin RCG, 2nd, Augenstein V, Reuter NP, Scoggins CR, McMasters KM. Simultaneous versus staged resection for synchronous colorectal cancer liver metastases. J Am Coll Surg. [Comparative Study]. 2009;208(5):842–50; discussion 50–2.
11. Buchs NC, Ris F, Majno PE, Andres A, Cacheux W, Gervaz P, et al. Rectal outcomes after a liver-first treatment of patients with stage IV rectal cancer. Ann Surg Oncol. [Research Support, Non-U.S. Gov't]. 22(3):931–7.
12. Gerard J-P, Azria D, Gourgou-Bourgade S, Martel-Lafay I, Hennequin C, Etienne P-L, et al. Clinical outcome of the ACCORD 12/0405 PRODIGE 2 randomized trial in rectal cancer. J Clin Oncol. 2012;30(36):4558–65.
13. Van Dijk TH, Tamas K, Beukema JC, Beets GL, Gelderblom AJ, De Jong KP, et al. Evaluation of short-course radiotherapy followed by neoadjuvant bevacizumab, capecitabine, and oxaliplatin and subsequent radical surgical treatment in primary stage IV rectal cancer. Ann Oncol. 2013;4(7):1762–9.
14. Thelen A, Jonas S, Benckert C, Spinelli A, Lopez-H Zinninen E, Rudolph B, et al. Simultaneous versus staged liver resection of synchronous liver metastases from colorectal cancer. Int J Colorectal Dis. 2007;22(10):1269–76.
15. Sauer R, Liersch T, Merkel S, Fietkau R, Hohenberger W, Hess C, et al. Preoperative versus postoperative chemoradiotherapy for locally advanced rectal cancer: results of the German CAO/ARO/AIO-94 randomized phase III trial after a median follow-up of 11 years. J Clin Oncol. 2012;30(16):1926–33.
16. Patel JA, Fleshman JW, Hunt SR, Safar B, Birnbaum EH, Lin AY, et al. Is an elective diverting colostomy warranted in patients with an endoscopically obstructing rectal cancer before neoadjuvant chemotherapy? Dis Colon Rectum. 2012;55(3):249–55.
17. Gall TMH, Basyouny M, Frampton AE, Darzi A, Ziprin P, Dawson P, et al. Neoadjuvant chemotherapy and primary-first approach for rectal cancer with synchronous liver metastases. Colorectal Dis. 2014;16(6):O197–205.
18. Ayez N, Burger JW, van der Pool AE, Eggermont AM, Grunhagen DJ, de Wilt JH, et al. Long-term results of the "liver first" approach in patients with locally advanced rectal cancer and synchronous liver metastases. Dis Colon Rectum. 2013;56(3):281–7.
19. Pettersson D, Holm T, Iversen H, Blomqvist L, Glimelius B, Martling A. Preoperative short-course radiotherapy with delayed surgery in primary rectal cancer. Br J Surg. 2012;99 (4):577–83.
20. Falcone A, Ricci S, Brunetti I, Pfanner E, Allegrini G, Barbara C, et al. Phase III trial of infusional fluorouracil, leucovorin, oxaliplatin, and irinotecan (FOLFOXIRI) compared with infusional fluorouracil, leucovorin, and irinotecan (FOLFIRI) as first-line treatment for metastatic colorectal cancer: the Gruppo Oncologico Nord Ovest. J Clin Oncol. 2007;25 (13):1670–6.
21. Lam VW, Spiro C, Laurence JM, Johnston E, Hollands MJ, Pleass HC, et al. A systematic review of clinical response and survival outcomes of downsizing systemic chemotherapy and

rescue liver surgery in patients with initially unresectable colorectal liver metastases. Ann Surg Oncol. 2012;19(4):1292–301.
22. Tol JAMG, Gouma DJ, Bassi C, Dervenis C, Montorsi M, Adham M, et al. Definition of a standard lymphadenectomy in surgery for pancreatic ductal adenocarcinoma: a consensus statement by the International Study Group on Pancreatic Surgery (ISGPS). Surgery. [Consensus Development Conference Practice Guideline]. 2014;156(3):591–600.
23. Adam R, de Gramont A, Figueras J, Kokudo N, Kunstlinger F, Loyer E, et al. Managing synchronous liver metastases from colorectal cancer: a multidisciplinary international consensus. Cancer Treat Rev. 2015;41(9):729–41.
24. Bensignor T, Brouquet A, Dariane C, Thirot-Bidault A, Lazure T, Julie C, et al. Pathological response of locally advanced rectal cancer to preoperative chemotherapy without pelvic irradiation. Colorectal Dis. 2015;17(6):491–8.
25. Boostrom SY, Vassiliki LT, Nagorney DM, Wolff BG, Chua HK, Harmsen S, et al. Synchronous rectal and hepatic resection of rectal metastatic disease. J Gastrointest Surg. 2011;15(9):1583–8.
26. Mayo SC, Shore AD, Nathan H, Edil BH, Hirose K, Anders RA, et al. Refining the definition of perioperative mortality following hepatectomy using death within 90 days as the standard criterion. HPB. 2011;13(7):473–82.

7 Laparoscopic Hemihepatectomy for Hepatocellular Carcinoma

Go Wakabayashi

Case Presentation

A 62-year-old man presented to his primary physician with a complaint of abdominal pain. Past history was hepatitis B infection and it was to be treated. Physical examination revealed a tender upper abdominal pain. The serum alpha-fetoprotein (AFP) level was 118.5 ng/mL, and PIVKA-II was 820 mAU/mL. Computed tomography (CT) evaluation revealed the images presented in Fig. 7.1, and magnetic resonance imaging (MRI) is presented in Fig. 7.2.

Diagnosis and Assessment

Our patient demonstrated common presentation of advanced HCC. HCC is the most frequent primary malignancy of the liver and one of the most common cancers in the world. Advanced HCC is associated with clinical manifestations of abdominal pain, weight loss, jaundice, hepatosplenomegaly, ascites, deranged liver function tests (LFTs), and elevated AFP [1]. We report here a patient with symptomatic advanced HCC, normal LFTs, and elevated AFP values. Protein induced by vitamin K absence or antagonist II (PIVKA-II) is also used as a diagnostic marker for HCC. The use of these two complementary markers (AFP and PIVKA-II) appears to be useful in the diagnosis of HCC. The frequencies of intrahepatic metastasis, portal vein tumor thrombus, hepatic vein tumor thrombus, and capsular infiltration are significantly higher in patients with positive PIVKA-II than in those with

G. Wakabayashi (✉)
Ageo Central General Hospital, 1-10-10 Kashiwaza,
Ageo 362-8588, Japan
e-mail: gowaka@ach.or.jp

T.M. Pawlik et al. (eds.), *Case-Based Lessons in the Management of Complex Hepato-Pancreato-Biliary Surgery*, DOI 10.1007/978-3-319-50868-9_7

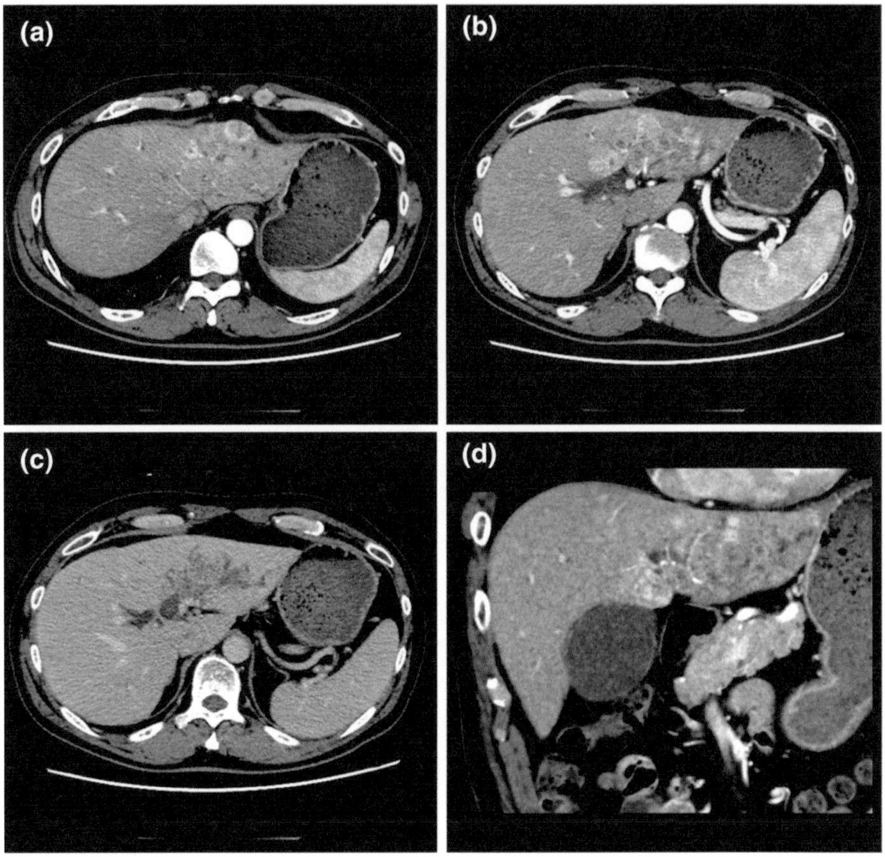

Fig. 7.1 Computed tomography imaging. **a** Arterial phase of multiple nodules; **b** arterial phase of diffuse area staining with bile duct dilatation; **c** delayed phase of washed-out area; **d** coronal view of arterial phase

negative-PIVKA-II. Therefore, PIVKA-II is one of the risk factors for recurrence of HCC after hepatectomy [2].

Diffuse-type HCC has been considered as an extensive and infiltrative tumor with poorly defined margins, frequently accompanied by portal venous tumor thrombosis and high level of AFP. Preoperative images of our patient showed small infiltrative diffuse-type HCC in segments II, III, IV (Fig. 7.1) and ill-defined lesions on segment IV with intermediate signal intensity and heterogeneous post-gadolinium enhancement (Fig. 7.2).

Assessment for the future-remnant liver function is the most important step to prevent postoperative liver failure. The Child-Pugh score consists of five clinical features and is used to assess the prognosis of chronic liver disease and cirrhosis. The score is also used to determine hepatic reserve for liver resection. The score considers five factors, three of which assess the synthetic function of the liver (i.e., total

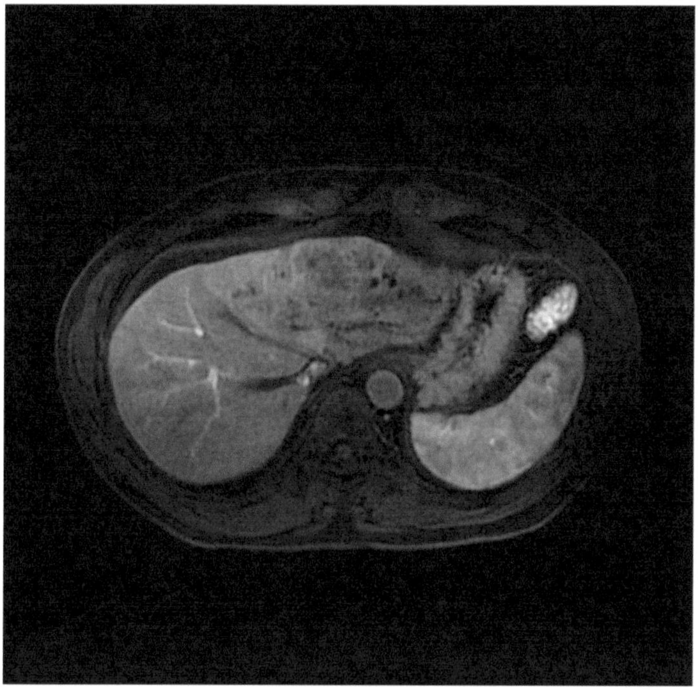

Fig. 7.2 Magnetic resonance imaging. Ill-defined lesions on segment IV with intermediate signal intensity and heterogeneous post-gadolinium

bilirubin level, serum albumin, and international normalized ratio, or INR) and two of which are based on clinical assessment (i.e., degree of ascites and degree of hepatic encephalopathy). Moreover, indocyanine green (ICG) clearance is one of the most reliable and easy-to-use tests for the preoperative dynamic assessment of liver function for resectability [3]. According to the decision tree that we use (Fig. 7.3), key points are: (1) contraindication to hepatic resection in presence of uncontrolled ascites or serum bilirubin > 1.9 mg/dL; (2) minor resections possible with serum bilirubin ranging between 1 and 1.9 mg/dL, the lower the bilirubin level, the larger the resection; and (3) according to ICGR15 intervals different types of hepatic resection possible in case of serum bilirubin < 1.1 mg/dL and no ascites [3].

Our patient was diagnosed as advanced HCC with possible infiltration to portal veins in the left hemi-liver. Small infiltrative diffuse-type HCC was confined in the left hemi-liver and the Child-Pugh score with ICGR15 allowed the left hemihepatectomy to remove all these HCC nodules.

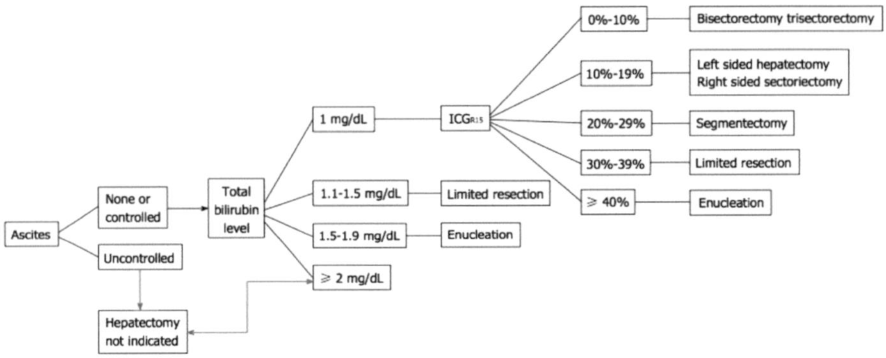

Fig. 7.3 Treatment algorithm for hepatectomy. Extent of hepatectomy in cirrhotic patients according to liver functional reserve. *ICGR15* Indocyanine green retention ratio at 15 min. Reprinted from De Gasperi A, Mazza E, Prosperi M. Indocyanine green kinetics to assess liver function: Ready for a clinical dynamic assessment in major liver surgery? World J Hepatol. 2016 Mar 8;8(7):355–67; with permission from Baishideng Publishing Group Inc.

Technical Pearls

1. Precise parenchymal transection is the key to perform high-quality LLR.
2. Expose MHV to keep transection plane and to avoid hepatic vein injury.
3. DO NOT touch tumors to avoid dissemination.
4. Isolate the tumor bearing area by inflow occlusion with outflow closure before manipulation.

Management

According to the BCLC algorithm, our patient is defined as stage B with intermediate HCC or stage C with advanced HCC, and resection is not recommended in either stages. The standard treatments are TACE or Sorafenib [1]. However, if hepatic reserve is preserved, we choose hepatectomy to remove all HCC with or without portal vein thrombus even in BCLC stage B/C patients. Resection will always give better effect on prognosis with better quality of life, if it is done safely.

We conducted a multi-institutional study using propensity score matching to compare the perioperative and long-term outcomes of LLR to OLR for HCC [4]. The study clearly showed clinical benefits of decreased estimated blood loss, shorter median length of stay, and less postoperative morbidity (6.7% vs. 13.0%) comparing LLR to OLR with comparable oncologic outcomes for HCC. With median follow-up of 47 months for LLR and 52 months for OLR, there were no differences in 1-, 2-, and 5-year disease-free or overall survival between the matched groups. Conversion from LLR to OLR or hybrid/hand-assisted procedure occurred in 25 of 387 (6.5%) patients [4].

LLR started with partial resection and left lateral sectionectomy in early 1990s [5–8]. The first formal laparoscopic hemihepatectomy was reported in 1998, using the pure laparoscopic method for left hepatectomies and the laparoscopy-assisted method for right hepatectomies [9]. After the laparoscopic left lateral sectionectomy became the standard of care for resection of lesions located in segments II and III, the laparoscopic left hemihepatectomy has also become a standard of care in expert hands [10, 11]. The surgical techniques for laparoscopic major hepatectomy include pure laparoscopic, hand-assisted laparoscopic, and laparoscopy-assisted methods [7, 12, 13]. Laparoscopic major hepatectomy is an innovative procedure that is still in the exploration phase [14]. Although new surgical techniques have learning curves, safety should be maintained from the onset [15]. We recommended at the second consensus that laparoscopic major hepatectomy should continue to be introduced cautiously [14].

Alternative left hepatectomy in minimally invasive way is laparoscopy-assisted/hybrid or hand-assisted procedure [16]. In the pure laparoscopic procedure, the entire resection is completed through laparoscopic ports. Hand-assisted laparoscopy was defined as the elective placement of a hand port during laparoscopic liver resection, to facilitate the procedure; and this technique is frequently called hand-assisted laparoscopic surgery (HALS). The hybrid technique is started as a pure or hand-assisted laparoscopic procedure, but the resection is performed through a mini-laparotomy incision. The hybrid technique is also frequently called the "laparoscopy-assisted" method. It is clear that HALS and the hybrid technique may overcome certain difficulties associated with pure laparoscopy, and may be less invasive than a traditional open laparotomy [16]. It is not clear that these minimally invasive liver resections would improve outcomes in patients with cirrhosis. According to our experience, it appears that LLR for selected HCC patients with cirrhosis is a feasible and promising procedure that is associated with less blood loss and fewer postoperative complications, especially the incidence of postoperative ascites. Further investigations are clearly warranted in this field [17].

Alternative Approaches

1. BCLC stage B or C HCC can be resected with R0 margin
2. Laparoscopy-assisted/hybrid or hand-assisted procedure are alternative way to perform left hemihepatectomy
3. HALS and the hybrid technique may overcome certain difficulties associated with pure laparoscopy.

Outcome

We chose to perform pure laparoscopic left hemihepatectomy on this patient. In our standardized LLR for left side liver, patients are placed in head-up supine position with legs closed, and the operator stands on the right side of patients [17]. A trocar for a laparoscope is inserted from the umbilical area to induce CO_2 pneumoperitoneum (10–12 mm Hg). Trocar placement is always the same as shown in Fig. 7.4. The operative procedures included: (1) cholecystectomy, (2) division of the left portal branch and the left hepatic artery, (3) division of the left hepatic vein (LHV), (4) parenchymal transection with exposure of the middle hepatic vein (MHV), and (5) removal of the resected left hemi-liver through supra-pubic incision. It is important to close LHV earlier to avoid tumor cells dissemination during manipulation of the left liver. We perform precise parenchymal transection under intermittent Pringle maneuver with slightly increased pneumoperitoneal pressure up to 12 mmHg. We use laparosonic coagulating shears for superficial parenchymal transection, and an ultrasonic dissector (CUSA Excel; Integra Lifesciences Corp., New Jersey, U.S.) for deeper parenchymal transection with exposure of MHV. Intraoperative images are shown in Figs. 7.5 and 7.6. Operative outcomes, pathological TNM staging, and postoperative course are summarized in Table 7.1. The resected left hemi-liver and its cut surface are shown in Fig. 7.7.

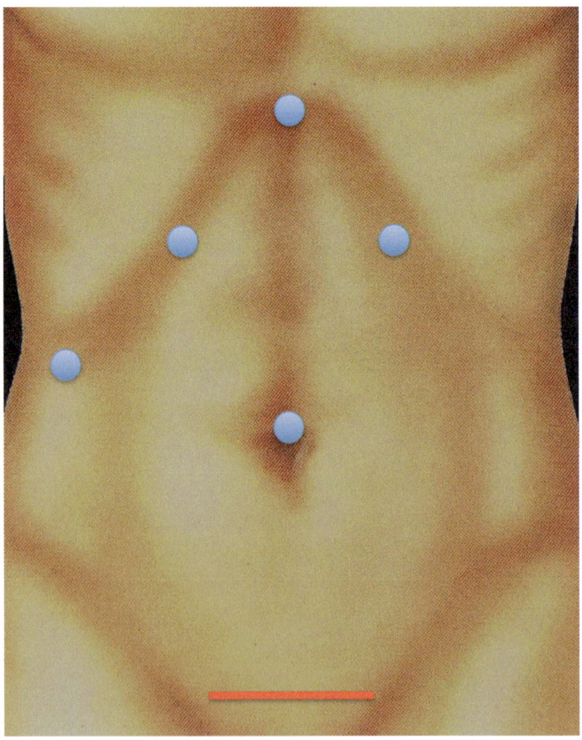

Fig. 7.4 Trocar position and retrieval site. All trocars are 12 mm. Laparoscope is inserted through umbilicus. The resected specimen is retrieved through supra-pubic incision

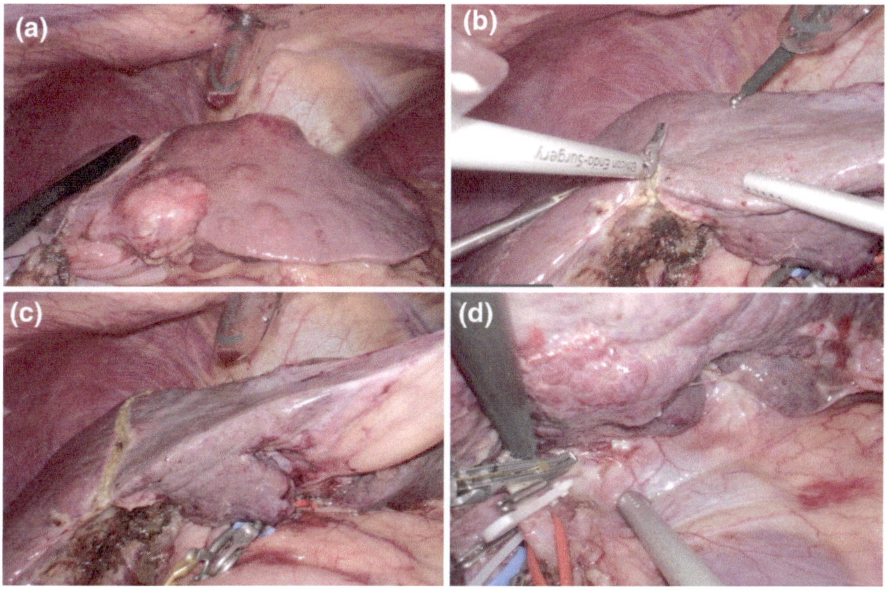

Fig. 7.5 Intraoperative view 1. **a** Multiple nodules are confined in the left liver; **b** superficial parenchymal transection with laparosonic coagulating shears along the demarcation line produced after inflow occlusion of the left hemi-liver; **c** demarcation line with superficial parenchymal transection; **d** division of the left hepatic artery (LHA) and clipping of the left portal vein (LPV)

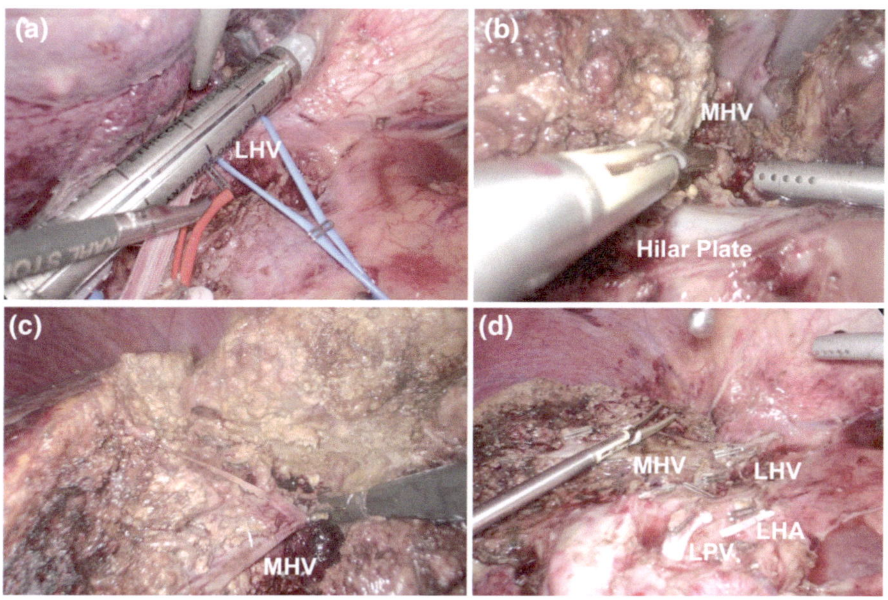

Fig. 7.6 Intraoperative view 2. **a** Division of the left hepatic vein (LHV) with an automatic stapler; **b** exposure of the middle hepatic vein (MHV) with an ultrasonic dissector over the hilar plate; **c** MHV is exposed and the hepatic vein from segment IV (V4) is divided; **d** final aspect of the cut surface of the right hemi-liver with exposed MHV, the stump of LHV, the stump of LHA, and the stump of LPV

Table 7.1 Summary data

Patient: 62y/o, Male, Hepatitis B virus infection Preoperative assessments: Child-Pugh Score: Class A (5 points), Bilirubin 0.6 mg/dL, Albumin 4.1 g/dL, Prothrombin time 86%, No ascites, No Encephalopathy ICGR15: 4% Tumor Markers: AFP 118.5 ng/mL, PIVKA-II 820 mAU/mL, CEA 1.2 ng/mL, CA19-9 6U/mL
Operative records: Pure Laparoscopic Left Hemihepatectomy (S2, 3, 4) Operative Time: 358 min Estimated Blood Loss: 290 ml Pringle Maneuver: 5 times (15 min clamp followed by 5 min reperfusion), total ischemic time 73 min Resected Liver Weight: 396 g
Pathological TNM staging: Multiple nodules with diffuse spread, Maximal size 5 cm, Microscopic invasions to the second bifurcation of portal veins, bile ducts, and peripheral hepatic veins, Stage 2 liver fibrosis (F2), Ishak staging scale 3 (F0 by AJCC/UICC), Negative surgical margin AJCC/UICC TNM stage: T3aN0M0, Stage IIIA LCSGJ TNM stage: T4N0M0, Stage IVA
Postoperative course: No complication, Diet started on 1POD, Drain removed on 2POD, Discharged on 6POD, No recurrence at 1POY

AFP alpha-fetoprotein; *PIVKA-II* protein induced by vitamin K absence or antagonist II; *CEA* Carcinoembryonic antigen; *CA-19-9* carbohydrate antigen 19-9; *TNM* Tumor-Node-Metastasis; *AJCC* American Joint Committee on Cancer; *UICC* International Union Against Cancer; *LCSGJ* The Liver Cancer Study Group of Japan

Clinical Pearls

1. Diffuse-type HCC confined to the left liver was totally resected by pure laparoscopic procedure.
2. LLR is associated with decreased estimated blood loss, shorter median length of stay, and less postoperative morbidity compared to OLR with comparable oncologic outcomes for HCC.
3. High-quality LLR is needed to treat advanced HCC with precise parenchymal transection and with oncological concerns.
4. Laparoscopic major hepatectomy should be introduced cautiously.

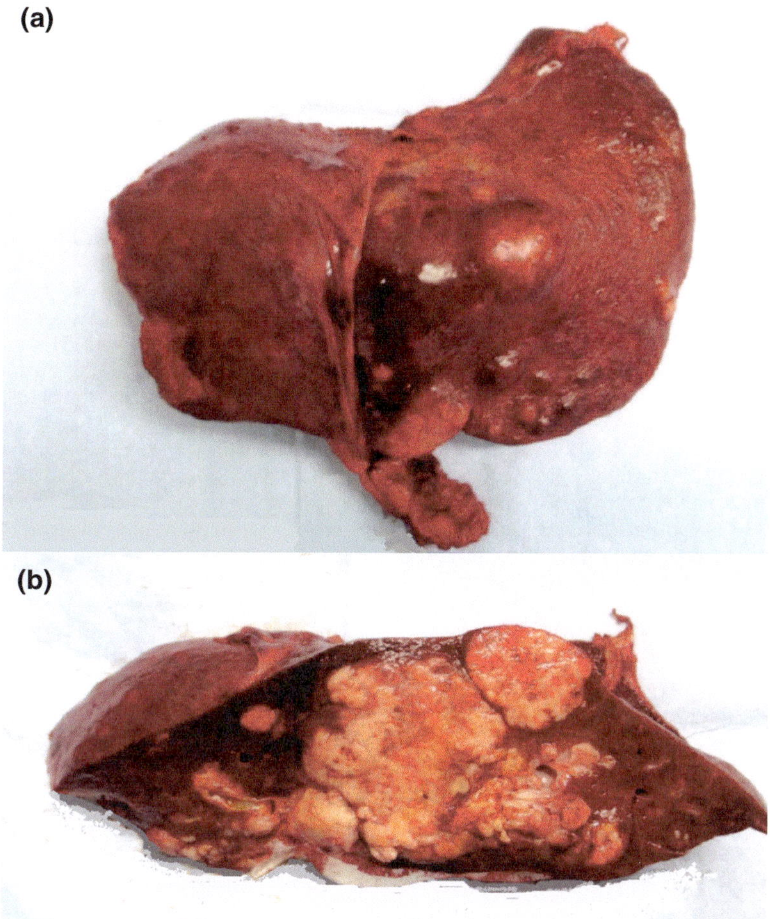

Fig. 7.7 The resected left hemi-liver with its cut surface. **a** Whole resected left liver **b** Its cut surface

References

1. Forner A, Llovet JM, Bruix J. Hepatocellular carcinoma. Lancet. 2012;379(9822):1245–55.
2. Suehiro T, Sugimachi K, Matsumata T, Itasaka H, Taketomi A, Maeda T. Protein induced by vitamin K absence or antagonist II as a prognostic marker in hepatocellular carcinoma. Comparison with alpha-fetoprotein. Cancer. 1994;73(10):2464–71.
3. De Gasperi A, Mazza E, Prosperi M. Indocyanine green kinetics to assess liver function: ready for a clinical dynamic assessment in major liver surgery? World J Hepatol. 2016;8(7):355–67.
4. Takahara T, Wakabayashi G, Beppu T, Aihara A, Hasegawa K, Gotohda N, et al. Long-term and perioperative outcomes of laparoscopic versus open liver resection for hepatocellular carcinoma with propensity score matching: a multi-institutional Japanese study. J Hepatobiliary Pancreat Sci. 2015;22(10):721–7.

5. Wakabayashi G. Laparoscopic liver resection: how far can we go? J Hepatobiliary Pancreat Surg. 2009;16(4):403–4.
6. Sasaki A, Nitta H, Otsuka K, Takahara T, Nishizuka S, Wakabayashi G. Ten-year experience of totally laparoscopic liver resection in a single institution. Br J Surg. 2009;96(3):274–9.
7. Buell JF, Cherqui D, Geller DA, O'Rourke N, Iannitti D, Dagher I, et al; World Consensus Conference on Laparoscopic Surgery. The international position on laparoscopic liver surgery: The Louisville Statement, 2008. Ann Surg. 2009;250(5):825–30.
8. Ciria R, Cherqui D, Geller DA, Briceno J, Wakabayashi G. Comparative short-term benefits of laparoscopic liver resection: 9000 cases and climbing. Ann Surg. 2016;263(4):761–77.
9. Huscher CG, Lirici MM, Chiodini S. Laparoscopic liver resections. Semin Laparosc Surg. 1998;5:204–10.
10. Belli G, Gayet B, Han HS, Wakabayashi G, Kim KH, Cannon R, et al. International Consensus Group for Laparoscopic Liver Surgery. Laparoscopic left hemihepatectomy a consideration for acceptance as standard of care. Surg Endosc. 2013;27(8):2721–6.
11. Dagher I, Gayet B, Tzanis D, Tranchart H, Fuks D, Soubrane O, et al. International experience for laparoscopic major liver resection. J Hepatobiliary Pancreat Sci. 2014;21 (10):732–6.
12. Nitta H, Sasaki A, Fujita T, Itabashi H, Hoshikawa K, Takahara T, et al. Laparoscopy-assisted major liver resections employing a hanging technique: the original procedure. Ann Surg. 2010;251(3):450–3.
13. Lin NC, Nitta H, Wakabayashi G. Laparoscopic major hepatectomy: a systematic literature review and comparison of 3 techniques. Ann Surg. 2013;257(2):205–13.
14. Wakabayashi G, Cherqui D, Geller DA, Buell JF, Kaneko H, Han HS, et al. Recommendations for laparoscopic liver resection: a report from the second international consensus conference held in Morioka. Ann Surg. 2015;261(4):619–29.
15. Hasegawa Y, Nitta H, Takahara T, Katagiri H, Baba S, Takeda D, et al. Safely extending the indications of laparoscopic liver resection: When should we start laparoscopic major hepatectomy? Surg Endosc. 2016 Jun 10 (Epub ahead of print).
16. Hasegawa Y, Koffron AJ, Buell JF, Wakabayashi G. Approaches to laparoscopic liver resection: a meta-analysis of the role of hand-assisted laparoscopic surgery and the hybrid technique. J Hepatobiliary Pancreat Sci. 2015;22(5):335–41.
17. Takahara T, Wakabayashi G, Nitta H, Hasegawa Y, Katagiri H, Takeda D, et al. Laparoscopic liver resection for hepatocellular carcinoma with cirrhosis in a single institution. Hepatobiliary Surg Nutr. 2015;4(6):398–405.

Minimally Invasive Resection of Colorectal Liver Metastases

8

Lee M. Ocuin and Allan Tsung

Case Presentation

A 49-year-old female presented to her primary care physician with several months of increasing fatigue, bright red blood per rectum, and a 10-lb weight loss. Her past medical history included only hypertension and she had no family history of colon cancer or other gastrointestinal malignancies. Rectal exam revealed a mass extruding from the anus that was fixed to the sphincter complex. Colonoscopy demonstrated an additional mass at the rectosigmoid junction. Biopsies of both masses were consistent with moderately differentiated adenocarcinoma that was microsatellite stable. Serum carcinoembryonic antigen (CEA) was < 4 ng/ml. A PET-CT scan (Fig. 8.1a, b) demonstrated increased SUV uptake in the distal sigmoid colon and rectum as well as a hypermetabolic mass in segment IVb/V of the liver, adjacent to the gallbladder.

L.M. Ocuin
Division of Surgical Oncology, Department of Surgery, University of Pittsburgh Medical Center, 5150 Centre Avenue, Suite 414, Pittsburgh, PA 15232, USA
e-mail: lee.ocuinmd@gmail.com

A. Tsung (✉)
Division of Hepatobiliary and Pancreatic Surgery, Department of Surgery, University of Pittsburgh Medical Center, Kauffman Buliding, 3471 Fifth Avenue Ste 300, Pittsburgh, PA 15213, USA
e-mail: tsunga@upmc.edu

T.M. Pawlik et al. (eds.), *Case-Based Lessons in the Management of Complex Hepato-Pancreato-Biliary Surgery*, DOI 10.1007/978-3-319-50868-9_8

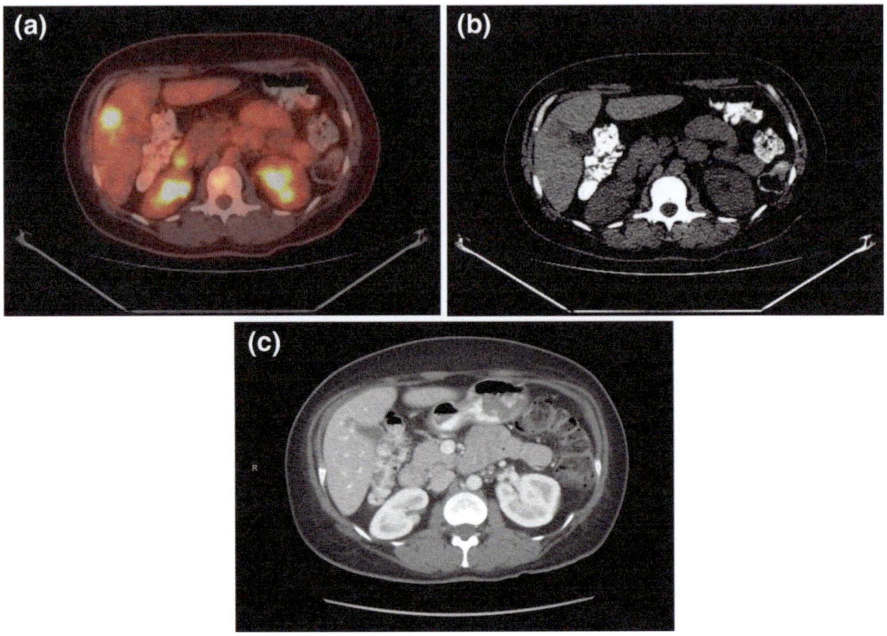

Fig. 8.1 Cross-sectional imaging demonstrating solitary hepatic metastatic disease. **a** and **b** Preoperative PET-CT showing segment IVb/V mass. **c** Restaging following four cycles of neoadjuvant 5-fluorouracil, leucovorin, oxaliplatin, and bevacizumab, showing decreased size of metastatic lesion

Epidemiology

Colorectal cancer is the fourth most frequently diagnosed cancer and the second leading cause of cancer death in the United States. In 2016, approximately 39,000 new cases of rectal cancer will be diagnosed and 49,000 patients will die from colorectal cancer combined [1]. Between 50 and 60% of patients diagnosed with colorectal cancer will develop metastatic disease [2] with 80–90% of patients having unresectable hepatic metastatic burden [3]. Most patients will present with metachronous liver metastatic disease. However, like our patient, 15–34% of patients with colorectal cancer present with synchronous liver metastatic disease [4–8].

Untreated patients have a median survival of 12 months or less [9]. Patients who undergo surgical resection in the context of multimodality therapy are the only patients with a chance at long-term cure, and 5-year survival is achieved in approximately 50% of patients [10].

Preoperative Planning

The management of patients who present with colorectal cancer with synchronous metastatic disease is complex. Decisions regarding timing of surgery, chemotherapy or chemoradiotherapy, and surgical approach are influenced by tumor biology, primary tumor location, extent of hepatic metastatic disease, and patient comorbidities. All patients should undergo a comprehensive history and physical examination. Prior abdominal surgery or the presence of underlying comorbidities, such as chronic obstructive pulmonary disease or congestive heart failure, should be kept in mind when choosing patients for minimally invasive hepatectomy.

Standard workup of patients with hepatic malignancy includes a triphasic CT scan (noncontrast, arterial, and portal venous phase) or contrast-enhanced MRI exam of the abdomen and pelvis. These imaging studies should be recent (within 4–6 weeks of surgery), and allow for evaluation of tumor size and location, extent of hepatic disease, assessment of the background liver for cirrhosis and hepatic steatosis, and the size of the future liver remnant. Evaluation for extrahepatic disease can be accomplished with a CT scan of the chest or CT/PET imaging. Routine labs include complete blood count, coagulation panel, and hepatic function panel. The serum CEA is useful as part of the diagnostic workup and postoperative surveillance.

Similar to open hepatectomy, we favor a low central venous pressure (CVP) anesthesia approach when performing minimally invasive hepatic resections [11]. This avoids distention of the inferior vena cava, facilitating mobilization of the liver and dissection of the retrohepatic cava and major hepatic veins. Low CVP anesthesia decreases bleeding during parenchymal transection and simplifies control of inadvertent venous injury. The incidence of gas embolism is rare during laparoscopic liver resection [12].

General Clinical Pearls

- The management of metastatic colorectal cancer should always involve a multidisciplinary team of physicians.
- The decision for synchronous versus staged resection and neoadjuvant therapy versus up-front resection should be guided by tumor biology and patient factors.
- Always perform intraoperative ultrasound
- The operative approach (minimally invasive vs. open, laparoscopic vs. robotic-assisted) is probably the least important decision in the comprehensive management of patients with Stage IV colorectal cancer. Decisions should be guided by surgeon experience and institutional resources.

Management

All patients with metastatic colorectal cancer should be discussed by a multidisciplinary panel of physicians, including colorectal and hepato-pancreato-biliary (HPB) surgeons, medical oncologists, radiation oncologists, interventional radiologists, gastroenterologists, pathologists, and palliative care providers. For our patient, the consensus of the multidisciplinary tumor board was to initiate systemic chemotherapy with 5-fluorouracil, leucovorin, oxaliplatin, and bevacizumab, with restaging after four cycles (2 months). There is no survival benefit to more than 2–3 months (four to six cycles) of preoperative chemotherapy, but liver-related posthepatectomy complications increase [13].

There is no consensus regarding the optimal management of patients with synchronous colorectal cancer and liver metastases. One option is the staged approach, addressing the primary first, followed by chemotherapy and hepatectomy at a later date. Theoretically, this approach eliminates potential complications from the primary tumor, such as bleeding, perforation, or obstruction. However, these complications arise in fewer than 10% of patients presenting with Stage IV colorectal cancer who receive systemic treatment in the setting of an intact primary [14]. Addressing the primary first delays the treatment of liver metastastic disease, which is of the greatest risk to long-term survival. Conversely, the liver metastatic disease can be addressed first, followed by colectomy and adjuvant chemotherapy. Alternatively, the patient can receive preoperative chemotherapy, followed by simultaneous or staged resection. A recent meta-analysis found that no single approach was superior to the others in terms of postoperative morbidity, mortality, or 5-year overall survival [6]. Given the lack of prospective data to guide decision-making, the order of therapy should be dictated by the extent of surgery that would be required to clear both the primary and the liver metastases [15]. For patients with less disease burden, consideration should be given to up-front simultaneous resection of both the primary and the liver metastatic diseases (i.e., solitary liver metastasis with a right colon cancer). Patients who would require extensive surgery to clear either the primary (i.e., proctosigmoidectomy or abdominoperineal resection) and/or the liver metastases (i.e., formal lobectomy or extended hepactectomy) warrant preoperative chemotherapy in an attempt to downstage disease and the extent of surgery required. Depending on the response, simultaneous or staged approaches can then be undertaken.

Minimally Invasive Hepatic Resection

Our patient completed 2 months of neoadjuvant chemotherapy and was restaged by contrast-enhanced CT scan. She had a partial clinical and radiographic response in both her primary rectal and rectosigmoid cancers (not shown) as well as in her solitary segment IVb/V liver metastasis (Fig. 8.1c). The decision was made to forgo neoadjuvant chemoradiotherapy for her distal rectal primary as the sphincter preservation was not an option; reducing the likelihood of pelvic recurrence was not a priority in the setting of end colostomy and the high risk of further distant disease recurrence. The patient underwent a robotic-assisted abdominoperineal resection with end colostomy and simultaneous cholecystectomy and segment IVb/V partial hepatectomy.

Our approach to robotic-assisted right and left anatomic lobectomy as well as left lateral sectionectomy has been previously described [16]. For robotic-assisted partial hepatectomy, patient positioning is generally supine, with arms tucked and in split-leg position. An orogastric tube and Foley catheter should be placed. In this specific case, the patient was in lithotomy with arms tucked because of the combined colorectal procedure. A cholecystectomy was performed and the gastrohepatic ligament was opened. A vessel loop was placed around the porta hepatis for control of vascular inflow (Fig. 8.2a). Intraoperative ultrasound (Fig. 8.2b) confirmed a solitary liver metastasis in segment IVb/V and no other lesions. Glisson's capsule was scored with cautery (Fig. 8.2c) and intraoperative ultrasound was repeated, confirming the target lesion was centered within the planned wedge resection. The vessel loop was tightened to perform a Pringle maneuver. A traction suture was placed through the specimen (Fig. 8.2d) to assist with exposure, and parenchymal transection was performed with bipolar forceps using the crush–clamp technique (Fig. 8.2e). The Pringle was released, the cut surface was inspected for bleeding, and hemostasis was achieved. The patient had an uneventful postoperative course and was discharged on postoperative day five. She has completed eight additional cycles (4 months) of 5-fluorouracil, leucovorin, oxaliplatin, and bevacizumab and currently has no evidence of recurrent disease.

Key Steps of Robotic-Assisted Partial Hepatectomy

- Creation of pneumoperitoneum
- Port placement
- Mobilization of target hemiliver from ligamentous attachments as needed
- Intraoperative ultrasound
- Score the liver capsule and confirm target on ultrasound
- Traction sutures on specimen
- Inflow control—Pringle maneuver
- Parenchymal transection and specimen retrieval
- Assess for hemostasis after Pringle released

The application of minimally invasive techniques has transformed the surgical landscape and has demonstrated benefit in surgical subspecialties including colorectal surgery [17, 18], gynecology [19], urology [20], and thoracic surgery [21]. Multiple studies have demonstrated reduced postoperative pain, reduced morbidity, decreased length of stay, improved cosmesis, and improved overall cost-effectiveness without

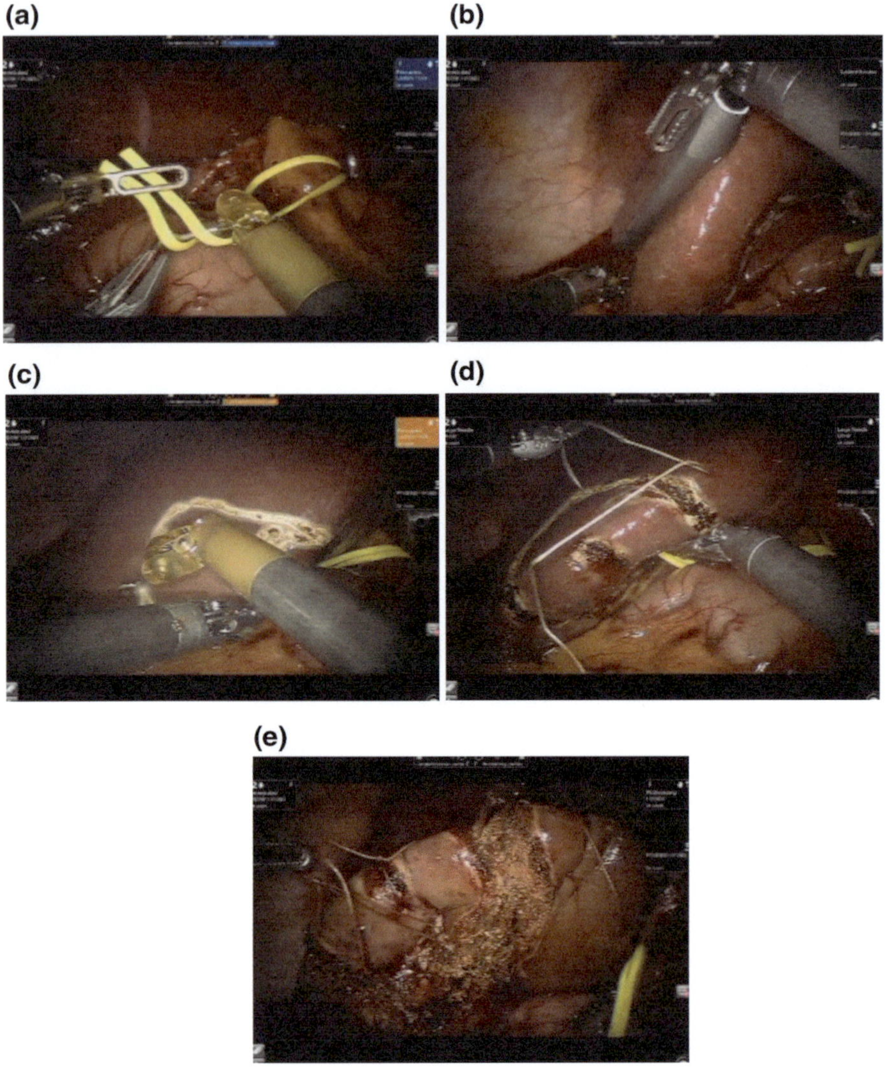

Fig. 8.2 Robotic-assisted partial hepatectomy. **a** The gastrohepatic ligament is opened and a vessel loop is placed around the hilar structures for control of vascular inflow. **b** Intraoperative ultrasound to confirm target lesion location and assess remaining liver. **c** The liver capsule is scored with cautery to declare the plane of transection and include the target lesion. **d** A traction suture is placed on the specimen to assist with exposure. Additional traction sutures may be placed on the remnant side as needed. **e** Parenchymal transection using bipolar forceps. A clamp crush technique is utilized. Larger pedicles can be ligated with endovascular staplers or electrothermal bipolar vessel sealing devices

compromising oncologic outcomes [17, 18, 22–24]. Limitations of conventional laparoscopic techniques include reduced visualization, amplification of physiologic tremor, and suboptimal ergonomics. Range of motion is restricted to four degrees of freedom, compared to the seven degrees of freedom of the human wrist [25, 26]. These limitations become increasingly apparent as the complexity of the procedure increases, and have likely slowed the application of minimally invasive approaches to HPB procedures, the majority of which are performed at high-volume tertiary care centers.

As the safety of HPB surgery has grown and outcomes have improved, minimally invasive approaches have been applied with increasing frequency to the field [27–37]. Laparoscopic liver surgery affords the same universal benefits of minimally invasive surgery elsewhere, including reduced postoperative pain and decreased length of hospital stay; and it has demonstrated safety in experienced hands [23]. However, the laparoscopic approach to the liver is challenging, due to complex vascular and biliary anatomy, risk of bleeding, fragile parenchyma, and difficult exposure secondary to size and deep, posterior retroperitoneal attachments. The minimally invasive approach is being utilized more frequently, but mainly for nonanatomic resections. Nguyen et al. reviewed more than 2,800 laparoscopic liver resections, and nonanatomic wedge resections and left lateral sectionectomy comprised nearly two-thirds of cases, while fewer than 10% of cases were formal right or left hepatic lobectomies [23].

In an effort to standardize and summarize the current position on laparoscopic liver surgery, an international conference was held in Louisville, Kentucky, USA in 2008 [38]. Consensus recommendations included: (1) the best indications for laparoscopic liver resection are in patients with solitary lesions, 5 cm or less, located in peripheral liver segments 2–6; (2) the laparoscopic approach to left lateral sectionectomy should be considered standard practice; and (3) although all types of liver resection can be performed laparoscopically, major liver resections (right or left hepatectomy) should be reserved for experienced surgeons already skilled at more complex laparoscopic hepatic resections. Lesions adjacent to major vessels or near the liver hilum were not considered appropriate for laparoscopic resection because of the potential risk of massive bleeding and need for biliary reconstruction. However, surgeons at high-volume centers may choose to operate beyond these criteria, provided that the surgeon is comfortable with minimally invasive methods to achieve hemostasis should significant bleeding be encountered. Despite the technical limitations of laparoscopy, malignant tumors are not a contraindication to minimally invasive resection, as demonstrated in many comparative studies; and laparoscopic resection does not appear to compromise the oncologic integrity of the procedure with regard to margin status and local recurrence rate when compared to the open approach [23, 33, 39, 40].

The inherent visual and ergonomic limitations of laparoscopy have played a major role in the development of robotic surgery, which allows surgeons to perform advanced laparoscopic procedures with greater ease. Currently, the da Vinci Surgical System (Intuitive Surgical, Inc, Sunnyvale, CA, USA) is the only commercially available robotic surgical system, approved by the United States Food and

Drug Administration (FDA) for use in surgery. Advantages include articulating instruments that recreate the seven degrees of freedom of the human wrist, three-dimensional view of the operative field in high definition, and complex algorithms that minimize physiologic tremor. These features allow for precise dissection and intracorporeal suturing, thus expanding the scope and complexity of procedures that can be performed in a minimally invasive fashion. Disadvantages include high cost, loss of haptic feedback, inability to operate in multiple fields, and need for a skilled bedside assistant. The lack of haptic feedback is generally overcome by enhanced three-dimensional visualization, which allows the operating surgeon to “see” how much tension or force is being applied to tissues and suture within the operative field [41].

The first major series reporting the use of robotics in general surgery was by Guilianotti et al. in 2003 [42]. The report included 207 procedures such as fundoplication, cholecystectomy, esophagectomy, colectomy, pancreatectomy, and hepatectomy. Morbidity and mortality rates were acceptable (8.3 and 1.5%, respectively), and the conversion rate was 2.1%. This report established that robotic surgery was both safe and feasible. Over the past decade, robotic-assisted surgery has been applied broadly in urological, gynecological, HPB, and cardiac surgery [36, 43–45]. The platform has controls and ergonomics that closely mimic the movements of open surgery, has improved three-dimensional visualization, and appears to shorten the learning curve for complex cases compared to conventional laparoscopy [42, 46, 47]. The multitude of technically challenging HPB procedures provides an ever-expanding and ideal application of this technology [34, 36, 48, 49].

Alternative Approaches and Controversies

- The robotic platform is an advanced laparoscopic tool—depending on surgeon experience and skill level, all robotic-assisted procedures can be performed with pure laparoscopy.
- Minimally invasive hepatectomy should only be performed by experienced HPB surgeons.
- Ablation techniques (radiofrequency or microwave) can be used in conjunction with partial hepatectomy for smaller lesions not amenable to partial hepatectomy. Local recurrence rates may be higher but overall survival does not appear to be different.

Outcomes

Minimally invasive hepatectomy is being performed with increasing frequency. In the largest review of laparoscopic liver resections to date, Nguyen et al. analyzed case series totaling more than 2,800 cases [23]. The overall findings suggest that minimally invasive liver resection is both safe and feasible. Nearly 75% of the cases were performed purely laparoscopic. Nearly 50% of resections were for malignancy, and the majority of cases (65%) were minor resections, including wedge hepatectomy or left lateral sectionectomy. Formal lobectomy was performed in 15% of cases, and fewer than 1% of the cases were extended lobectomies. Perioperative death occurred in 0.3% of the patients. The overall complication rate was 11%, with the most common complications being bile leak (1.5%) and transient hepatic dysfunction (1%).

Several series have compared laparoscopic to open major liver resection [50–53]. Laparoscopic resections appear to be associated with less blood loss, fewer postoperative complications, and shorter hospital length of stay, with the trade-off being slightly longer operative times. Short- and long-term oncologic outcomes of laparoscopic liver resections are comparable to disease-matched open outcomes [54, 55].

There are eight series in the literature that compare robotic-assisted liver resection to laparoscopic liver resection [34, 49, 56–61]. Data are summarized in Table 8.1. The largest experience belongs to the group of Tsung et al. at the University of Pittsburgh [34]. Each of the 57 patients who underwent robotic hepatectomy were retrospectively matched in a 1:2 ratio to patients that underwent laparoscopic liver resection, with emphasis on background liver disease, extent of resection, diagnosis, American Society of Anesthesiologists (ASA) score, age, body mass index (BMI), and gender. There was no difference in blood loss, transfusion requirements, conversion rate, complication rate, or length of stay. Robotic-assisted procedures took significantly longer (253 vs. 199 min). There appeared to be a learning curve effect when comparing the initial 13 robotic procedures to the subsequent 44, as there were significant reductions in blood loss (300 vs. 100 ml), operative times (381 vs. 232 min), and length of stay (5 vs. 4 days). However, the comparison of robotic-assisted to surgery to conventional laparoscopy may not be worthwhile, because the robotic platform should be looked at as an advanced tool to overcome the inherent limitations of conventional laparoscopy, thus expanding the repertoire of complex minimally invasive procedures that can be applied to the liver, pancreas, and biliary tract.

Table 8.1 Perioperative outcomes of robotic-assisted hepatectomy versus laparoscopic hepatectomy

	Tsung et al. (2014)			Tranchart et al. (2014)			Troisi et al. (2013)			Wu et al. (2014)			Yu et al. (2014)			Spampinato et al. (2014)			Packiam et al. (2012)			Berber et al. (2010)		
	LA	RA	*p*	LA	RA	*p*	LA	RA	*p*	LA	RA	*p*	LA	RA	*p*	LA	RA	*p*	LA	RA	p	LA	RA	p
Major resection (n)	42	21	NS	0	0	NS	37	0	**<0.05**	10	20	NR	11	3	NR	25	25	NS	0	0	NR	0	0	NR
Minor resection (n)	72	36		28	28		186	40	NR	59	32	NR	6	10		0	0	NS	18	11	NR	23	9	NS
Operative time (min)	199	253	**<0.05**	176	210	NS	262	271	NS	227	380	**<0.05**	241	292	NS	360	430	NS	188	175	NS	234	259	NS
EBL (ml)	100	200	NS	150	200	NS	174	330	**<0.05**	173	325	**<0.05**	343	389	NS	400	250	NS	30	30	NS	155	136	NS
Transfusion (%)	7	4	NS	4	14	NS	NR			NR			0	0	NS	44	16	**<0.05**	0	0	NS	NR		
Conversion (%)	9	7	NS	7	14	NS	8	20	**<0.05**	12.2	5	NS	0	0	NS	4	4	NS	0	0	NS	0	11	NR
Morbidity (%)	26	20	NS	18	18	NS	13	13	NS	10	8	NS	12	0	NS	36	16	NS	0	27	**<0.05**	17	11	NR
Length of stay (days)	4	4	NS	6	6	NS	6	6	NS	7	8	NS	10	8	NS	7	8	NS	3	4	**<0.05**	NR		

LA laparoscopic-assisted; *RA* robotic-assisted; *NR* not reported; *NS* not significant

Conclusion

In conclusion, the literature demonstrates that in properly selected patients, minimally invasive liver resection is a feasible and safe option, best performed by surgeons trained in open liver surgery who are skilled in minimally invasive techniques. Available data suggest that open, laparoscopic, and robotic approaches have similar perioperative outcomes. Short- and long-term oncologic outcomes appear to be equivalent. Currently, the majority of minimally invasive hepatectomies are nonanatomic resections, and therefore there is no clear-cut advantage to the robotic approach over laparoscopy in minor hepatectomy. There exists no high-quality, prospective data analyzing minimally invasive hepatectomy. Therefore, it is difficult to draw any definitive conclusions at this time with regard to overall efficacy and benefits in both immediate (length of stay, postoperative pain, morbidity, mortality, and cost-effectiveness) and long-term (quality of life, oncologic recurrence) patient outcomes. Existing data are promising and warrant further investigation.

References

1. Siegel RL, Miller KD, Jemal A. Cancer statistics, 2016. CA Cancer J Clin. 2016;66(1):7–30. doi:10.3322/caac.21332.
2. Yoo PS, Lopez-Soler RI, Longo WE, Cha CH. Liver resection for metastatic colorectal cancer in the age of neoadjuvant chemotherapy and bevacizumab. Clin Colorectal Cancer. 2006;6 (3):202–7. doi:10.3816/CCC.2006.n.036.
3. Alberts SR, Horvath WL, Sternfeld WC, Goldberg RM, Mahoney MR, Dakhil SR, et al. Oxaliplatin, fluorouracil, and leucovorin for patients with unresectable liver-only metastases from colorectal cancer: a North Central Cancer Treatment Group phase II study. J Clin Oncol. 2005;23(36):9243–9. doi:10.1200/JCO.2005.07.740.
4. Muratore A, Zorzi D, Bouzari H, Amisano M, Massucco P, Sperti E, et al. Asymptomatic colorectal cancer with un-resectable liver metastases: immediate colorectal resection or up-front systemic chemotherapy? Ann Surg Oncol. 2007;14(2):766–70. doi:10.1245/s10434-006-9146-1.
5. Hayashi M, Inoue Y, Komeda K, Shimizu T, Asakuma M, Hirokawa F, et al. Clinicopathological analysis of recurrence patterns and prognostic factors for survival after hepatectomy for colorectal liver metastasis. BMC Surg. 2010;27(10):27. doi:10.1186/1471-2482-10-27.
6. Kelly ME, Spolverato G, Le GN, Mavros MN, Doyle F, Pawlik TM, et al. Synchronous colorectal liver metastasis: a network meta-analysis review comparing classical, combined, and liver-first surgical strategies. J Surg Oncol. 2015;111(3):341–51. doi:10.1002/jso.23819.
7. Leporrier J, Maurel J, Chiche L, Bara S, Segol P, Launoy G. A population-based study of the incidence, management and prognosis of hepatic metastases from colorectal cancer. Br J Surg. 2006;93(4):465–74. doi:10.1002/bjs.5278.
8. Manfredi S, Lepage C, Hatem C, Coatmeur O, Faivre J, Bouvier AM. Epidemiology and management of liver metastases from colorectal cancer. Ann Surg. 2006;244(2):254–9. doi:10.1097/01.sla.0000217629.94941.cf.
9. Bird NC, Mangnall D, Majeed AW. Biology of colorectal liver metastases: a review. J Surg Oncol. 2006;94(1):68–80. doi:10.1002/jso.20558.
10. de Jong MC, Pulitano C, Ribero D, Strub J, Mentha G, Schulick RD, et al. Rates and patterns of recurrence following curative intent surgery for colorectal liver metastasis: an international

multi-institutional analysis of 1669 patients. Ann Surg. 2009;250(3):440–8. doi:10.1097/SLA.0b013e3181b4539b.
11. Cunningham JD, Fong Y, Shriver C, Melendez J, Marx WL, Blumgart LH. One hundred consecutive hepatic resections. Blood loss, transfusion, and operative technique. Arch Surg. 1994;29(10):1050–6.
12. Lin NC, Nitta H, Wakabayashi G. Laparoscopic major hepatectomy: a systematic literature review and comparison of 3 techniques. Ann Surg. 2013;257(2):205–13. doi:10.1097/SLA.0b013e31827da7fe.
13. Karoui M, Penna C, Amin-Hashem M, Mitry E, Benoist S, Franc B, et al. Influence of preoperative chemotherapy on the risk of major hepatectomy for colorectal liver metastases. Ann Surg. 2006;243(1):1–7.
14. Poultsides GA, Servais EL, Saltz LB, Patil S, Kemeny NE, Guillem JG, et al. Outcome of primary tumor in patients with synchronous stage IV colorectal cancer receiving combination chemotherapy without surgery as initial treatment. J Clin Oncol. 2009;27(20):3379–84. doi:10.1200/JCO.2008.20.9817.
15. Siriwardena AK, Mason JM, Mullamitha S, Hancock HC, Jegatheeswaran S. Management of colorectal cancer presenting with synchronous liver metastases. Nat Rev Clin Oncol. 2014;11(8):446–59. doi:10.1038/nrclinonc.2014.90.
16. Ocuin LM, Tsung A. Minimally invasive hepatic surgery. Surg Clin North Am. 96(2): 299–313. doi:10.1016/j.suc.2015.12.004.
17. Clinical Outcomes of Surgical Therapy Study Group. A comparison of laparoscopically assisted and open colectomy for colon cancer. N Engl J Med. 2004;350(20):2050–9. doi:10.1056/NEJMoa032651.
18. Guillou PJ, Quirke P, Thorpe H, Walker J, Jayne DG, Smith AM, et al. Short-term endpoints of conventional versus laparoscopic-assisted surgery in patients with colorectal cancer (MRC CLASICC trial): multicentre, randomised controlled trial. Lancet. 2005;365(9472):1718–26. doi:10.1016/S0140-6736(05)66545-2.
19. Ghezzi F, Cromi A, Ditto A, Vizza E, Malzoni M, Raspagliesi F, et al. Laparoscopic versus open radical hysterectomy for stage IB2-IIB cervical cancer in the setting of neoadjuvant chemotherapy: a multi-institutional cohort study. Ann Surg Oncol. 2013;20(6):2013;2007–15. doi:10.1245/s10434-012-2777-5.
20. Trabulsi EJ, Hassen WA, Touijer AK, Saranchuk JW, Guillonneau B. Laparoscopic radical prostatectomy: a review of techniques and results worldwide. Minerva Urol Nefrol. 2003;55(4):239–50.
21. Luketich JD, Pennathur A, Awais O, Levy RM, Keeley S, Shende M, et al. Outcomes after minimally invasive esophagectomy: review of over 1000 patients. Ann Surg. 2012;256(1):95–103. doi:10.1097/SLA.0b013e3182590603.
22. Martel G, Boushey RP. Laparoscopic colon surgery: past, present and future. Surg Clin N Am. 2006;86(4):867–97. doi:10.1016/j.suc.2006.05.006.
23. Nguyen KT, Gamblin TC, Geller DA. World review of laparoscopic liver resection—2,804 patients. Ann Surg. 2009;250(5):831–41. doi:10.1097/SLA.0b013e3181b0c4df.
24. Jayne DG, Guillou PJ, Thorpe H, Quirke P, Copeland J, Smith AM, et al. Randomized trial of laparoscopic-assisted resection of colorectal carcinoma: 3-year results of the UK MRC CLASICC Trial Group. J Clin Oncol. 2007;25(21):3061–8. doi:10.1200/JCO.2006.09.7758.
25. Berguer R, Rab GT, Abu-Ghaida H, Alarcon A, Chung J. A comparison of surgeons' posture during laparoscopic and open surgical procedures. Surg Endosc. 1997;11(2):139–42.
26. Cadiere GB, Himpens J, Germay O, Izizaw R, Degueldre M, Vandromme J, et al. Feasibility of robotic laparoscopic surgery: 146 cases. World J Surg. 2001;25(11):1467–77.
27. Wakabayashi G, Cherqui D, Geller DA, Buell JF, Kaneko H, Han HS, et al. Recommendations for laparoscopic liver resection: a report from the second international consensus conference held in Morioka. Ann Surg. 2015;261(4):619–29. doi:10.1097/SLA.0000000000001180.

28. Croome KP, Farnell MB, Que FG, Reid-Lombardo K, Truty MJ, Nagorney D, et al. Pancreaticoduodenectomy with major vascular resection: a comparison of laparoscopic versus open approaches. J Gastrointest Surg. 2015;19(1):189–94. doi:10.1007/s11605-014-2644-8.
29. Croome KP, Farnell MB, Que FG, Reid-Lombardo KM, Truty MJ, Nagorney DM, et al. Total laparoscopic pancreaticoduodenectomy for pancreatic ductal adenocarcinoma: oncologic advantages over open approaches? Ann Surg. 2014;260(4):633–8; discussion 638–40. doi:10.1097/SLA.0000000000000937.
30. Kendrick ML. Laparoscopic and robotic resection for pancreatic cancer. Cancer J. 2012;18(6):571–6. doi:10.1097/PPO.0b013e31827b8f86.
31. Kendrick ML, Cusati D. Total laparoscopic pancreaticoduodenectomy: feasibility and outcome in an early experience. Arch Surg. 2010;145(1):19–23. doi:10.1001/archsurg.2009.243.
32. Kendrick ML, Sclabas GM. Major venous resection during total laparoscopic pancreaticoduodenectomy. HPB. 2011;13(7):454–8. doi:10.1111/j.1477-2574.2011.00323.x.
33. Nguyen KT, Marsh JW, Tsung A, Steel JJ, Gamblin TC, Geller DA. Comparative benefits of laparoscopic vs open hepatic resection: a critical appraisal. Arch Surg. 2011;146(3):348–56. doi:10.1001/archsurg.2010.248.
34. Tsung A, Geller DA, Sukato DC, Sabbaghian S, Tohme S, Steel J, et al. Robotic versus laparoscopic hepatectomy: a matched comparison. Ann Surg. 2014;259(3):549–55. doi:10.1097/SLA.0000000000000250.
35. Zeh HJ 3rd, Bartlett DL, Moser AJ. Robotic-assisted major pancreatic resection. Adv Surg. 2011;45:323–40.
36. Zureikat AH, Moser AJ, Boone BA, Bartlett DL, Zenati M, Zeh HJ 3rd. 250 robotic pancreatic resections: safety and feasibility. Ann Surg. 2013;258(4):554–9; discussion 559–62. doi:10.1097/SLA.0b013e3182a4e87c.
37. Zureikat AH, Nguyen KT, Bartlett DL, Zeh HJ, Moser AJ. Robotic-assisted major pancreatic resection and reconstruction. Arch Surg. 2011;146(3):256–61. doi:10.1001/archsurg.2010.246.
38. Buell JF, Cherqui D, Geller DA, O'Rourke N, Iannitti D, Dagher I, et al. The international position on laparoscopic liver surgery: The Louisville Statement, 2008. Ann Surg. 2009;250(5):825–30.
39. Cai XJ, Yang J, Yu H, Liang X, Wang YF, Zhu ZY, et al. Clinical study of laparoscopic versus open hepatectomy for malignant liver tumors. Surg Endosc. 2008;22(11):2350–6. doi:10.1007/s00464-008-9789-z.
40. Mirnezami R, Mirnezami AH, Chandrakumaran K, Abu Hilal M, Pearce NW, Primrose JN, et al. Short- and long-term outcomes after laparoscopic and open hepatic resection: systematic review and meta-analysis. HPB. 2011;13(5):295–308. doi:10.1111/j.1477-2574.2011.00295.x.
41. Amodeo A, Linares Quevedo A, Joseph JV, Belgrano E, Patel HR. Robotic laparoscopic surgery: cost and training. Minerva Urol Nefrol. 2009;61(2):121–8.
42. Giulianotti PC, Coratti A, Angelini M, Sbrana F, Cecconi S, Balestracci T, et al. Robotics in general surgery: personal experience in a large community hospital. Arch Surg. 2003;138(7):777–84. doi:10.1001/archsurg.138.7.777.
43. Coelho RF, Rocco B, Patel MB, Orvieto MA, Chauhan S, Ficarra V, et al. Retropubic, laparoscopic, and robot-assisted radical prostatectomy: a critical review of outcomes reported by high-volume centers. J Endourol. 2010;24(12):2003–15. doi:10.1089/end.2010.0295.
44. O'Neill M, Moran PS, Teljeur C, O'Sullivan OE, O'Reilly BA, Hewitt M, et al. Robot-assisted hysterectomy compared to open and laparoscopic approaches: systematic review and meta-analysis. Arch Gynecol Obstet. 2013;287(5):907–18. doi:10.1007/s00404-012-2681-z.
45. Tatooles AJ, Pappas PS. Gordon PJ, Slaughter MS. Minimally invasive mitral valve repair using the da Vinci robotic system. Ann Thorac Surg. 2004;77(6):1978–82; discussion 1982–74. doi:10.1016/j.athoracsur.2003.11.024.

46. Bokhari MB, Patel CB, Ramos-Valadez DI, Ragupathi M, Haas EM. Learning curve for robotic-assisted laparoscopic colorectal surgery. Surg Endosc. 2011;25(3):855–60. doi:10.1007/s00464-010-1281-x.
47. Buchs NC, Pugin F, Bucher P, Hagen ME, Chassot G, Koutny-Fong P, Morel P. Learning curve for robot-assisted Roux-en-Y gastric bypass. Surg Endosc. 2012;26(4):1116–21. doi:10.1007/s00464-011-2008-3.
48. Daouadi M, Zureikat AH, Zenati MS, Choudry H, Tsung A, Bartlett DL, et al. Robot-assisted minimally invasive distal pancreatectomy is superior to the laparoscopic technique. Ann Surg. 2013;257(1):128–32. doi:10.1097/SLA.0b013e31825fff08.
49. Packiam V, Bartlett DL, Tohme S, Reddy S, Marsh JW, Geller DA, et al. Minimally invasive liver resection: robotic versus laparoscopic left lateral sectionectomy. J Gastrointest Surg. 2012;16(12):2233–8. doi:10.1007/s11605-012-2040-1.
50. Martin RC, Scoggins CR, McMasters KM. Laparoscopic hepatic lobectomy: advantages of a minimally invasive approach. J Am Coll Surg. 2010;210(5):627–34. doi:10.1016/j.jamcollsurg.2009.12.022.
51. Cai XJ, Wang YF, Liang YL, Yu H, Liang X. Laparoscopic left hemihepatectomy: a safety and feasibility study of 19 cases. Surg Endosc. 2009;23(11):2556–62. doi:10.1007/s00464-009-0454-y.
52. Dagher I, Di Giuro G, Dubrez J, Lainas P, Smadja C, Franco D. Laparoscopic versus open right hepatectomy: a comparative study. Am J Surg. 2009;198(2):173–7. doi:10.1016/j.amjsurg.2008.09.015.
53. Abu Hilal M, Di Fabio F, Teng MJ, Lykoudis P, Primrose JN, Pearce NW. Single-centre comparative study of laparoscopic versus open right hepatectomy. J Gastrointest Surg. 2011;15(5):818–23. doi:10.1007/s11605-011-1468-z.
54. Takahara T, Wakabayashi G, Beppu T, Aihara A, Hasegawa K, Gotohda N, et al. Long-term and perioperative outcomes of laparoscopic versus open liver resection for hepatocellular carcinoma with propensity score matching: a multi-institutional Japanese study. J Hepatobiliary Pancreat Sci. 2015;22(10):721–7. doi:10.1002/jhbp.276.
55. Beppu T, Wakabayashi G, Hasegawa K, Gotohda N, Mizuguchi T, Takahashi Y, et al. Long-term and perioperative outcomes of laparoscopic versus open liver resection for colorectal liver metastases with propensity score matching: a multi-institutional Japanese study. J Hepatobiliary Pancreat Sci. 2015;22(10):711–20). doi:10.1002/jhbp.261.
56. Berber E, Akyildiz HY, Aucejo F, Gunasekaran G, Chalikonda S, Fung J. Robotic versus laparoscopic resection of liver tumours. J Hepatobiliary Pancreat Sci. 2010;12(8):583–6. doi:10.1111/j.1477-2574.2010.00234.x.
57. Spampinato MG, Coratti A, Bianco L, Caniglia F, Laurenzi A, Puleo F, et al. Perioperative outcomes of laparoscopic and robot-assisted major hepatectomies: an Italian multi-institutional comparative study. Surg Endosc. 2014;28(10):2973–9. doi:10.1007/s00464-014-3560-4.
58. Tranchart H, Ceribelli C, Ferretti S, Dagher I, Patrit A. Traditional versus robot-assisted full laparoscopic liver resection: a matched-pair comparative study. World J Surg. 2014;38(11):2904–9. doi:10.1007/s00268-014-2679-8.
59. Troisi RI, Patriti A, Montalti R, Casciola L. Robot assistance in liver surgery: a real advantage over a fully laparoscopic approach? Results of a comparative bi-institutional analysis. MRCAS. 2013;9(2):160–6. doi:10.1002/rcs.1495.
60. Wu YM, Hu RH, Lai HS, Lee PH. Robotic-assisted minimally invasive liver resection. Asian J Surg. 2014;37(2):53–7. doi:10.1016/j.asjsur.2014.01.015.
61. Yu YD, Kim KH, Jung DH, Namkoong JM, Yoon SY, Jung SW, et al. Robotic versus laparoscopic liver resection: a comparative study from a single center. Langenbecks Arch Surg. 2014;399(8):1039–45. doi:10.1007/s00423-014-1238-y.

Totally Laparoscopic Right Hepatectomy Combined with En-Bloc Partial Resection of the Inferior Vena Cava

9

Christophe Bourdeaux, David Fuks and Brice Gayet

Introduction

The practice of laparoscopic liver surgery has grown steadily during the last years, and many liver resections are now performed laparoscopically[1 - 6].

Laparoscopic liver surgery does not allow the same exposure as performed by laparotomy, as some areas of the liver are more accessible than others, especially the most anterior segments. Thus, anatomic resections initially included mainly the left lobe (segments 2, 3, and 4) and segments 5 and 6 of the right liver [5, 6]. Later, all types of resections were considered (anatomical segmentectomy and major hemihepatectomies), and left lobe resection from living related donors in the context of pediatric transplants [7].

Currently, laparoscopic liver resection is feasible and safe when performed in centers where surgeons are experienced in both liver surgery and laparoscopic surgery [8]. Further studies, however, seem necessary, especially to determine long-term oncological results and for major hepatectomy [9]. Regarding colorectal liver metastasis, laparoscopic resection yields better operative outcomes without impairing disease-free and long-term survival, and with no difference in terms of resection margins [10].

C. Bourdeaux · D. Fuks · B. Gayet (✉)
Department of Digestive Diseases, Institut Mutualiste Montsouris,
Université Paris Descartes, 42 Boulevard Jourdan, 75014 Paris, France
e-mail: brice.gayet@imm.fr

C. Bourdeaux
e-mail: christophebourdeaux@hotmail.com; c.bourdeaux@cdle.be

D. Fuks
e-mail: david.fuks@imm.fr

T.M. Pawlik et al. (eds.), *Case-Based Lessons in the Management of Complex Hepato-Pancreato-Biliary Surgery*, DOI 10.1007/978-3-319-50868-9_9

Laparoscopic right hepatectomy is still a challenging abdominal surgical procedure [11], but has become standard in specialized centers [3]. In this setting, we performed 80 totally laparoscopic right hepatectomies by an anterior approach between January 2009 and January 2016. While tumor involvement of the inferior vena cava (IVC) is still considered a contraindication to laparoscopy. We have a short experience of 4 cases. The last case is a patient with bilateral colorectal liver metastases involving the right anterior wall of the retrohepatic IVC who underwent successful laparoscopic right hepatectomy extended to segment 1 with lateral resection of the IVC [12]. The case described here illustrates this procedure.

Case Description

A 58-year-old male (BMI 23.24 kg/m^2) without previous medical history presented with synchronous bilateral colorectal liver metastases involving the right anterior wall of the retrohepatic IVC. Because the primary tumor was symptomatic, a right colectomy was first performed laparoscopically and the lesion was staged pT4N1M1. The patient was treated then with nine cycles of chemotherapy (FOLFOX) with a decrease in the size of the liver metastases. Indeed, after four cycles, imaging response was adequate for surgery, but chemotherapy was pursued during the whole strategy.

A contrast-enhanced CT showed one lesion involving segments 8 and 9, with infiltration of the right anterior wall of the adjacent vena cava (Fig. 9.1). A second lesion was located in segments 2 and 3 near the root of the left hepatic vein, as shown in Fig. 9.2.

Because right hepatectomy with en-bloc resection of the involved portion of IVC would have been required for the first lesion, a two-stage procedure was deemed necessary as an initial approach, with subsequent left lateral sectionectomy planned for the second lesion at a second stage.

We will describe here a safe surgical procedure of purely laparoscopic right hepatectomy extended to segment 1 using an anterior approach with partial IVC resection.

Patient Positioning

A low lithotomy, i.e., “French position,” with both the legs abducted at the hip and flexed at the knees and the patient in reverse Trendelenburg position was used (Fig. 9.3). Other routine precautions like adequate padding of the pressure points and thermal covers for the exposed limbs should be followed, and were applied to the case described here.

Trocar Placement

It is difficult to describe a universally acceptable trocar position because of minor variations needed pertaining to each case. Nevertheless, five trocars are usually introduced for standard laparoscopic right hepatectomy. The optical trocar should

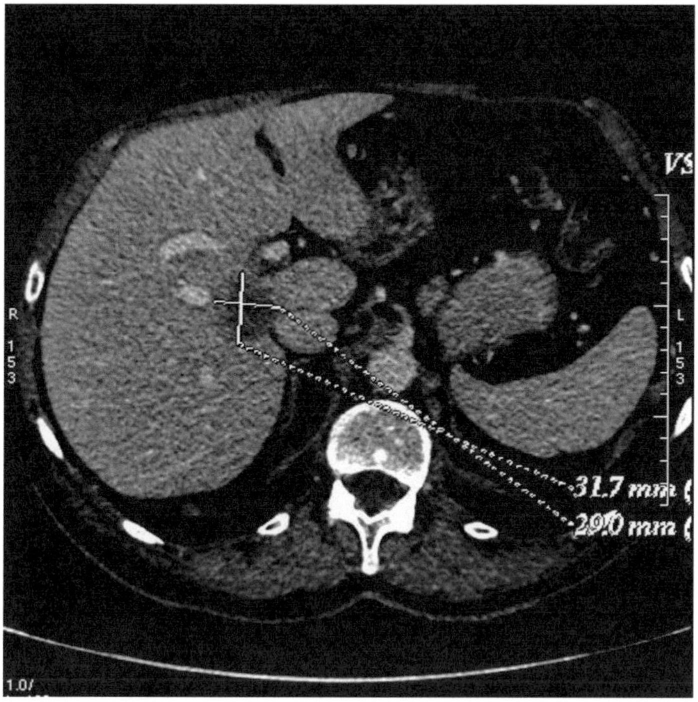

Fig. 9.1 A contrast–enhanced CT showed the metastatic lesions of the right lobe, involving segments 8 and 9, infiltrating the right anterior wall of the adjacent vena cava

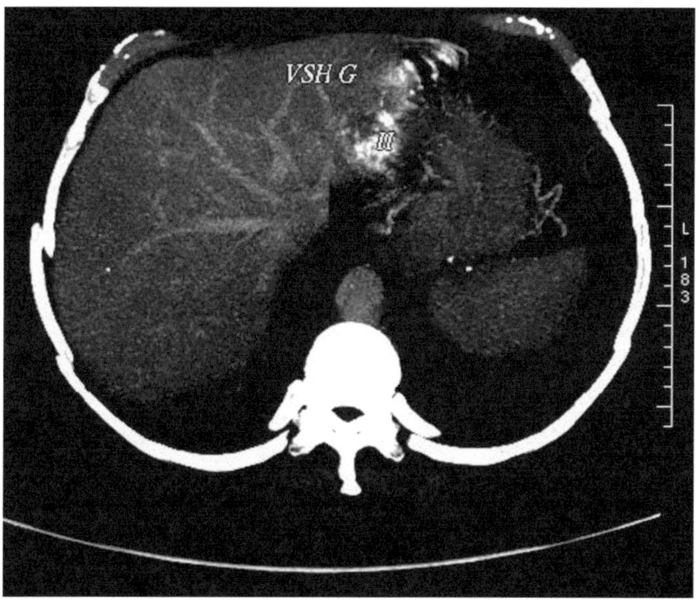

Fig. 9.2 A contrast–enhanced CT showed the second metastatic lesion in the left lobe, in segments 2 and 3 near the root of the left hepatic vein

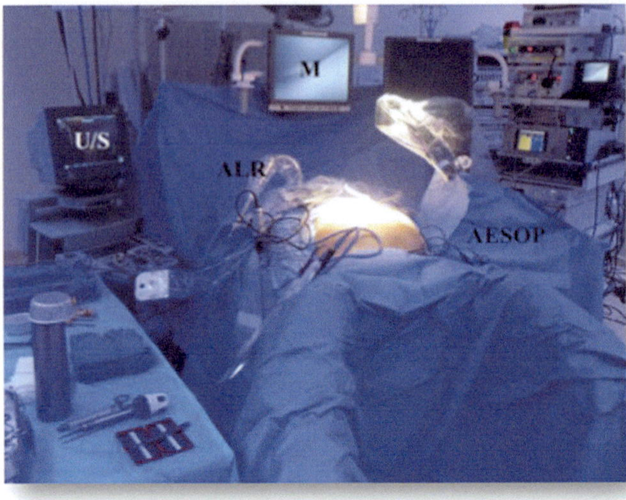

Fig. 9.3 Shows the patient positioning, a low lithotomy, i.e., "French position," with both the legs abducted at the hip and flexed at the knees and the patient in reverse Trendelenburg position

be located high enough to access the hepatic dome, with two trocars just under the rib, introduced after the establishment of the pneumoperitoneum.

Hand-assist ports can be helpful, especially in case of emergency situations like bleeding, for surgeons with minimal expertise in advanced laparoscopic procedures [13]. In patients with colorectal liver metastases, if there is a previous colostomy then it can be used for gel-ports. In the case described here, the three main working ports were sited subcostally in the right upper quadrant, and a hand-assisted device

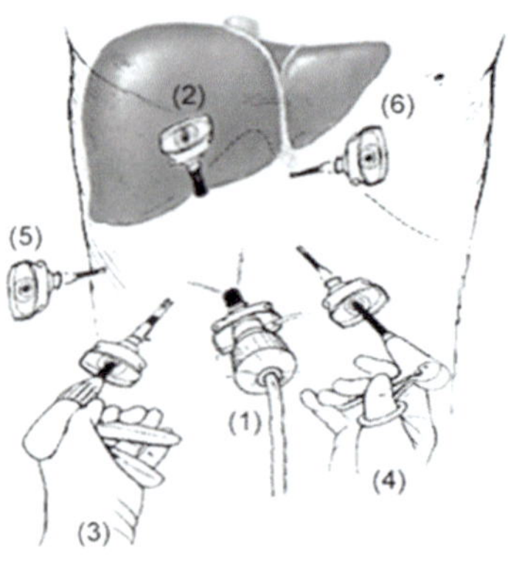

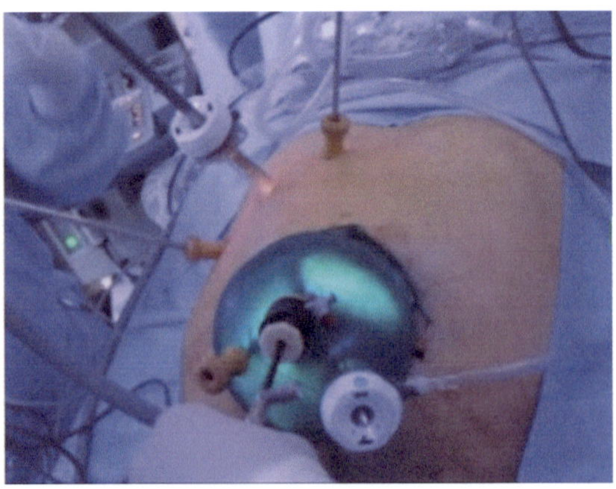

Fig. 9.4 Shows the trocar placement; the three main working ports were sited subcostally in the *right upper quadrant* and a hand-assisted device was inserted at the site of the original colectomy scar. The illustration shows the trocar placement we use for a right hepatectomy

was inserted at the site of the original colectomy scar, as shown in Fig. 9.4. Apart from use for specimen retrieval, this port proved very useful in the event of major hemorrhage.

Surgery

Following insufflation, the abdominal cavity was explored to confirm the absence of disseminated disease. Intra-abdominal pressure was maintained at 12 mmHg. Of note, a higher intra-abdominal pressure was avoided due to a potentially higher risk of gas embolism. A large gauze was placed intra-abdominally, should a compression for haemostasis be necessary in emergency. This can be done through the hand-assist system without losing intra-abdominal pressure. Intraoperative ultrasound was performed to define the extent of the lesion located at the junction of segments 8 and 9 involving IVC. The surgery began with the dissection on the hilum. Cholecystectomy was performed, without removing of the gallbladder, so as to allow a simple way to grasp and retract the liver. Helped by retraction of the cystic duct stump, the hilar region was carefully dissected. The posterior right branches of the bile duct were divided. The hepatic artery and portal vein were isolated and divided between clips, which was usually performed in this order.

Next, the anterior right branches were divided. Hilar dissection was completed to allow access to the IVC. Further dissection was continued in this area by dividing the short hepatic veins and small caudate branches. Here the laparoscopy enabled a very clear view of the anterior surface of IVC from the caudate side. With the line of demarcation established on the liver surface following division of the right hepatic inflow, parenchymal transection via bipolar electrocautery was commenced along Cantlie's line using an ultrasonic scalpel. The tributaries of the middle vein to segments 5 and 8 were identified, and blood loss was controlled by bipolar electrocautery. Because in this particular case a subsequent left lateral sectionectomy was planned, the middle hepatic vein was not exposed during the right hepatectomy in order to prevent potential injury. The location of the second lesion necessitated the sacrifice of the left hepatic vein, thus leaving the middle hepatic vein as the sole venous outflow of the remnant liver. The parenchymal transection was continued to the hepatic vein/IVC junction. This junction was completely cleared with scissor before the vein was cut using the Endo GIA™ Universal Stapling System.

After the right hepatic vein was divided, the space above the retrohepatic IVC was opened to allow close inspection, in order to delineate whethere there was macroscopic involvement of tumor growth or fibrosis. Partial resection of the IVC was performed by serial applications of the endovascular stapler (Fig. 9.5). Caval resection can be alternatively accomplished with a non-absorbable monofilament whipstitch and vascular clamp. All remaining bands tethering the resected specimen to the diaphragm and retroperitoneum were divided. Haemostasis was verified and the resected margin was carefully inspected for bile leakage, which was controlled with monofilament sutures. The specimen was extracted through the hand-assist system placed on the previous incision.

No drainage was used. The surgical duration was 270 min and the blood loss was 50 ml.

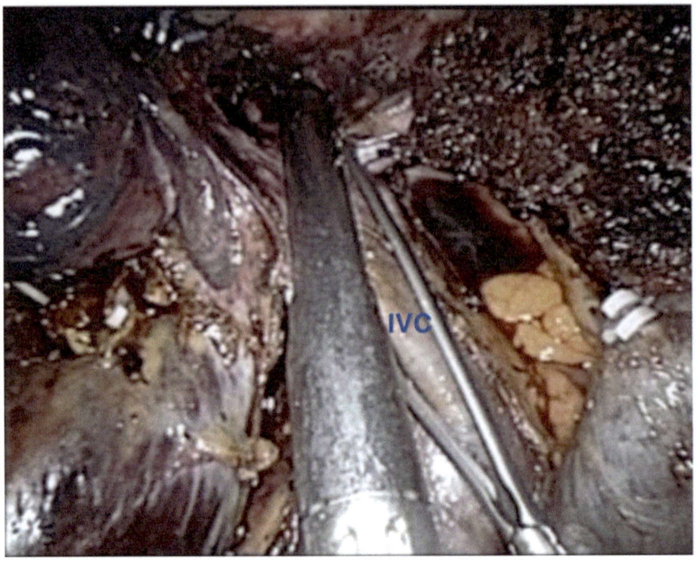

Fig. 9.5 Shows an intraoperative picture of the partial resection of IVC performed by serial applications of the endovascular stapler. A vascular clamp is always ready and under vision intracorporeally when using the stapler devices for hepatic veins or IVC

Histological Analysis and Postoperative Course

Histological analysis revealed moderately differentiated adenocarcinoma with a 2 mm surgical margin. The surrounding liver parenchyma showed steatosis. The postoperative period was uneventful and the patient was discharged after 9 days. After a selective portal embolization of segment 2 and 3, the segment 4 showed a volume 515 cc and a full laparoscopic left lateral sectionectomy was performed 7 weeks after the first liver resection. The resection was complete and no adjuvant chemotherapy was used.

Tips and Tricks of the Experienced Surgeon

Specific instrumentation for laparoscopic hepatectomy

The laparoscopic liver surgery requires the following specific hardware (besides the standard equipment of laparoscopic surgery, and open surgery equipment available if conversion is required):

- Optical at 0° or 30°, or, better, one flexible 3D optical [14]
- Laparoscopic intraoperative ultrasound
- Liver retractor

- Adjustable cutting linear stapler with vascular several refills
- Clips (metal clips, locked clips)
- Plastic bag for extraction

To ensure the dissection of the vessels and bile ducts and parenchymal transection, various specific methods can be used (new instruments using different types of energy to dissect the parenchyma, or coagulate vessels in the closing time of hepatic transection) [15].

Coagulator argon should not be recommended in laparoscopy, although some new-generation devices allow a stream of argon at a pressure 10 times lower than the first devices, because of the risk of air embolism [16]. The mechanical fastening clips can be used for elements of the section of the pedicle and the hepatic veins, but also parenchymal transection.

Ultrasound

An important instrument in liver resection is an intraoperative ultrasound [17]. Both in open and laparoscopic liver surgery, ultrasound of the liver is performed for identification of other lesions, to confirm the relationship of the lesion with the portal and hepatic veins [18] and to analyze the distance between the segment 8 vein and IVC.

In laparoscopic approach, until the 3D camera becomes easily available, one of the main risks during the hepatic transection phase is struggling to maintain the correct plane, making intraoperative ultrasonography (IOUS) absolutely mandatory. Although the use of a 3D camera may make this transection phase easier, it will not replace IOUS. Performing a laparoscopic ultrasound of the liver can be a challenging procedure if one has only a rigid device. Thus, a modern ultrasound device should be flexible and should have a guidance system for an RFA-needle.

For right hemi-hepatectomy, IOUS is useful in confirming the position of segment VIII draining vein into either MHV or directly into IVC (Fig. 9.6), which might avoid unnecessary bleeding [17].

Technical Alternatives

If the surgeon is not experienced, we recommend a first manually assisted laparoscopic right hepatectomy. The arguments in favor of hand-assisted technique are the possibility of liver palpation, easier exposure, especially in the first and lower posterior segments and speed and efficiency in control of bleeding [13].

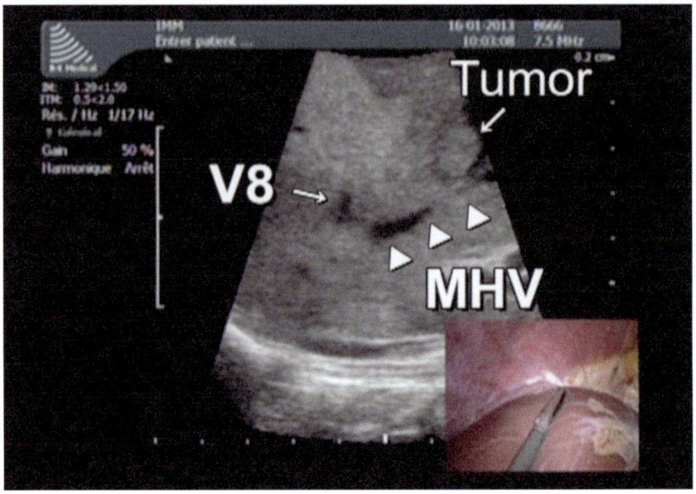

Fig. 9.6 Shows a picture of IOUS showing the position of segment VIII draining vein into either MHV or directly into IVC; in laparoscopic right hepatectomy, the position of this vein is systematically checked before the hepatic transection

Control of Hemorrhage

In open liver surgery, inflow control (Pringle maneuver) is a tool to decrease blood loss. It is mainly used for major resections. In laparoscopic liver resection, it is feasible to obtain inflow control by performing a similar Pringle maneuver [19]. Although it can be useful, it is not a standard procedure. However, we advise becoming experienced performing a Pringle maneuver, at least in the beginning of laparoscopic liver surgery [13]. After opening the pars flaccida of the lesser omentum, a traumatic forceps or a dissector passed through the hiatus of Winslow and tape is placed around the hepatic pedicle (inserted into a rubber tube for pedicle clamping lakes).

If used, the clamping is preferably intermittent (15 min clamping and 5 min of unclamping). In cases of cirrhotic, steatotic, or blue liver (post chemotherapy), which cannot tolerate prolonged ischaemia, isolated arterial Pringle could be also a useful maneuver [20].

Pneumoperitoneum with an intra-abdominal pressure of 12 mmHg itself will decrease hemorrhage during parenchymal transection, which can also be increased up to 15 mm of Hg if needed [21].

Bipolar devices can be used to stop minor bleeding from the hepatic veins [19]. Vascular and bile structures over 3 mm are controlled by clips, then sectioned.

A hand-assist system and gauze in the abdominal cavity will also help in immediate control of bleeding. Other routine measures that are useful in open surgery like haemostatic agents (oxidized cellulose), suturing devices, and vascular clamps are also helpful.

Parenchymal Dissection

In both open and laparoscopic surgery, different techniques are described for parenchymal transection: electrosurgical devices, bipolar, thermofusion, ultrasound scissors, ultrasound dissector, the clamp-and-crush method (so-called Kelly clamping) and staplers. No single method has proven to be superior for parenchymal dissection and as in open surgery there is no consensus on the preferred technique [6]. However, in laparoscopic surgery electrosurgical, CUSA and stapler devices are mainly used. All have their advantages and disadvantages; after our experience with the first 100 cases with ultrasound dissector (CUSA) and bipolar we have moved to ultrasound scissors and bipolar. When using bipolar forceps, avoid contact of the bile duct with both the limbs of the forceps together, to prevent bile duct injury.

When using the ultrasound scissors, i.e., Harmonic, Sonosurg, or Thunderbeat, always remember to keep the active blade away from major vascular structures and bile duct [15].

Transection Without Mobilization of the Right Lobe or the Anterior Approach Technique

The anterior approach is the standard procedure for open right hepatectomy [22]. The advantages of this procedure are first, the reduced risk of tumor rupture and dissemination resulting from liver mobilization, and second, the limited possibility of ischemic reperfusion injury resulting from rotating the right lobe during mobilization and parenchymal transection [23, 24]. In contrast, this approach has the disadvantage of increased risk of major bleeding from the deep parenchymal plane. The major advantages of laparoscopy in the anterior approach are the superior unparalleled views of the posteroinferior aspects of the liver and caudate lobe, thereby allowing easier and safer deep parenchymal transection and dissection along the anterior caval plane [3].

The hanging maneuver was not considered in this particular situation [25],as obliteration of the plane between the liver and vena cava from tumor infiltration. Previous surgery may sometimes also be a contraindication for this technique [24].

Control of Hepatic Outflow

In our experience, we have never had to control the outflow and dissection of the suprahepatic area before the transection. It seems quite dangerous, with a risk of vascular tear especially between the vein and the IVC.

The right hepatic vein is approached intraparenchymally. Vascular staplers are used with the vascular clamp present after circumferential dissection of the vein is complete [26]. At the end of the procedure when using vascular staplers, there is always a chance of error leading to unnecessary exsanguination. A few safety tips to avoid such events:

1. Create adequate space around the major veins before introducing the vascular staplers.
2. When using the staplers, never pull on the hepatic veins that might avulse the vein from the IVC.
3. Always have the vascular clamp ready and under vision intracorporeally when using the stapler devices for hepatic veins (Fig. 9.5).

Haemostasis, Drain and Specimen Extraction

The best way to have proper haemostasis is to control the bleeding points rather than to use too much haemostatic agents [19]. Too much haemostatic agents can also mimic an abscess in the follow-up CT scans or a false recurrence in the PET-CT. We use drains only in cases with a high risk for postoperative bleed or bile leak, which is decided by a difficult intraoperative course [27]. The procedure ends by extraction of the specimen using retrieval bags through a suprapubic or peri-umbilical incision if a hand-assist system is placed. Releasing the intra-abdominal adhesions at the beginning of the procedure will ease the specimen retraction at the end of the procedure.

A conversion is indicated in case of technical difficulties (difficult exposure, inadequate vision or poor, weak tumor, uncertainty about the distance between tumor and resection margin) and uncontrolled bleeding [28].

Postoperative Complication

The postoperative course of the case presented here was uneventful, and the patient was discharged at postoperative day nine. After major laparoscopic resection, the potential risks cited by the experts are uncontrollable bleeding, biliary leak, air embolism, deep-vein thrombosis, and infection. In our experience, the most frequent complications after major laparoscopic liver resections are pulmonary complications, biliary leak, liver failure, and ascites. In a previous series, the major risk factor identified for global postoperative complications were intraoperative simultaneous radiofrequency ablation, intraoperative blood transfusion, and bilobar resection [29]. The potential benefits of the use of the laparoscopic approach for liver resection correspond to "traditional" benefits of this surgical approach: reduction of postoperative pain, faster recovery of transit, decreased lung [30] and parietal morbidity, improved quality of life, and decreased length of hospitalization.

Alternative Approaches/Controversies

If the surgeon is not experienced enough, we recommend a first manually assisted laparoscopic right hepatectomy. The arguments in favor of hand-assisted technique is the possibility of liver palpation, easier exposure—

especially in the first and lower posterior segments—and speed and efficiency in control of bleeding with the finger.

- *Transection with mobilization of the right lobe*: Transection after laparoscopic mobilization of the right lobe has been proposed for hybrid technic in order to reduce the abdominal wall incision. However, this approach is of relatively little value and should not be routinely performed in standard case.
- *Laparoscopic resection with a curative intent for liver malignancies*: During laparoscopic resection of liver malignancies, the same oncologic principles should be applied as in open surgery: radical resection, and achievement of free surgical margin. Inadequate margins are potential disadvantages of the laparoscopic approach. The lack of digital palpation during laparoscopic resection makes determining the appropriate surgical margin challenging. However, intraoperative ultrasonography should be used as a direct guide for localizing tumors and division of the liver parenchyma.

Conclusion

Historically, the main barriers to the use of laparoscopy in liver surgery were, in addition to the technical complexity of interventions and lack of suitable instrumentation, the risk of air embolism associated with pneumoperitoneum, the difficulty of locating intraparenchymal lesions, and difficulties in achieving hemostasis. The development of new techniques and new instruments has gradually allowed the evolution of laparoscopic hepatectomy techniques, allowing major liver resection even as described here in case of IVC involvement.

We devised here a safe and secure procedure to perform totally laparoscopic right hepatectomy using an anterior approach combined with partial resection of IVC. The anterior approach presents a safe and useful technique to perform a purely laparoscopic right hepatectomy.

References

1. Gumbs AA, Gayet B. Totally laparoscopic central hepatectomy. J Gastrointest Surg. 2008;12(7):1153.
2. Gumbs AA, Gayet B. Totally laparoscopic left hepatectomy. Surg Endosc. 2007;21(7):1221.
3. Gayet B, Cavaliere D, Vibert E, Perniceni T. Totally laparoscopic right hepatectomy. Am J Surg. 2007;194(5):685–9.

4. Dagher I, O'Rourke N, Geller DA, Cherqui D, Belli G, Gamblin TC, et al. Laparoscopic major hepatectomy: an evolution in standard of care. Ann Surg. 2009;250(5):856–60.
5. Buell JF, Cherqui D, Geller DA, O'Rourke N, Iannitti D, Dagher I, et al. The international position on laparoscopic liver surgery: the Louisville Statement, 2008. Ann Surg. 2009;250 (5):825–30.
6. Wakabayashi G, Cherqui D, Geller DA, Buell JF, Kaneko H, Han HS, et al. Recommendations for laparoscopic liver resection: a report from the second international consensus conference held in Morioka. Ann Surg. 2015;261(4):619–29.
7. Soubrane O, de Rougemont O, Kim KH, Samstein B, Mamode N, Boillot O, et al. Laparoscopic living donor left lateral sectionectomy: a new standard practice for donor hepatectomy. Ann Surg. 2015;262(5):757–61.
8. Simillis C, Constantinides VA, Tekkis PP, Darzi A, Lovegrove R, Jiao L, Antoniou A. Laparoscopic versus open hepatic resections for benign and malignant neoplasms a meta-analysis. Surgery. 2007;141(2):203–11.
9. Cherian PT, Mishra AK, Kumar P, Sachan VK, Bharathan A, Srikanth G, et al. Laparoscopic liver resection: wedge resections to living donor hepatectomy, are we heading in the right direction? World J Gastroenterol. 2014;20(37):13369–81.
10. Allard MA, Cunha AS, Gayet B, Adam R, Goere D, Bachellier P, et al. Early and long-term oncological outcomes after laparoscopic resection for colorectal liver metastases: a propensity score-based analysis. Ann Surg. 2015;262(5):794–802.
11. Cai X, Li Z, Zhang Y, Yu H, Liang X, Jin R, et al. Laparoscopic liver resection and the learning curve: a 14-year, single-center experience. Surg Endosc. 2014;28(4):1334–41.
12. Nomi T, Fuks D, Agrawal A, Kawaguchi Y, Ogiso S, Gayet B. Totally laparoscopic right hepatectomy combined with resection of the inferior vena cava by anterior approach. Ann Surg Oncol. 2015;22(3):851.
13. Nomi T, Fuks D, Kawaguchi Y, Mal F, Nakajima Y, Gayet B. Learning curve for laparoscopic major hepatectomy. Br J Surg. 2015;102(7):796–804.
14. Velayutham V, Fuks D, Nomi T, Kawaguchi Y, Gayet B. 3D visualization reduces operating time when compared to high-definition 2D in laparoscopic liver resection: a case-matched study. Surg Endosc. 2016;30(1):147–53.
15. Scatton O, Brustia R, Belli G, Pekolj J, Wakabayashi G, Gayet B. What kind of energy devices should be used for laparoscopic liver resection? Recommendations from a systematic review. J Hepatobiliary Pancreat Sci. 2015;22(5):327–34.
16. Ikegami T, Shimada M, Imura S, Nakamura T, Kawahito S, Morine Y, et al. Argon gas embolism in the application of laparoscopic microwave coagulation therapy. J Hepatobiliary Pancreat Surg. 2009;16(3):394–8.
17. Araki K, Conrad C, Ogiso S, Kuwano H, Gayet B. Intraoperative ultrasonography of laparoscopic hepatectomy: key technique for safe liver transection. J Am Coll Surg. 2014;218 (2):37–41.
18. Viganò L, Ferrero A, Amisano M, Russolillo N, Capussotti L. Comparison of laparoscopic and open intraoperative ultrasonography for staging liver tumours. Br J Surg. 2013;100 (4):535–42.
19. Kawaguchi Y, Nomi T, Fuks D, Mal F, Kokudo N, Gayet B. Hemorrhage control for laparoscopic hepatectomy: technical details and predictive factors for intraoperative blood loss. Surg Endosc. 2016;30(6):2543–51.
20. Nomi T, Fuks D, Agrawal A, Govindasamy M, Araki K, Gayet B. Modified Pringle maneuver for laparoscopic liver resection. Ann Surg Oncol. 2015;22(3):852.
21. Eiriksson K, Fors D, Rubertsson S, Arvidsson D. High intra-abdominal pressure during experimental laparoscopic liver resection reduces bleeding but increases the risk of gas embolism. Br J Surg. 2011;98(6):845–52.
22. Lai E, Fan ST, Lo CM, Chu KM, Liu CL. Anterior approach for difficult major right hepatectomy. World J Surg. 1996;20(3):314–7.

23. Liu CL, Fan ST, Cheung ST, Lo CM, Ng IO, Wong J. Anterior approach versus conventional approach right hepatic resection for large hepatocellular carcinoma: a prospective randomized controlled study. Ann Surg. 2006;244(2):194–203.
24. Liddo G, Buc E, Nagarajan G, Hidaka M, Dokmak S, Belghiti J. The liver hanging manoeuvre. HPB. 2009;11(4):296–305.
25. Nitta H, Sasaki A, Fujita T, Itabashi H, Hoshikawa K, Takahara T, et al. Laparoscopy-assisted major liver resections employing a hanging technique: the original procedure. Ann Surg. 2010;251(3):450–3.
26. Buell JF, Gayet B, Han HS, Wakabayashi G, Kim KH. Evaluation of stapler hepatectomy during a laparoscopic liver resection. HPB. 2013;15(11):845–50.
27. Ishizawa T, Zuker NB, Conrad C, Lei HJ, Ciacio O, Kokudo N, Gayet B. Using a "no drain"policy in 342 laparoscopic hepatectomies: which factors predict failure? HPB. 2014;16 (5):494–9.
28. Cauchy F, Fuks D, Nomi T, Schwarz L, Barbier L, Dokmak S, et al. Risk factors and consequences of conversion in laparoscopic major liver resection. Br J Surg. 2015;102 (7):785–95.
29. Nomi T, Fuks D, Govindasamy M, Mal F, Nakajima Y, Gayet B. Risk factors for complications after laparoscopic major hepatectomy. Br J Surg. 2015;102(3):254–60.
30. Fuks D, Cauchy F, Ftériche S, Nomi T, Schwarz L, Dokmak S, et al. Laparoscopy decreases pulmonary complications in patients undergoing major liver resection: a propensity score analysis. Ann Surg. 2016;263(2):353–61.

Liver Cancer Necessitating Ex Vivo Resection and Reconstruction

10

Jennifer Berumen and Alan Hemming

Introduction

Chemotherapy options for primary and metastatic cancers to the liver have improved over the last decade; however curative options remain limited with surgery, if possible, being the only route to cure. With the limitations of treatment with chemotherapy and interventional radiology, more aggressive and creative surgical resection options have been developed. Non-anatomical and anatomical liver resections have become standard practice, including the removal of 75% of the liver in various extended hepatectomies. However, when tumors are in difficult locations, surgeons have employed vascular resection with portal vein or arterial reconstructions when needed [1]. Outcomes for this have improved with experience, with at least portal vein reconstruction results being similar to the same hepatic resections not requiring portal vein resection. Arterial resection and reconstruction is not widely employed, is considered to have an increased technical risk, and suggests more advanced disease [2–4]. Tumors that invade the inferior vena cava (IVC) or hepatic veins can make standard techniques for resection impossible. While tumors involving the IVC needing complex vein resection and reconstruction have high morbidity and 10–15% mortality [5–14], long-term survival has been achieved [5, 6, 15, 16].

J. Berumen (✉) · A. Hemming
Department of Surgery, University of California, San Diego,
9300 Campus Point Dr., #7745, La Jolla, CA 92037, USA
e-mail: jberumen@ucsd.edu

A. Hemming
e-mail: ahemming@ucsd.edu

T.M. Pawlik et al. (eds.), *Case-Based Lessons in the Management of Complex Hepato-Pancreato-Biliary Surgery*, DOI 10.1007/978-3-319-50868-9_10

Ex Vivo Resection

In the more complex situations, liver resection techniques have been ported from liver transplantation and applied to resect these complicated lesions. Ex vivo resection remains the most dramatic of these complex resection techniques, and is used for the most difficult tumor locations involving IVC and hepatic veins, with or without involvement of the portal structures. During ex vivo liver resection, the entire liver, tumor, and its vasculature are removed, flushed on the back table with cold preservation solution. The tumor is resected in a bloodless field allowing unhurried, precise resection along with the ability to perform complex intrahepatic vascular anastomoses in a time period that is not hurried by issues of warm ischemia. Ex vivo liver resection has been used for malignant disease such as hepatocellular carcinoma, cholangiocarcinoma, and colorectal metastasis, as well as echinococcal cysts and benign obstructive disease [7–9, 15–22].

The chosen technique for resection depends on tumor location and vessel involvement, which should be assessed with high-resolution CT or MR preoperative imaging. If the tumor only involves the vena cava, the IVC can be resected and reconstructed with a patch of bovine pericardium or GoreTex, or completely replaced using a synthetic tube graft. This resection may only require partial side clamping of the IVC if a very small area is involved, or may require clamping the IVC above and below the tumor but below the level of the hepatic veins, allowing continuous portal venous inflow and hepatic vein outflow [23–28].

Clinical Pearls

- Plan potential need for vascular grafts whether synthetic, cryopreserved, or autologous source prior to surgery. It is easier to have them available and not need them than need them and not have them.
- Decide on if the ex vivo technique is needed as early in the case as possible, and proceed in a stepwise fashion. Persisting in an alternative technique may lead to massive hemorrhage and not allow continuing on with resection.
- Median sternotomy provides excellent access to the suprahepatic IVC. Do not hesitate to use it if needed. Exposure in this operation is key.
- IVC grafts should be sized much shorter than what visibly appears needed. When the separation caused by retractors is removed, a graft that seems the right length initially will be too long with the retractors out, leading to potential kinking and thrombosis of the graft. The top end of the graft can be sutured in standard fashion, with the lower anastomosis parachuted in place.

When the hepatic vein confluence is involved, the need for the exclusion of portal and hepatic vein blood flow is clear. Tumors in this location require total vascular exclusion (TVE) for safe resection. The hilum is clamped, and the hepatic vein outflow clamped, with no arterial or portal inflow present. This is clearly detrimental to the liver for long periods, since there is no blood flow through the liver with TVE. While liver surgeons often use portal inflow occlusion alone during liver resection, periods of inflow occlusion are ideally limited to 15 min, with 5-min intervals of reperfusion followed by reapplication of occlusion. Depending on the complexity of the vascular reconstruction, periods in excess of an hour may be needed for the reconstruction alone, in addition to whatever time is needed to transect the liver. In order to avoid ischemic damage to the liver, as much of the liver resection and exposure of the IVC that can be done should be done prior to placing the clamps, to minimize time with TVE [6, 29–31].

For tumors involving the hepatic vein confluence and vena cava, where simple resection is not possible in an acceptably short time period with TVE, options include in situ cold perfusion, *ante situm*, and ex vivo techniques. These procedures involve TVE in different forms and may necessitate the use of veno-venous bypass if the patient has hemodynamic instability, with clamping of the vena cava after volume resuscitation, or if prolonged portal occlusion is likely to result in splanchnic venous congestion. In situ cold perfusion is recommended if the length of ischemia is expected to extend past 45 min to an hour [6, 23, 29–31]. For in situ perfusion, the liver is flushed with cold solution via the portal vein, and drained typically via a venotomy in the IVC or hepatic veins. Solutions used include University of Wisconsin (UW) solution or histidine–tryptophan–ketoglutarate (HTK). This has been shown to decrease the ischemic injury to the liver and may be used for in situ and ex vivo resection while the resection is carried out in a bloodless field. The *ante situm* technique involves dividing the suprahepatic vena cava while using TVE and rotating the liver forward for better access to the hepatic vein/caval confluence [6]. This can also be combined with division of the infrahepatic inferior vena cava below for even more rotation of the liver up into the operative field, and improved access without requiring division of the portal structures and ex vivo resection.

Ex vivo resection may be considered if tumors have more extensive hepatic vein involvement, involve the hilum and hepatic veins, or create outflow obstruction that makes transection of the liver tissue dangerous or prohibits mobilization. Adequate preoperative imaging and planning must be completed to consider the ex vivo technique. MRIs and 3-D imaging assist with complete imaging and significantly contribute to operative planning. Although for most standard hepatic procedures a 20–25% future liver remnant is recommended, in this case where the liver will undergo significant ischemic injury, a future liver remnant of 40% is recommended, and preoperative portal vein embolization is used liberally [32–34]. If preoperative biliary obstruction is present, our practice is to percutaneously drain the liver prior to resection until the bilirubin is 2 mg/dl or less [34–38].

The ex vivo technique is developed from techniques used in liver transplant, and involves removing the liver completely from the abdomen in order to complete the resection and necessary vascular reconstruction on the back table [8, 17]. This gives the ideal access for resection and reconstruction. Intraoperatively, the tumor is first assessed for resectability prior to committing to resection. If the tumor is resectable, the hilum is then dissected out and cholecystectomy is performed. The bile duct is divided approximately mid-bile duct, and common hepatic artery and portal vein skeletonized. The intrahepatic IVC is dissected out and short hepatic veins are transected if they are accessible without undue torsion. The suprahepatic IVC is dissected, and the phrenic veins are divided into gain additional length on the suprahepatic IVC. Control of the suprahepatic IVC may be possible below the diaphragm, but with bulky tumors often must be encircled at its intrapericardial portion, which can be accessed either from below through the pericardium, or via a median sternotomy.

A vascular clamp is then placed on the infrahepatic IVC and, if bypass is to be used, the caval limb of the bypass circuit placed. The portal vein is divided approximately 2 cm below the bifurcation after placing the portal limb of the bypass circuit. When stable on bypass, the hepatic artery is divided at the level of the gastroduodenal artery. A clamp is placed on the suprahepatic IVC above the confluence, or within the pericardial space if needed. If the tumor does not involve the IVC, the hepatic vein confluence can be clamped without clamping the entire IVC. The IVC or caval confluence is then transected, and the liver removed from the patient and taken to the back table [8].

On removal of the liver, it is placed in an ice bath, and cold perfusion is introduced to the liver via the transected portal vein. Solutions used include University of Wisconsin (UW) solution or histidine–tryptophan–ketoglutarate (HTK). UW solution has high potassium content, and should be flushed out of the liver prior to reperfusion of the liver during reimplantation. At our institution we use UW as our perfusion solution and then flush with chilled 5% albumin or Ringers lactate solution prior to reimplantation. The hepatic artery and bile duct are also flushed with solution prior to resection.

If there is concern about cardiac return or hemodynamic instability of the patient with removal of the liver and clamping of the IVC and portal vein, veno-venous bypass can be used. Inflow cannulas are typically placed in the femoral vein and portal vein, and one outflow cannula is placed in the right jugular or axillary vein. The portal cannula can be left out of the circuit to use only systemic and not portal bypass, with the option to place a temporary porta-caval shunt if needed for the portal system. Some surgeons prefer to place cannulas percutaneously and others open, but both are accepted practices. If a patient is hemodynamically stable, veno-venous bypass may be avoided with several methods. One possibility is to place a temporary porta-caval shunt and IVC graft during the ex vivo period, removing this upon reimplantation of the liver. If the IVC does not require resection with the ex vivo specimen or there is adequate systemic collateral flow, only the temporary porta-caval shunt may need to be used, or only an IVC graft if the portal circulation has collaterals. Avoiding bypass may decrease the risk of potential complications such as venous thromboembolic events, and the potential for vascular complications or air embolus. Bypass is associated with increased length of stay and need for blood transfusions, but does not appear to increase the risk of renal injury or need for dialysis over clamping, and may help in more complex cases [39–42]. The potential need for bypass should be anticipated in preoperative planning.

After cold perfusion on the back table and confirming patient stability, the resection is completed using individually preferred techniques, which may include sharp knife dissection, Kelly clamp/crush, ultrasonic, or water jet dissection. Our current preference is to use the water jet dissector. The liver can be flushed again after resection to evaluate for leaks, which can be controlled with clips or sutures. Once the resection is done, vascular reconstruction is performed as needed to restore routes of inflow and outflow to the liver remnant. Multiple options are available for reconstructions depending on what is needed. Hepatic veins can be directly reimplanted into the IVC, plastied together for reconstruction, or reconstructed using various vein grafts or synthetic grafts. If the IVC has had a large portion resected, it can be reconstructed using a 20-mm GoreTex tube graft [8].

After completion of resection and reconstruction, the resultant liver segment is reimplanted in a similar manner as a standard partial liver transplant. The suprahepatic anastomosis is completed first, and then the infrahepatic anastomosis if needed. Prior to the completion of the IVC anastomoses, the liver is flushed free of UW solution via the portal vein if UW was used. After this, the portal vein is re-anastomosed. The IVC clamps are removed, starting with the suprahepatic clamp. The portal clamp is then opened to return portal blood flow to the liver. The hepatic artery is then anastomosed once hemostasis is obtained. Finally, the biliary anastomosis is completed, typically as an end-to-end choledocho-choledochostomy; however, if this cannot be completed without tension, a roux-en-Y choledochojejunostomy is created.

Alternative Approaches

- In situ cold perfusion with or without *ante situm* rotation is an alternative technique for some cases that can be applied, and has the advantage of not requiring division of the portal structures.
- The role of ex vivo resection remains controversial given the high mortality and relatively poor disease-free survival in the setting of advanced malignancy. Long-term survival is possible, however.

Case 1

A 63-year-old woman presented with abdominal discomfort and bilateral mild lower limb edema. She was otherwise asymptomatic. Her past medical history was unremarkable with no history of jaundice, weight loss, or other pertinent history. On presentation to an outside hospital her physical examination was described as having had no positive findings apart from 2+ pitting edema in both legs. Blood work demonstrated normal electrolytes and renal function, with Hepatitis B and C serologies negative. Serum aspartate and alanine aminotransferases (AST, ALT) were within normal limits; however, the alkaline phosphatase (ALK) was elevated at 240 IU/L. The serum bilirubin was normal. Tumor markers demonstrated a normal carcinoembryonic antigen (CEA) and alpha-fetoprotein (AFP), and however demonstrated an elevated cancer antigen 19-9 (CA 19-9) of 160 U/ml, approximately four times the upper limit of normal reference value. Imaging showed a 7-cm mass located in the caudate lobe with IVC and hepatic vein involvement. A percutaneous biopsy of the lesion was reported as adenocarcinoma with features and a cytokeratin staining pattern consistent with cholangiocarcinoma. Chest CT, mammogram, and upper and lower endoscopy were negative. The patient was felt to be unresectable by an outside surgical team, and she was started on gemcitabine/cisplatinum. After four cycles of chemotherapy, the patient was referred for a second opinion regarding surgical resection. Imaging showed no response of tumor to therapy, but also showed no evidence of progression. CA19-9 remained unchanged. Repeat staging showed disease limited to the primary lesion. Assessing the imaging for resectability revealed circumferential involvement of the inferior vena cava at and below the hepatic veins with complete involvement of the left and middle hepatic veins (Fig. 10.1). The right hepatic vein was involved with

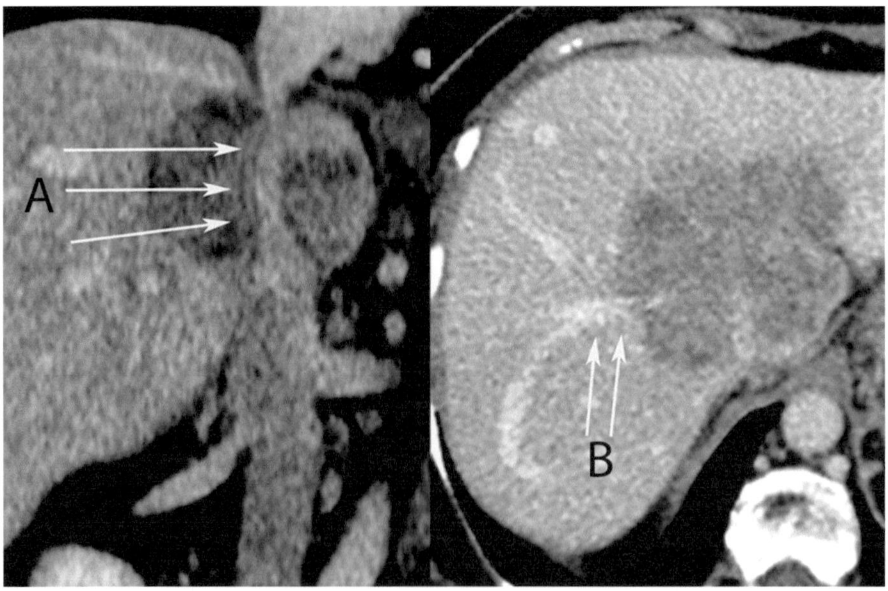

Fig. 10.1 CT images of the cholangiocarcinoma involving the IVC and all hepatic veins. *A* IVC involvement. *B* Patient right hepatic vein extending up to the tumor margin. Reprinted from Journal of the American College of Surgeons Jul;217(1). Hemming AW, Mekeel KL, Zendejas I, Kim RD, Sicklick JK, Reed AI. Resection of the liver and inferior vena cava for hepatic malignancy; p.115–24; © 2013, with permission from Elsevier

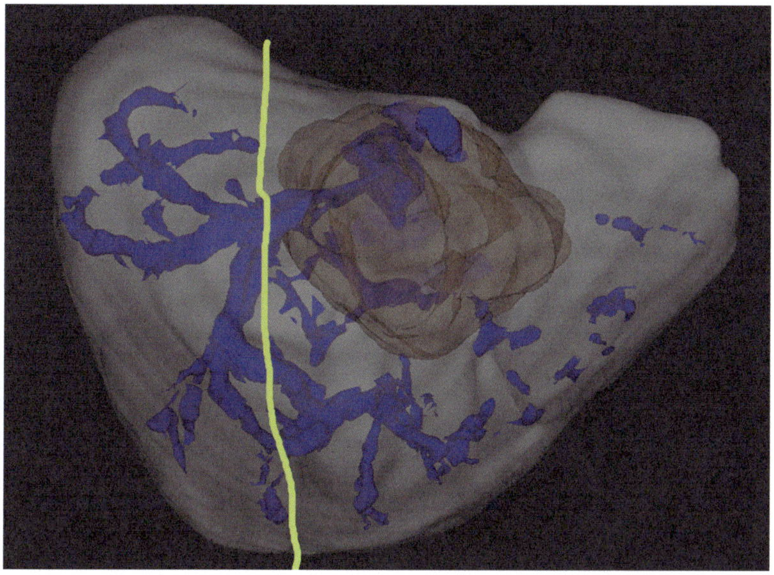

Fig. 10.2 CT volumetry of the cholangiocarcinoma indicated a future liver remnant of 41% with a line of resection (*yellow line*) along the right hepatic vein

tumor at its entry to the IVC, but was patent. The proximal extent of tumor along the right hepatic vein appeared to end just prior to a trifurcated branch point draining segments 6 and 7. There was hypertrophy of the right liver, with CT volumetry calculating a standardized future liver remnant of 41% based on a transection line along the right hepatic vein (Fig. 10.2).

The surgical assessment was that the tumor was unresectable using standard techniques, but an ex vivo approach with cold perfusion, resection, and replacement of the inferior vena cava, and resection and reimplantation of the right hepatic vein into the replaced IVC would be possible. Surgical planning included securing the availability of veno-venous bypass given the need for IVC replacement, and potential prolonged time required for back table reconstruction of the IVC and hepatic veins. Options for venous grafts were considered with the planned IVC reconstruction using a 20 mm GoreTex tube graft and possibly left renal vein or bovine pericardium for hepatic vein reconstruction.

Surgery was initiated with a negative staging laparoscopy and subsequently a right upper quadrant "hockey stick" incision was made. This was later extended with a median sternotomy to provide access to the intrapericardial IVC, which in this patient was poorly accessed through the pericardium from below (Fig. 10.3). The liver was obviously venous congested. The falciform and left and right triangular ligaments were divided and the liver mobilized to the IVC. Intraoperative ultrasound was used to assess the position of the tumor, which was as demonstrated

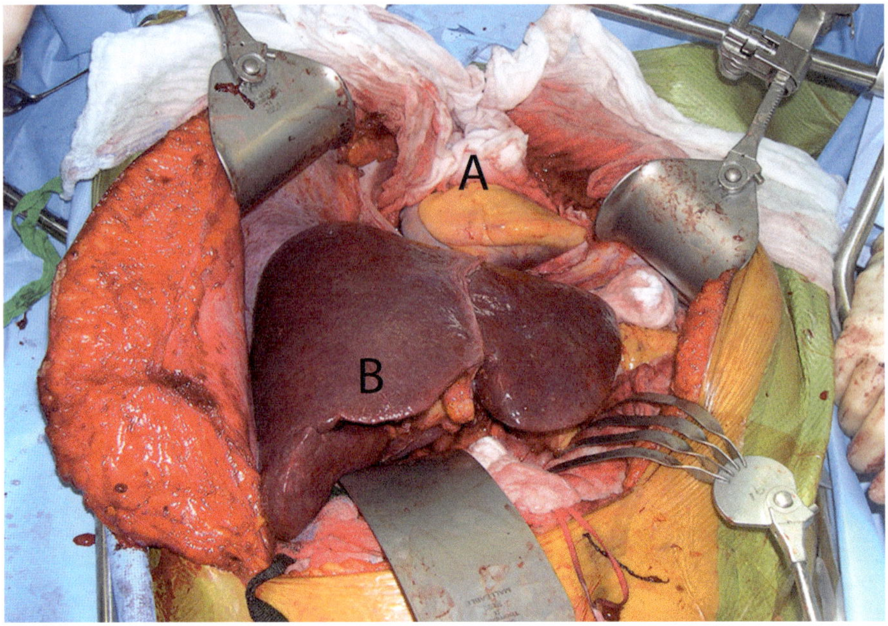

Fig. 10.3 Intraoperative photo of the exposure used for the cholangiocarcinoma resection. A sternotomy had been performed to increase exposure to the suprahepatic IVC and hepatic veins. *A* pericardial space and heart; *B* liver

on CT extending to the trifurcated branching of the right hepatic vein. The common and proper hepatic arteries were dissected out, the bile duct transected at mid common duct, and portal vein cleared of lymphatic tissue from the bifurcation to the neck of the pancreas. The retrohepatic IVC was freed up and the pericardium opened to control the intrapericardial IVC. The patient was placed on the caval portion of veno-venous bypass via percutaneous femoral and internal jugular vein cannulas. The infrahepatic IVC was clamped and then the portal limb of the veno-venous bypass placed and portal vein divided. The hepatic artery was divided just above the gastroduodenal artery, maintaining flow through the gastroduodenal artery. The intrapericardial IVC was clamped and the IVC divided above and below the liver, and the liver was removed and placed in an ice bath on the back table.

The liver was flushed with 1 L of chilled UW solution through the portal vein, with the hepatic artery and bile duct subsequently hand-flushed with the same solution. The left hepatic artery, left portal vein, and left hepatic duct were divided and oversewn on the back table. The liver was divided along the line of the right hepatic vein using the water jet dissector. A long tonsil clamp was placed in the right hepatic vein from the caval side as a guide to the line of resection. The right hepatic vein was transected at the trifurcation, leaving three branches of the vein to be reconstructed. The IVC was removed en bloc with the specimen. The three

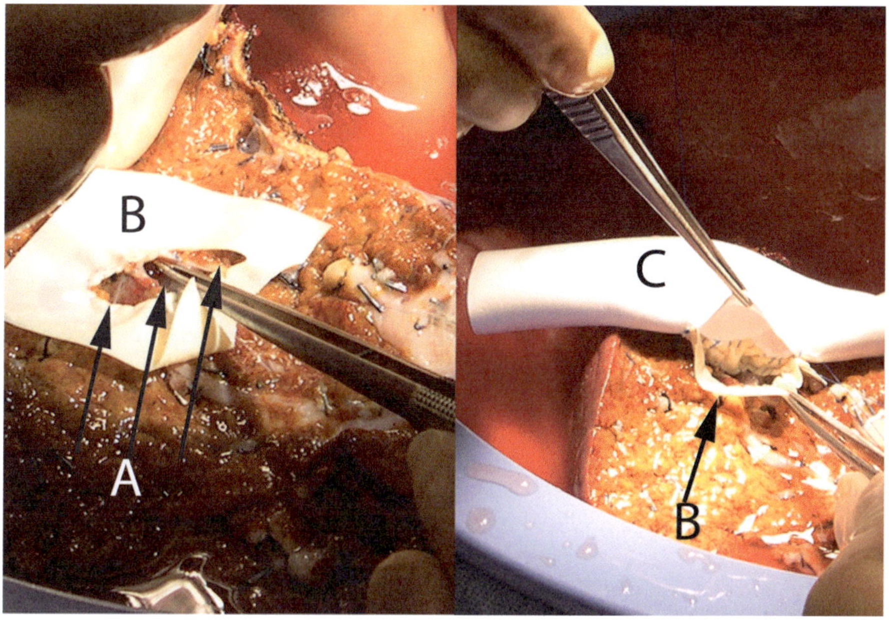

Fig. 10.4 Reconstruction of the right hepatic vein branches using bovine pericardial graft fashioned to recreate a right hepatic vein orifice. *A* Branches of the right hepatic vein; *B* bovine pericardial patch; *C* implantation of the right hepatic vein graft into a GoreTex IVC graft. Reprinted from Journal of the American College of Surgeons Jul;217(1). Hemming AW, Mekeel KL, Zendejas I, Kim RD, Sicklick JK, Reed AI. Resection of the liver and inferior vena cava for hepatic malignancy; p. 115–24; © 2013, with permission from Elsevier

branches of the right hepatic vein were plastied together and then a cuff of bovine pericardium anastomosed to the outer circumference of the plastied veins to from a longer, wider common outflow tract. The bovine pericardium outflow tract was then anastomosed to a 20-mm non-ringed GoreTex graft (Fig. 10.4). The entire graft was then reimplanted into the patient with first the suprahepatic IVC anastomosis, and second, the infrahepatic IVC. Prior to completing the lower IVC anastomosis, the graft was flushed via the portal vein with chilled ringers lactate to remove the UW solution. The portal limb of the bypass circuit was discontinued and the portal anastomosis performed. The autograft was reperfused with portal flow and after hemodynamic stability achieved, the veno-venous bypass was discontinued. The arterial anastomosis was performed after ligating and dividing the gastroduodenal artery and creating a branch patch at that site. The bile duct was reconstructed with a Roux-en-Y choledochojejunostomy.

The patient received six units of packed red blood cells and four units of fresh frozen plasma (FFP) during the procedure. Cold ischemic time was 115 min. Total operative time was approximately 6 h. The patient had a peak bilirubin of 8 mg/dl and required FFP for the first 3 days to maintain an INR < 2.0. She was discharged from hospital on postoperative day 15. Final pathology revealed an 8 cm cholangiocarcinoma with negative margins but vascular invasion. The patient received 6 months of postoperative gemcitabine and cisplatinum, and at 1 year had no evidence of disease. The patient did well for 2.5 years, at which point she developed pulmonary metastases and went on to succumb from her disease by 3 years post-resection.

Case 2

A 28-year-old woman presented with abdominal swelling and bilateral leg edema. She was otherwise asymptomatic. Her past medical history was unremarkable, with no history of jaundice, weight loss, or other pertinent history. On presentation her physical examination was notable for a palpable upper abdominal mass and bilateral leg edema. There were no obvious venous collaterals in the abdominal wall. Blood work demonstrated normal electrolytes and renal function with hepatitis B and C serologies negative. Serum AST and ALT were within normal limits; however, the alkaline phosphatase was elevated at 200 IU/L. Serum bilirubin was normal. Tumor markers demonstrated a normal CEA and AFP, Beta HCG, and CA 19-9. Imaging demonstrated a 16-cm mass located in the caudate lobe with IVC and hepatic vein compression, and subsequent displacement of the normal hilar anatomy (Figs. 10.5, 10.6, and 10.7). A percutaneous biopsy of the lesion was reported

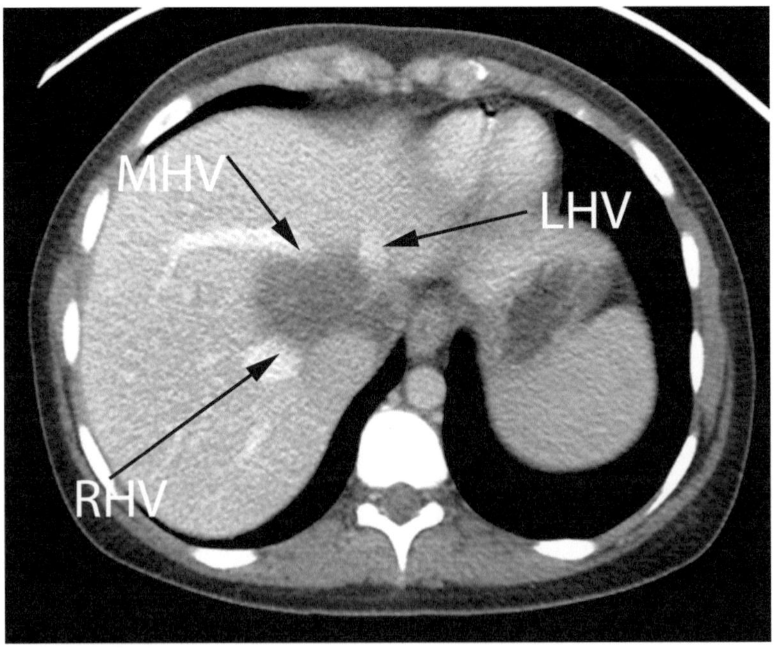

Fig. 10.5 CT imaging demonstrating abutting and compression of the hepatic veins from the caudate lobe tumor. *RHV* Right Hepatic Vein, *MHV* Middle Hepatic Vein, *LHV* Left Hepatic Vein

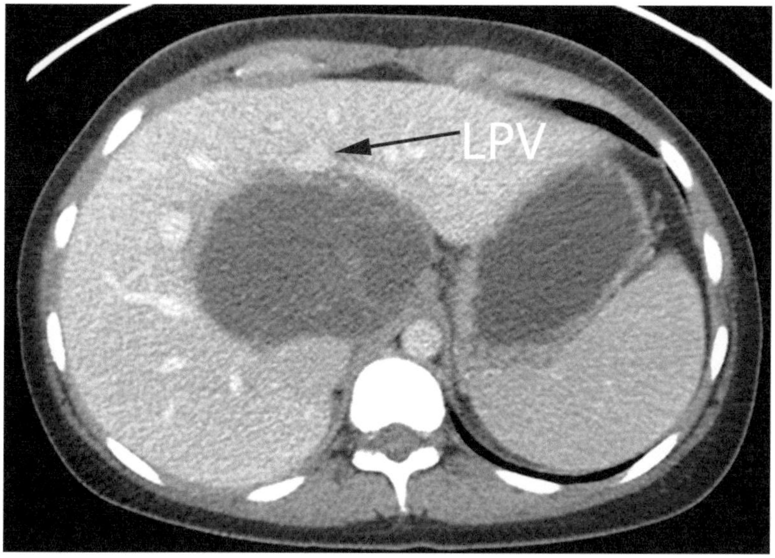

Fig. 10.6 Further CT imaging demonstrating displacement of the normal hilar anatomy from the caudate lobe mass. *LPV* Left Portal Vein

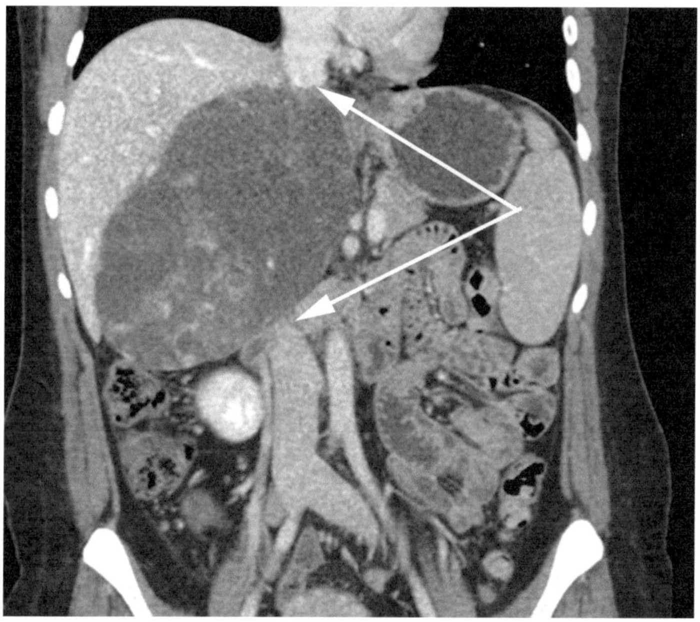

Fig. 10.7 CT imaging demonstrating complete caudate lobe replacement from the tumor, with compression of the IVC. *Arrows* are pointing to the supra- and infrahepatic IVC at the areas of compression

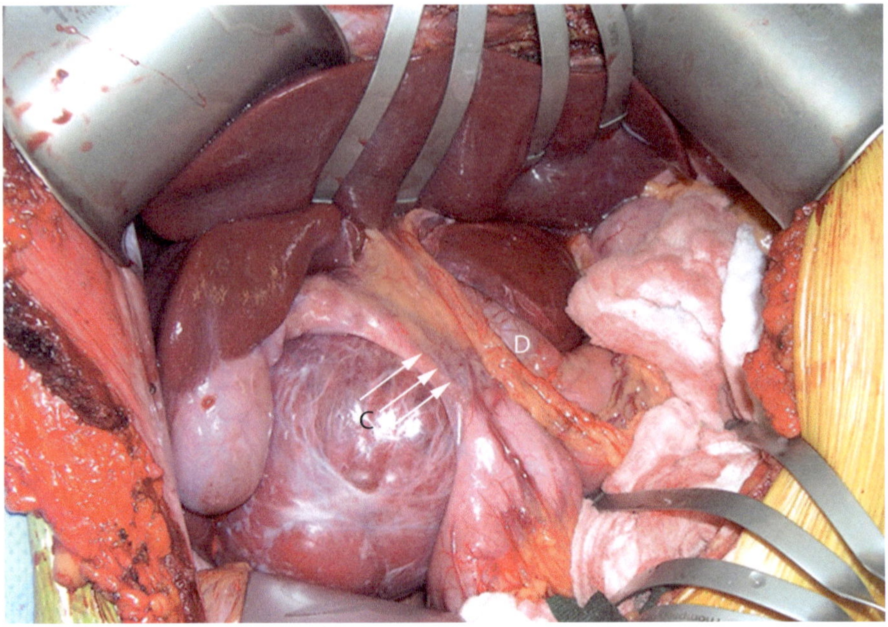

Fig. 10.8 Intraoperative images prior to ex situ resection. The hilum was displaced by the large caudate lobe tumor. *C* Caudate Lobe of the Liver (replaced here by tumor). *D* Common Hepatic Artery. *Arrows* point to the Common Bile Duct

as consistent with embryonal sarcoma. Further staging revealed no evidence of extrahepatic spread. Planning for surgery included extended resection with vascular reconstruction of hepatic veins under either in situ or ex vivo cold perfusion, and liver transplantation was considered as a potential salvage option should resection with clear margins not felt to be an option after intraoperative assessment.

At surgery the liver had venous congestion and hilar displacement was visualized (Fig. 10.8). A wedge biopsy of the tumor confirmed the diagnosis of embryonal sarcoma. The falciform and triangular ligaments were divided, and intraoperative ultrasound demonstrated the tumor compressing the IVC and all three hepatic veins. Attempts to rotate the liver proved unsuccessful due to large tumor size and the required torsion on the IVC and hepatic veins. An initial attempt to dissect the tumor away from liver parenchyma even under hepatic inflow occlusion led to impressive hemorrhage, presumably from outflow obstruction. The infrahepatic IVC was encircled. The suprahepatic IVC could not be safely dissected within the abdomen; therefore, the pericardium was opened from below and the intrapericardial IVC encircled. The bile duct was transected at the cystic duct entry. The hepatic artery was dissected out from the common hepatic artery to its right and left branches, and the portal vein cleared of lymphatic tissue from the head of the

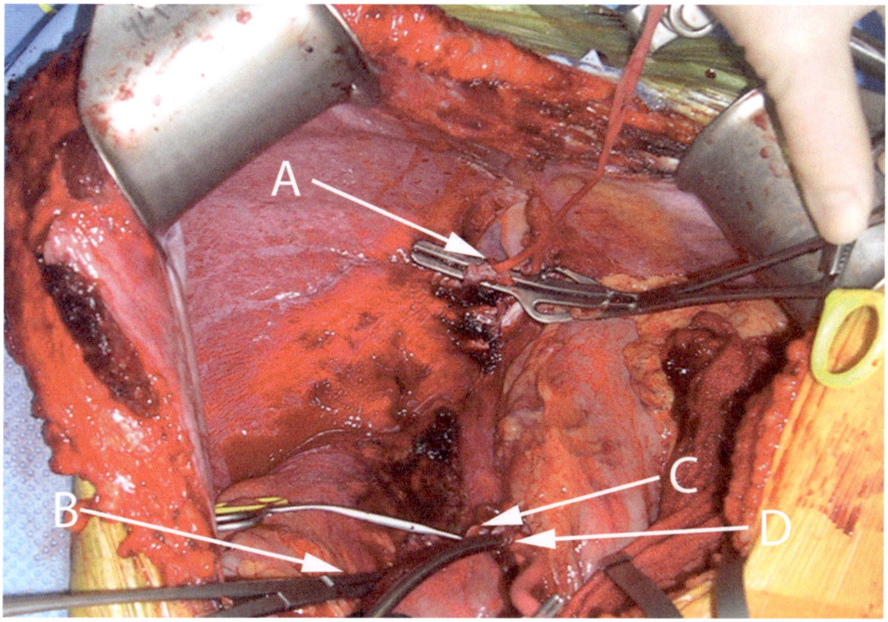

Fig. 10.9 Intraoperative imaging after the liver was removed. *A* Suprahepatic clamp placed in the intrapericardial IVC/right atrium; *B* the infrahepatic IVC clamp; *C* the hepatic artery clamp and site of transection; *D* portal cannula for the portal portion of veno-venous bypass

pancreas to the portal bifurcation. Percutaneous catheters were placed in femoral and internal jugular veins and the patient placed on the caval portion of veno-venous bypass. The infrahepatic IVC was clamped. The portal circulation was then added to the bypass. The hepatic artery was controlled and divided just above the gastroduodenal artery takeoff, maintaining flow through the gastroduodenal artery. The intrapericardial IVC was clamped and the liver removed after dividing the suprahepatic and infrahepatic IVC. The liver was lifted forward and the remaining posterior attachments to IVC divided (Fig. 10.9).

The liver was then flushed on the back table with 1 L of chilled UW solution (Fig. 10.10). The water jet dissector was then used to separate the tumor from both portal, hepatic veins, and IVC. The resection performed was an isolated caudate lobectomy (Fig. 10.11). The liver was then reimplanted with an end-to-end bi-caval anastomosis without need for graft. The liver was flushed with 1 L of chilled ringers lactate through the portal vein prior to completing the infrahepatic caval anastomosis. The patient was taken off the portal component of bypass, and a standard portal venous anastomosis was performed and the liver reperfused. The patient was then taken off the caval portion of bypass and the arterial anastomosis completed. The biliary anastomosis was performed in end-to-end fashion over an 8 French internal stent. The cold ischemic time was 90 min, with total operative time

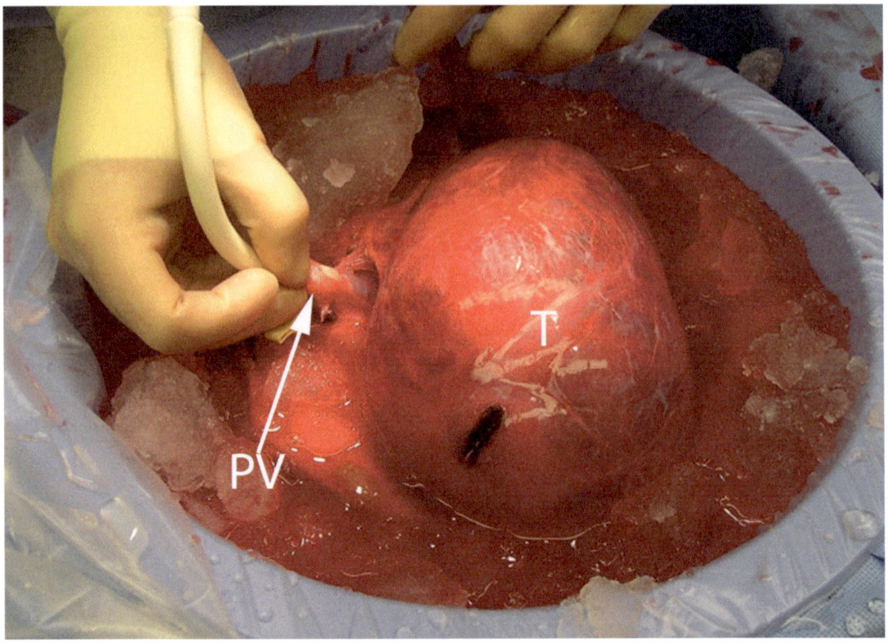

Fig. 10.10 Intraoperative photo of the ex vivo perfusion of the liver after placement in the ice bath. *PV* the portal vein. Cold perfusion solution is flushed through the liver to preserve the liver during resection. *T* tumor. The wedge biopsy is visible on the tumor

of 5.5 h. The patient received five units of packed red cells and four units of FFP. Peak bilirubin was 3.5 mg/dl, and she was discharged home on postoperative day eight. She is alive and free of disease 2 years post-resection.

Overall Management

- Patient selection is key. Patients with underlying co-morbidities are unlikely to have successful outcomes.
- Ex vivo liver resection should be the last option considered. There are very few candidates for liver surgery who cannot be managed with a lesser magnitude procedure.
- Excellent anesthesia and critical care support are also required. Intra- and perioperative management is very similar to liver transplantation, and similar resources are required.

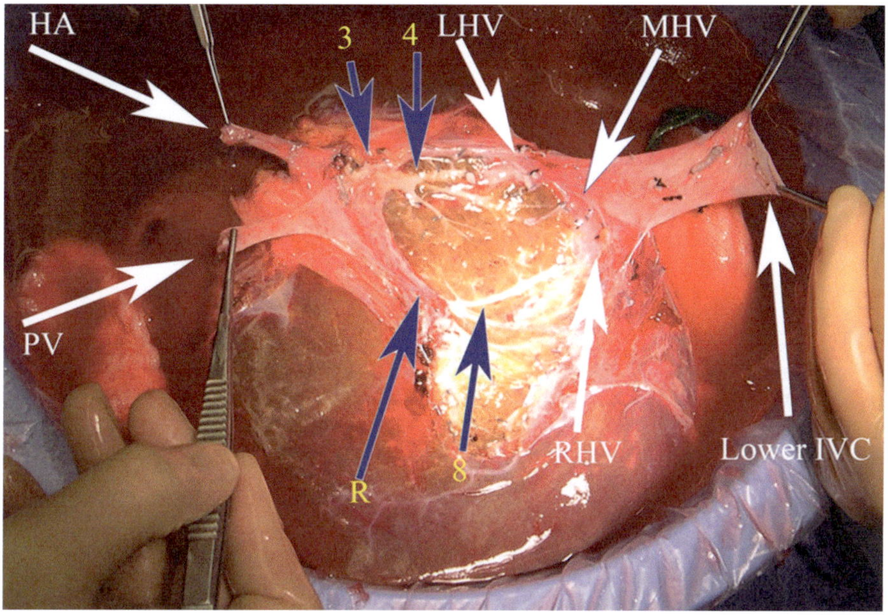

Fig. 10.11 Dissection of the hepatic structures around the tumor after resection. The caudate lobe has been removed with an isolate caudate lobectomy including the tumor. *HA* Hepatic Artery, *PV* Portal Vein, *R* Right Portal Vein *3, 4, 8* Individual Segmental Bile Duct Branches to 3, 4, 8, *LHV* Left Hepatic Vein, *RHV* Right Hepatic Vein. *MHV* Main Hepatic Vein, *Lower IVC* Infrahepatic IVC. Ties are visible where short hepatic veins were removed off the caudate lobe

Conclusion

Ex vivo resection is a dramatic technique, used only when all other techniques have been considered and rejected. The procedure is associated with an approximately 15% mortality and considerable morbidity, including postoperative liver failure, but at centers that have experience with the technique, it remains an option for the unusual tumor that cannot be resected using more standard liver resection techniques. Successful long-term survival has been demonstrated and is perhaps not surprisingly more common in benign disease such as echinococcus [15]. Patient selection is an important part of improving survival. Unfortunately, if postoperative liver failure develops, options are limited. Molecular Adsorbents Recirculating System (MARS) therapy may help decrease or alleviate some of the liver failure while patients recover [16]. Salvage liver transplantation is not typically an option, given the initial advanced malignant indication for the resection, but would be considered on an individual basis.

References

1. Nuzzo G, Giuliante F, Ardito F, Giovannini I, Aldrighetti L, Belli G, et al. Improvement in perioperative and long-term outcome after surgical treatment of hilar cholangiocarcinoma: results of an Italian multicenter analysis of 440 patients. Arch Surg. 2012;147(1):26–34.
2. Hemming AW, Reed AI, Fujita S, Zendejas I, Howard RJ, Kim RD. Role for extending hepatic resection using an aggressive approach to liver surgery. J Am Coll Surg. 2008; 206(5):870–5.
3. Berumen J, Hemming A. Vascular reconstruction in hepatic malignancy. Surg Clin North Am. 2016;96(2):283–98.
4. Mekeel K, Hemming A. Evolving role of vascular resection and reconstruction in hepatic surgery for malignancy. Hepatic Oncol. 2014;1(1):53–65.
5. Lin DX, Zhang QY, Li X, Ye QW, Lin F, Li LL. An aggressive approach leads to improved survival in hepatocellular carcinoma patients with portal vein tumor thrombus. J Cancer Res Clin Oncol. 2011;137(1):139–49.
6. Yamamoto Y. Ante-situm hepatic resection for tumors involving the confluence of hepatic veins and IVC. J Hepatobiliary Pancreat Sci. 2013;20(3):313–23.
7. Hemming AW, Reed AI, Langham MR Jr, Fujita S, Howard RJ. Combined resection of the liver and inferior vena cava for hepatic malignancy. Ann Surg. 2004;239(5):712–9.
8. Hemming AW, Mekeel KL, Zendejas I, Kim RD, Sicklick JK, Reed AI. Resection of the liver and inferior vena cava for hepatic malignancy. J Am Coll Surgeons. 2013;217(1):115–24.
9. Malde DJ, Khan A, Prasad KR, Toogood GJ, Lodge JP. Inferior vena cava resection with hepatectomy: challenging but justified. HPB (Oxford). 2011;13(11):802–10.
10. Lin DX, Zhang QY, Li X, Ye QW, Lin F, Li LL. An aggressive approach leads to improved survival in hepatocellular carcinoma patients with portal vein tumor thrombus. J Cancer Res Clin Oncol. 2011;137(1):139–49.
11. Kondo K, Chijiiwa K, Kai M, Otani K, Nagaike K, Ohuchida J, et al. Surgical strategy for hepatocellular carcinoma patients with portal vein tumor thrombus based on prognostic factors. J Gastrointest Surg. 2009;13(6):1078–83.
12. Xu JF, Liu XY, Wang S, Wen HX. Surgical treatment for hepatocellular carcinoma with portal vein tumor thrombus: a novel classification. World J Surg Oncol. 2015;13:86.
13. Shi J, Lai EC, Li N, Guo WX, Xue J, Lau WY, et al. Surgical treatment for hepatocellular carcinoma with portal vein tumor thrombus. Hepatogastroenterology. 2006;53(69):415–9.
14. Peng ZW, Guo RP, Zhang YJ, Lin XJ, Chen MS, Lau WY. Hepatic resection versus transcatheter arterial chemoembolization for the treatment of hepatocellular carcinoma with portal vein tumor thrombus. Cancer. 2012;118(19):4725–36.
15. Wen H, Dong J-H, Zhang J-H, Duan W-D, Zhao J-M, Liang Y-R, et al. Ex vivo liver resection and autotransplantation for end-stage alveolar echinococcosis: a case series. Am J Transplant. 2016;16(2):615–24.
16. Baker MA, Maley WR, Needleman L, Doria C. Ex vivo resection of hepatic neoplasia and autotransplantation: a case report and review of the literature. J Gastrointest Surg. 2015; 19(6):1169–76. doi:10.1007/s11605-015-2806-3.
17. Oldhafer KJ, Lang H, Schlitt HJ, Hauss J, Raab R, Klempnauer J, et al. Long-term experience after ex situ liver surgery. Surgery. 2000;127(5):520–7.
18. Lodge JP, Ammori BJ, Prasad KR, Bellamy MC. Ex vivo and in situ resection of inferior vena cava with hepatectomy for colorectal metastases. Ann Surg 2000;231(4):471–9.
19. Forni E, Meriggi F. Bench surgery and liver autotransplantation. Personal experience and technical considerations. G Chir. 1995;16(10):407–13.
20. Gruttadauria S, Marsh JW, Bartlett DL, Gridelli B, Marcos A. Ex situ resection techniques and liver autotransplantation: last resource for otherwise unresectable malignancy. Dig Dis Sci. 2005;50(10):1829–35.

21. Zhang KM, Hu XW, Dong JH, Hong ZX, Wang ZH, Li GH, et al. Ex-situ liver surgery without veno-venous bypass. World J Gastroenterol. 2012;18(48):7290–5.
22. Wang H, Liu Q, Wang Z, Zhang F, Li X, Wang X. Clinical outcomes of Ex Vivo liver resection and liver autotransplantation for hepatic alveolar echinococcosis. J Huazhong Univ Sci Technolog Med Sci. 2012;32(4):598–600.
23. Azoulay D, Andreani P, Maggi U, Salloum C, Perdigao F, Sebagh M, et al. Combined liver resection and reconstruction of the supra-renal vena cava: the Paul Brousse experience. Ann Surg. 2006;244(1):80–8.
24. Sarmiento JM, Bower TC, Cherry KJ, Farnell MB, Nagorney DM. Is combined partial hepatectomy with segmental resection of inferior vena cava justified for malignancy? Arch Surg 2003;138(6):624–30; discussion 630–1.
25. Johnson ST, Blitz M, Kneteman N, Bigam D. Combined hepatic and inferior vena cava resection for colorectal metastases. J Gastrointest Surg. 2006;10(2):220–6.
26. Delis SG, Madariaga J, Ciancio G. Combined liver and inferior vena cava resection for hepatic malignancy. J Surg Oncol. 2007;96(3):258–64.
27. Bower TC, Nagorney DM, Cherry KJ Jr, Toomey BJ, Hallett JW, Panneton JM, et al. Replacement of the inferior vena cava for malignancy: an update. J Vasc Surg. 2000;31 (2):270–81.
28. Azoulay D, Eshkenazy R, Andreani P, Castaing D, Adam R, Ichai P, et al. In situ hypothermic perfusion of the liver versus standard total vascular exclusion for complex liver resection. Ann Surg. 2005;241(2):277–85.
29. Dubay D, Gallinger S, Hawryluck L, Swallow C, McCluskey S, McGilvray I. In situ hypothermic liver preservation during radical liver resection with major vascular reconstruction. Br J Surg. 2009;96(12):1429–36.
30. Azoulay D, Lim C, Salloum C, Andreani P, Maggi U, Bartelmaos T, et al. Complex liver resection using standard total vascular exclusion, venovenous bypass, and in situ hypothermic portal perfusion: an audit of 77 consecutive cases. Ann Surg. 2015;262(1):93–104.
31. Smyrniotis V, Kostopanagiotou G, Lolis E, Theodoraki K, Farantos C, Andreadou I, et al. Effects of hepatovenous back flow on ischemic reperfusion injuries in liver resections with the Pringle maneuver. J Am Coll Surg. 2003;197(6):949–54.
32. Shindoh J, Tzeng CW, Aloia TA, Curley SA, Huang SY, Mahvash A, et al. Safety and efficacy of portal vein embolizationbefore planned major or extended hepatectomy: an institutional experience of 358 patients. J Gastrointest Surg. 2014;18(1):45–51.
33. Hemming AW, Reed AI, Howard RJ, Fujita S, Hochwald SN, Caridi JG, et al. Preoperative portal vein embolization for extended hepatectomy. Ann Surg. 2003;237(5):686–91; discussion 691–3.
34. Sano T, Shimizu Y, Senda Y. Assessing resectability in cholangiocarcinoma. Hepatic Oncol. 2014;1(1):39–51.
35. Nimura Y. Preoperative biliary drainage before resection for cholangiocarcinoma (Pro). HPB (Oxford). 2008;10(2):130–3.
36. Neuhaus P, Thelen A. Radical surgery for right-sided Klatskin tumor. HPB (Oxford). 2008;10 (3):171–3.
37. Nimura Y. Radical surgery: vascular and pancreatic resection for cholangiocarcinoma. HPB (Oxford). 2008;10(3):183–5.
38. Hemming A, Mekeel K, Khanna A, Baquerizo A, Kim RD. Portal vein resection in the management of hilar cholangiocarcinoma. J Am Coll Surg. 2011;212(4):604–13.
39. Gurusamy KS, Koti R, Pamecha V, Davidson BR. Veno-venous bypass versus none for liver transplantation. Cochrane Database Syst Rev. 2011;(3):CD007712.
40. Glebova NO, Hicks CW, Piazza KM, Lum YW2, Abularrage CJ, Black JH 3rd. Outcomes of bypass support use during inferior vena cava resection and reconstruction. Ann Vasc Surg. 2016;30:12–21.

41. Jackson P, Jankovic Z. Veno-venous bypass catheters for hepatic transplant risk unique complications. Anaesth Intensive Care. 2007;35(5):805–6.
42. Khoury GF, Mann ME, Porot MJ, Abdul-Rasool IH, Busuttil RW. Air embolism associated with veno-venous bypass during orthotopic liver transplantation. Anesthesiology. 1987;67:848–51.

Resection of Renal Cell Carcinoma Involving the Liver with Tumor Thrombus Extending into Inferior Vena Cava Requiring Venovenous Bypass

11

Chetana Lim, Chady Salloum, Eylon Lahat, Michael Ossesis, Concepcion Gomez Gavara, Philippe Compagnon and Daniel Azoulay

First Case Presentation

Right Renal Cell Carcinoma with Tumor Thrombus Extending into the Retrohepatic Inferior Vena Cava

A 66-year-old man presented to his general practitioner with a complaint of dyspnea. He did not have any significant past medical history. Physical examination did not reveal any symptoms such as hematuria, abdominal pain or mass, ascites or lower extremity edema.

C. Lim · C. Salloum · E. Lahat · M. Ossesis · C. Gomez Gavara · P. Compagnon · D. Azoulay (✉)
Department of HPB Surgery and Liver Transplant Unit, Henri Mondor Hospital,
51 Avenue du Marechal de Lattre de Tassigny, Creteil 94010, France
e-mail: daniel.azoulay@aphp.fr

C. Lim
e-mail: Chetana.lim@gmail.com

C. Salloum
e-mail: chady.salloum@gmail.com

E. Lahat
e-mail: eylonlahat@yahoo.com

M. Ossesis
e-mail: osseis@hotmail.com

C. Gomez Gavara
e-mail: imgoga@hotmail.com

P. Compagnon
e-mail: Philippe.compagnon@aphp.fr

T.M. Pawlik et al. (eds.), *Case-Based Lessons in the Management of Complex Hepato-Pancreato-Biliary Surgery*, DOI 10.1007/978-3-319-50868-9_11

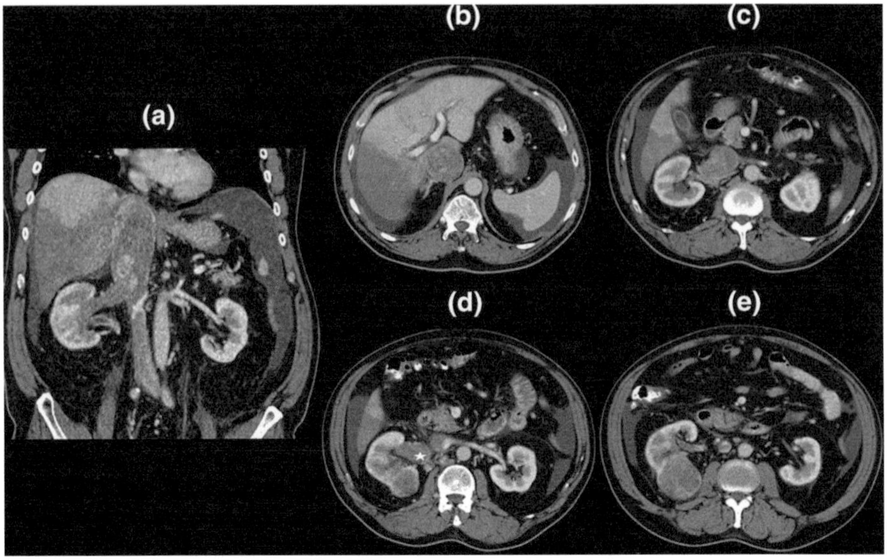

Fig. 11.1 Computed tomography scan revealed the presence of right renal cell carcinoma with tumor thrombus extending into the retrohepatic inferior vena cava and right hepatic vein. **a** Coronal view showing the tumor thrombus extending into the retrohepatic inferior vena cava and right hepatic vein with liver congestion. **b–d** Transversal views showing the right renal cell carcinoma with tumor thrombus in the right renal vein extending into the inferior vena cava

Laboratory explorations showed moderate cytolysis (aspartate aminotransferase = 126 IU/L and alanine aminotransferase = 133 IU/L). Multi-detector computed tomography (MDCT) revealed pulmonary embolism and the images presented in Fig. 11.1.

Clinical Presentation

A more liberal use of imaging techniques is associated with increased incidental detection of asymptomatic renal cell carcinoma (RCC). But more than 90% of patients with tumor thrombus extending into inferior vena cava (IVC) present with symptoms [1]. The symptoms of patients with RCC extending into the IVC include hematuria (35%), abdominal pain (17%), and abdominal mass (2%) [2]. Other symptoms such as lower extremity edema, right varicocele, dilated superficial abdominal veins (caput medusae), or diagnosis such as pulmonary embolism, can reveal the diagnosis of RCC with caval tumor thrombus. When the tumor thrombus obstructs the hepatic veins, this may lead to abdominal pain, hepatomegaly, and ascites (Budd-Chiari syndrome) [3]. Also, paraneoplastic syndromes including hypertension, non-metastatic hepatic dysfunction (Stauffer's syndrome), polycythemia, and hypercalcemia may have been observed in these patients [4].

Diagnosis and Assessment

RCC is the third most frequent genitourinary cancer and its prevalence is estimated to be between 2 and 3% of all malignant tumors in adults [5]. Due to its particular tropism for the venous system, there is a potential for extension into the renal vein, IVC (4–10%) and the right atrium (1%) [6, 7].

Assessment should be initiated with ultrasonography and MDCT, which are the primary methods for diagnosis of RCC with tumor thrombus. These two imaging techniques have demonstrated good specificity in detecting the presence of tumor thrombus, with a sensitivity of 65–90%, reaching 87% when used in combination.

Doppler ultrasound provides an estimate of the direction and speed of the blood flow within the IVC. However, the infrarenal portion of the IVC is imperfectly visualized in obese patients and when there is some gas interposition. Also, ultrasonography does not allow performing vessel reconstruction. MDCT is usually required for diagnosis of RCC, staging of IVC tumor thrombus, and surgical strategy [8]. It allows simultaneous thoracic screening. Magnetic resonance imaging (MRI) is usually considered as the gold standard for thrombus evaluation [9]. Fluorine 18-fluorodeoxyglucose (18F-FDG) PET-CT is commonly used in cancer staging disease. It can also be used to detect avid fluorodeoxyglucose thrombus, reflecting malignant thrombus. In our case, the patient demonstrates common presentation of right RCC with IVC tumor thrombosis.

Chronic obstruction of IVC by a tumor thrombus may lead to collateral vein development through deep and superficial venous collateral vessels. Four major collateral pathways have been described [10]: (i) The deep pathway, the most common, concerns the ascending lumbar veins, anastomosing with the azygos vein on the right side and the hemiazygos vein on the left side. Blood flow can also join vertebral, paraspinal, and extravertebral plexus. (ii) In the intermediate pathway, blood flow returns through the periureteric plexus bilaterally and the left gonadal vein to the left renal vein. (iii) The superficial pathway is constituted with the inferior epigastric and the abdominal wall veins, anastomosing with the superior epigastric veins and internal mammary veins to join the subclavians veins and the superior vena cava. (iv) The portal pathway concerns blood arising from lower extremities through the internal iliac veins to the hemorrhoidal plexus to join the inferior mesenteric vein and the portal system. The extent of development of these collateral veins may help in the decision whether to proceed or not to IVC reconstruction.

Staging of Intracaval Extension

The classification proposed by Neves and Zincke (i.e., Mayo Classification) [11] is the most widely used classification staging system of intracaval extension. This latter describes four levels of IVC extension: level I when extension only concerns the renal vein and/or the IVC < 2 cm; level II corresponds to extension within the

IVC > 2 cm below the hepatic veins; level III corresponds to retrohepatic IVC and/or hepatic veins involvement; and level IV corresponds to extension above the diaphragm with or without atrial thrombus. The anatomic level of the tumor thrombus within the IVC dictates surgical strategy.

Surgical Strategy

This complex surgery requires a multidisciplinary management including experienced anesthesiologists and liver surgeons. This also requires an accurate preoperative imaging assessment by experienced radiologists.

In our patient, the level and extent of tumor thrombus was established preoperatively with MDCT and MRI. The patient had a tumor originated from the right kidney with an IVC tumor thrombus involving more than half of the circumference of the IVC, and extending into the retrohepatic IVC and the ostia of the right hepatic vein. There was no lymph node involvement or metastasis upon preoperative imaging. The relationship of the tumor thrombus to the liver, hepatic veins, diaphragm, and right atrium determined its staging as a level III tumor, according to the classification by Neves and Zincke.

For this case, we discussed three potential scenarios according to the preoperative clinical and radiological findings: (i) to perform right nephrectomy and IVC thrombectomy; (ii) to perform right nephrectomy and IVC resection; or (iii) to perform right nephrectomy, right hepatectomy and IVC resection. In all cases, it is necessary to perform the surgery under standard total vascular exclusion (TVE) of the liver. In case of hemodynamics instability at the moment of TVE, a venovenous bypass would be installed to maintain hemodynamics and prevent kidney and splanchnic venous congestion (see below) [12, 13]. This case of level III thrombus (extension to the right hepatic vein) did not theoretically require a combined abdominal-thoracic and sternotomy approach with a cardiopulmonary bypass. In addition, if TVE was predicted to last potentially longer than 60 min, the patient would have TVE of the liver with in situ hypothermic portal perfusion and venovenous bypass (usually cavo-porto-jugular, see below).

Intraoperative anesthesia was specifically adapted to the risks of massive bleeding, general hypothermia, rapid hemodynamic changes, and coagulation disorders subsequent to ischemia-reperfusion injury. Intraoperative monitoring and management included the following modifications in addition to standard noninvasive techniques: (1) two large-bore intravenous cannulas or a large-bore central catheter (a cordis with a triple-lumen central catheter); (2) an arterial catheter; (3) a Swann-Ganz catheter; (4) a rapid infusion device; (5) body and fluids warmers. Transesophageal echocardiography was used to provide real-time staging and surveillance of the cranial part and mobility of the thrombus.

Technical Aspects

Surgical Incisions

Surgical incision should be performed according to the anticipated level of tumor thrombus and the type of vascular control. A large number of different incisions are possible for the treatment of right renal tumors with retrohepatic IVC thrombosis. For our case, a transabdominal approach (J-shaped or bi-subcostal incision) or a thoracophrenolaparotomy using an oblique incision along the eighth or ninth intercostal space may be performed. The goal of these incisions was to facilitate proximal control of the suprahepatic IVC. This latter might be achieved either via an abdominal approach with or without pericardial incision, a transdiaphragmatic extrapericardial approach [14], or by sternotomy. In our patient, we performed a J-shaped incision with an intrapericardial approach of the IVC (Fig. 11.2).

Surgery of the IVC and Hepatic Veins

The type of IVC surgery varied according to the location and the extent of the tumor thrombus, which was decided during surgery. If less than 30% of the

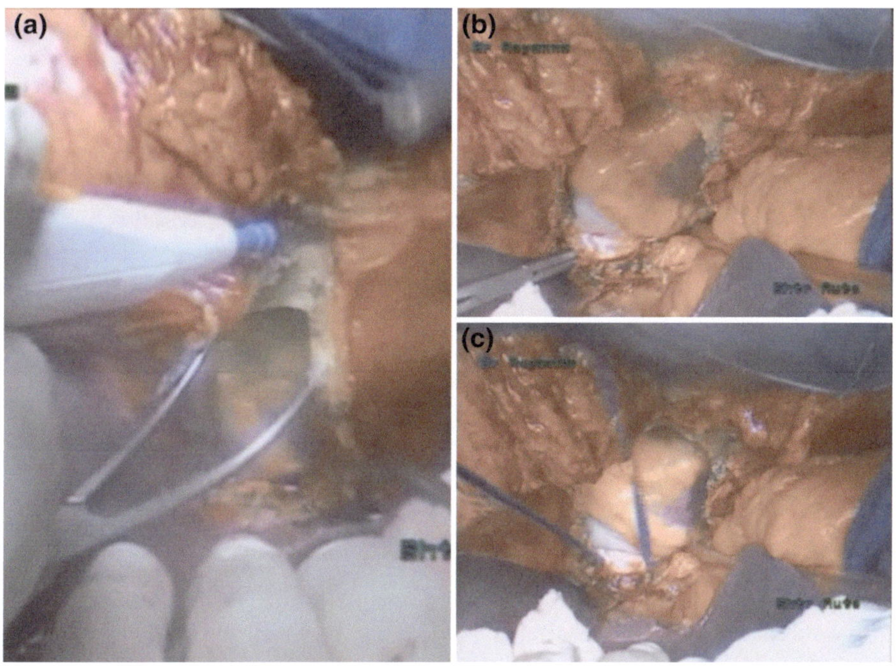

Fig. 11.2 Control of the suprahepatic inferior vena cava. **a** Pericardiotomy. **b**, **c** Control of intrapericardiac inferior vena cava

circumference of the IVC wall was involved, it was sutured longitudinally. If wall involvement was between 30 and 50%, the IVC was sutured transversally to prevent stenosis of the vein. If the circumference of the wall was involved, the IVC was resected and replaced by a 20-mm-diameter external ring-reinforced PTFE.

In our patient, intraoperative ultrasonography was first performed to confirm the presence of tumor thrombus in the retrohepatic IVC extending into the right hepatic vein and to rule out for any occult liver metastases. The surgical treatment of this patient required at least a radical right nephrectomy with en bloc resection of the retrohepatic IVC. It was not possible in our case to preserve the IVC because the thrombus was adherent to the caval wall and completely obstructed the IVC lumen.

Vascular Control of the IVC

The type of vascular control was planned following preoperative morphologic analysis. It was then adapted during surgery according to the intraoperative ultrasonography's findings, with the aim of (1) minimizing the need for transfusion; (2) shortening ischemia time as much as possible; (3) maintaining stable systemic hemodynamics; and (4) to improve the tolerance of the remnant liver to ischemia-reperfusion injury in case of liver resection.

Two different vascular control techniques were possible: standard vascular exclusion of the liver, or two-step vascular exclusion of the liver. The standard TVE involved mobilization of the liver, and isolation of the suprahepatic and infrahepatic vena cava and the hepatic pedicle. The infrahepatic vena cava, hepatic pedicle, and suprahepatic vena cava were serially clamped following systematic ligation and division of the adrenal vein. After specimen removal, circulation was restored by unclamping successively the suprahepatic vena cava, the infrahepatic vena cava, and the portal triad. In the two-step TVE technique, TVE was performed, leaving a sufficiently long IVC stump below the confluence of the hepatic veins for replacement of the suprahepatic caval clamp by another clamp on the replaced retrohepatic vena cava, below the confluence of the hepatic veins (seen in Fig. 11.1c). En bloc resection of the specimen and of a segment of the vena cava could then be completed, with revascularization of the liver.

In our patient, we decided to control the vena cava in the pericardium (Fig. 11.2) for the following two reasons: (i) a safer control of the suprahepatic vena cava and (ii) to ensure that a sufficiently long stump of suprahepatic vena cava was available for secondary IVC reconstruction. The first strategic surgical step was to prepare the standard TVE by controlling the vena caval portion below (infrahepatic/renal IVC) and above the thrombus (supradiaphragmatic/intrapericardial IVC), particularly to avoid an embolism during preparation of the tumor-bearing kidney.

After complete mobilization of the right colon, liver, and a Kocher Maneuver, the right kidney and infrahepatic/infrarenal IVC were fully exposed. Kidney mobilization and control of the right renal artery was performed as usual (through either an

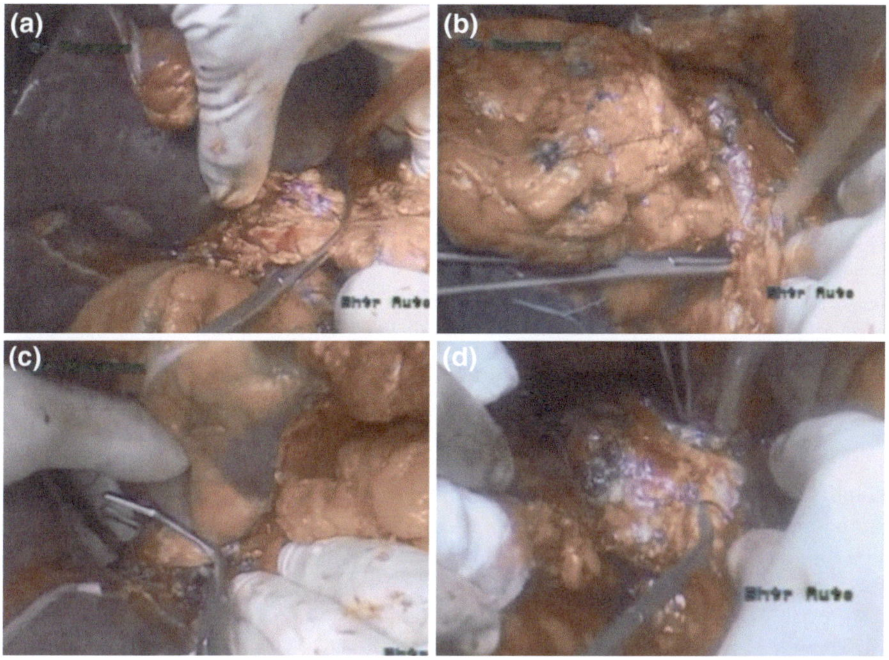

Fig. 11.3 Vascular control of the inferior vena cava. **a** Clamping of the portal triad. **b** Control of the infrahepatic/infrarenal inferior vena cava. **c** Clamping of the intrapericardiac inferior vena cava. **d** Control of the left renal vein

anterior or posterior approach). The infrahepatic segment was dissected and encircled with a tourniquet. Left renal and gonadal veins were controlled and clamped before opening the IVC. The posterior surface of the infrahepatic/infrarenal IVC needs to be dissected carefully from the posterior abdominal wall by ligating and dividing all the lumbar veins found at this level, thus allowing complete circumferential control of this segment. The retrohepatic/suprahepatic infradiaphragmatic IVC segment should be circumferentially controlled. Exposure of this segment requires full liver mobilization. Then, the supradiaphragmatic IVC segment was controlled by opening the central tendon of the diaphragm. The pericardium was then opened so that the intrapericardial IVC can be encircled and taped below the confluence into the right atrium (Fig. 11.2).

Vascular exclusion of the IVC was then achieved (superior and inferior to the thrombus and the left renal vein). An opening to the lesser omentum allowed control of the hepatic pedicle with a tourniquet and vascular exclusion of the liver was also achieved (Fig. 11.3).

Adjunct Procedures: The Venovenous Bypass and Hypothermic Perfusion Techniques [12–14]

Caval occlusion at the suprahepatic or intrapericardial segments can compromise venous return to the heart in cases of partially occluding tumor thrombi, which results in decreased cardiac output, hemodynamic instability, and hypoperfusion. Extracorporeal circulation (i.e., venovenous or cardiopulmonary bypass) is indicated when resection followed by complex reconstruction of the inferior vena cava is performed (see second case presentation) or if caval-cross clamping is not hemodynamically tolerated despite adequate fluid loading (if cardiac output fell by more than 50% or a decrease in mean arterial pressure > 30%). The conventional technique for establishing vascular access for bypass involves cannulation of the portal (or inferior mesenteric vein) and right femoral veins to provide pump inflow and cannulation of the left axillary vein to accept pump outflow. This procedure implies a surgical dissection of the inferior mesenteric or portal veins that can be technically demanding in case of portal cavernoma, can prolong operating time, and can be associated with significant complications such as hematoma or bleeding. The puncture and cannulation of femoral and left axillary vein is then done under ultrasonography control as described by Oken et al. in 1994 [15].

If TVE was predicted to last potentially longer than 60 min, we advocate the use of hypothermia technique as an adjunct to increase the tolerance of the liver to prolonged ischemia. It has been demonstrated that every 10 °C fall in temperature of liver parenchyma decreases the liver enzyme activity by 1.5- to 2-fold. The principle of hypothermia approach is to perfuse the liver with conservation liquid used in organ transplantation and refrigerated at 4 °C. The temperature of the liver decreased then to 20 °C. The most popular methods of cooling for liver surgery include hypothermia portal perfusion and topical cooling (see second case presentation).

In our patient, we used neither venovenous bypass nor hypothermic portal perfusion techniques.

IVC Resection and Reconstruction

Risk factors for IVC resection include (i) complete obstruction of the caval lumen; (ii) densely adherent intracaval tumor; (iii) encasement of the great vessels by bulky disease; and (iv) direct caval wall invasion [16]. This has been the case in our patient.

In our patient we performed a two-step TVE. When complete IVC control is achieved, the first step is started, the infrarenal vena cava is resected by stapling. The left renal vein could be completely ligated and divided. Then, an extended longitudinal cavotomy allowed complete thrombus removal along the retrohepatic IVC (Fig. 11.4a, b). Then the IVC anterior wall was opened to a level of the right hepatic vein, and the IVC and right hepatic vein lumens were flushed with heparin and completely cleared of thrombus fragments. The retrohepatic IVC was resected

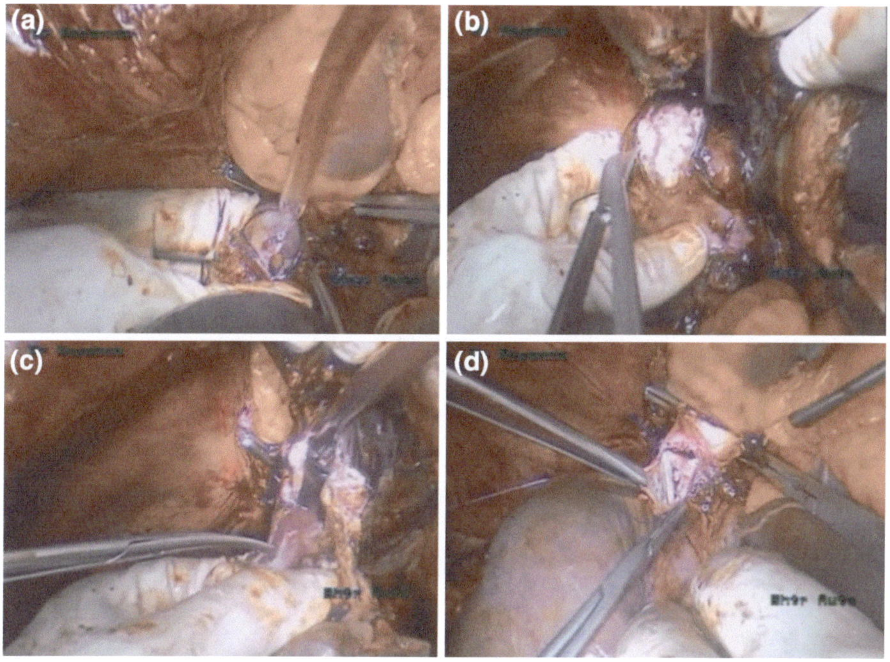

Fig. 11.4 Resection of the inferior vena cava. **a** Cavotomy at a level above the hepatic vein. **b** Cavotomy at a level below the hepatic vein. **c** Resection of the inferior vena cava. **d** Reconstruction of the inferior vena cava

to a level below the ostia of the right hepatic vein (Fig. 11.4c, d). Some centers did not perform IVC replacement, as chronic venous obstruction had created spontaneous retroperitoneal collaterals. In our case, we performed IVC replacement and reimplanted left renal vein into the prosthetic graft.

To re-establish IVC reconstruction, we used a 20-mm diameter external ring-reinforced PTFE (polytetrafluoroethylene). PTFE is the preferred synthetic material when replacement is considered, as it has low thrombogenic potential and a high reported patency rate. Once the upper part of the graft was anastomosed to the proximal end of the cavotomy, the cranial clamp is then repositioned at a level below the hepatic veins (Fig. 11.5).

Thereafter, the Pringle maneuver is released, and liver perfusion is restored. In a second step, radical en bloc resection of the right kidney and IVC was then performed. Then the resected caval segment is replaced with a synthetic graft in an end-to-end fashion.

In our case, the left renal vein stump was reconstructed by joining its free end to the interposition graft in an end-to-side fashion (Fig. 11.5c). Some other centers do not perform left renal vein reconstruction due to the presence of collateral veins development via the azygos-hemiazygos system that may preserve adequate drainage.

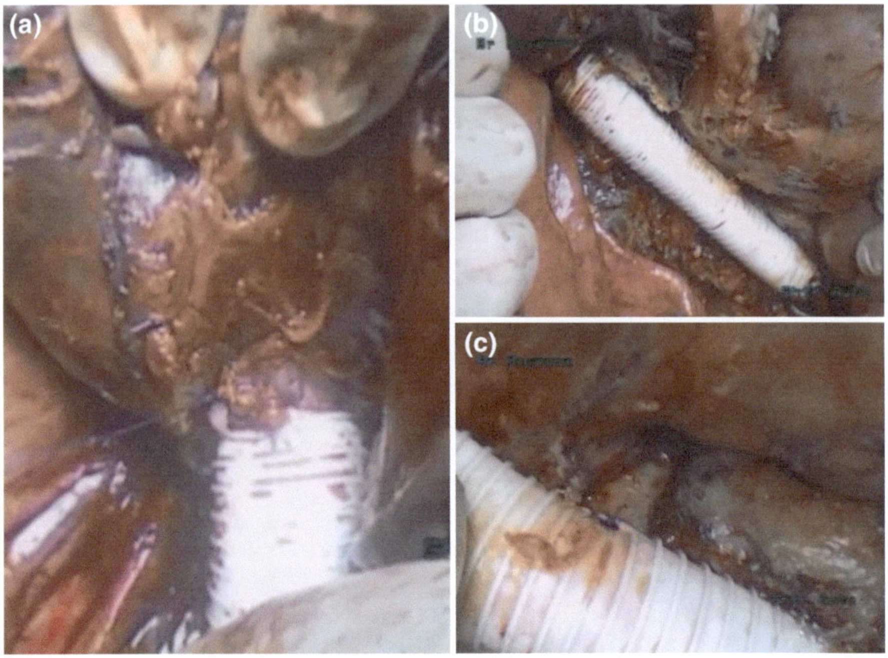

Fig. 11.5 Inferior vena cava reconstruction using a PTFE. **a**, **b** Inferior vena cava reconstruction. **c** Reimplantation of the left renal vein

As for the right hepatic vein, two scenarios were possible: (i) the root of the right hepatic vein in the native vena cava remained untouched and this latter is patent, or (ii) the right hepatic vein was resected and its stump is reimplanted into the replaced vena cava. In our case, the root of the right hepatic vein in the native IVC was not resected and the right hepatic vein was completely patent after thrombus extraction.

The patient received seven units of packed red blood cells and three units of fresh frozen plasma.

Technical Pearls

- In case of level III tumors, the control of the suprahepatic/infradiaphragmatic or transdiaphragmatic/extrapericardial IVC rather than intrapericardial IVC should be preferred because of the risk of postoperative pericardial tamponade.
- If intrapericardial IVC is planned to be controlled, all the diaphragmatic veins should be ligated to ensure that a sufficiently long stump of suprahepatic vena cava was available for secondary IVC reconstruction.
- Sternotomy is in most of cases useless for surgical management of level III tumors.

- Autologous or cadaveric graft should be preferred to prosthetic grafts because of the lower risk of secondary infections.
- In case of IVC reconstruction, arterio-venous fistula has not been shown to decrease the rate of postoperative thrombosis.
- When the venovenous is planned to be performed, vascular exclusion of the IVC including the tumor thrombus must be performed before the extracorporeal circulation starts because of the risks of the migration of fragments of tumor thrombus into the systemic circulation.

Short-Term Outcome

This surgery is technically demanding and is associated with potential life-threatening complications, including massive hemorrhage and pulmonary embolism. Nearly 8% of patients experience uncontrollable bleeding. Risk factors include the level and degree of occlusion, and the presence and extent of collateral vein circulation in response to obstruction. Also the level of IVC thrombus was associated with an increase in complications rates (nearly 15, 14, 18, and 30%, respectively, for levels I–IV) [17]. Up to 3.4% of patients develop pulmonary embolism due to embolization of dislodged thrombus fragments to pulmonary circulation secondary to excessive IVC manipulation. The occurrence of a pulmonary embolism has been associated with a high mortality rate of 75%. The anatomic thrombus level is the main risk factor for pulmonary embolism.

Postoperative mortality rate following nephrectomy with tumor thrombectomy is less than 5% and has been directly associated with tumor thrombus level [18, 19] (22% for level IV).

The postoperative course of the patient was uneventful. He did not develop postoperative blood thrombus emboli or liver insufficiency. Liver and renal functions tests were within normal limits at discharge. Postoperative MDCT showed patency of the IVC prosthetic graft, reconstructed left renal vein and a partial thrombosis of the right hepatic vein (Fig. 11.6).

Histopathological examination of the resected specimen showed that the vena cava was obstructed by a tumoral thrombus and its wall was involved by the tumor. Resections margins of the vena cava and right kidney were free for tumor.

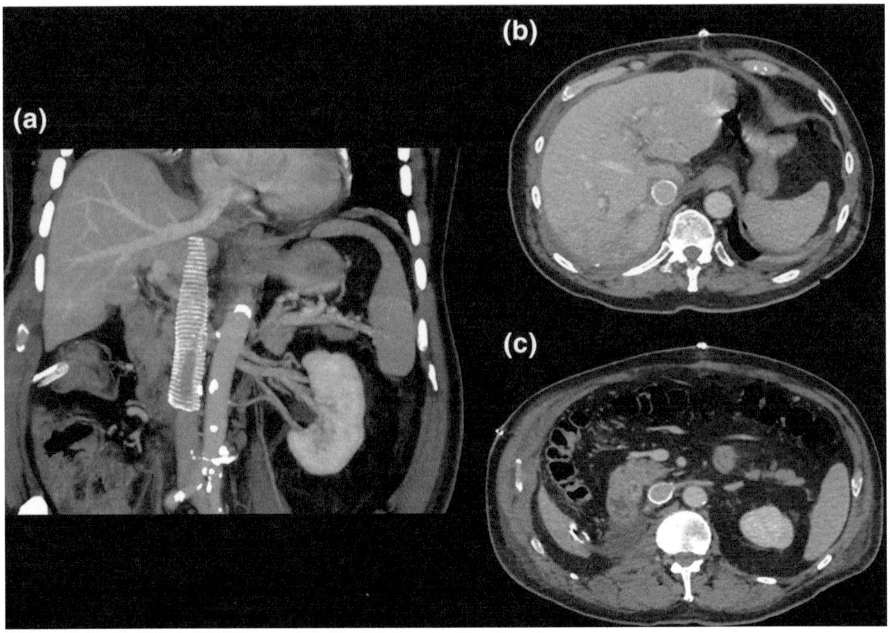

Fig. 11.6 Postoperative computed tomography showed the patency of the prosthetic graft (**a**, **c**) and a partial thrombosis of the right hepatic vein (**b**)

Long-Term Outcome

More than half of the patients with IVC tumor thrombus present with simultaneous distant metastases. The spontaneous prognosis of such patients with metastatic disease at presentation is poor, with a five-year overall survival of 0–10% and a mean survival of 4 to 6 months [20, 21].

Radical nephrectomy with tumor thrombectomy for renal tumors with isolated IVC invasion without distant metastasis achieved five-year disease-free survival rates between 40 and 65%, with median disease-free survival rate between 38 and 116 months. The same procedure in patients with renal tumors with metastatic disease achieved five-year disease-free survival rates between 6 and 28%, with median disease-free survival rate between 11 and 20 months [20–24]. The long-term results obtained can be considered good as compared with the poor prognosis from nonoperative management of the patients.

Second Case Presentation

Liver Metastases from Renal Cell Carcinoma Following Right Nephrectomy and Inferior Vena Cava Tumor Resection

Fifteen months later, a surveillance MRI showed a solitary hypervascular 9-cm mass located in the segment 6 of the liver (Fig. 11.7). The PET scan revealed avid fluorodeoxyglucose activity in this hepatic mass (SUV 13.6). Percutaneous biopsy of this lesion revealed liver recurrence of RCC. Preoperative imaging assessment showed that there was no caval recurrence and no distant metastasis. Our patient had a metachronous solitary liver metastasis which developed 15 months later after right nephrectomy with IVC resection for locally advanced RCC.

Surgical Strategy

Preoperative imaging evaluation showed that the lesion was in contact with the replaced IVC but did not seem to involve it. The volume of the remnant left liver and segment 1 was more than 40% of the total volume of the liver. Liver function tests were normal and the indocyanine retention rate at 15 min was 3.6%. Based on the preoperative assessment of the vascular relationship, right hepatectomy was planned to be performed safely under standard TVE. Redo resection of the replaced IVC would be decided intraoperatively based on intraoperative findings (Fig. 11.8). Therefore, the TVE was predicted to last longer than 60 min. Thus, to ensure safe resection, the patient was planned to have TVE of the liver with in situ hypothermic portal perfusion and venovenous bypass.

Technical Aspects

Anesthetic Management

The anesthetic management was the same as described above. A low central venous pressure of 5 mm Hg was maintained before and during resection simultaneously with stable systemic hemodynamic and adequate (>0.5 mL/kg/h) urine output. Once the resection was completed, normovolemia was restored by fluid expansion using warmed colloid-hetastarch solutions (to a maximum of 35 mL/kg body weight) and 5% albumin rather than crystalloid solutions.

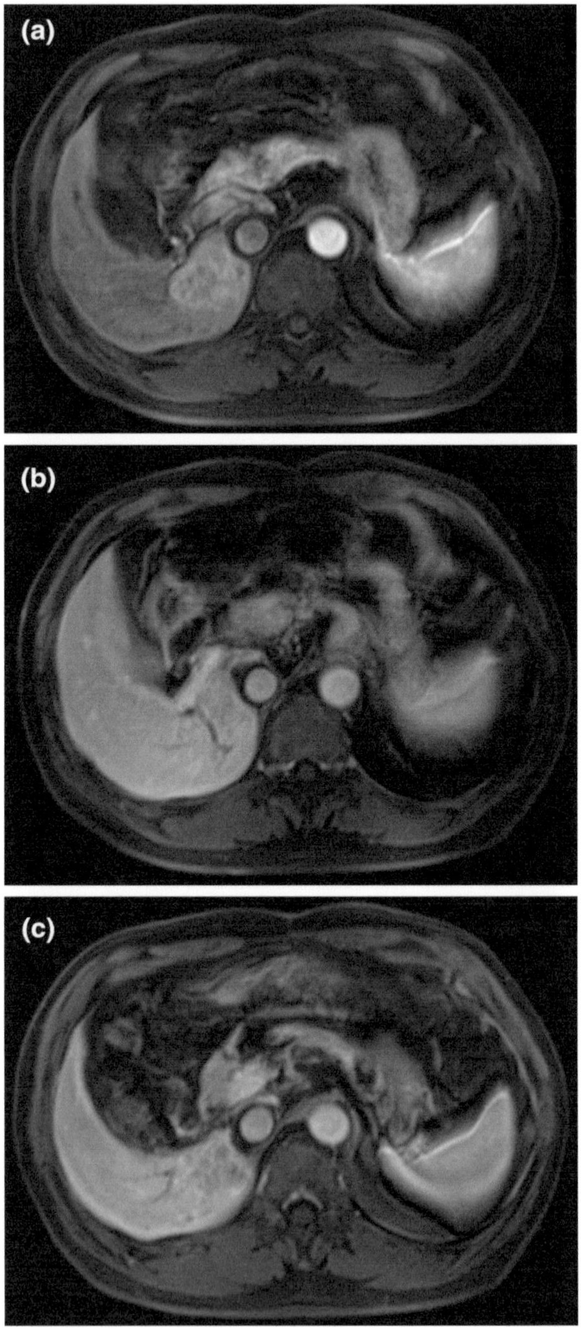

Fig. 11.7 Magnetic resonance imaging scan revealed the presence of metachronous liver metastasis from renal cell carcinoma 17 months later following right nephrectomy and inferior vena cava resection. The tumor was located in the segment 6 of the liver

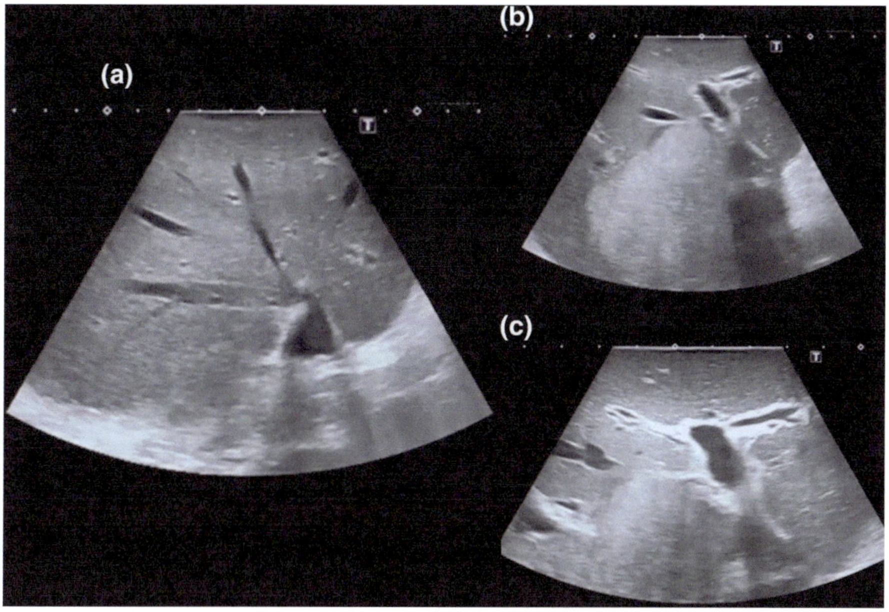

Fig. 11.8 Intraoperative ultrasonography. **a** The right hepatic vein was not involved by the tumor. **b**, **c** The right portal branch and the middle hepatic vein were involved by the tumor. There was a thrombus in the right portal branch

TVE, Venovenous Bypass, and In Situ Hypothermic Perfusion of the Liver

The same surgical incision as performed in the first surgery was used (Figs. 11.9, 11.10, and 11.11). In situ hypothermic perfusion of the liver was initiated early in the procedure before hepatic transection. The first step was to install the venovenous bypass from the inferior mesenteric vein and the femoral vein to the left internal jugular vein or the left axillary vein. The femoral vein and the left axillary vein were punctured under ultrasound guidance, and percutaneous catheters were installed. The second step was to gain vascular control at two different levels: infrahepatic/infrarenal at the junction of the lower part of the replaced IVC and the infrarenal IVC, and supradiaphragmatic/intrapericardic as described above. The portal triad was control as usual. After venovenous bypass and TVE, the portal vein was catheterized above the portal triad clamp, and Custodiol solution cooled to 4 °C was used for in situ hypothermic perfusion of the liver (Fig. 11.10b, c). The volume of infusion ranged from 2 to 4 L, which was placed at 50 cm above the level of the operating table. The right hepatic vein was dissected extrahepatic ally and a veinotomy was made in the right hepatic vein between the two caval clamps for placement of a 30-French catheter to drain the effluent perfusate. The effluent perfusate was used to prevent induced systemic hypothermia, particularly when the diaphragm was opened. The liver temperature was measured by deep insertion of a

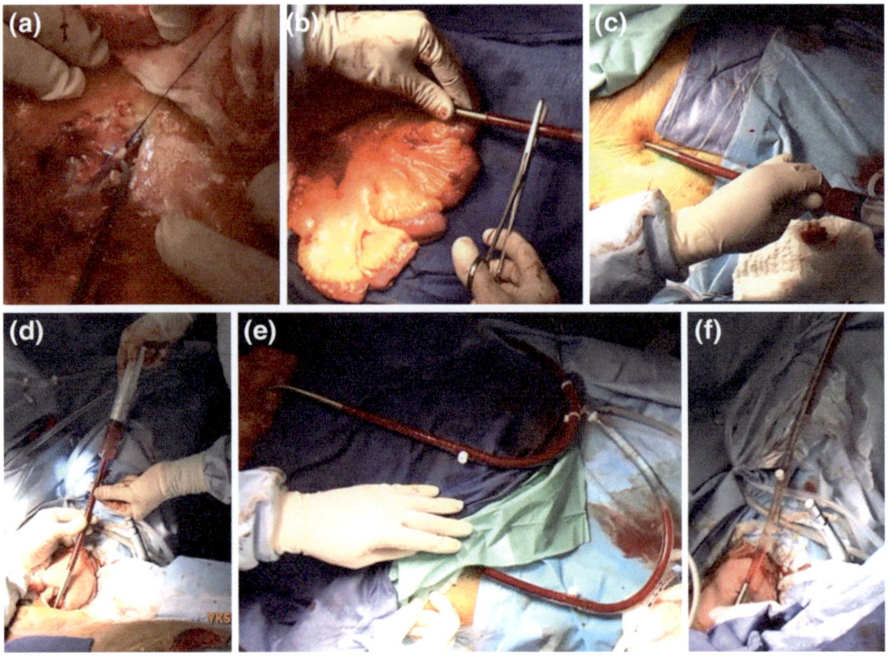

Fig. 11.9 Venovenous bypass. **a**, **b** Dissection and cannulation of the inferior mesenteric vein. **c** Percutaneous cannulation of the right femoral vein. **d** Percutaneous cannulation of the left axillary vein. **e**, **f** Extracorporeal circulation

thermistor probe thermometer into the future liver remnant. Topical cooling of the liver remnant was also applied.

In our patient, an anterior approach technique was performed because of the potential adherence between the posterior mass and the replaced IVC. Then, the right liver was fully mobilized to expose the root of the right hepatic vein, which was ligated and divided. When the liver transection was completed, the liver was flushed with serum albumin (500 mL) via the portal vein. The cannula of portal perfusion and the caval drainage were then removed. The portal vein hole was rinsed with heparin and sutured transversally with interrupted vascular sutures to prevent stenosis. Circulation was then restored as for standard TVE. The portal cannula of the bypass was clamped quickly upon revascularization of the remaining left liver to optimize portal reperfusion. The bypass was stopped and removed when hemodynamic stability was confirmed by the anesthesiologists. Doppler ultrasonography was used to assess the patency of vessels. The Doppler imaging also helped optimize the position of the remaining liver by preventing any vascular kinking of the hepatic veins or the suprahepatic vena cava. The venovenous bypass lasted 120 min and TVE 55 min. Blood loss was 1000 ml. The patient received two units of packed red blood cells.

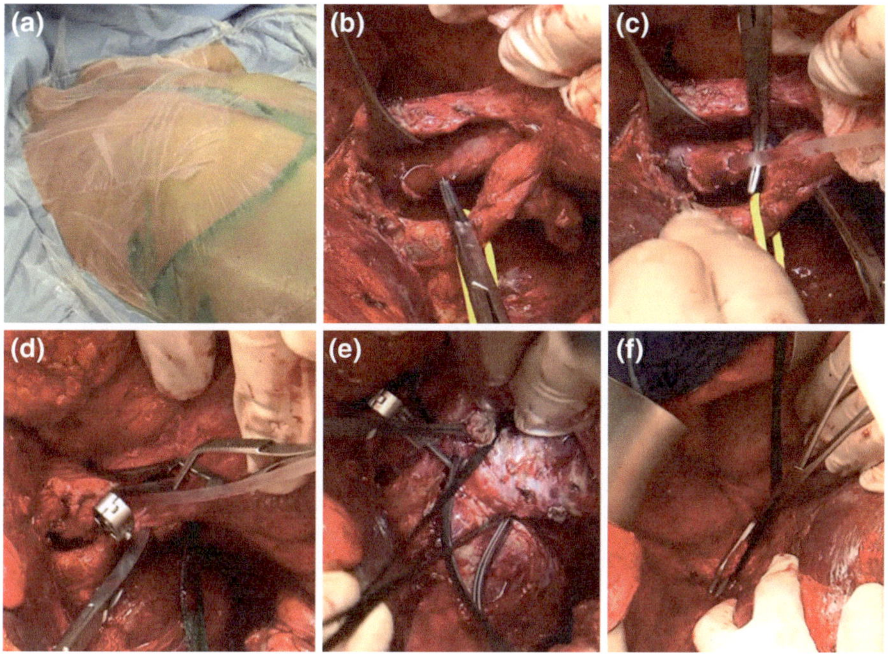

Fig. 11.10 **a** Right subcostal incision combined to midline incision. **b**, **c** The portal vein was catheterized above the portal triad clamp. **d** Clamping of the portal triad. **e** Infrahepatic inferior vena cava clamping (below the prosthetic graft). **f** Intrapericardial vena cava clamping

Fig. 11.11 The clamp was located below the prosthetic graft

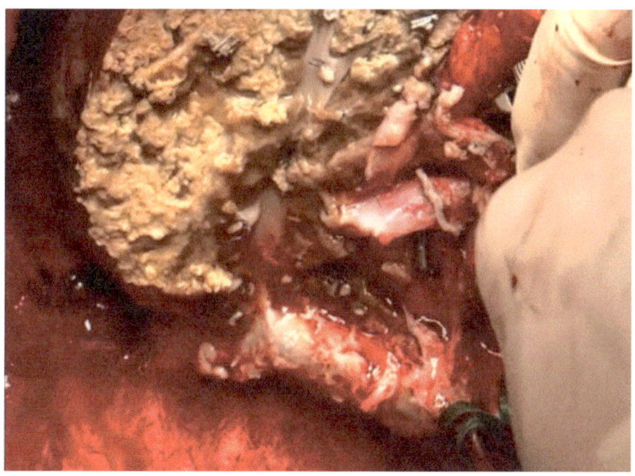

Discussion

The main technical aspect which is the in situ hypothermic technique with the use of venovenous bypass of this procedure could be discussed. With the advance in surgical technique, liver resection under hypothermic perfusion remains rare (3% in our experience). It is mainly indicated for tumors invading the cavo-hepatic junction and if complex vascular reconstruction is required for the remnant liver. The majority of patients with "limited vascular invasion or contact" can nowadays be operated on safely with intermittent occlusion of the hepatic pedicle. Another possibility could be to start the hepatic transection under intermittent clamping of the hepatic pedicle and apply short TVE when approaching the vascular contact with the replaced IVC. In this case, isolated occlusion of the replaced IVC should be avoided to limit postoperative IVC thrombosis.

Alternatives Approaches

- The decision to proceed for IVC reconstruction should depend upon preoperative criteria (lower extremity edema, collateral venous pathways on the radiological imaging).
- The IVC reconstruction is not without postoperative risks, including thrombosis and sepsis.
- In case of IVC resection combined with right nephrectomy, left renal vein reconstruction is not mandatory. But in case of IVC resection with left nephrectomy, right renal vein reconstruction is mandatory.

Short-Term Outcome

The postoperative course was uneventful. The patient did not experience postoperative liver failure or acute kidney injury. The liver tests were normal at discharge. Postoperative MDCT was normal and show patency of the replaced IVC (Fig. 11.12).

In our reported experience, this complex procedure performed for primary and secondary liver tumors achieved a five-year survival rate of 30.4% and a high 90-day mortality of 19.5% [13]. Risk factors for postoperative mortality include Charlson comorbidity index ≥ 3 (indicating at least 2 comorbid conditions), maximum tumor diameter ≥ 10 cm, and the presence of 50/50 criteria on postoperative day 5 were independent predictors of surgical mortality measured at 90 days.

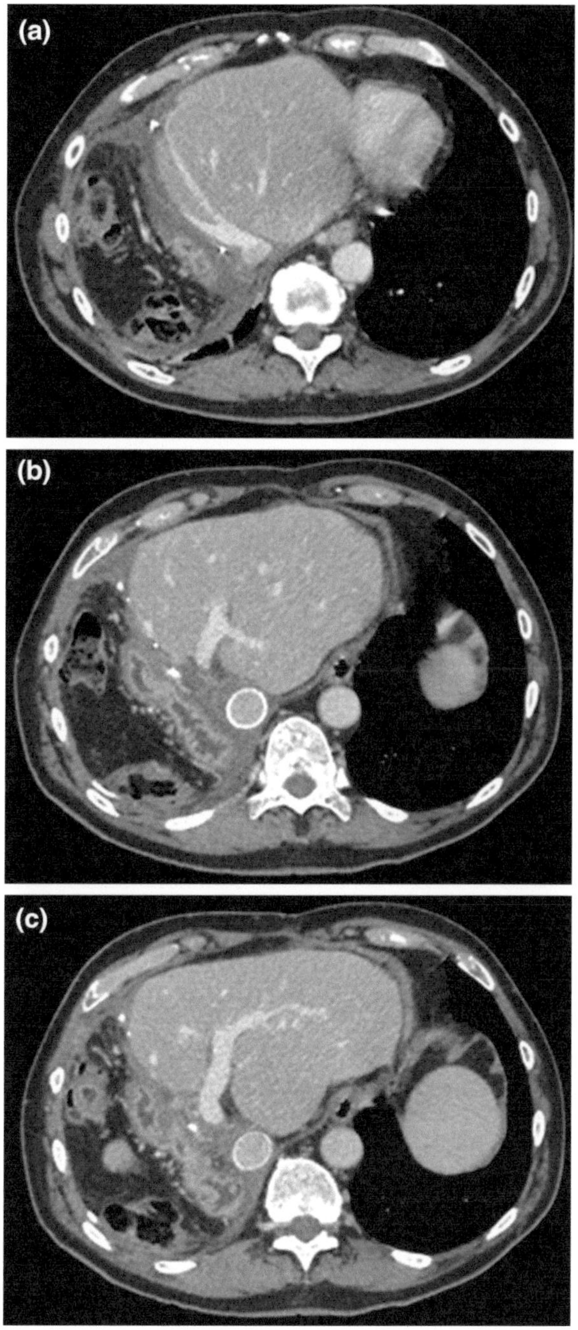

Fig. 11.12 Postoperative computed tomography after right hepatectomy

Long-Term Outcome

RCC can metastasize to almost every organ. Metastatic RCC represent 30% of RCC at diagnosis and occur in 15–30% following nephrectomy [25–27]. The most common metastatic sites include lung (50–60%), bone (30–40%), liver (30–40%), and brain (5%). Unusual sites of metastases include thyroid, pancreas, muscle, and skin [28]. To date, the European Association of Urology recommended in their guidelines that surgical resection of metastases from RCC should be considered for most metastatic sites, with the exception of brain and bones. To date, surgical resection remains the only curative treatment of metastases from RCC with a five-year survival rate of 30–45% for patients who underwent surgical resection of metastases whatever the sites [29–32]. Surgery for the metastases from RCC can be proposed if it concerns an isolated metastatic site and if complete resection can be achieved regardless of the length of the disease-free interval (synchronous vs. metachronous) [33]. Of course, a longer disease-free interval following nephrectomy has been shown to be a positive prognostic factor [34].

Survival data reported from targeted therapy clinical trials showed a median overall survival between 26.4 and 32 months for patients who received sunitinib or combined sunitinib and everolimus [35, 36].

Liver metastases from RCC, like any other metastatic lesions, can be treated by surgery, systemic chemotherapy, radiotherapy, percutaneous ablation, and transarterial chemoembolization. Surgical resection of liver metastases from RCC achieved survival rates of 26–54% at 3 years with a median survival time reaching 48 months. The three-year survival rates for patients treated by chemotherapy and interferon were 15 and 48%, respectively [28]. Although TACE can result in a favorable local tumor response, survival rates are less favorable than those achieved by surgery with one- and two-year survival rates (from the start of treatment) for patients treated with TACE of 31 and 6%, respectively, with a median survival time of 8.8 months [37].

In our case, the patient recurred in the liver 15 months later following right nephrectomy and IVC thrombectomy for a RCC with tumor thrombus extending into the retrohepatic IVC.

Global Pearls

- The anatomic level of the tumor thrombus within the inferior vena cava according to the classification by Neves and Zincke dictates the surgical strategy.
- Surgery of the IVC requiring infrahepatic and retrohepatic inferior vena cava (below the level of the hepatic veins) control are usually well tolerated in terms of hemodynamics, especially when the inferior vena cava is completely obstructed by the thrombus. While surgery of the IVC combined with standard total vascular exclusion of the liver can induce hemodynamic consequences with a risk of postoperative liver failure.

- Use of venovenous bypass and hypothermic perfusion of the liver can decrease the risk of postoperative liver failure, particularly when a vascular reconstruction is needed or standard vascular exclusion of the liver is planned to last >60 min.

References

1. Zisman A, Pantuck AJ, Chao DH, Wieder JA, Dorey F, Said JW, et al. Renal cell carcinoma with tumor thrombus: is cytoreductive nephrectomy for advanced disease associated with an increased complication rate? J Urol. 2002;168(3):962–7.
2. Lambert EH, Pierorazio PM, Shabsigh A, Olsson CA, Benson MC, McKiernan JM. Prognostic risk stratification and clinical outcomes in patients undergoing surgical treatment for renal cell carcinoma with vascular tumor thrombus. Urology. 2007;69(6):1054–8.
3. Ciancio G, Soloway M. Renal cell carcinoma invading the hepatic veins. Cancer. 2001;92 (7):1836–42.
4. Parekh DJ, Cookson MS, Chapman W, Harrell F Jr, Wells N, Chang SS, et al. Renal cell carcinoma with renal vein and inferior vena caval involvement: clinicopathological features, surgical techniques and outcomes. J Urol. 2005;173(6):1897–902.
5. Gupta K, Miller JD, Li JZ, Russell MW, Charbonneau C. Epidemiologic and socioeconomic burden of metastatic renal cell carcinoma (mRCC): a literature review. Cancer Treat Rev. 2008;34(3):193–205.
6. Boorjian SA, Blute ML. Surgery for vena caval tumor extension in renal cancer. Curr Opin Urol. 2009;19(5):473–7.
7. Pouliot F, Shuch B, Larochelle JC, Pantuck A, Belldegrun AS. Contemporary management of renal tumors with venous tumor thrombus. J Urol. 2010;184(3):833–41; quiz 1235.
8. Calero A, Armstrong PA. Renal cell carcinoma accompanied by venous invasion and inferior vena cava thrombus: classification and operative strategies for the vascular surgeon. Semin Vasc Surg. 2014;26(4):219–25.
9. Lawrentschuk N, Gani J, Riordan R, Esler S, Bolton DM. Multidetector computed tomography vs magnetic resonance imaging for defining the upper limit of tumour thrombus in renal cell carcinoma: a study and review. BJU Int. 2005;96(3):291–5.
10. Sonin AH, Mazer MJ, Powers TA. Obstruction of the inferior vena cava: a multiple-modality demonstration of causes, manifestations, and collateral pathways. Radiographics. 1992;12(2): 309–22.
11. Neves RJ, Zincke H. Surgical treatment of renal cancer with vena cava extension. Br J Urol. 1987;59(5):390–5.
12. Azoulay D, Andreani P, Maggi U, Salloum C, Perdigao F, Sebagh M, et al. Combined liver resection and reconstruction of the supra-renal vena cava: the Paul Brousse experience. Ann Surg. 2006;244(1):80–8.
13. Azoulay D, Lim C, Salloum C, Andreani P, Maggi U, Bartelmaos T, et al. Complex Liver resection using standard total vascular exclusion, venovenous bypass, and in situ hypothermic portal perfusion: an audit of 77 consecutive cases. Ann Surg. 2014;262(1):93–104.
14. Le Treut YP, Fara R, Barbier L, Delpero JR, Arellano N, Hardwigsen J. Transdiaphragmatic extrapericardial approach of the inferior vena cava. J Am Coll Surg. 2013;217(5):e41–3.

15. Oken AC, Frank SM, Merritt WT, Fair J, Klein A, Burdick J, et al. A new percutaneous technique for establishing venous bypass access in orthotopic liver transplantation. J Cardiothorac Vasc Anesth. 1994;8(1):58–60.
16. Gonzalez J, Gorin MA, Garcia-Roig M, Ciancio G. Inferior vena cava resection and reconstruction: technical considerations in the surgical management of renal cell carcinoma with tumor thrombus. Urol Oncol. 2013;32(1):34.e19–26.
17. Blute ML, Leibovich BC, Lohse CM, Cheville JC, Zincke H. The Mayo Clinic experience with surgical management, complications and outcome for patients with renal cell carcinoma and venous tumour thrombus. BJU Int. 2004;94(1):33–41.
18. Boorjian SA, Sengupta S, Blute ML. Renal cell carcinoma: vena caval involvement. BJU Int. 2007;99(5 Pt B):1239–44.
19. Karnes RJ, Blute ML. Surgery insight: management of renal cell carcinoma with associated inferior vena cava thrombus. Nat Clin Pract Urol. 2008;5(6):329–39.
20. Klatte T, Pantuck AJ, Riggs SB, Kleid MD, Shuch B, Zomorodian N, et al. Prognostic factors for renal cell carcinoma with tumor thrombus extension. J Urol. 2007;178(4 Pt 1):1189–95; discussion 1195.
21. Moinzadeh A, Libertino JA. Prognostic significance of tumor thrombus level in patients with renal cell carcinoma and venous tumor thrombus extension. Is all T3b the same? J Urol. 2004;171(2 Pt 1):598–601.
22. Sweeney P, Wood CG, Pisters LL, Slaton JW, Vaporciyan A, Munsell M, et al. Surgical management of renal cell carcinoma associated with complex inferior vena caval thrombi. Urol Oncol. 2003;21(5):327–33.
23. Rini BI, Campbell SC, Escudier B. Renal cell carcinoma. Lancet. 2009;373(9669):1119–32.
24. Wagner B, Patard JJ, Mejean A, Bensalah K, Verhoest G, Zigeuner R, et al. Prognostic value of renal vein and inferior vena cava involvement in renal cell carcinoma. Eur Urol. 2009;55(2):452–9.
25. Pantuck AJ, Zisman A, Belldegrun AS. The changing natural history of renal cell carcinoma. J Urol. 2001;166(5):1611–23.
26. Kattan MW, Reuter V, Motzer RJ, Katz J, Russo P. A postoperative prognostic nomogram for renal cell carcinoma. J Urol. 2001;166(1):63–7.
27. Sorbellini M, Kattan MW, Snyder ME, Reuter V, Motzer R, Goetzl M, et al. A postoperative prognostic nomogram predicting recurrence for patients with conventional clear cell renal cell carcinoma. J Urol. 2005;173(1):48–51.
28. Motzer RJ, Bander NH, Nanus DM. Renal-cell carcinoma. N Engl J Med. 1996;335(12):865–75.
29. Eggener SE, Yossepowitch O, Kundu S, Motzer RJ, Russo P. Risk score and metastasectomy independently impact prognosis of patients with recurrent renal cell carcinoma. J Urol. 2008;180(3):873–8; discussion 878.
30. Kavolius JP, Mastorakos DP, Pavlovich C, Russo P, Burt ME, Brady MS. Resection of metastatic renal cell carcinoma. J Clin Oncol. 1998;16(6):2261–6.
31. Kierney PC, van Heerden JA, Segura JW, Weaver AL. Surgeon's role in the management of solitary renal cell carcinoma metastases occurring subsequent to initial curative nephrectomy: an institutional review. Ann Surg Oncol. 1994;1(4):345–52.
32. Motzer RJ, Bacik J, Schwartz LH, Reuter V, Russo P, Marion S, et al. Prognostic factors for survival in previously treated patients with metastatic renal cell carcinoma. J Clin Oncol. 2004;22(3):454–63.
33. Jakubowski CD, Vertosick EA, Untch BR, et al. Complete metastasectomy for renal cell carcinoma: comparison of five solid organ sites. J Surg Oncol. 2016;114(3):375–9.
34. Hofmann HS, Neef H, Krohe K, Andreev P, Silber RE. Prognostic factors and survival after pulmonary resection of metastatic renal cell carcinoma. Eur Urol. 2005;48(1):77–81; discussion 81–2.
35. Motzer RJ, Hutson TE, Tomczak P, Michaelson MD, Bukowski RM, Oudard S, et al. Overall survival and updated results for sunitinib compared with interferon alfa in patients with metastatic renal cell carcinoma. J Clin Oncol. 2009;27(22):3584–90.

36. Motzer RJ, Barrios CH, Kim TM, Falcon S, Cosgriff T, Harker WG, et al. Phase II randomized trial comparing sequential first-line everolimus and second-line sunitinib versus first-line sunitinib and second-line everolimus in patients with metastatic renal cell carcinoma. J Clin Oncol. 2014;32(25):2765–72.
37. Nabil M, Gruber T, Yakoub D, Ackermann H, Zangos S, Vogl TJ. Repetitive transarterial chemoembolization (TACE) of liver metastases from renal cell carcinoma: local control and survival results. Eur Radiol. 2008;18(7):1456–63.

Part II
Gallbladder/Bile Duct

Hilar Cholangiocarcinoma with Portal Vein Involvement

12

Ryan T. Groeschl and David M. Nagorney

Case Presentation

A 64-year-old man with several years of diarrhea and crampy abdominal pain underwent CT enterography. Assessment of the liver demonstrated severe atrophy of the left lobe, with the absence of a visible left portal vein (Fig. 12.1). He was not jaundiced. Serum bilirubin was normal and CA 19-9 was 76 U/mL. His past medical and surgical history was non-contributory.

A contrast-enhanced MRI with MRCP was obtained to further characterize the liver and bile ducts, particularly at the hepatic hilus. MRI revealed a distinct 2.7 cm mass in the left lobe that caused a tight stenosis of the main left hepatic duct without visualization of the left portal vein (Fig. 12.2). There was also irregular contour of the common hepatic duct on MRCP. The clinical diagnosis was type IIIb HC. There was no evidence of distant disease on either CT or MRI. No effort was made to obtain a tissue diagnosis preoperatively.

The complete absence of a visible left portal vein supported the preoperative assumption of malignant obstruction of the left portal vein. The presence of lobar hepatic atrophy and the absence of jaundice and cholangitis obviated the need for any preoperative intervention. An en-bloc left hepatectomy, extrahepatic bile duct resection, regional lymphadenectomy, and Roux-en-Y hepaticojejunostomy were performed. Intraoperatively, the malignant involvement of the left portal vein

R.T. Groeschl (✉) · D.M. Nagorney
Department of Surgery, Mayo Clinic, 200 First Street SW, Rochester, MN 55905, USA
e-mail: groeschl.ryan@mayo.edu

D.M. Nagorney
e-mail: nagorney.david@mayo.edu

T.M. Pawlik et al. (eds.), *Case-Based Lessons in the Management of Complex Hepato-Pancreato-Biliary Surgery*, DOI 10.1007/978-3-319-50868-9_12

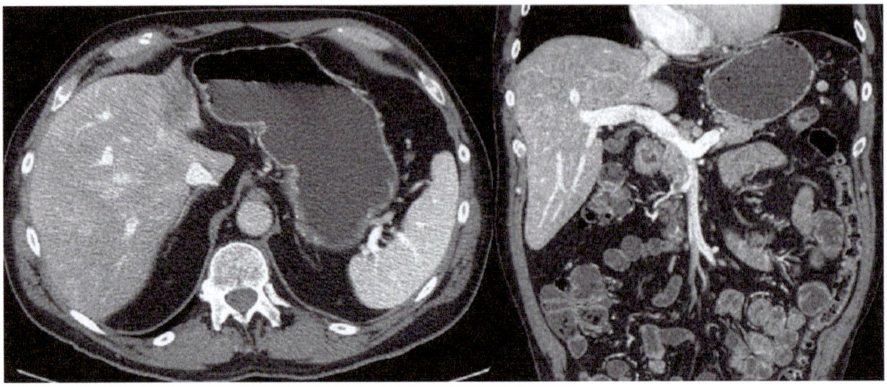

Fig. 12.1 CT showing incidental finding of significant left liver atrophy, and question of mass in remaining left lobe (*left*). The portal vein appears patent and normal into the right lobe, but there is no apparent origin of any remaining left portal vein (*right*)

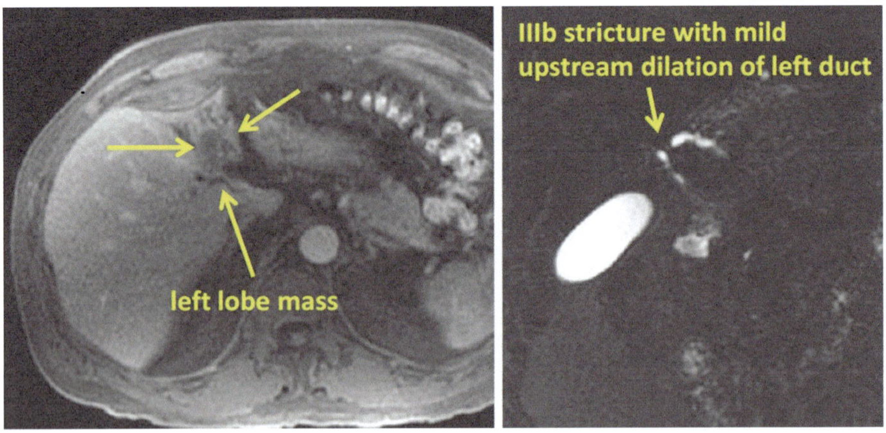

Fig. 12.2 MRI demonstrates a more obvious mass with upstream biliary dilation in the remaining left lobe (*left*). MRCP illustrates a dominant central IIIb stricture, with complete stenosis of the main left hepatic duct, and irregularity of the common hepatic duct (*right*)

extended into the right portal vein. Accordingly, a 2-cm segment of portal vein inclusive of the right portal venous origin was resected and reconstructed by an end-to-end veno-venostomy.

Final pathology showed a single focus of moderately differentiated HC with mixed mass-forming ($4.0 \times 3.5 \times 1.9$ cm) and periductal infiltrating components involving the common hepatic and left hepatic ducts. Margins were negative, with the closest margin 1 mm from the cut liver parenchyma. The tumor invaded periductal adipose tissue (T4). Seven lymph nodes were identified, all negative for tumor. Fourteen months after surgery, he has no evidence of recurrent cancer.

Diagnosis and Assessment

Our patient presented with atypical nonspecific symptoms for HC. The diagnosis was made incidentally on imaging performed for other reasons. More typically, symptoms of HC include jaundice, anorexia, fatigue, right upper quadrant pain, or occasionally cholangitis. The majority (50–60%) of cholangiocarcinomas develop at the confluence of the lobar bile ducts in the hepatic hilum. HC has several growth patterns, including mass-forming (exophytic), sclerosing (infiltrative growth along involved ducts), papillary (intraductal-growing), or any combination of the above [1, 2]. Nearly 80% of HC have a locally infiltrative component [3]. The primary differential diagnosis includes primary sclerosing cholangitis (PSC), IgG-4 cholangiopathy, HCC with an atypical periductal extension, and idiopathic biliary strictures. Risk factors for the development of HC include advanced age, PSC, longstanding choledocholithiasis, biliary adenoma or papillomatosis, Caroli's disease, choledochal cysts, smoking, parasitic infestation of the biliary tract, and chronic carriers of typhoid [2].

Serologic testing will often (but not always) reveal evidence of biliary obstruction: increased total and direct bilirubin levels with or without mild transaminase elevation or a rise in alkaline phosphatase or gamma-glutamyl transferase. Of all tumor markers studied to date, carbohydrate antigen 19-9 (CA 19-9) is the most sensitive and specific [2]. Jaundice from bile duct obstruction additionally increases CA 19-9. The degree of serum elevation of CA 19-9 correlates adversely with prognosis, particularly after jaundice is resolved [4].

Noninvasive imaging with ultrasonography, CT, and, increasingly, MRI/MRCP, are the most useful studies to evaluate the presence and extent of HC. These modalities can identify the site and size of HC, define transitions from dilated to non-dilated biliary trees, and often define fully the involvement of the adjacent lobar hepatic arteries and portal veins. Endoscopic retrograde cholangiography (ERC) and percutaneous transhepatic cholangiography (PTC) are commonly employed to clarify the anatomy of the biliary system. PTC better defines the intrahepatic ductal system. Both methods provide access for biliary intubation and decompression to resolve jaundice preoperatively. This access to the bile ducts also allows for brushings for cytology and fluorescence in situ hybridization (FISH) and direct biopsy for diagnosis. Endoscopic ultrasound (EUS) can be used to characterize and sample tissue in the hepatic hilus or regional lymph nodes.

Cytology alone with a clear diagnosis of HC has a sensitivity of only 15%, and even when combined with samples suspicious for malignancy, the sensitivity only rises to 48% [5]. The addition of FISH to assess for aneusomy, particularly polysomy, increases sensitivity to 58% and specificity up to 93% [5].

Technical Pearls for Portal Vein Reconstruction after Resection of HC

- For type IIIa HC requiring portal vein resection, anticipate the need for interposition grafting as primary end-to-end repair is often not feasible.

- For type IIIb HC, mobilize the main portal vein to its origin behind the pancreatic neck—this will allow primary end-to-end anastomosis in almost all cases.
- During primary end-to-end anastomosis, spatulate of the distal lobar portal vein if size mismatch is present, and parachute the anastomosis (avoid pulling tension on the suture and approximating the vessel ends until all throws for the back wall of the anastomosis have been completed).

Management and Outcomes

Candidacy for operation depends on patient features as well as cancer characteristics on imaging. Surgical candidates must have an adequate clinical performance status (>50% of normal) and compensated comorbidity. Exclusion of clinical frailty is mandatory. In fact, even modern resection for HC (hepatectomy and en-bloc radical bile duct resection with hepaticojejunostomy) is associated with a 5–10% mortality rate, and 40–50% morbidity rate. The primary goal of surgical resection must be an R0 resection. Invasive HC at the resection margin consistently has been the factor most associated with adverse long-term survival. Consequently, in planning R0 resections, a clear definition of portal venous and hepatic arterial involvement is mandatory before resection and reconstruction is undertaken [3]. Failure to recognize and define vascular involvement preoperatively can lead to aborting potentially curative attempts at resection in some patients. Vascular reconstruction of the portal vein is undertaken most frequently. Although primary end-to-end reconstruction is preferable, various conduits including autologous vein (saphenous, left renal, internal jugular, internal iliac), cadaveric vein, polytetrafluoroethylene grafts, bovine pericardium, and even peritoneum can be used. No current evidence strongly favors a superior conduit.

The management of HC should always be multidisciplinary. Regardless, non-surgical therapies have had limited efficacy, and resection remains key to cure. Due to the low incidence of HC, neither neoadjuvant nor adjuvant therapy has been evaluated in randomized clinical trials. Although not specific for HC, the ABC-02 trial (n = 410 patients) conducted in the United Kingdom has established combination gemcitabine and cisplatin (Gem/Cis) as the chemotherapeutic standard of care for locally advanced and metastatic biliary tract cancer [6]. Median progression-free survival on Gem/Cis was 8.0 months compared to 5.0 months on gemcitabine alone ($p < 0.001$), and median overall survival was 11.7 months versus 8.1 months, respectively ($p < 0.001$). Unfortunately, all patients progressed and there were no survivors beyond 32 months. Some patients with locally unresectable HC have been treated selectively by external beam radiation, but long-term survival is rare even with boost intraoperative irradiation. Concurrent chemoradiotherapy may afford longer overall survival and progression-free survival compared to radiotherapy alone [7].

As stated previously, surgical treatment for HC is preferred, and several hepatobiliary factors must be addressed for proper patient selection. Importantly, an adequate liver remnant must be expected. The expected hepatic remnant volume should exceed 30% and must provide adequate hepatic function. Jaundice in the remnant should be resolved by stenting of the remnant duct. Cholangitis, whether present at diagnosis or occurring after stenting, is treated with antibiotics and stent exchange as necessary before resection. Inadequate remnant volume dictates portal venous embolization of the contralateral lobe. With R0 resection, long-term (5 to 8 years) recurrence-free survival can be achieved in 20–25% of patients [8, 9].

Current Controversies Regarding Resection of HC

- The "no-touch" technique:
  - Proponents of this technique do not dissect portal venous or hepatic arterial branches away from the bile duct hilum, and resect the portal vein en-bloc with an extended right hepatectomy. This approach has claimed a 5-year survival rate of 61%.
  - Opponents of this approach argue a low rate of radial margin involvement during routine dissection, and cite the 8% perioperative mortality associated with "no-touch" resections.

- Questions related to liver transplantation for HC:
  - Generally, if a resection can technically be performed, it is favored over transplantation. Are there some patients with de novo HC who would benefit more from transplantation?
  - Transplantation for HC in the setting of PSC yields a better 5-year survival than transplantation for de novo HC (79% vs. 63%, respectively). In countries with tight organ allocation pressure, is continued transplantation for de novo HC justified?

The Bismuth–Corlette classification stratifies HC conceptually into four primary types and broadly guides hepatobiliary resection (Fig. 12.3). This classification

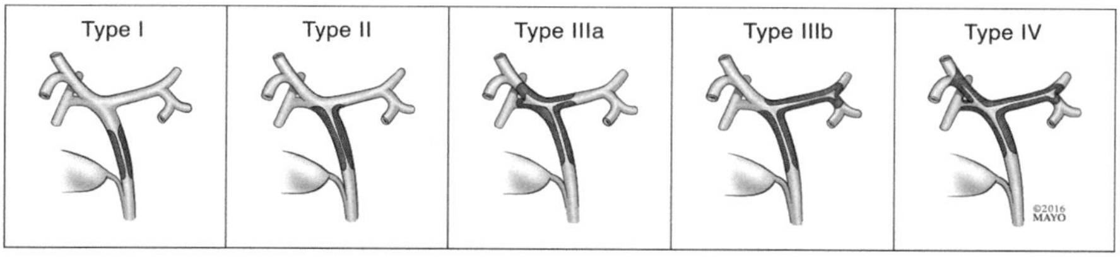

Fig. 12.3 Bismuth–Corlette classification for bile duct involvement by hilar cholangiocarcinoma. Used with permission of Mayo Foundation for Medical Education and Research. All rights reserved

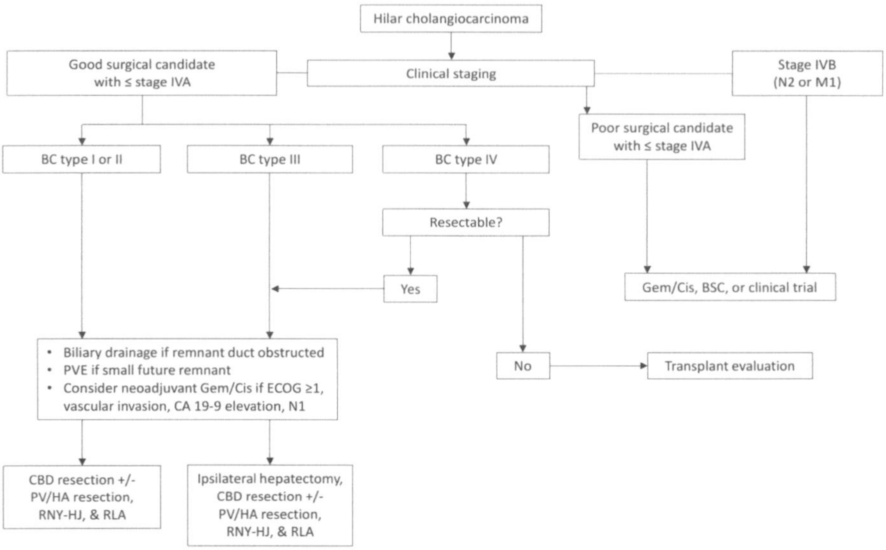

Fig. 12.4 Flow diagram depicting approach to management of patients with hilar cholangiocarcinoma. *BC* Bismuth–Corlette; Gem/Cis gemcitabine and cisplatin; *BSC* best supportive care; *PVE* portal vein embolization; *ECOG* Eastern Cooperative Oncology Group; *CBD* common bile duct; *PV* portal vein; *HA* hepatic artery; *RNY-HJ* Roux-en-Y hepaticojejunostomy; *RLA* regional lymphadenectomy

addresses biliary site and extent only and does not address vascular involvement. Other attempts to classify HC by its specific degree of vascular involvement have been described [10], but are not commonly used in clinical practice. Patients with type I, II, or III HC without distant metastases are candidates for resection. Type IV HC is resectable less frequently than other types of HC (Fig. 12.4). Typically, Roux-en-Y hepaticojejunostomy is used for biliary reconstruction. Because malignant extension into intrahepatic lobar or segmental bile ducts frequently is present and difficult to define intraoperatively, an ipsilateral hemihepatectomy or extended hepatectomy has been recommended over extended proximal bile duct resection alone to improve the chance of R0 resection. Some patients with type IV HC are candidates for resection provided preoperative imaging does not show radial extension into the liver or vasculature at the periphery of the HC and the sectional bile duct is accessible for reconstruction. Moreover, the volume and function of the planned hepatic remnant liver must be adequate with preserved vasculature or vasculature that can be reconstructed. Such patients may be candidates for liver transplantation [11]. Liver transplantation for HC is highly selective and requires the absence of transperitoneal biopsy or prior operative attempts at resection, completion of neoadjuvant chemotherapy and radiation, preoperative exclusion of regional nodal metastases at pretransplant operative staging, and donor availability.

Portal venous and hepatic arterial involvement by HC previously was considered a contraindication to resection. However, from lessons learned regarding resection and reconstruction of these vessels during liver transplantation, portal venous, and hepatic arterial resection and reconstruction have been employed increasingly in selected patients with HC to obtain an R0 resection [3]. Portal venous resection increases the risk of vessel-specific morbidity (odds ratio: 8.8), but does not significantly impact mortality. In contrast, hepatic arterial resection is associated with greater mortality (odds ratio: 4.5) [12]. However, as experience has increased, particularly at referral centers for HC, morbidity and mortality from vascular resection and reconstruction have decreased substantially [13]. The current literature on operative safety for resection of HC with concurrent vascular resection and reconstruction is too heterogeneous to fully interpret, as details of the extent of vascular resection and reconstruction are unclear. Whether small, tangential vein resections (<360° circumference involvement) add significant risk, or whether segmental resections requiring an interposition graft (2 circumferential anastomoses) are more likely to thrombose than end-to-end venous anastomosis is unknown. Common options for patch or interposition graft include left renal vein, internal jugular vein, saphenous vein, internal iliac vein, bovine pericardium, and non-biologic vascular conduits such as polytetrafluoroethylene.

Portal venous reconstruction differs between Bismuth–Corlette types of HC. For any portal vein reconstruction, the main portal vein should be mobilized to its origin behind the neck of the pancreas with ligation of the coronary vein and superior pancreaticoduodenal vein if necessary. Type I and II usually dictate resection and reconstruction of the main portal vein near the bifurcation. Usually a direct end-to-end anastomosis is feasible. For type IIIa HC with portal vein involvement, reconstruction with a direct veno-venostomy usually is feasible and is technically simple to perform for several reasons. First, the biliary hilum is on the right side of the porta hepatis, often sparing the left portal vein. Second, the extrahepatic portion of the left portal vein is also generally longer, providing greater mobility for a primary reconstruction. Usually the caudate lobe branches are divided as the caudate lobe is resected and the commonly encountered parenchymal bridge between segments 4B and 3 under the left portal vein can be divided to increase mobility. Finally, the left portal vein bifurcates from the right portal vein at nearly a right angle. Consequently, resecting the origin or proximal portion of the left portal vein allows the transected main portal vein to directly bridge the resected portion as a hypotenuse to that right angle, allowing an end-to-end anastomosis.

In contrast, involvement of the portal vein by type IIIb HC more often requires interposition grafting, as the main right portal vein is short before its bifurcation and lies in a direct line with the main portal vein. Moreover, right sectional portal veins may arise separately (portal vein trifurcation) which may further preclude mobilization for a direct venous anastomosis. Figure 12.5 provides an illustration of portal vein reconstruction after left trisectionectomy.

Figure 12.6 shows type IIIa HC involving the right portal vein and the portal vein bifurcation. There is size mismatch between the main portal vein and a more

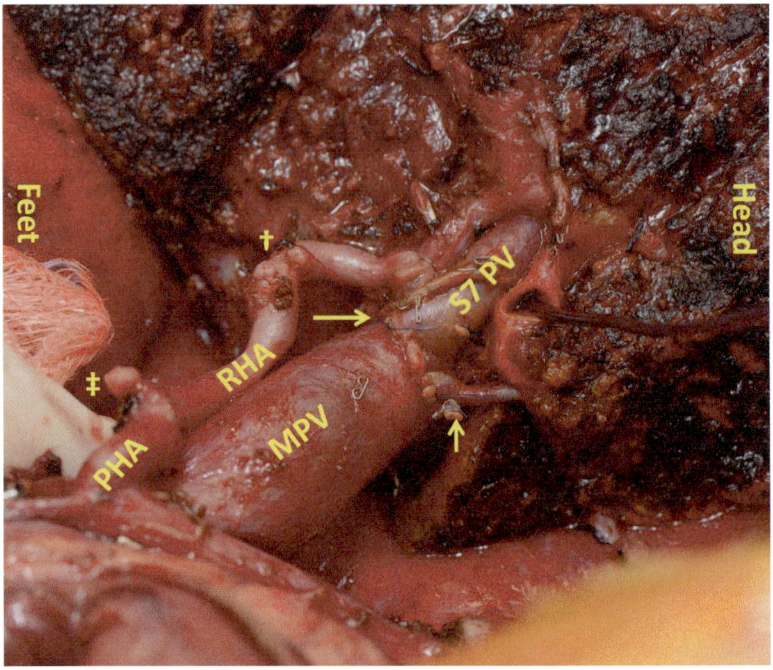

Fig. 12.5 Photograph of vascular inflow to remnant liver (segments 6 & 7) after left trisectionectomy for type IV HC involving the left and right anterior systems. The figure is oriented such that the *right border* represents the cranial direction. *PHA* proper hepatic artery; *RHA* right hepatic artery; ‡ ligated stump of left hepatic artery; † ligated segment 5 & 8 arterial branches; *MPV* main portal vein; *S7 PV* segment 7 portal vein. A large right portal vein branch extends primarily into segment 6, and to a lesser extent segment 7. An anomalous segment 7 portal vein from the right anterior system was preserved during dissection, and reimplanted into the former origin of the left portal vein (*arrows*). The right posterior sectional duct is shown with a probe in its lumen

distal lobar branch that must be addressed at reconstruction. In these instances, spatulation of the distal target vein and parachuting of the main portal vein to the remnant vein can simplify the reconstruction. Although portal venous anatomy is fairly consistent, two main variations are noteworthy: (1) a portal "trifurcation," where the left main, right anterior, and right posterior sectional branches all arise simultaneously; and (2) an early takeoff of the right posterior sectional branch, with the left main and right anterior sectional branches subsequently bifurcating. These anomalies should be anticipated by review of preoperative cross-sectional imaging.

Tumor abutment of the portal vein can be hard to differentiate from true invasion of the portal vein. The authors frequently will make at least a gentle effort to dissect the portal vein free of the tumor, particularly in patients undergoing preoperative PVE where inflammatory reactions develop around the orifice of the embolized vein. Given that R0 resection is the primary goal, these efforts are aborted and

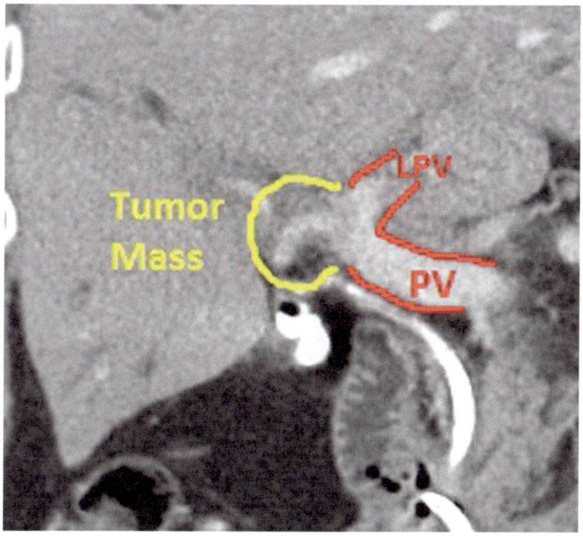

Fig. 12.6 Bismuth–Corlette type IIIa tumor, with occlusion of the main right portal vein and left liver hypertrophy. The left portal vein (LPV) is patent, but stenosed where tumor abuts its origin. The left hepatic artery and a middle hepatic artery (not demonstrated in this image) are uninvolved by tumor. As anticipated, this tumor was resectable with en-bloc full-circumference excision of the main portal vein (PV), with a primary end-to-end reconstruction. Due to size mismatch, the distal vein was spatulated to simplify reconstruction

portal vein resection is undertaken if this dissection proves difficult. Alternatively, to avoid the potential for transection and disseminating HC by such dissection, a "no-touch" resection has been proposed with routine en-bloc resection of the portal vein for type IIIa or right-side predominant type IV HC [14]. The merits of each approach remain controversial. Notably, the survival of patients undergoing portal vein resection has not been affected adversely whether or not the portal vein is histologically invaded by tumor [12].

Preservation of arterial flow to the remnant liver is vital to ensure integrity of the bilioenteric anastomosis. When tumor arterial involvement is present, it is almost always the right lobar hepatic artery, which typically courses immediately posterior to the biliary hilus. For type IIIa HC, this rarely poses a problem unless tumor extends proximally along the artery to compromise left lobar branches. It is generally type IIIb tumors with arterial involvement that will require a reconstruction to preserve arterial flow to a right-sided remnant. As hepatic arterial anatomy is highly variable [15], review of contrast-enhanced cross-sectional imaging is crucial to anticipate the presence of replaced or accessory arteries, assess tumor-vessel involvement, and study the course of the right hepatic artery either anterior or posterior to the bile duct and tumor.

Important preoperative Considerations before Resection of HC

- When a small remnant is anticipated during initial evaluation, PVE of the contralateral liver lobe should be performed.
- If jaundice is present in conjunction with biliary dilation in the remnant, then ductal system must be decompressed with either endobiliary or percutaneous transhepatic stenting.
- Type IV HC can be resected, provided that sectoral target ducts are available for reconstruction.

References

1. Groeschl RT, Gamblin TC. Resection of hilar cholangiocarcinoma. In: Hughes SJ, Mulholland MW, editors. Operative techniques in hepato-pancreato-biliary surgery. Philadelphia: Wolters Kluwer Health; 2015. p. 72–9.
2. Malhi H, Gores GJ. The modern diagnosis and therapy of cholangiocarcinoma. Aliment Pharmacol Ther. 2006;23(9):1287–96.
3. Groeschl RT, Nagorney DM. Portal vein reconstruction during surgery for cholangiocarcinoma. Curr Opin Gastroenterol. 2016;32(3):216–24.
4. Bergquist JR, Ivanics T, Storlie CB, Groeschl RT, Tee MC, Habermann EB, et al. Implications of CA19-9 elevation for survival, staging, and treatment sequencing in intrahepatic cholangiocarcinoma: a national cohort analysis. J Surg Oncol. 2016;114(4):475–82.
5. Razumilava N, Gores GJ. Classification, diagnosis, and management of cholangiocarcinoma. Clin Gastroenterol Hepatol. 2013;11(1):13–21.e1; quiz e3–4.
6. Valle J, Wasan H, Palmer DH, Cunningham D, Anthoney A, Maraveyas A, et al. Cisplatin plus gemcitabine versus gemcitabine for biliary tract cancer. N Engl J Med. 2010;362(14):1273–81.
7. Chen SC, Chen MH, Li CP, Chang PM, Liu CY, Tzeng CH, et al. External beam radiation therapy with or without concurrent chemotherapy for patients with unresectable locally advanced hilar cholangiocarcinoma. Hepatogastroenterology. 2015;62(137):102–7.
8. Croome KP, Rosen CB, Heimbach JK, Nagorney DM. Is liver transplantation appropriate for patients with potentially resectable de novo hilar cholangiocarcinoma? J Am Coll Surg. 2015;221(1):130–9.
9. Groot Koerkamp B, Wiggers JK, Allen PJ, Besselink MG, Blumgart LH, Busch OR, et al. Recurrence rate and pattern of perihilar cholangiocarcinoma after curative intent resection. J Am Coll Surg. 2015;221(6):1041–9.
10. Deoliveira ML, Schulick RD, Nimura Y, Rosen C, Gores G, Neuhaus P, et al. New staging system and a registry for perihilar cholangiocarcinoma. Hepatology. 2011;53(4):1363–71.
11. Heimbach JK, Gores GJ, Haddock MG, Alberts SR, Nyberg SL, Ishitani MB, et al. Liver transplantation for unresectable perihilar cholangiocarcinoma. Semin Liver Dis. 2004;24(2):201–7.
12. Abbas S, Sandroussi C. Systematic review and meta-analysis of the role of vascular resection in the treatment of hilar cholangiocarcinoma. HPB (Oxford). 2013;15(7):492–503.
13. Wu XS, Dong P, Gu J, Li ML, Wu WG, Lu JH, et al. Combined portal vein resection for hilar cholangiocarcinoma: a meta-analysis of comparative studies. J Gastrointest Surg. 2013;17(6):1107–15.

14. Neuhaus P, Jonas S, Settmacher U, Thelen A, Benckert C, Lopez-Hanninen E, et al. Surgical management of proximal bile duct cancer: extended right lobe resection increases resectability and radicality. Langenbecks Arch Surg. 2003;388(3):194–200.
15. Michels NA. Newer anatomy of the liver and its variant blood supply and collateral circulation. Am J Surg. 1966;112(3):337–47.

Hilar Cholangiocarcinoma with Hepatic Artery Involvement

13

Junichi Shindoh and Yoshihiro Sakamoto

Case Presentation

A 56-year-old woman presented to her primary physician with a complaint of jaundice and was referred to a tertiary hepatobiliary center. Computed tomography (CT) revealed a low density mass measuring 2 cm in diameter at the hepatic hilum, obstructing the bifurcation of the hepatic ducts and involving the right hepatic artery (Fig. 13.1a). Serum total bilirubin level was 24.2 mg/dL and she accompanied hepatic dysfunction and cholangitis because of biliary obstruction (AST, 570 IU/L; ALT, 623 IU/L; alkaline phosphatase, 3,332 IU/L; and C-reactive protein, 5.3 mg/dL). Serum level of carcinoembryonic antigen was 2.6 ng/dL and CA19-9 was 3,457 U/mL, respectively.

Percutaneous transhepatic biliary drainage (PTBD) was emergently performed from the biliary branch for Segment III with initial planning of subsequent extended right hepatectomy considering the tumor location and involvement of the right hepatic artery by the tumor. At 14 days after the PTBD, however, obstructive jaundice sustained with serum biliary level of 11 mg/dL. Contrast-enhanced CT for reevaluation revealed further extension of the tumor toward the left hepatic duct and the right paramedian biliary branch (Fig. 13.1b). Because only the right lateral biliary branch seemed to be intact at this point, the surgical plan needed to be

J. Shindoh (✉)
Hepatobiliary-Pancreatic Surgery Division, Department of Gastroenterological Surgery, Toranomon Hospital, 2-2-2 Toranomon, Minato-Ku, Tokyo 105-8470, Japan
e-mail: shindou-tky@umin.ac.jp

Y. Sakamoto
Hepato-Biliary-Pancreatic Surgery Division, University of Tokyo Hospital, 7-3-1 Hongo, Bunkyo-Ku, Tokyo 113-8655, Japan
e-mail: yosakamo-tky@umin.ac.jp

T.M. Pawlik et al. (eds.), *Case-Based Lessons in the Management of Complex Hepato-Pancreato-Biliary Surgery*, DOI 10.1007/978-3-319-50868-9_13

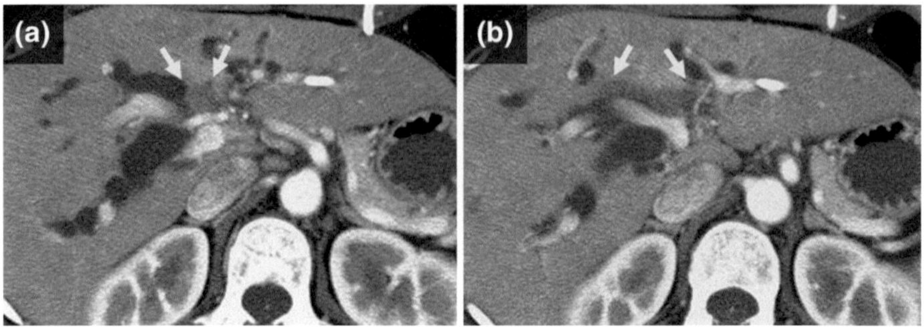

Fig. 13.1 Preoperative computed tomography. **a** at presentation; **b** at re-evaluation

changed to left trisectionectomy with reconstruction of the right hepatic artery to achieve R0 resection.

After an additional PTBD for the right biliary branches, serum bilirubin level gradually decreased. Percutaneous transhepatic portal vein emblization (PTPE) was subsequently performed when serum bilirubin level reached below 5 mg/dL, and the left and right paramedian portal branches were completely embolized (Fig. 13.2). At 19 days after the PTPE, sufficient hypertrophy of the future liver remnant (i.e., the right lateral sector) was obtained from 34 to 47% to the total liver volume, and the patient proceeded to surgery.

Technical Pearls

- Given the high invasiveness of the surgical procedures for hilar cholangiocarcinoma, careful inspection of distant metastases at laparotomy and intraoperative ultrasonography for exploring the extension of tumor are essential during the initial assessment of resectability.
- Start from a step which can be converted to palliative procedure (e.g., hilar dissection) and leave the "point of no return" (e.g., ligations of major hepatic vessels) until confirming the resectability of tumor.
- Dissect the intact part of the artery as long as possible on either side of the involved part before determining the points to cut the arteries.
- Check the arterial flow with Doppler ultrasound just after arterial anastomosis. If a Doppler pulse is weak, try to drip lidocaine on the arterial wall to relief the vascular spasm. If no improvement is confirmed in the arterial flow, do not hesitate to redo anastomosis.

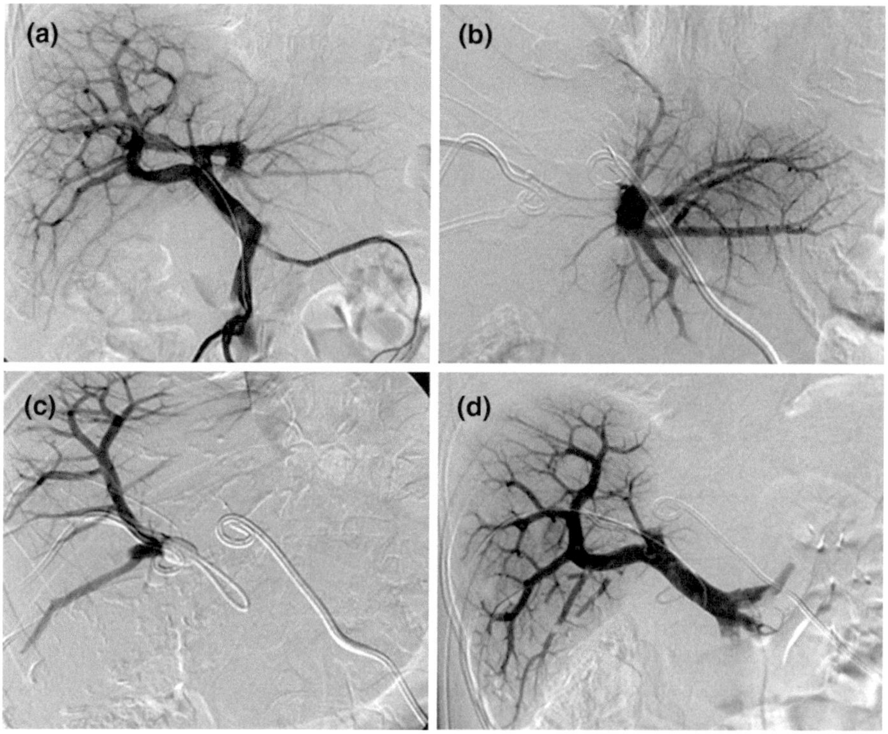

Fig. 13.2 Percutaneous transhepatic portal embolization. **a** Portogram before embolization; **b** embolization of the left portal pedicle; **c** embolization of the right paramedian portal pedicle; **d** portogram after embolization

Surgery and Outcomes

The abdominal cavity was entered with inverted L-shaped incision. No ascites or evidence of peritoneal dissemination was confirmed. Intraoperative ultrasound revealed that the tumor was located at the confluence of bilateral hepatic duct. The left hepatic duct and the root of the right paramedian duct were invaded by the tumor. The right paramedian portal pedicle and the left portal vein were also suspected to be involved by the tumor. The right lateral portal pedicle was independently branched from the main portal trunk and it was free from tumor invasion. Encasement of the right hepatic artery was confirmed as expected on preoperative CT scan (Fig. 13.3).

First, to confirm the resectability of the tumor, the surgical procedure was started from hilar dissection. The common bile duct was divided at the level of the cranial border of the pancreatic body. Frozen section confirmed that the stump of the common bile duct was negative for cancer. With dissecting the hepatoduodenal nodes, the right hepatic artery, the left hepatic artery, and the main portal vein were taped. By flipping up the bile duct and the hepatoduodenal lymphatic basin, the

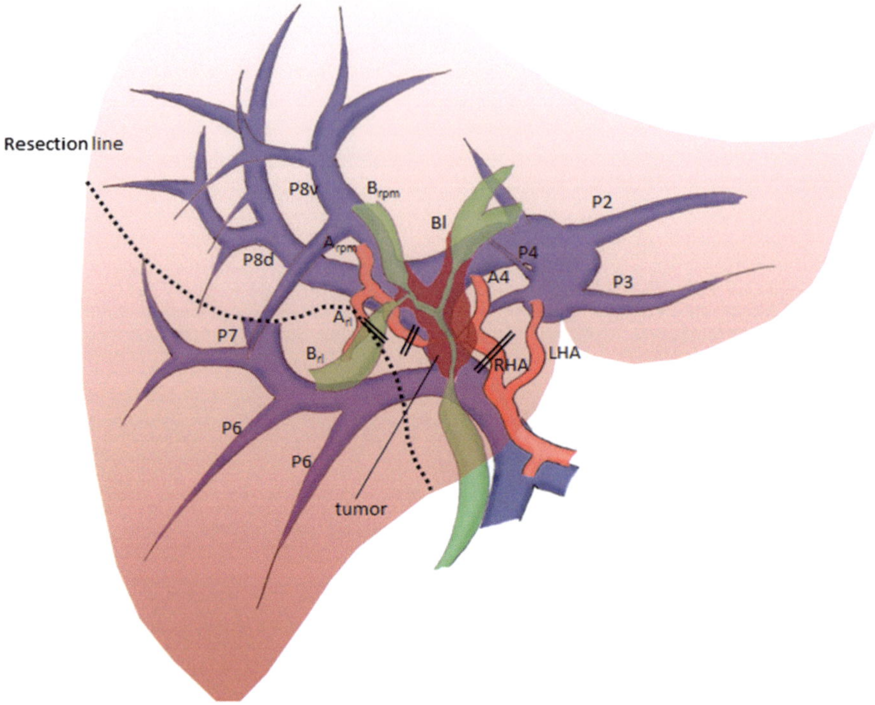

Fig. 13.3 Location of tumor and its relation with intrahepatic vascular structures. *RHA* Right hepatic artery; *LHA* left hepatic artery; A_{rpm} right paramedian arterial branch; A_{rl} right lateral arterial branch; *Bl* left hepatic duct; B_{rpm} right paramedian biliary branch; B_{rl} right lateral biliary branch

exposure of the portal vein was continued toward the hepatic hilum, and the common trunk of the left portal pedicle and the right paramedian portal pedicle was ligated and divided (Fig. 13.4a). Then, the right paramedian arterial branch and the right lateral arterial branch were exposed and taped separately at right border of the hepatic hilum (Fig. 13.4b). After a clamping test, the right paramedian arterial branch was ligated and divided. Demarcation line for the left trisectionectomy was marked with cautery on the surface of the liver.

The liver was completely mobilized. The common trunk of the left and the middle hepatic vein was divided and the stump was closed with running suture. A thick inferior right hepatic vein was preserved to secure the venous drainage for segment VI. Parenchymal transection was then started under vascular occlusion at the hepatic hilum. The liver parenchyma was transected with clamp-crushing method and thin vascular branches were sealed with energy devices. After completion of the hepatic parenchymal transection, the hilar plate was divided at the root of the right lateral sector. Finally, the right hepatic artery and the right lateral

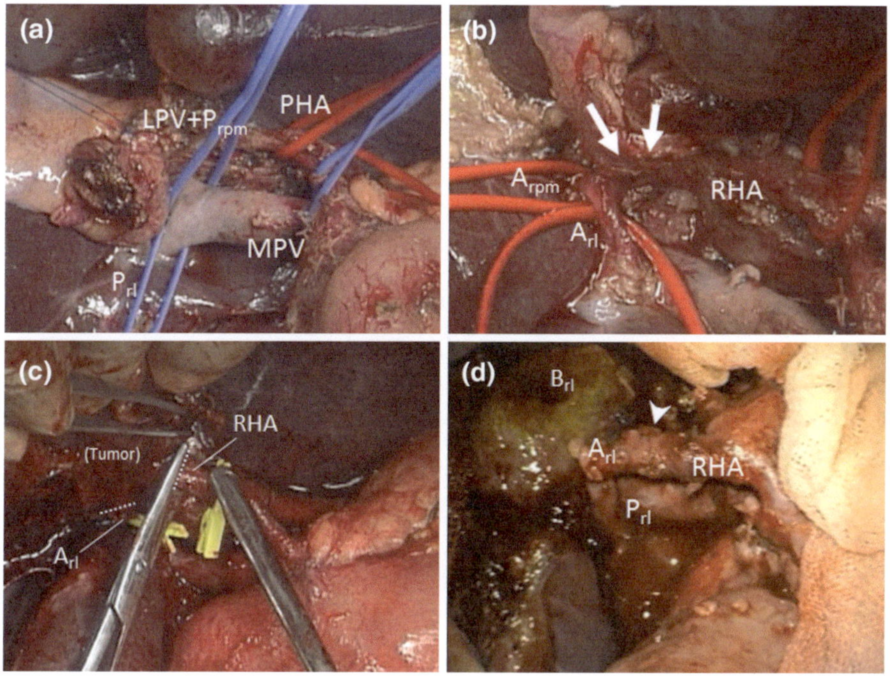

Fig. 13.4 Intraoperative pictures. **a** Dissection of hepatoduodenal ligament and ligation of the common trunk of left portal pedicle and right paramedian portal pedicle. **b** Dissection of right hepatic artery and 2nd-order arterial branches. Center part of the right hepatic artery was encased with the tumor (*arrows*). **c** The right hepatic artery and the right lateral arterial branch were cut at the end of liver resection. **d** Anastomosis between the right hepatic artery and the right paramedian arterial branch was performed (*arrowhead*). *MPV* Main portal vein; *LPV* left portal vein; P_{rpm} right paramedian portal pedicle; P_{rl} right lateral portal pedicle; *PHA* proper hepatic artery; *RHA* right hepatic artery; A_{rpm} right paramedian arterial branch; A_{rl} right lateral arterial branch; B_{rl} right lateral biliary branch

arterial branch were clamped and divided, and the specimen was removed (Fig. 13.4c). Frozen section revealed negative cancer margin at the stump of the right lateral biliary branch. Arterial reconstruction was performed with direct anastomosis between the right hepatic artery and the right lateral arterial branch by a plastic surgeon (Fig. 13.4d). Hepaticojejunostomy was then performed with a Roux-en Y loop (Fig. 13.5).

Operation time was 580 min and blood loss was 1650 ml. Vascular occlusion time for the parenchymal transection was 50 min and no transfusion was performed. Postoperative course was uneventful, and the patient was discharged on postoperative day 18. Pathology revealed hilar cholangiocarcinoma involving the right hepatic artery and the portal vein. Surgical margin was histologically negative for cancer, and no lymph node metastases was observed. The patient developed recurrence in a distant lymph node and bones at nine months after surgery and died

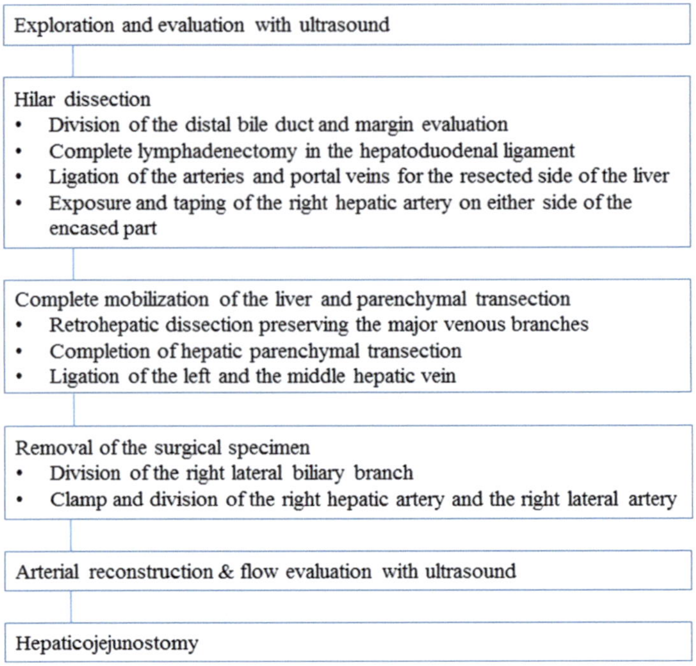

Fig. 13.5 Summary of the procedure

from cancer at 26 months. The reconstructed artery was patent throughout the clinical course.

Alternative Approaches

- If a long segment of the hepatic artery is involved and direct anastomosis between the arterial branches are difficult, the right gastroepiploic artery, the gastroduodenal artery, or the splenic artery can be used as an *in situ* graft. If these arteries are not appropriate for reconstruction, interposition graft should be considered using the saphenous vein or the radial artery, as appropriate.
- If the arterial reconstruction is technically impossible, the artery can be anastomosed with the portal vein as a rescue procedure until arterial collaterals will develop around the hepatic hilum after surgery. The arterioportal shunt should be embolized by interventional radiology approximately one month after surgery to avoid portal hypertension.

Conclusion

Given the common location of tumor and anatomical relation with the right hepatic artery, right-sided hepatectomy is usually adopted in surgical treatment for hilar cholangiocarcinoma. However, left-sided hepatectomy is sometimes required to obtain R0 resection margin according to the distribution of tumor. For such cases, involvement of the right hepatic artery can be an obstacle for resectability of tumor because (1) the right hepatic artery is the primary artery for the right hemiliver (i.e., future liver remnant after left-sided hepatectomy), and (2) it is difficult to expect arterial feeding through the arterial communications in hilar plate after complete dissection and division of the hilar plate.

The efficacy and safety of left-sided hepatectomy for hilar cholangiocarcinoma have been reported in two large series. [1, 2] Natsume et al. reported that left trisectionectomy can be performed with similar mortality rates as left hepatectomy, and it can be a choice for advanced perihilar cholangiocarcinoma, if required. [1] Although left trisectionectomy is a technically demanding procedure, adequate preoperative management can reduce the risk of surgery and such extended procedure would offer higher chance of R0 resection.

Although surgical indications of arterial reconstruction for biliary malignancy remain controversial, feasibility and potential prognostic advantage of the extended hepatectomy with arterial reconstruction for hilar cholangiocarcinoma have recently been reported. [3–6] As presented in this chapter, long-term patency of the reconstructed arteries have been confirmed in a large series reported by Nagino et al. [6]

From a technical standpoint, the choice of arterial branches for reconstruction should be made according to the caliber of the artery and the distance for the arterial branches to be reconstructed. When multiple arterial branches are noted in the remnant liver, the largest branch should be chosen for the anastomosis. [3] The candidates of donor artery include the right hepatic artery, the left hepatic artery, the gastroduodenal artery, [7] the right gastroepiploic artery, [8] or the splenic artery. [9] However, when arterial reconstruction is technically impossible, arterioportal shunt [10] can be a rescue procedure. The temporal shunt between the artery and the portal vein can function as an oxygen supply route for the liver until perihilar collaterals will develop after surgery. The created arterioportal shunt should be embolized by interventional radiology at approximately one month after surgery to avoid secondary portal hypertension.

Overall Management

- Preoperative biliary drainage (preferably endoscopic approach) is needed to manage cholangitis and decrease the risk of extensive hepatectomy.
- Volumetry of the liver is mandatory and portal vein embolization should be performed prior to surgery when estimated future liver remnant volume is relatively small.

- Detailed vascular mapping and surgical planning based on the preoperative imaging studies are important to adopt the optimal surgical approach.

References

1. Natsume S, Ebata T, Yokoyama Y, Igami T, Sugawara G, Shimoyama Y, et al. Clinical significance of left trisectionectomy for perihilar cholangiocarcinoma: an appraisal and comparison with left hepatectomy. Ann Surg. 2012;255(4):754–62.
2. Shimizu H, Kimura F, Yoshidome H, Ohtsuka M, Kato A, Yoshitomi H, et al. Aggressive surgical resection for hilar cholangiocarcinoma of the left-side predominance: radicality and safety of left-sided hepatectomy. Ann Surg. 2010;251(2):281–6.
3. Sakamoto Y, Sano T, Shimada K, Kosuge T, Kimata Y, Sakuraba M, et al. Clinical significance of reconstruction of the right hepatic artery for biliary malignancy. Langenbecks Arch Surg. 2006;391(3):203–8.
4. Shimada H, Endo I, Sugita M, Masunari H, Fujii Y, Tanaka K, et al. Hepatic resection combined with portal vein or hepatic artery reconstruction for advanced carcinoma of the hilar bile duct and gallbladder. World J Surg. 2003;27(10):1137–42.
5. Yamanaka N, Yasui C, Yamanaka J, Ando T, Kuroda N, Maeda S, et al. Left hemihepatectomy with microsurgical reconstruction of the right-sided hepatic vasculature. A strategy for preserving hepatic function in patients with proximal bile duct cancer. Langenbecks Arch Surg. 2001;386(5):364–8.
6. Nagino M, Nimura Y, Nishio H, Ebata T, Igami T, Matsushita M, et al. Hepatectomy with simultaneous resection of the portal vein and hepatic artery for advanced perihilar cholangiocarcinoma: an audit of 50 consecutive cases. Ann Surg. 2010;252(1):115–23.
7. Sarmiento JM, Panneton JM, Nagorney DM. Reconstruction of the hepatic artery using the gastroduodenal artery. Am J Surg. 2003;185(4):386–7.
8. Ikegami T, Kawasaki S, Hashikura Y, Miwa S, Kubota T, Mita A, et al. An alternative method of arterial reconstruction after hepatic arterial thrombosis following living-related liver transplantation. Transpl. 2000;69(9):1953–5.
9. Figueras J, Pares D, Aranda H, Rafecas A, Fabregat J, Torras J, et al. Results of using the recipient's splenic artery for arterial reconstruction in liver transplantation in 23 patients. Transpl. 1997;64(4):655–8.
10. Noji T, Tsuchikawa T, Okamura K, Nakamura T, Tamoto E, Shichinohe T, et al. Resection and reconstruction of the hepatic artery for advanced perihilar cholangiocarcinoma: result of arterioportal shunting. J Gastrointest Surg. 2015;19(4):675–81.

Gallbladder Cancer with Common Bile Duct Invasion

14

Russell C. Langan and Michael I. D'Angelica

Case Presentation

Our patient was a 47-year-old woman who came to consultation following an episode of right upper quadrant and epigastric pain associated with laboratory values consistent with biliary obstruction. These findings prompted ultrasound imaging followed by magnetic resonance cholangiopancreatography (MRCP). Contrast-enhanced MRCP revealed a malignant-appearing gallbladder mass with narrowing of the cystic duct and soft tissue infiltration of the porta hepatis, suggestive of common bile duct (CBD) involvement (Fig. 14.1). This was corroborated with contrast-enhanced computed tomography (CT) which confirmed the gallbladder mass with contiguous soft tissue encasing the CBD (Fig. 14.2). Additionally, a hepatic duplex ultrasound was obtained and denoted abutment of the main portal vein (Fig. 14.3). Of note, imaging did not show any obvious arterial involvement.

Subjectively, the patient only complained of nonspecific abdominal discomfort. Objectively, the patient's performance status was an ECOG 0. On physical exam, the patient was mildly jaundiced with scleral icterus, however she had no abdominal tenderness and a negative Murphy's sign. Pertinent laboratory values

R.C. Langan
Department of Surgery, Division of Surgical Oncology,
Memorial Sloan Kettering Cancer Center, 1275 York Avenue,
New York, NY 10065, USA
e-mail: langanr@mskcc.org

M.I. D'Angelica (✉)
Department of Surgery, Division of Hepatopancreatobiliary Surgery,
Memorial Sloan Kettering Cancer Center, 1275 York Avenue,
New York, NY 10065, USA
e-mail: dangelim@mskcc.org

T.M. Pawlik et al. (eds.), *Case-Based Lessons in the Management of Complex Hepato-Pancreato-Biliary Surgery*, DOI 10.1007/978-3-319-50868-9_14

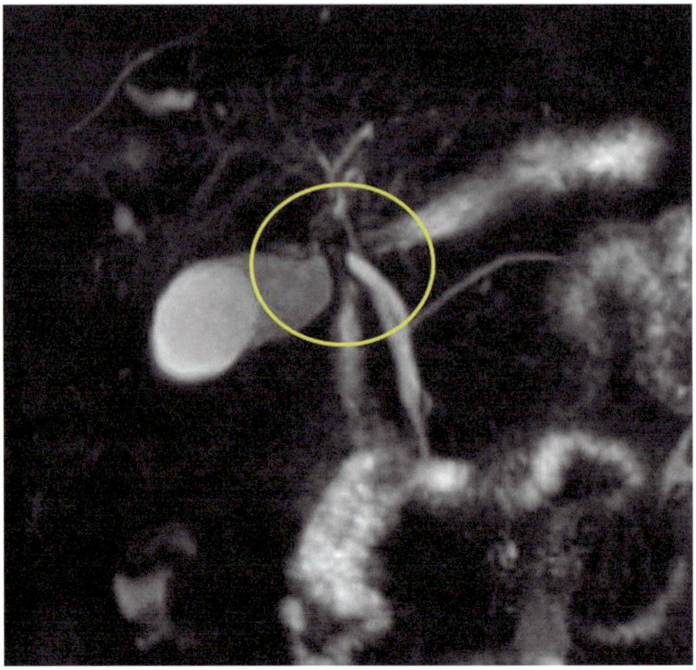

Fig. 14.1 Magnetic resonance cholangiopancreatography denoting locally advanced gallbladder cancer with common bile duct involvement (*yellow circle*)

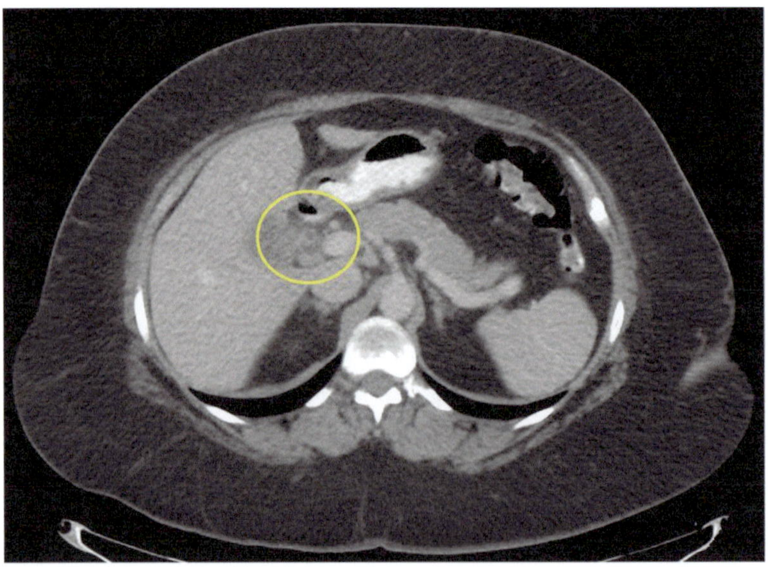

Fig. 14.2 Computed tomography imaging denoting locally advanced gallbladder cancer with common bile duct involvement (*yellow circle*)

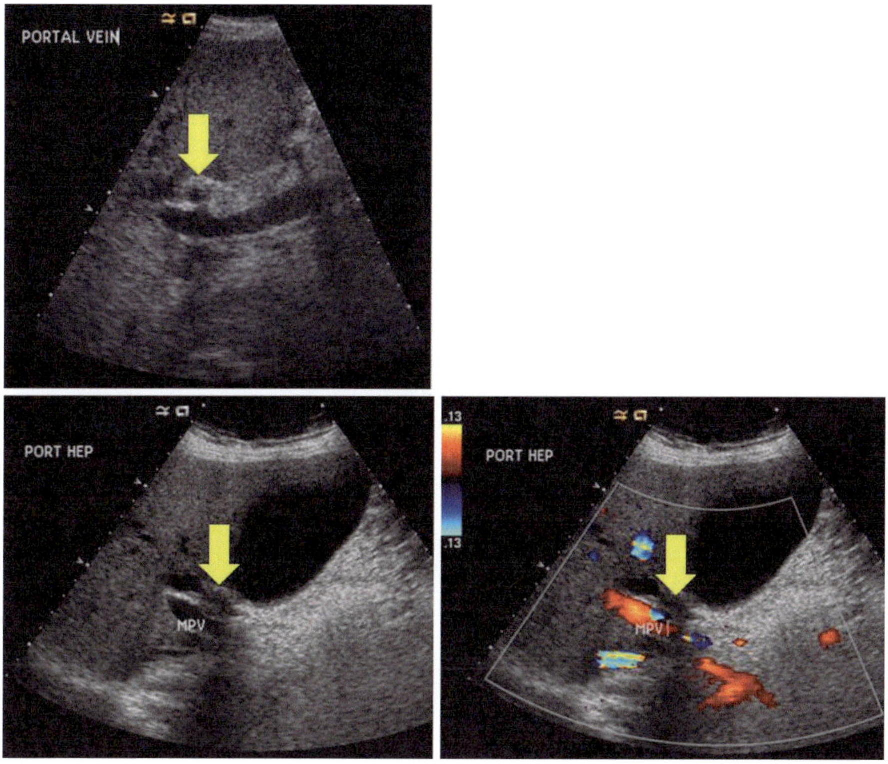

Fig. 14.3 Abutment of the main portal vein by locally advanced gallbladder cancer (*yellow arrow*)

included a WBC of 14.7 K/mcL, hematocrit of 44%, platelet count of 271 K/mcL, Cancer Antigen 19-9 level of 314 U/mL, total bilirubin of 4.4 mg/dL, direct bilirubin 3.5 mg/dL, aspartate aminotransferase 132 U/L, alanine aminotransferase 275 U/L, alkaline phosphatase 250 U/L, creatinine 0.7 mg/dL, and an albumin level of 4.0 g/dL.

Endoscopic retrograde cholangiopancreatography (ERCP) was performed at an outside institution and a CBD stricture was identified and biopsied. Cytology was consistent with adenocarcinoma. The patient then presented for surgical consultation and multidisciplinary discussion ensued.

Due to the previously documented high rate of irresectability and early oncologic failure (see below) in the setting of gallbladder cancer presenting with jaundice, consensus favored commencement of systemic chemotherapy with gemcitabine and cisplatin. Radiographic reassessment was then performed after three months of therapy. Cross-sectional imaging with contrast-enhanced CT along with ultrasonography found no progression of disease, stable CBD involvement, and decreased abutment of the portal vein. This was interpreted to be a modest response to therapy.

The patient was then taken for diagnostic laparoscopy and potential resection. At operation, there was no evidence of distant disease. There was a firm mass arising from the gallbladder extending into the porta hepatis. Within the porta hepatis, the portal vein along with the CBD were involved with tumor. Therefore, complete resection required an extended right hepatectomy, bile duct resection, portal vein resection and regional lymphadenectomy. Final pathology found a 90% treatment response within a 2.3 cm gallbladder neck tumor with no evidence of vascular or perineural invasion. All margins including the distal common bile duct, left hepatic duct, hepatic parenchymal margin, and soft tissue margin were negative for carcinoma. All regional lymph nodes were also negative for carcinoma and the patient was staged as an ypT2N0 stage II gallbladder adenocarcinoma. Of note, the patient had an initial clinical stage of T4 prior to the administration of systemic therapy. The patient subsequently recovered without sequelae and is alive without disease seven months from the date of surgery.

Clinical Pearls

- Preoperative staging should be aimed not only at the exclusion of distant metastases but also at the assessment of local extent of disease. Cross-sectional, contrast-enhanced imaging (computed tomography [CT] and/or MRCP) is the mainstay of investigation. Selective use of hepatic duplex ultrasound imaging can add valuable information in patients with locally advanced tumors.
- Staging laparoscopy should be employed in all patients with suspected CBD involvement in order to avoid non-therapeutic laparotomy.
- At the time of resection, we recommend a diligent search for metastatic disease, including assessment of distant lymph nodes at the celiac axis, as well as in the aortocaval and retropancreatic spaces. If identified, intraoperative frozen section should be obtained and the case aborted for positive results.
- Achievement of a negative pathologic margin (R0) is of paramount importance (survival in those with residual disease is synonymous to those with stage IV disease).
- At times, en bloc resection of segments IVb/V (with or without resection of the CBD) would result in an inadequate margin. In this situation, major hepatic resection with or without bile duct resection (extended right hepatectomy) is required.

Radiographic Assessment of Locally Advanced Gallbladder Carcinoma

Preoperative staging should be aimed not only at the exclusion of distant metastases but also at the assessment of local extent of disease. Cross-sectional, contrast-enhanced imaging (computed tomography [CT] and/or MRCP) is the mainstay of investigation. Multi-phasic CT of the chest, abdomen, and pelvis to include portal venous and arterial phases should be used to assess the extent of disease in the liver and porta hepatis, while also evaluating for metastatic disease.

Imaging should include thin cuts through the liver and porta hepatis to elucidate detailed relationships between the tumor and porta hepatis structures. With respect to the local assessment of disease, one study of 118 patients with gallbladder carcinoma found CT to be 79% accurate for differentiating T1 versus T2 tumors, 93% accurate for differentiating T2 versus T3 tumors, and 100% accurate for differentiating T3 versus T4 tumors [1]. Further, the overall accuracy improved from 72% to 85% when multiplanar reconstructions were added to conventional axial imaging [1].

MRCP with intravenous contrast is a valuable radiologic modality to assess the extent of the primary tumor. Specifically, analyses of MRI for the assessment of gallbladder carcinoma have shown sensitivities of 70–100% for hepatic invasion, 100% for vascular involvement, and 75% for lymph node metastases [2, 3]. That being said, it remains unclear and relatively unstudied as to whether MRI has added benefit to that of CT. The two studies are likely complimentary and should be used in such a manner. Lastly, selective use of hepatic duplex ultrasound imaging can add valuable information in patients with locally advanced tumors. Our experience has found duplex ultrasonography to act as an excellent adjunct to assess the extent of transmural tumoral invasion into hepatic parenchyma or biliary structures (87% accuracy), while simultaneously assessing for involvement of portal venous or hepatic arterial structures, which can be challenging to assess on cross-sectional imaging [4]. It should be noted that initial imaging studies should be performed prior to biliary stenting (if it is to be performed), as stenting will cause local inflammation, making assessment of tumor extent difficult.

Additionally, FDG-PET imaging may be helpful in the identification of distant disease, as depicted by retrospective reviews. In a study of 61 patients with biliary tract malignancies, PET/CT had a sensitivity of 100%, as compared to 25% for CT alone, ($p < 0.001$) in the identification of distant metastases [5] Moreover, PET results changed surgical management in 17% of cases [5]. In an analysis of 41 patients with gallbladder carcinoma at Memorial Sloan Kettering Cancer Center (MSKCC), preoperative PET results altered surgical management in 23% of patients (for either the initial operation or re-resection after an incidental finding following cholecystectomy) [6]. Lastly, in a recent analysis of the efficacy of PET imaging as compared to CT and MRI, PET identified occult distant metastatic disease and also proved findings suspicious on CT to be negative; therefore altering surgical decision-making in 17% of patients [7]. Although the evidence is limited to small retrospective reviews, one should consider PET imaging when evaluating newly diagnosed, locally advanced gallbladder carcinoma, largely to evaluate for distant metastatic disease or to confirm/refute questionable findings on cross-sectional imaging.

General Principles of Surgical Management

Although uncertainty remains as to whether resection offers oncologic benefit for patients with locally advanced gallbladder carcinoma, the possibility of long-term survival after complete resection has been shown. As a baseline, documented 5-year survival rates for resected gallbladder carcinoma range from approximately 20–50% [8–16]. Specifically, in a review of 410 gallbladder carcinoma patients who presented to MSKCC between 1986 and 2000, the median and 5-year survivals for resected patients were 26 months and 38% respectively, with 14% of T3 patients and 19% of T4 patients alive at 5 years [8].

Yet, until recently, the optimal extent of resection was unknown and often debated. However, an analysis of the impact of the extent of resection on disease-specific survival (DSS) in 104 patients with gallbladder cancer at MSKCC found tumor biology and stage, rather than the extent of resection, to predict DSS. Empiric major hepatic resections and bile duct excision for early-stage tumors resulted in higher morbidity, and were not associated with prolonged survival as compared to lesser hepatic resections. However, major hepatic resections, including extended hepatectomy and CBD excision, are appropriate when necessary to clear disease and achieve negative margins. These larger resections, when necessary, were associated with acceptable long-term survival [9]. Therefore, the extent of resection should be dictated by what is necessary to achieve a negative margin.

Additionally, regional (portal) lymphadenectomy should be performed for accurate staging information [17, 18]. The chance of nodal involvement increases with increasing T stage. Bartlett et al. found nodal disease was associated with 46% of resected T2 tumors and 54% of resected T3 tumors [14]. Others have found that on progression of T stage from T2 to T4, nodal and distant metastases increased from 16% to 79% and from 33% to 69%, respectively [8]. Although the impact of node dissection on survival is controversial (rare 5-year survivors with N1 disease), the diagnostic information gained regarding node positivity may help in determining adjuvant therapies [19–23].

As stated, if resection is undertaken, the goal is the achievement of a pathologically margin negative (R0) resection. In an analysis of 135 patients subjected to definitive resection following an incidentally diagnosed gallbladder carcinoma, the presence of residual disease at any site was associated with significantly worse survival [24]. The median disease-free survival (DFS) (11.2 vs. 93.4 months, $p < 0.0001$) and disease-specific survival (DSS) (25.2 months vs. not reached, $p < 0.0001$) were dramatically lower than in patients without residual disease [24]. Moreover, residual disease identified at any particular site predicted DFS (HR 3.3,

95% CI 1.9–5.7, $p = 0.0003$) and DSS (HR 2.4, 95% CI 1.2–4.6, $p = 0.01$) and was independent of all other tumor-related variables [24]. In essence, survival among patients with residual disease at any site was not significantly different than those with stage IV disease [24]. Importantly, and relevant to our discussion of resecting T3/T4 lesions, the T stage of the gallbladder specimen was the only independent predictor of residual disease (T1b = 35.7%, T2 = 48.3%, T3 = 70%; $p = 0.015$) [24].

Alternative Approaches/Controversies

- In patients with invasion into the common bile duct, consideration should be made for neoadjuvant chemotherapy prior to surgical exploration in an attempt to best select patients for potentially curative resection.
- Although uncertainty remains, the possibility of long-term survival after complete resection of gallbladder carcinoma has been shown. To date, documented 5-year survival rates for resected gallbladder carcinoma in all comers range from 20% to 50%.
- Specifically, in a review of 410 gallbladder carcinoma patients who presented to MSKCC between 1986 and 2000, the median and 5-year survivals for resected patients were 26 months and 38% respectively, with 14% of T3 patients and 19% of T4 patients alive at 5 years.
- Although the survival benefits of node dissection are unproven and unlikely (rare 5-year survivors with N1 disease), the diagnostic information gained regarding node positivity is important and can inform decisions about adjuvant therapy.

Management of Gallbladder Cancer with CBD Invasion

Except for the uncommon patient with concomitant common bile duct stones, patients with gallbladder carcinoma presenting with obstructive jaundice have tumor involvement of the porta hepatis by either direct extension of the tumor, diffuse invasion of the porta hepatis, or extensive nodal disease. These patients are rarely resectable and have an associated poor prognosis [25]. Therefore, upfront attempts at resection are hard to justify. Although theoretically, local extension should not necessarily affect oncologic outcome, studies have found jaundice to be an indicator of advanced malignancy and portends a poor survival.

An analysis of 240 patients with gallbladder carcinoma from Memorial Sloan Kettering Cancer Center compared oncologic outcomes between those who presented with obstructive jaundice and those who did not [25]. Overall, 34% (82/240) of patients within the cohort presented with obstructive jaundice [25]. Causes of obstructive jaundice included CBD involvement in 89% (73/82), common hepatic duct involvement in 9% (7/82) and obstructing gallstones in 2% (2/82) [25]. Among the jaundiced patients, 67% (55/82) underwent operative exploration [25]. Patients were excluded from exploration for the following reasons: 14 radiographically documented liver metastasis, 6 radiographically unresectable invasion of the portal vein, and 12 with peritoneal metastases [25]. In the 55 patients who were explored, diagnostic laparoscopy was performed in 45% (25/55) and found peritoneal metastases in 68% (17/25), precluding further exploration [25]. Ultimately, exploratory laparotomy was undertaken in 37 patients. Among these 37 patients, distant peritoneal and liver metastases were found in 8 (22%) patients, and locally unresectable disease in the porta hepatis was found in an additional 10 (27%). In summary, 52% (19/37) of jaundiced patients who underwent exploratory laparotomy were resected with curative intent, however this represented only 7% (6/82) of all patients presenting with jaundice.

As compared to their non-jaundiced counterparts, jaundiced patients were more likely to have advanced-stage disease (Stage III/IV) at the time of presentation, 96% versus 60%, respectively ($p < 0.001$). With respect to survival, the median disease-specific survival was significantly lower in those with jaundice as compared to the non-jaundiced patients, 6 versus 16 months, respectively ($p < 0.0001$). Moreover, there were no disease-free survivors at 2 years in the jaundiced group, whereas 21% of the non-jaundiced patients were alive without disease at this time-point [25].

These results have been recently corroborated. In an analysis of 192 patients with gallbladder carcinoma, who underwent resection with curative intent, 25% (47/192) presented with obstructive jaundice [26]. As compared to their non-jaundiced counterparts, those with jaundice had increased perioperative complications as well as worse survival. Specifically, preoperative jaundice was associated with longer operative times ($p < 0.001$), higher intraoperative blood loss ($p < 0.001$), increased multi-visceral resections (23.4% vs. 2.8%, $p = 0.001$), and increased post-operative complications (34 vs. 12%, $p = 0.001$). Predicted 5-year overall survival in jaundiced versus non-jaundiced patients was 6% versus 36% ($p < 0.001$), respectively [26]. However, in disagreement with the MSKCC data presented above, 77% (36/47) of jaundiced patients within this cohort underwent an R0 resection.

While difficult to ascertain from studies, it is important to assess patients for the uncommon but favorable patient with gallbladder cancer and jaundice. Occasionally, the patient will have stones causing jaundice, which do not preclude surgical treatment. Additionally, sometimes a small tumor in an unfortunate location will involve the bile duct simply by proximity rather than extensive local invasion. These patients are sometimes hard to discern, but should be considered for upfront surgical therapy.

It is clear that obstructive jaundice is a poor prognostic indicator and a marker of advanced disease in patients with gallbladder adenocarcinoma. Although there is no proven correct approach to those with obstructive jaundice in the setting of gallbladder carcinoma, we recommend a multidisciplinary discussion and consideration of systemic therapy, prior to undertaking surgical exploration. Given the low yield of surgery in terms of resectability and early recurrence, a course of systemic therapy to assess response and improve patient selection is reasonable. gemcitabine in combination with a platinum agent (cisplatin/oxaliplatin) remains the standard of care [27]. In a randomized prospective trial in patients with metastatic biliary cancers (including gallbladder cancer), which assessed overall survival as the primary endpoint, Valle et al. found that as compared with gemcitabine alone, cisplatin plus gemcitabine was associated with a significant advantage in overall survival (8.1 vs. 11.7 months, $P < 0.001$) along with an improvement in median progression-free survival (5.0 vs. 8.0 months, $P < 0.001$) [27]. Following two to three months of systemic therapy, repeat imaging should be carried out and resection considered, if technically feasible and if there has been no evidence of progressive disease.

Gallbladder carcinoma can also present with involvement of the CBD without obstructive jaundice. There is a paucity of data on this particular clinical scenario. That being said, our group has retrospectively assessed 104 patients who underwent resection for gallbladder carcinoma and found clinical involvement of the CBD to be associated with higher T ($p = 0.01$) and overall stage ($p = 0.007$). Additionally, as compared to a cohort of patients without CBD involvement, median overall survival (62 vs. 19 months) and predicted 5-year survival (49% vs. 21%) were both found to be inferior in those with involvement of the CBD, at a median follow up of 58 months ($p = 0.01$) (Fig. 14.4). On multivariate analysis of clinicopathologic factors associated with survival, CBD involvement was found to be an independent

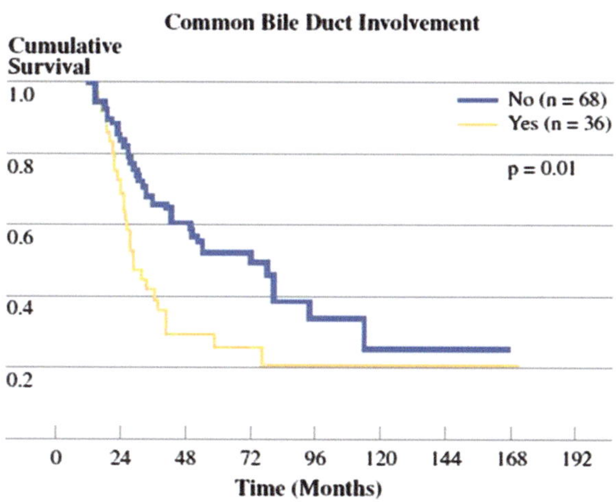

Fig. 14.4 Disease-specific survival for 104 patients who underwent resection for locally advanced gallbladder adenocarcinoma at Memorial Sloan Kettering Cancer Center, stratified by common bile duct involvement or lack thereof. Reproduced from Annals of Surgical Oncology, 2008; Vol.16. p. 806–16. Michael D'Angelica. Analysis of the Extent of Resection for Adenocarcinoma of the Gallbladder. © 2008; with permission of Springer

predictor of worse DSS ($p = 0.02$, 95% CI 0.30–0.90). While upfront resection can certainly be considered, given the relatively poor survival in this patient population, we recommend strong consideration for neoadjuvant chemotherapy in all patients with gallbladder carcinoma and known or suspected involvement of the CBD. Again, the rationale for this approach, while unproven, is to exclude patients with particularly poor tumor biology from surgery and to maximize the success of surgical exploration.

Operative Principles

In patients with suspicious gallbladder masses, a preoperative tissue diagnosis is not required. Biopsies can result in false negative findings and may spread tumor into the peritoneum. However, staging laparoscopy should be considered for all malignant-appearing gallbladder masses in an attempt to avoid non-therapeutic laparotomy [28]. If there is no evidence of peritoneal or hepatic metastases, laparotomy should be performed and resection undertaken, with the paramount goal being negative margins.

Generally, the recommended surgical approach for gallbladder carcinoma greater than T1a utilizes an extended cholecystectomy to include resection of segments IVb & V of the liver along with a portal lymph node dissection. The only reason to extend an operation beyond this (such as major hepatectomy or bile duct resection) would be an inability to obtain a negative margin. At operation, prior to proceeding with resection, we recommend a complete search for metastatic disease that would preclude resection. Mobilization of the duodenum and assessment for aortocaval, retropancreatic and/or celiac lymphadenopathy should be performed. If the nodes in these areas are suspicious for metastatic disease, intraoperative frozen section should be obtained and the case aborted for positive results, as these nodes would be representative of distant metastatic disease. Regional lymphadenectomy for gallbladder carcinoma should include removal of nodes in the porta hepatis, gastrohepatic ligament and retroduodenal space [17, 29, 30]. Specific to cases of CBD involvement, division of the CBD should occur at the junction of the duodenum/pancreas and the circumferential nodal tissue swept cranially, skeletonizing the vasculature of the porta hepatis; therefore ensuring that all soft tissue surrounding portal structures is removed.

In the case of CBD involvement, such as the one depicted above, the extrahepatic bile duct must be incorporated into the resection in order to achieve a negative margin. Proximal transection should be dictated by the extent of the tumor. Many cases will require division of the left hepatic duct and excision of the biliary confluence along with an extended right hepatectomy. In rare cases, a local excision of the common hepatic/bile duct may be possible. If the right hepatic duct and/or biliary confluence is involved, an extended right hepatectomy is mandatory for complete resection of the tumor. The distal bile duct, which is typically divided first, should be divided at the level of the duodenum. Intraoperative frozen section should be obtained on the proximal and distal bile duct margins. If a negative margin cannot be obtained on the left bile duct or the distal bile duct, the operation should be abandoned. Combined hepatic and pancreatic resections for tumors involving the distal bile duct has been reported, but it is a controversial operation and is beyond the scope of this review. Reconstruction is typically via a roux-en-y hepaticojejunostomy.

In summary, if resection of segments IVb/V (with or without resection of the CBD) as described above would result in an inadequate margin, major hepatic resections (extended right hepatectomy) are required. These extended operations may be required for tumors invading the right portal pedicle or tumors originating from the infundibulum of the gallbladder which encroach upon the porta hepatis. For example, if a tumor is adherent to the right-sided hepatic inflow structures, an extended right hepatectomy would be mandated for a complete resection. In most cases, it is the involvement of major hepatic vascular structures rather than tumoral depth into liver parenchyma that dictates the extent of hepatic resection needed to be performed (Fig. 14.5).

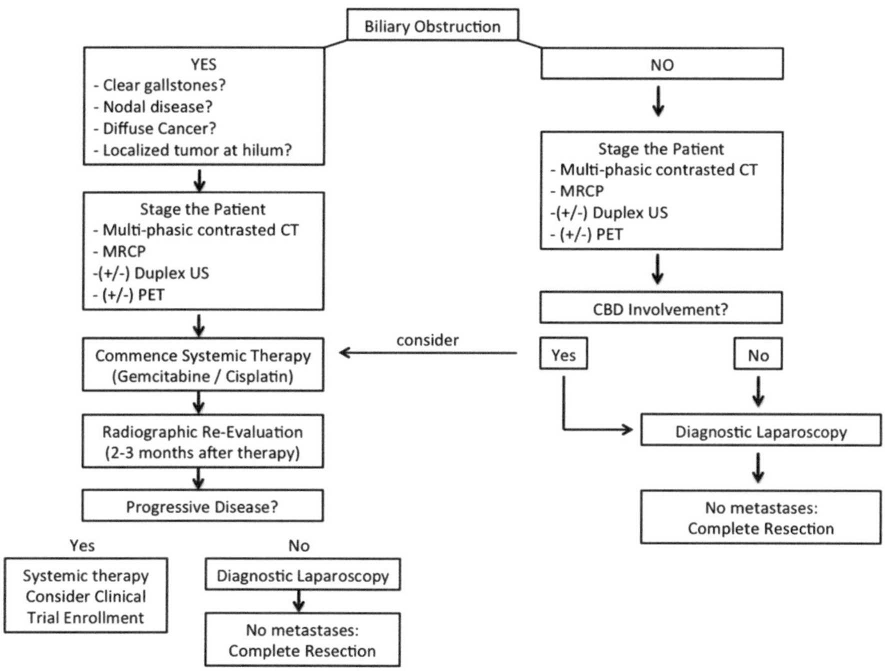

Fig. 14.5 Proposed algorithmic flow of management for patients with gallbladder carcinoma

Overall Management

- Common bile duct involvement is an indicator of advanced disease and is associated with a worse survival.
- Obstructive jaundice in the setting of gallbladder carcinoma portends poor survival, and systemic therapy should commence prior to entertaining surgical resection.
- Following systemic therapy (gemcitabine/cisplatin), cross-sectional imaging along with duplex ultrasonography should be repeated after three months of therapy, and surgical resection entertained if there has been no progression of disease.

Conclusion

The gallbladder is the most common site of biliary tract malignancy, and up to 35% of patients have been reported to have extrahepatic bile duct involvement [9]. Generally speaking, involvement of the CBD is a marker of advanced disease and portends poor survival. Survival is particularly poor in those who present with jaundice. Due to the high rate of oncologic failure, in patients with gallbladder cancer and involvement of the common bile duct we recommend the use of neoadjuvant chemotherapy prior to undertaking surgical exploration.

Acknowledgements This study was supported in part by NIH/NCI P30 CA008748 (Cancer Center Support Grant)

References

1. Kim SJ, Lee JM, Lee JY, Choi JY, Kim SH, Han JK, et al. Accuracy of preoperative T-staging of gallbladder carcinoma using MDCT. Am J Roentgenol. 2008;190(1):74–80.
2. Kim JH, Kim TK, Eun HW, Kim BS, Lee MG, Kim PN, et al. Preoperative evaluation of gallbladder carcinoma: efficacy of combined use of MR imaging, MR cholangiography, and contrast-enhanced dual-phase three-dimensional MR angiography. J Magn Reson Imaging. 2002;16(6):676–84.
3. Schwartz LH, Black J, Fong Y, Jarnagin W, Blumgart L, Gruen D, et al. Gallbladder carcinoma: findings at MR imaging with MR cholangiopancreatography. J Comput Assist Tomogr. 2002;26(3):405–10.
4. Rodriguez-Fernandez A, Gómez-Río M, Medina-Benítez A, Moral JV, Ramos-Font C, Ramia-Angel JM, et al. Application of modern imaging methods in diagnosis of gallbladder cancer. J Surg Oncol. 2006;93(8):650–64.

5. Petrowsky H, Wildbrett P, Husarik DB, Hany TF, Tam S, Jochum W, et al. Impact of integrated positron emission tomography and computed tomography on staging and management of gallbladder cancer and cholangiocarcinoma. J Hepatol. 2006;45(1):43–50.
6. Corvera CU, Blumgart LH, Akhurst T, DeMatteo RP, D'Angelica M, Fong Y, et al. 18F-fluorodeoxyglucose positron emission tomography influences management decisions in patients with biliary cancer. J Am Coll Surg. 2008;206(1):57–65.
7. Leung U, Pandit-Taskar N, Corvera CU, D'Angelica MI, Allen PJ, Kingham TP, et al. Impact of pre-operative positron emission tomography in gallbladder cancer. HPB (Oxford). 2014;16 (11):1023–30.
8. Fong Y, Jarnagin W, Blumgart LH. Gallbladder cancer: comparison of patients presenting initially for definitive operation with those presenting after prior noncurative intervention. Ann Surg. 2000;232(4):557–69.
9. D'Angelica M, Dalal KM, DeMatteo RP, Fong Y, Blumgart LH, Jarnagin WR. Analysis of the extent of resection for adenocarcinoma of the gallbladder. Ann Surg Oncol. 2009;16 (4):806–16.
10. Goetze TO, Paolucci V. Adequate extent in radical re-resection of incidental gallbladder carcinoma: analysis of the German Registry. Surg Endosc. 2010;24(9):2156–64.
11. Foster JM, Hoshi H, Gibbs JF, Iyer R, Javle M, Chu Q, et al. Gallbladder cancer: defining the indications for primary radical resection and radical re-resection. Ann Surg Oncol. 2007;14 (2):833–40.
12. Onoyama H, Yamamoto M, Tseng A, Ajiki T, Saitoh Y. Extended cholecystectomy for carcinoma of the gallbladder. World J Surg. 1995;19(5):758–63.
13. Donohue JH, Nagorney DM, Grant CS, Tsushima K, Ilstrup DM, Adson MA. Carcinoma of the gallbladder. Does radical resection improve outcome? Arch Surg. 1990;125(2):237–41.
14. Bartlett DL, Fong Y, Fortner JG, Brennan MF, Blumgart LH. Long-term results after resection for gallbladder cancer. Implications for staging and management. Ann Surg. 1996;224(5):639–46.
15. Matsumoto Y, Fujii H, Aoyama H, Yamamoto M, Sugahara K, Suda K. Surgical treatment of primary carcinoma of the gallbladder based on the histologic analysis of 48 surgical specimens. Am J Sur. 1992;163(2):239–45.
16. Gall FP, Köckerling F, Scheele J, Schneider C, Hohenberger W. Radical operations for carcinoma of the gallbladder: present status in Germany. World J Surg. 1991;15(3):328–36.
17. Shirai Y, Wakai T, Hatakeyama K. Radical lymph node dissection for gallbladder cancer: indications and limitations. Surg Oncol Clin N Am. 2007;16(1):221–32.
18. Kelly KJ, Dukleska K, Kuk D, Kingham TP, D'Angelica MI, DeMatteo RP, et al. Prognostic significance of the highest peripancreatic lymph node in biliary tract adenocarcinoma. Ann Surg Oncol. 2014;21(3):979–85.
19. Paquet KJ. Appraisal of surgical resection of gallbladder carcinoma with special reference to hepatic resection. J Hepatobiliary Pancreat Surg. 1998;5(2):200–6.
20. Muratore A, Polastri R, Bouzari H, Vergara V, Capussotti L. Radical surgery for gallbladder cancer: a worthwhile operation? Eur J Surg Oncol. 2000;26(2):160–3.
21. Taner CB, Nagorney DM, Donohue JH. Surgical treatment of gallbladder cancer. J Gastrointest Surg. 2004;8(1):83–9. discussion 89.
22. Dixon E, Vollmer CM Jr, Sahajpal A, Cattral M, Grant D, et al. An aggressive surgical approach leads to improved survival in patients with gallbladder cancer: a 12-year study at a North American Center. Ann Surg. 2005;241(3):385–94.
23. Pitt HA. Gallbladder cancer: what is an aggressive approach? Ann Surg. 2005;241(3):395–6.
24. Butte JM, Kingham TP, Gönen M, D'Angelica MI, Allen PJ, Fong Y, et al. Residual disease predicts outcomes after definitive resection for incidental gallbladder cancer. J Am Coll Surg. 2014;219(3):416–29.
25. Hawkins WG, DeMatteo RP, Jarnagin WR, Ben-Porat L, Blumgart LH, Fong Y. Jaundice predicts advanced disease and early mortality in patients with gallbladder cancer. Ann Surg Oncol. 2004;11(3):310–5.

26. Yang XW, Yuan JM, Chen JY, Yang J, Gao QG, Yan XZ, et al. The prognostic importance of jaundice in surgical resection with curative intent for gallbladder cancer. BMC Cancer. 2014;14:652.
27. Valle J, Wasan H, Palmer DH, Cunningham D, Anthoney A, Maraveyas A, et al. Cisplatin plus gemcitabine versus gemcitabine for biliary tract cancer. N Engl J Med. 2010;362 (14):1273–81.
28. Butte JM, Gönen M, Allen PJ, D'Angelica MI, Kingham TP, Fong Y, et al. The role of laparoscopic staging in patients with incidental gallbladder cancer. HPB (Oxford). 2011;13 (7):463–72.
29. Ito H, Ito K, D'Angelica M, Gonen M, Klimstra D, Allen P, et al. Accurate staging for gallbladder cancer: implications for surgical therapy and pathological assessment. Ann Surg. 2011;254(2):320–5.
30. Pandey D. Technical description of a regional lymphadenectomy in radical surgery for gallbladder cancer. HPB (Oxford). 2012;14(3):216–9.

15 Management of the Gangrenous Gallbladder

Jean-Michel Aubin, Chad G. Ball and Henry A. Pitt

Case Presentation

A 68-year-old male presented to the Emergency Department (ED) with a two-day history of significant right upper quadrant pain. Although he had also presented to the ED two weeks earlier for similar symptoms, these were thought to be pleuritic in origin at the initial visit. An electrocardiogram, chest X-ray, and computed tomography (CT) examination of the thorax had been obtained. Pericholecystic fluid and a very small volume of air was noted on the CT. The ED physician thought that these findings were "incidental" and suggested that they be followed.

During the current visit, the patient describes a history of post-prandial indigestion, which had become increasingly symptomatic, persisting for 48 h and associated with rigors and chills. He did not display or endorse signs or symptoms suggestive of obstructive jaundice. His past medical history included hypertension, dyslipidemia, diabetes mellitus, coronary artery disease, and central obesity.

On physical assessment, he appeared unwell but was hemodynamically stable. Examination revealed focal right upper quadrant pain, with a positive Murphy's sign. Further investigations revealed a leukocytosis of 16,000, mild increases in

J.-M. Aubin · C.G. Ball
Department of Surgery, Foothills Medical Centre, University of Calgary,
1403 29 St. NW, Calgary, AB T2N 2T9, Canada
e-mail: jmraubin@gmail.com

C.G. Ball
e-mail: ball.chad@gmail.com

H.A. Pitt (✉)
Department of Surgery, Temple University Health System,
3509 N. Broad St. Boyer Pavilion E938, Philadelphia, PA 19140, USA
e-mail: Henry.Pitt@tuhs.temple.edu

T.M. Pawlik et al. (eds.), *Case-Based Lessons in the Management of Complex Hepato-Pancreato-Biliary Surgery*, DOI 10.1007/978-3-319-50868-9_15

liver transaminase and alkaline phosphatase levels, as well as normal bilirubin and lipase levels. The serum creatinine was slightly above the normal laboratory range.

Due to a large body habitus, the ultrasound evaluation of the abdomen was technically difficult, and the ultrasonographer could not comment on the presence of a sonographic Murphy's sign. Cholelithiasis, mild gallbladder wall thickening, possible discontinuity of the posterior gallbladder wall, and a fatty liver were noted. The intra-luminal air identified on the prior CT scan appeared to have decreased in volume.

Antibiotic therapy was instituted and intravenous fluids were administered. A consultation by the General Surgery service was obtained, prompting patient admission. Cross-sectional imaging was requested to further characterize the integrity of the gallbladder. The CT now identified pericholecystic fluid, gallbladder wall hyper-enhancement and focal discontinuity, as well as intra-luminal air (Figs. 15.1 and 15.2). This constellation of symptoms and image finding were concerning for GC.

Surgical management in the form of cholecystectomy was recommended to the patient. A laparoscopic approach was attempted; however conversion to an open cholecystectomy ensued, due to the finding of a thin-walled necrotic gallbladder,

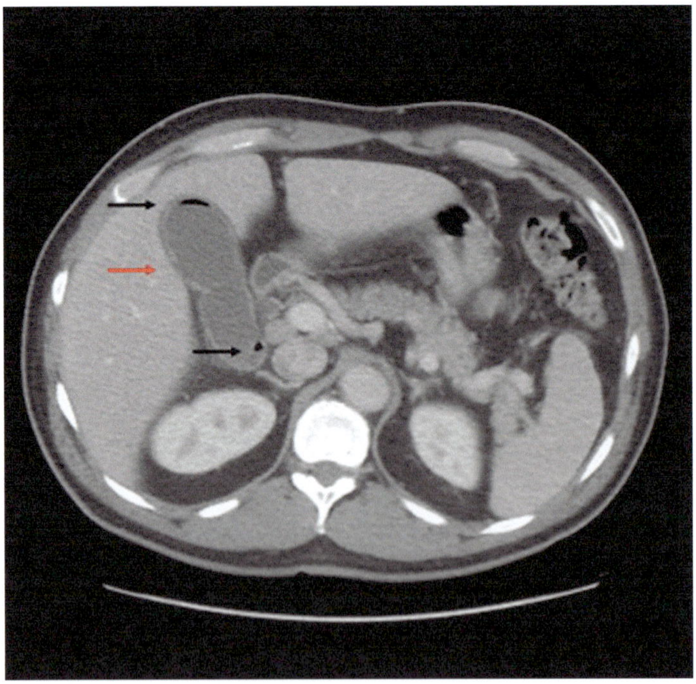

Fig. 15.1 Axial CT scan slice showing gallbladder wall enhancement, suspected wall discontinuity (*red arrow*) and intra-luminal air (*black arrows*)

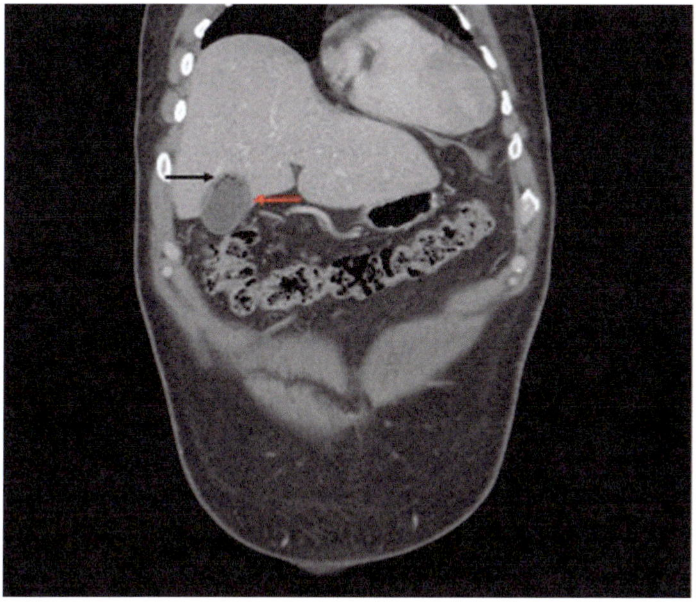

Fig. 15.2 Coronal CT scan slice showing gallbladder wall enhancement, suspected wall discontinuity (*red arrow*), and intra-luminal air (*black arrow*)

poor handling of the organ rendering dissection challenging, in combination with poor visualization due to the patient's body habitus.

The gallbladder was removed, and a closed-suction drain was placed within the gallbladder fossa. Postoperatively, the patient required ongoing aggressive fluid therapy to address an acute kidney injury, maintain urine output, and optimize hemodynamics. As expected, the inflammatory response moderated itself between 48 and 72 h, allowing clinical amelioration. Other minor complications such as atelectasis and poor glycemic control were improved via standard therapies. The patient was discharged home on postoperative day 5. His drain was removed prior to discharge in light of the low-volume, sero-sanguinous effluent.

Our Approach

Although acute cholecystitis (AC) represents a common diagnosis within any General Surgery practice, GC often causes significantly more angst due to the technical challenges and increased complications [1]. GC is typically defined as necrosis with possible perforation of the gallbladder wall caused by ischemia following progressive vascular insufficiency [2]. GC has also long plagued general surgeons (first reported in 1894 [3]) and continues to be encountered in up to 40% of patients presenting with AC [2–5].

Acute GC should be viewed as a surgical emergency. This recommendation is especially true given its association with increased morbidity, including bile duct injuries [4]. Furthermore, delays in management result in inferior outcomes [1]. "Gangrene" of the gallbladder wall reflects the duration of the inflammatory and ischemic process. More specifically, obstruction of the cystic duct results in prolonged increased intra-luminal pressure, to the point where this pressure exceeds the arterial inflow pressure, causing ischemia of the organ [1, 5].

Given this well-defined pathophysiology, timely diagnosis and treatment must be engaged to limit morbidity [1]. We present a case of GC to highlight the salient features of this disease, notably the challenges and delays surrounding its diagnosis in at-risk patients. We also review optimal management strategies, and offer insight into approaching this onerous clinical scenario. With a relative paucity of current literature on this topic, combined with the decreased comfort of contemporary general surgeons performing open cholecystectomy (which is more frequently required in this scenario), surgeons facile with the liver and extra-hepatic biliary tree will not infrequently be called upon to assist in the care of these patients.

Initial Presentation

As outlined in the preceding case, delays in presentation, and further delays in obtaining diagnostic imaging and consultation by a surgical service, are more frequent among individuals with GC [6]. Numerous risk factors of varying significance, listed below, have been reported to predispose patients to progress to GC [1, 2, 5, 7–13]. Abnormalities in laboratory values often include [5] leukocytosis, and an elevation in alkaline phosphatase and GGT. Increases in transaminases can also be noted, driven by hepatocyte necrosis in the liver tissue adjacent to the gallbladder bed. [2] As the inflammatory process progresses, the edematous or hydropic gallbladder can display a mass effect on surrounding structures, such as the bile duct, and trigger a rise in bilirubin [2]. This situation further complicates the clinical picture and may delay treatment as investigations are pursued to clarify the hyperbilirubinemia. Despite, and in light of, these various changes and patient-related factors, preoperative prediction of GC remains as low as 9% [6].

Risk Factors for Gangrenous Cholecystitis
Increased age
Male sex
Diabetes mellitus
Coronary artery disease
Steroid use
Dependent functional status
SIRS (systemic inflammatory response syndrome) at presentation
Gallbladder wall thickening, pericholecystic fluid on ultrasound

Diabetes is consistently associated with GC [1, 2, 4, 5, 8–13]. The pathophysiology of this association is thought to be two-fold. Diabetes leads to micro-vascular disease [3] and therefore, smaller caliber, atherosclerotic vessels may have increased susceptibility to the increased pressure stemming from cystic duct occlusion and frank ischemia may take place earlier in the process of cholecystitis. Second, diabetes has a known associated neuropathy, which may limit the sensory perception of an inflamed gallbladder [3]. These combined diabetes-related issues subsequently cascade into delayed presentation, as well as altered presenting symptoms, typical of patients with GC. Not surprisingly, diabetic patients also may be subject to higher rates of perioperative morbidity and mortality [5].

Elderly patients tend to present in a similar fashion. Impaired sensation of symptoms, relative inability to mount an inflammatory response, combined with possible changes in cognition and communication all contribute to delayed or missed diagnosis and treatment [2]. Institutional reviews of elderly patients with GC have identified higher rates of mortality [5, 8]. Patients for whom mortality occurred also were noted to have increased delays in time to admission (54 vs. 21 h) [2]. As exemplified in this case, the typical patient at risk of GC is male, diabetic, and of advanced age. These three factors are simply surrogates for less healthy patients who present later in the course of their disease, and consequently with a more severe cholecystitis [3].

Diagnostic Imaging

Patients suspected to have cholecystitis will typically have a leukocytosis, and often abnormalities in liver enzymes [1, 5, 7]. The diagnostic imaging modality of choice remains the ultrasound (readily available, safe, and low in cost) [14, 15]. Despite the user dependence associated with ultrasonography, its sensitivity in detecting acute inflammation of the gallbladder is reported to be 90–95% [5]. However, the ability of ultrasound to discriminate between gangrenous and non-gangrenous cholecystitis is quite limited [6]. This inability to differentiate these two entities is true of diagnostic imaging in general [1]. Gallbladder wall thickening, pericholecystic fluid, and a positive sonographic Murphy's sign are all reported to be associated with GC [4, 5]. These findings are also present in simple acute cholecystitis, and comprise the diagnostic criteria in the revised Tokyo guidelines [16].

Although ultrasonography remains the gold standard for acute cholecystitis, CT may offer a diagnostic advantage over ultrasound in detecting GC. The presence of a perfusion defect, or discontinuous/irregular enhancement of the gallbladder mucosa, has a high positive predictive value (94–100%), sensitivity of 30–70%, specificity of up to 100%, and accuracy of 80% [7, 17, 18]. Often, the diagnosis of acute cholecystitis will be suspected clinically, and confirmed by ultrasound. However, a minority of patients will undergo cross-sectional imaging, which may explain the relatively high intraoperative, rather than preoperative, discovery of GC.

Magnetic resonance (MR) has proven to be an effective modality for imaging of the biliary tree. MR can identify features of GC, such as ulceration, hemorrhage, necrosis, or micro-abscesses, to a greater degree than US or CT, notably when intravenous contrast is employed [18]. As with the previous modalities, the finding of inhomogeneous wall enhancement or disrupted mucosal enhancement on MR is characteristic of GC [18]. While air in the gallbladder lumen, emphysematous cholecystitis (EC), was observed in our case, this finding is unusual in patients with GC.

Given that most patients undergo ultrasound assessment as their sole imaging modality, clinical acumen must be relied upon to suspect GC and avoid missing or delaying the diagnosis. If suspicion is high, other modalities such as CT or MR can be utilized to confirm the diagnosis. However, treatment options may not be altered by these additional tests, as these patients typically require surgical intervention. The sagacious surgeon will expedite surgery, anticipate an intraoperative diagnosis of GC, and prepare the perioperative team accordingly. Furthermore, if GC poses a challenging resection, involvement of a hepatobiliary surgeon may be helpful.

Tokyo Guidelines

An international group of experts has published guidelines to better characterize and guide the management of cholecystitis and cholangitis. These Tokyo Guidelines (TG) highlight the process of cholecystitis as it evolves from an edematous stage (1st stage), to necrotizing cholecystitis (2nd stage), and then finally to suppurative cholecystitis (3rd stage) [19]. The diagnosis of GC lies between the second and third stages, where findings such as hemorrhage and necrosis result from vascular occlusion, which then progresses to necrosis, breakdown of the gallbladder wall, and development of intra-mural or pericholecystic abscesses [20].

These stages are either established intraoperatively or via pathologic confirmation. Preoperatively, patients are categorized according to clinical grade. As part of the 2012 Tokyo Guidelines, [16] proposed severity assessment criteria identify three grades (mild, moderate, severe) based on presentation and duration of symptoms, laboratory values, and associated organ/system dysfunction. Management options are tailored to the presence of these grades. As previously mentioned, predicting GC is challenging and, as such, management should be responsive to the patient's clinical picture.

In the presented case, the presence of leukocytosis above 18,000/mm^3, duration of symptoms >72 h, and the presence of marked inflammatory changes on imaging categorize the patient as Grade II—moderate cholecystitis. This prompted early cholecystectomy, in accordance with current (TG 13) guidelines [21].

Clinical Pearls

1. If clinically appropriate, surgical management should be expedited if GC is suspected (with a surgeon facile in challenging biliary diseases and anatomy).
2. Perform a bile duct time-out in the setting of ambiguity (B.E. S.A.F.E.).

3. Possess a low threshold to convert to an open procedure for safety and to ensure a total cholecystectomy.
4. Beware of nearby hepatic venous branches.
5. Follow curve of gallbladder to decrease risk of injury to bile duct.

Management

Initial management is directed toward fluid resuscitation, and the institution of antimicrobial therapy if sepsis is suspected. Antibiotic regimens, such as a broad-spectrum penicillin, should treat common biliary organisms including Enterococcus and Gram-negative rods. Up to one-third of patients with GC and EC also are likely to harbor anaerobes including *Clostridia perfringens*. Patients are nil per os (npo), provided with adequate analgesia, and urgent steps are taken to treat the cholecystitis [14].

The clinical picture dictates management for patients with Grade III cholecystitis, with or without underlying GC. Aggressive medical therapy is essential. If organ dysfunction persists or the patient is a poor surgical candidate, percutaneous drainage may be preferred as a temporizing measure to control sepsis and allow stabilization. However, the likelihood that percutaneous cholecystostomy will be successful is reduced in patients with GC.

The Tokyo Guidelines suggest consideration of percutaneous gallbladder drainage for Grades II and III cholecystitis. However, when a gangrenous gallbladder is present, cholecystectomy should be strongly considered, as these patients are more likely to require gallbladder removal (81 vs. 61%, $p < 0.001$) [12]. This observation suggests that despite the presence of a percutaneous drain, patients still require surgery during the initial admission. The development of GC may also reflect the delay that occurs in attempting alternative diagnostic imaging and interventions, such as percutaneous drainage (i.e., prolonging the ischemic insult to the gallbladder). Consequently, recommendations to proceed with surgery instead of nonoperative treatment are typical, notably in patients at risk of gangrenous degeneration [5, 12, 22].

Patient stability permitting, the increased morbidity and mortality associated with GC leads the authors to prefer proceeding with cholecystectomy. Considering all patients, cholecystitis has a reported mortality rate of less than 1% [1, 20]. Mortality rates rise to 1.5–15% in the setting of GC, notably in at-risk populations such as the elderly, immunocompromised, or diabetic patients [1–3, 5, 12]. Consequently, optimal preparedness is imperative. Members of the perioperative team, including anesthesiologists and operative nurses, as well as the patient, need to be aware of the higher likelihood of conversion to an open approach (75% compared to 17% in acute cholecystitis) [3, 8].

Surgical Considerations

The following comments apply to both laparoscopic and open cholecystectomy. Proper visualization and understanding of nearby landmarks is imperative to avoid iatrogenic complications. With a wide view of the subhepatic space, the surgeon must lift the liver off the porta hepatis and identify the umbilical fissure, base of segment IV, and portal structures such as the hepatic artery and bile duct, duodenum, sulcus of Rouvier, and gallbladder. Performing this check at the beginning of the procedure helps ensure proper orientation and guide safe dissection. This safety maneuver, referred to as the "bile duct time-out," should be periodically repeated. This step is particularly important when ambiguity of the anatomy is encountered, and prior to clipping and transecting structures. The mnemonic "B.E. S.A.F.E." has been established to remind the surgeon of important landmarks (Fig. 15.3). In the setting of a gangrenous gallbladder, the associated cholecystectomy is expected to be more challenging, [3] but understanding the local-regional anatomy will allow safe progression through the procedure.

Prior to starting the dissection, tissue handling in this setting is of utmost importance. The gallbladder wall can be thin and friable, depending on location and duration of the ischemic process. During a laparoscopic approach, atraumatic graspers should be utilized, and pushing on the gallbladder to create countertraction can be employed instead of grasping and retracting, which may easily tear the organ. Pushing the gallbladder is more easily done if the structure is distended. Alternatively, the gallbladder can also be decompressed, in a controlled fashion with suction, if this maneuver provides better exposure.

We often begin the cholecystectomy by mobilizing the lateral leaflet of peritoneum (back of the triangle). This step allows mobilization of the infundibulum, helps unravel a folded cystic duct, and may create space within the triangle of Calot. If the expected location of the triangle is obscured or thought to be fraught with risk, then gaining the angle at the junction of the infundibulum and cystic duct may

B – Bile duct
E – Enteric (Duodenum) position

S – Sulcus of Rouvier
A – Artery (hepatic artery)
F – Fissure (umbilical fissure)
E – Environment (back the camera out for improved perspective)

Fig. 15.3 Bile Duct "Time-Out" (B.E. S.A.F.E)

help identify the location of the inferior border of the gallbladder. Caution must be exercised, as approximation of the gallbladder and bile duct may have occurred, leading to the increased risk of iatrogenic bile duct injury [4]. Anatomic ambiguity should prompt the surgeon to slow down his/her cadence, obtain a wide view, and perform a safety maneuver such as the bile duct time-out prior to proceeding.

If dissection at this anatomic level is not deemed safe, a top-down approach can be attempted, dissecting the gallbladder away from the cystic plate in a hemostatic fashion with electrocautery. When performing a retrograde cholecystectomy, one must be wary to follow the natural curve of the gallbladder as the dissection is carried toward the infundibulum, and not continue in a linear, posterior direction that risks injury to the extra-hepatic biliary tree at a proximal level. The significant inflammatory process associated with GC may fuse the gallbladder to the bile duct. Obscure and distorted nearby anatomy should prompt continuous reassessment of the proximity of portal structures, all the while "hugging" the gallbladder wall during dissection.

A pitfall associated with dissecting the gallbladder from the cystic plate lies in carrying the dissection into the hepatic parenchyma and injuring the superficial branch of the middle hepatic vein. The back wall of the gallbladder may be quite thickened, contain intra-mural abscesses, or have become thin and gangrenous. These changes render a typically easy step of the cholecystectomy into a tedious dissection. Many patients (15–30%) will have sizeable branches from the middle hepatic vein within 1 mm of the gallbladder bed [23]. These venous injuries are a clear risk and can result in substantial bleeding. This particular hemorrhage can be addressed by applying high-intensity cautery directly to the site and compressing the vein into the liver, in order to appose the walls of the bleeding vein, thereby occluding and sealing it with cautery. Apposition of the walls of the vein is imperative, otherwise the flow of the bleed will exceed the capacity of the cautery.

In the setting of challenging cholecystectomies, subtotal cholecystectomy, with or without closure of the remnant and closed-suction drainage, is acceptable [24]. While resultant complications from long cystic ducts, remnant gallbladders, and retained cholelithiasis are possible, these delayed problems are less morbid than a bile duct injury. While we aim to achieve total cholecystectomy, even in the setting of GC, to fully control the source of sepsis and avoid leaving non-viable tissue, this goal should be balanced against biliary and/or vascular injuries. As such, if a necrotic/gangrenous gallbladder is encountered and there is significant concern regarding the proximity of the portal structures (or progression of the laparoscopic procedure is hindered), we prefer to convert to an open cholecystectomy. Clearly, total cholecystectomy should not be pursued if it risks injury to portal structures. In these cases, the gallbladder should be opened and all stones and debris removed. The portion of gallbladder that can be safely accessed is resected. Fenestration or reconstitution (endoloops, suturing, or stapling) of the remnant is then performed, according to surgeon preference [24].

Alternative Approaches

1. Percutaneous cholecystostomy drains can be employed, but often only temporize and bridge the patient to cholecystectomy.
2. Subtotal cholecystectomy can be employed in select cases to avoid injury to portal structures.

Due to varying definitions of gangrenous or severe cholecystitis, establishing precise rates of open cholecystectomy within this population is challenging. Expert surgeons will recognize when a laparoscopic approach is futile, and conversion will result in a more rapid conclusion of the procedure. Conversion allows for ongoing resuscitation and medical management of the patient. The astute surgeon also will recognize that open cholecystectomies are challenging in patients at higher risk of GC, such as the obese, diabetic male who may have a thick abdominal wall, high intra-abdominal visceral fat phenotype, and poor healing capacity. Another high-risk group are frail elderly patients who will struggle with respiratory toilet and ventilation due to the cephalad location of the incision. Recognizing these clinical situations is an important piece of intraoperative decision-making.

Though we prefer an upper midline incision, a right subcostal (Kocher) incision can be employed to expose the area, especially when the gallbladder is in a lateral position. The ligamentum teres and falciform ligaments are taken down to allow mobilization. Sponges can be placed above the liver in order to bring the liver and gallbladder into view. A fixed retractor is placed to optimize exposure. The abdominal wall is a dynamic structure; retracting blades on a fixed retractor can gradually be pushed further to continue to increase exposure. A malleable blade is placed over the base of segment IV to expose the anterior aspect of the porta hepatis and medial side of the gallbladder.

We approach open cholecystectomies in a similar fashion as the laparoscopic counterpart. Open cholecystectomy often allows improved visualization and palpation of nearby landmarks and portal structures, which helps identify their location and proximity. The cautery can be used as a dissection instrument, to bluntly displace tissues and develop planes. The initial objective should remain to identify the cystic duct and artery. Once this goal is achieved, dissection of the gallbladder from the cystic plate ensures the absence of structures returning to the liver, and improves the safety of the procedure. In these arduous cases, we often take the cystic artery early, which allows further opening of the triangle of Calot. We then proceed with retrograde cholecystectomy, ensuring that we are left with the cystic duct as the sole structure attached to the gallbladder. Considerations of proximity of hepatic veins and portal structures remain true in open cholecystectomy. The cystic duct is then occluded with clips and/or ties, and transected.

Cholangiography is reported to be used at similar rates in patients with acute or GC, [12] but this adjunct should be considered if the anatomy remains obscured or the integrity of the extra-hepatic biliary tree is questioned. Placement of closed-suction drains can be used to monitor for postoperative bile leaks, which may result from cystic duct stumps that undergo resolution of the inflammatory process, leading to reconstitution of a lumen previously occluded by thick, inflamed cystic duct walls. Management of these complications is beyond the scope of this chapter.

Conclusion

Gangrenous cholecystitis occurs uncommonly; however, surgeons must remain vigilant to identify at-risk patients, who often present atypically and later in the course of their disease. When the inflammatory process reaches this degree of severity, it poses significant intraoperative challenges and increases rates of morbidity and mortality. With the aging population, we can anticipate the potential for an increasing incidence of GC. Thus, new generations of surgeons must remain facile with the management of severe forms of cholecystitis. In an era when cholecystectomies are almost exclusively performed laparoscopically, surgeons must maintain skills and comfort with the open counterpart of the procedure, to avoid iatrogenic complications and offer optimal management for these patients. Though the ability to perform increasingly complicated surgeries via laparoscopy is growing, persistence with a laparoscopic approach may be detrimental in a patient whose physiology is impacted by ongoing sepsis.

This chapter has presented safety maneuvers and approaches to this arduous scenario, gangrenous cholecystitis. Various techniques can be used to resolve the cholecystitis, always with the safety of the patient in mind. Multidisciplinary institutional pathways bridging the emergency department, diagnostic imaging, and surgical services may expedite the assessment, diagnosis, and management of these patients, in whom undue delays may alter their clinical course.

Overall Pearls

1. Male sex, advanced age, and diabetes are key risk factors.
2. Delayed presentation and diagnosis plague these patients; a high index of suspicion should be maintained to achieve timely diagnosis and proceed to management.
3. The finding of inhomogeneous wall enhancement or disrupted mucosal enhancement is characteristic of gangrenous cholecystitis.
4. Gangrenous cholecystitis is associated with increased morbidity and mortality; involvement of a hepatobiliary surgeon may help optimize outcomes.

References

1. Bourikian S, Anand RJ, Aboutanos M, Wolfe LG, Ferrada P. Risk factors for acute gangrenous cholecystitis in emergency general surgery patients. Am J Surg. 2015;210(4):730–3.
2. Onder A, Kapan M, Ulger BV, Oguz A, Turkoglu A, Uslukaya O. Gangrenous cholecystitis: mortality and risk factors. Int Surg. 2015;100(2):254–60.
3. Ganapathi AM, Speicher PJ, Englum BR, Perez A, Tyler DS, Zani S. Gangrenous cholecystitis: a contemporary review. J Surg Res. 2015;197(1):18–24.
4. Wu B, Buddensick TJ, Ferdosi H, Narducci DM, Sautter A, Setiawan L, et al. Predicting gangrenous cholecystitis. HPB (Oxford). 2014;16(9):801–6.
5. Aydin C, Altaca G, Berber I, Tekin K, Kara M, Titiz I. Prognostic parameters for the prediction of acute gangrenous cholecystitis. J Hepatobiliary Pancreat Surg. 2006; 13(2):155–9.
6. Yeh DD, Cropano C, Fagenholz P, King DR, Chang Y, Klein EN, et al. Gangrenous cholecystitis: deceiving ultrasounds, significant delay in surgical consult, and increased postoperative morbidity! J Trauma Acute Care Surg. 2015;79(5):812–6.
7. Wu CH, Chen CC, Wang CJ, Wong YC, Wang LJ, Huang CC, et al. Discrimination of gangrenous from uncomplicated acute cholecystitis: accuracy of CT findings. Abdom Imaging. 2011;36(2):174–8.
8. Merriam LTK, Dawes LG, Angelos P, Prystowsky JB, Rege RV, Joehl RJ. Gangrenous cholecystitis: analysis of risk factors and experience with laparoscopic cholecystectomy. Surgery. 1999;126(4):680–6.
9. Fagan SP, Awad SS, Rahwan K, Hira K, Aoki N, Itani KMF, et al. Prognostic factors for the development of gangrenous cholecystitis. Am J Surg. 2003;186(5):481–5.
10. Nguyen L, Fagan SP, Lee TC, Aoki N, Itani KM, Berger D, et al. Use of a predictive equation for diagnosis of acute gangrenous cholecystitis. Am J Surg. 2004;188(5):463–6.
11. Yacoub WN, Petrosyan M, Sehgal I, Ma Y, Chandrasoma P, Mason RJ. Prediction of patients with acute cholecystitis requiring emergent cholecystectomy: a simple score. Gastroent Res Pract. 2010;2010:901739.
12. Nikfarjam M, Niumsawatt V, Sethu A, Fink MA, Muralidharan V, Starkey G, et al. Outcomes of contemporary management of gangrenous and non-gangrenous acute cholecystitis. HPB (Oxford). 2011;13(8):551–8.
13. Falor AE, Zobel M, Kaji A, Neville A, De Virgilio C. Admission variables predictive of gangrenous cholecystitis. Am Surg. 2012;78(10):1075–8.
14. Butte JM, Hameed M, Ball CG. Hepato-pancreato-biliary emergencies for the acute care surgeon: etiology, diagnosis and treatment. World J Emerg Surg. 2015;10:13.
15. Strasberg SM. Acute calculous cholecystitis. N Eng J Med. 2008;358(26):2804–11.
16. Yokoe M, Takada T, Strasberg SM, Solomkin JS, Mayumi T, Gomi H, et al. New diagnostic criteria and severity assessment of acute cholecystitis in revised Tokyo Guidelines. J Hepatobiliary Pancreat Sci. 2012;19(5):578–85.
17. Singh AK, Sagar P. Gangrenous cholecystitis: prediction with CT imaging. Abdom Imaging. 2005;30(2):218–21.
18. Watanabe Y, Nagayama M, Okumura A, Amoh Y, Katsube T, Suga T, et al. MR imaging of acute biliary disorders. RadioGraphics. 2007;27(2):477–95.
19. Kimura Y, Takada T, Strasberg SM, Pitt HA, Gouma DJ, Garden OJ, et al. TG13 current terminology, etiology, and epidemiology of acute cholangitis and cholecystitis. J Hepatobiliary Pancreat Sci. 2013;20(1):8–23.
20. Kimura Y, Takada T, Kawarada Y, Nimura Y, Hirata K, Sekimoto M, et al. Definitions, pathophysiology, and epidemiology of acute cholangitis and cholecystitis: Tokyo Guidelines. J Hepatobiliary Pancreat Surg. 2007;14(1):15–26.

21. Miura F, Takada T, Strasberg SM, Solomkin JS, Pitt HA, Gouma DJ, et al. TG13 flowchart for the management of acute cholangitis and cholecystitis. J Hepatobiliary Pancreat Sci. 2013;20(1):47–54.
22. Borzellino G, Sauerland S, Minicozzi AM, Verlato G, Di Pietrantonj C, de Manzoni G, et al. Laparoscopic cholecystectomy for severe acute cholecystitis. A meta-analysis of results. Surg Endosc. 2008;22(1):8–15.
23. Ball CG, MacLean AR, Kirkpatrick AW, Bathe OF, Sutherland F, Debru E, et al. Hepatic vein injury during laparoscopic cholecystectomy: the unappreciated proximity of the middle hepatic vein to the gallbladder bed. J Gastrointest Surg. 2006;10(8):1151–5.
24. Strasberg SM, Pucci MJ, Brunt LM, Deziel DJ. Subtotal cholecystectomy-"Fenestrating" vs "Reconstituting" subtypes and the prevention of bile duct injury: definition of the optimal procedure in difficult operative conditions. J Am Coll Surg. 2016;222(1):89–96.

Surgical Resection of a Type IVa Choledochal Cyst

16

J. Robert O'Neill and Rowan W. Parks

Case Presentation

A 17-year-old female presented with a history of recurrent upper abdominal pain. On detailed questioning, intermittent symptoms had been present since childhood, but she had not previously been admitted to hospital and had no previous episodes of cholangitis. She had no other past medical history and was not on any regular medications. Her liver function tests at presentation were as follows: Bilirubin 14 μmol/l (Normal range 3–21 μmol/l); ALP 109 iU/L (Normal range 40–125 iU/L); ALT 232 iU/L (Normal range 10–50 iU/L); Albumin 44 g/L (Normal range 36–47 g/L).

An abdominal ultrasound demonstrated a bright liver echo-texture consistent with fatty infiltration, and a partially contracted and thick-walled gallbladder with no evidence of gallstones. The intrahepatic ducts were moderately dilated around the porta measuring 15 mm at the level of the common hepatic duct (CHD) and 30 mm in the mid common bile duct (CBD), tapering distally down to normal calibre with an abrupt termination within the pancreas (Fig. 16.1). The other visualised abdominal organs were normal and there was no evidence of free fluid.

Electronic supplementary material

The online version of this chapter (doi:10.1007/978-3-319-50868-9_16) contains supplementary material, which is available to authorized users.

J. Robert O'Neill · R.W. Parks (✉)
Department of Clinical Surgery, University of Edinburgh, Royal Infirmary of Edinburgh, 51 Little France Crescent, Edinburgh EH16 4SA, UK
e-mail: R.W.Parks@ed.ac.uk

J. Robert O'Neill
e-mail: Robert.o'neill@ed.ac.uk

T.M. Pawlik et al. (eds.), *Case-Based Lessons in the Management of Complex Hepato-Pancreato-Biliary Surgery*, DOI 10.1007/978-3-319-50868-9_16

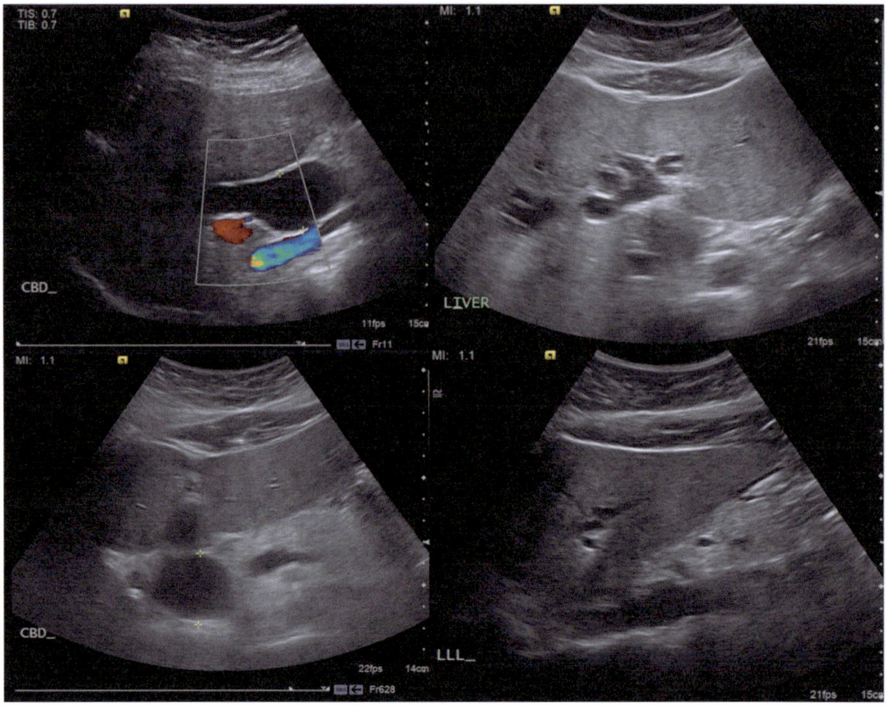

Fig. 16.1 Abdominal ultrasound images demonstrating a grossly dilated CBD (3 cm between *yellow* cross-hairs) (*upper left* and *lower left* images). Duplex colour-flow imaging of the portal vein (*blue*) and hepatic artery (*red*) adjacent to the dilated CBD (*upper left image*). Centrally dilated intrahepatic ducts were also seen tapering within the hepatic parenchyma (*upper right* and *lower right* images). *CBD* common bile duct; *LLL* left lobe of liver

These ultrasound findings raised the possibility of a choledochal cyst, and therefore the patient proceeded to magnetic resonance cholangiopancreatography (MRCP). This demonstrated centrally dilated intrahepatic ducts which tapered to normal calibre beyond the secondary order division. The cystic duct, CHD, and CBD were all dilated, with gross fusiform dilatation of the proximal CBD up to a maximum diameter of 3.5 cm (Fig. 16.2, and supplemental video).

The pancreaticobiliary segment of the common duct was long, with the pancreaticobiliary junction identified proximal to the usual site. There was no sign of intrahepatic or extrahepatic ductal calculi, no evidence of intrahepatic or extrahepatic strictures, and no other abnormalities in the liver parenchyma, spleen, kidneys, adrenals, or pancreas. These findings confirmed the diagnosis of a Type IVa choledochal cyst.

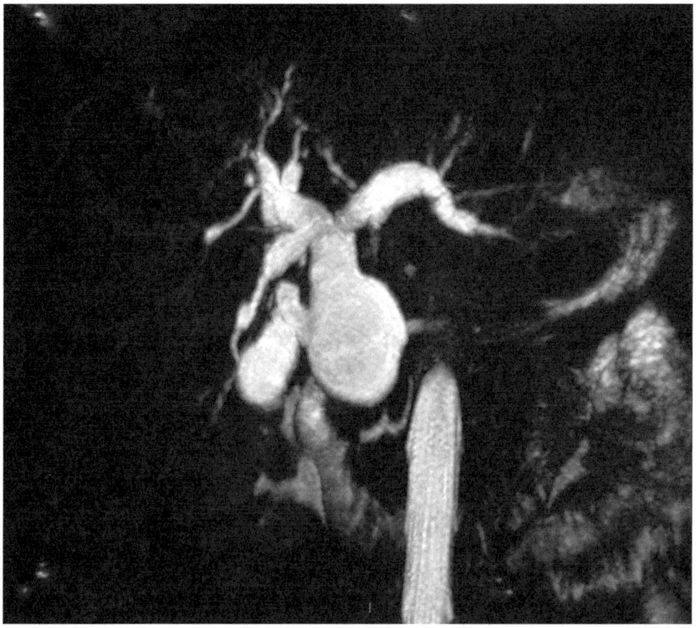

Fig. 16.2 Representative image of the 3D cholangiography reconstruction from the MRCP. The full reconstruction can be viewed online (A supplementary video has been submitted)

Diagnosis and Assessment

Choledochal cysts are rare developmental malformations of the biliary tree, comprising 1% of all benign biliary conditions [1]. The classical presentation is of a female child with abdominal pain, jaundice, and an abdominal mass, although up to a quarter of patients present as adults [2]. Perhaps due to the increasing availability of high-quality noninvasive imaging, patients are more frequently being diagnosed in adulthood [3].

An abdominal ultrasound would be the commonest initial investigation for patients with abdominal pain and deranged liver function tests, and this test is sensitive for the detection of intrahepatic cystic disease. Delineating the extent of choledochal cystic disease is best accomplished by magnetic retrograde cholangiopancreatography MRCP [4]. A triple-phase contrast-enhanced CT can be complementary in determining the relationship of extrahepatic cystic disease to neighbouring vascular structures. If MRI is contraindicated, direct cholangiography either by endoscopic retrograde cholangiography (ERC) or percutaneous transhepatic cholangiography (PTC) is recommended, but this is associated with a greater risk to the patient.

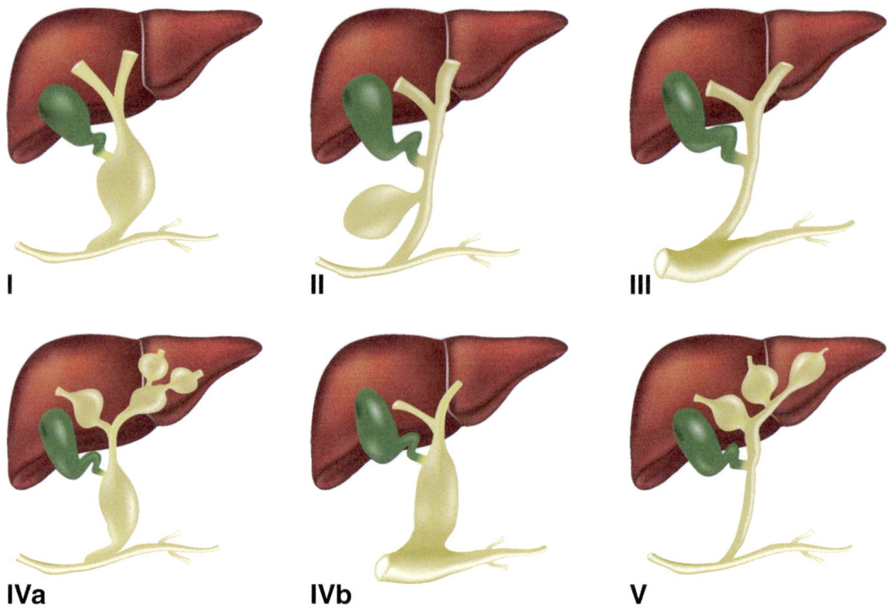

Fig. 16.3 Todani classification of choledochal cysts, adapted from [5]. **Type I** solitary extrahepatic cyst (can be subclassified according to fusiform (If) or cystic (Ic) type); **Type II** extrahepatic bile duct diverticulum; **Type III** cyst of the common pancreaticobiliary channel (choledochocele); **Type IVa** extrahepatic and intrahepatic cysts; **Type IVb** multiple extrahepatic cysts; **Type V** intrahepatic cysts (Caroli's disease)

Our own experience is that patients commonly present with abdominal pain, and most have at least one episode of cholangitis, with many having intermittently deranged liver function tests.

The modified Todani classification is the most widely established in clinical practice, and segregates patients on the anatomical distribution of the abnormalities (Fig. 16.3) [5]. Across published series, approximately 80% of patients have type I cysts, 15% have type IVa cysts, and the remainder are classified as types II, III, IVb, and V [6]. Type IVa cysts are more common in adults.

Clinical Pearls

- Cyst drainage procedures (e.g. cyst-duodenostomy) have poor long-term success rates due to complications with the cyst remnant and should be avoided in favour of primary extrahepatic cyst excision and biliary reconstruction.

- The risk of cholangiocarcinoma remains for all patients with choledochal cysts even after cyst excision and this appears higher in patients with an APBJ or residual intrahepatic disease. These patients should remain under long-term follow-up. The frequency and mode of follow-up are largely down to surgical preference but those patients developing cholangiocarcinoma following cyst excision currently have a poor prognosis.

Incidence and Aetiology

Choledochal cysts are rare globally, with an estimated incidence of 1 in 100,000 live births in Western countries, but they are more common in Asian countries and up to 100-fold more frequent in Japan [7]. Several studies report a strong association between an abnormal pancreatico-biliary junction (APBJ) and choledochal cysts [8, 9]. A report of monozygotic twins provides further support of the direct association. One sibling presented at 2 years of age with abdominal pain and abnormal liver function tests, and was demonstrated to have an anomalous pancreatico-biliary junction and associated type I choledochal cyst. The other twin was asymptomatic and had a normal pancreaticobiliary junction and biliary tree [10].

Reflux of pancreatic exocrine secretions into the biliary tree due to an APBJ has been proposed as the central aetiological factor in choledochal cyst development. The finding of a long common pancreaticobiliary duct in our case further supports the association of APBJ and choledochal cysts and the long common channel hypothesis [11].

The in utero finding of a choledochal cyst prior to the development of the exocrine pancreas, however, casts doubt on the necessity of reflux of exocrine secretions in cystic degeneration, and an alternative hypothesis is that neonatal biliary obstruction is the central factor [12].

Clinical Course

Regardless of the underlying aetiology, choledochal cysts are associated with multiple complications. Impaired biliary drainage and cholestasis predispose to stone development, and infectious sequelae are common, including cholecystitis, cholangitis, and hepatic abscess [13]. Pancreatitis is also common and may be secondary to stones, causing pancreatic duct obstruction, a direct result of the APBJ, or as a consequence of ERCP undertaken for biliary drainage [14]. Recurrent cholangitis and biliary obstruction can lead to cirrhosis and portal hypertension, and patients should be thoroughly assessed for these complications prior to operative intervention [13, 15, 16].

Up to 75% of patients with type I cysts have ductal stones, and the prevalence is even higher in patients with type IVa cysts [17]. It is important to establish the extent of intrahepatic disease and the presence of abscesses, stones, or strictures pre-operatively, as these pathologies may not be adequately treated by hepatico-jejunostomy and may result in recurrent stone formation and sepsis [17].

Patients with choledochal cysts have up to a 100-fold higher risk of developing cholangiocarcinoma than the general population [18]. The incidence of malignancy increases with age, with the majority of cancers presenting by the fourth decade of life. The overall incidence of malignancy is 11%, [2, 19, 20] and those patients with type I or type IVa cysts appear to be at highest risk [21, 22].

The risk of cholangiocarcinoma remains following resection of extrahepatic cystic disease, with a 10% reported cumulative incidence in one Japanese series up to 25 years post-excision, although the risk appears lower in Western populations [18, 23]. Patients at higher risk include those with an APBJ or those with incomplete cyst excision, such as patients with type IVa cysts and residual intrahepatic disease [22].

A key principle in the treatment of choledochal cysts is complete excision of the extrahepatic disease, as patients who have undergone a cyst drainage procedure—such as transduodenal sphincteroplasty, choledochoduodenostomy, or choledochojejunostomy—have a higher risk of cholangiocarcinoma than those patients who have undergone cyst excision [23, 24].

Interestingly, drainage procedures in patients without choledochal cysts are also associated with an increased risk of cholangiocarcinoma, and this may reflect the carcinogenic effect of chronic enteric reflux on the biliary epithelium [25].

Alternative Approaches and Controversies

- Patients with Type IVa choledochal cysts have both intra and extrahepatic disease. One approach is to only resect the extrahepatic disease. An alternative is to resect both the intrahepatic and extrahepatic components, with a greater risk of post-operative morbidity but potentially a reduced risk of future intrahepatic complications.
- Our approach is to undertake excision of the extrahaptic disease only, reserving synchronous resection for selected patients with predominantly unilobar disease and evidence of intrahepatic strictures or multiple intrahepatic stones at high risk of recurrent biliary sepsis.

Operative Management

Our patient underwent laparotomy with intraoperative ultrasonography, confirming dilated intrahepatic and extrahepatic ducts with no evidence of ductal stones, liver abscess, or other parenchymal lesions. The extrahepatic biliary tree was excised from the confluence of the hepatic ducts to the superior border of the pancreas with an en-bloc cholecystectomy. On-table choledochoscopy was performed and confirmed no intrahepatic ductal stones or strictures (See **Technical Elements** box below).

A Roux-en-Y hepaticojejunostomy was performed for reconstitution of biliary drainage. This would be our favoured approach for both type I and type IVa choledochal cysts, and is increasingly recognised as the established standard in the literature [26]. Cyst excision and reconstruction should be performed in all cases, including those patients who have previously undergone a primary cyst drainage procedure, as post-operative complication rates are low and longer term outcomes are superior [24]. If the gallbladder is present, a cholecystectomy should always be performed as part of the procedure [27].

Our practice would be to perform the biliary-enteric anastomosis at the confluence of right and left hepatic ducts. Spatulation of the left hepatic duct allows a wide anastomosis to be constructed in most patients, reducing the risk of a post-operative anastomotic stricture and therefore reducing the need for revisional surgery [28]. If the intrahepatic component of the choledochal cyst involves the confluence of the hepatic ducts, we would still recommend excision of the extra-hepatic component and anastomosis to an epithelial-lined portion of the intrahepatic cyst. In patients with distal extrahepatic disease, complete excision of the extra-hepatic ducts and anastomosis at the biliary confluence should still be performed.

The feasibility of laparoscopic resection and reconstruction for a Type IVa choledochal cyst has been reported with outcomes from case series comparable to those after open surgery [29]. However, previous recurrent attacks of cholangitis and pancreatitis can make these cases particularly challenging, and this approach should only be attempted by surgeons with advanced laparoscopic skills and experience in complex hepatobiliary surgery.

Partial hepatectomy to excise the intrahepatic cystic disease has been proposed for patients with type IVa choledochal cysts [30–32]. Advocates of this approach suggest there are fewer long-term complications with intrahepatic stone disease and cholangitis, [2] however, the higher post-operative morbidity rates have been cited as justification for a more conservative approach. The optimal approach remains an area of controversy, with only case series to guide recommendations [33, 34].

Our approach would be to consider synchronous hepatic resection and extra-hepatic cyst excision if the intrahepatic disease is predominantly unilobar, with a dominant intrahepatic ductal stricture or extensive intrahepatic stones, either of which may predispose to cholestasis and recurrent cholangitis. Hepatic resection should be anatomical and undertaken as for other indications, preserving sufficient future liver remnant volume, adjusting for underlying liver disease if biliary cirrhosis is suspected.

Outcome

Our patient made an uncomplicated post-operative recovery with no septic complications, and was discharged on the fifth post-operative day with normal liver function tests. She remains well, with normal liver function at last follow-up, 3 years after her procedure.

Post-operative cholangitis has been reported after primary excision of the extrahepatic portion of Type IVa cysts [2, 28]. The risk of post-operative complications, specifically cholangitis or anastomotic stricture, appears higher in patients with previous surgery, especially cyst drainage procedures.

Due to the risk of post-operative stricture, stone formation, and development of cholangiocarcinoma, it is recommended that patients should undergo routine follow-up [33, 35]. Cases of cholangiocarcinoma have been reported over 30 years after the primary resection of a choledochal cyst, and therefore this monitoring should continue lifelong [18, 36]. Patients with choledochal cysts are at risk of developing malignancy throughout their biliary tree, and this risk, although lower, persists post-operatively. Therefore, even those patients with type I cysts who have undergone complete cyst excision should remain under surveillance [37].

It is unclear from published series what the optimal follow-up interval should be and whether serial imaging is required to detect complications. It is also not clear if follow-up improves outcome, as the median survival in a series of 32 patients who developed cholangiocarcinoma during follow-up after cyst excision was just 15 months [18].

In the absence of evidence, our pragmatic approach is to follow patients who are otherwise well by annual clinical review and routine blood tests. If patients become symptomatic or liver function tests become abnormal, then an MRCP is undertaken to identify evidence of intrahepatic stones, strictures, abscesses or pancreaticobiliary malignancy.

Technical Elements

- Pre-operative imaging is essential to plan the extent of resection and identify aberrant anatomy.
- Dissection can be challenging, as most adult patients will have had previous episodes of pancreatitis, cholangitis and/or operative drainage procedures.
- Intraoperative ultrasound should be used to confirm the distribution of cystic disease and ductal stones, and can identify occult intrahepatic masses or abscesses.

- During resection the hilar plate should be lowered to allow access to the confluence of hepatic ducts. Our standard approach would be to only excise the extrahepatic cyst, and this would generally denote the superior limit of the resection.
- Intraoperative choledochoscopy should be performed to confirm there are no residual intrahepatic stones or strictures.
- Reconstruction with a Roux-en-Y hepaticojejunostomy at the biliary confluence should be performed to minimise the risk of post-operative stricture. Our favoured method is to perform an end-to-side, single layer, mucosa-to-mucosa, hepaticojejunostomy using interrupted 4/0 polydioxanone (PDS®) suture.
- Some surgeons advocate a hepaticoduodenostomy for reconstruction, predominantly in the paediatric setting. This offers the advantage of providing endoscopic access to the biliary tree.

References

1. Jabłońska B. Biliary cysts: etiology, diagnosis and management. World J Gastroenterol. 2012;18(35):4801–10.
2. Lenriot JP, Gigot JF, Ségol P, Fagniez PL, Fingerhut A, Adloff M. Bile duct cysts in adults: a multi-institutional retrospective study. French Associations for Surgical Research. Ann Surg. 1998;228(2):159–66.
3. Dhupar R, Gulack B, Geller DA, Marsh JW, Gamblin TC. The changing presentation of choledochal cyst disease: an incidental diagnosis. HPB Surg. 2009;2009:103739.
4. Kim SH, Lim JH, Yoon HK, Han BK, Lee SK, Kim YI. Choledochal cyst: comparison of MR and conventional cholangiography. Clin Radiol. 2000;55(5):378–83.
5. Todani T, Watanabe Y, Narusue M, Tabuchi K, Okajima K. Congenital bile duct cysts: classification, operative procedures, and review of thirty-seven cases including cancer arising from choledochal cyst. Am J Surg. 1977;134(2):263–9.
6. Söreide K, Körner H, Havnen J, Söreide JA. Bile duct cysts in adults. Br J Surg. 2004;91(12):1538–48.
7. Yamaguchi M. Congenital choledochal cyst. Analysis of 1,433 patients in the Japanese literature. Am J Surg. 1980;140(5):653–7.
8. Rattner DW, Schapiro RH, Warshaw AL. Abnormalities of the pancreatic and biliary ducts in adult patients with choledochal cysts. Arch Surg. 1983;118(9):1068–73.
9. Sugiyama M, Atomi Y, Kuroda A. Pancreatic disorders associated with anomalous pancreaticobiliary junction. Surgery. 1999;126(3):492–7.
10. Uchida M, Tsukahara M, Fuji T, Fujihara T, Ueki K, Kajii T. Discordance for anomalous pancreaticobiliary ductal junction and congenital biliary dilatation in a set of monozygotic twins. J Pediatr Surg. 1992;27(12):1563–4.
11. Babbitt DP. Congenital choledochal cysts: new etiological concept based on anomalous relationships of the common bile duct and pancreatic bulb. Ann Radiol (Paris). 1969;12(3):231–40.

12. Schroeder D, Smith L, Prain HC. Antenatal diagnosis of choledochal cyst at 15 weeks' gestation: etiologic implications and management. J Pediatr Surg. 1989;24(9):936–8.
13. Nicholl M, Pitt HA, Wolf P, Cooney J, Kalayoglu M, Shilyansky J, et al. Choledochal cysts in western adults: complexities compared to children. J Gastrointest Surg. 2004;8(3):245–52.
14. Komuro H, Makino SI, Yasuda Y, Ishibashi T, Tahara K, Nagai H. Pancreatic complications in choledochal cyst and their surgical outcomes. World J Surg. 2001;25(12):1519–23.
15. Rao KL, Chowdhary SK, Kumar D. Choledochal cyst associated with portal hypertension. Pediatr Surg Int. 2003;19(11):729–32.
16. Martin LW, Rowe GA. Portal hypertension secondary to choledochal cyst. Ann Surg. 1979;190(5):638–9.
17. Cetta F, Montalto G, Nuzzo G. Recurrent hepatolithiasis after primary excision of choledochal cysts. J Am Coll Surg. 1997;185(2):198–200.
18. Ohashi T, Wakai T, Kubota M, Matsuda Y, Arai Y, Ohyama T, et al. Risk of subsequent biliary malignancy in patients undergoing cyst excision for congenital choledochal cysts. J Gastroenterol Hepatol. 2013;28(2):243–7.
19. Komi N, Tamura T, Miyoshi Y, Kunitomo K, Udaka H, Takehara H. Nationwide survey of cases of choledochal cyst. Analysis of coexistent anomalies, complications and surgical treatment in 645 cases. Surg Gastroenterol. 1984;3(2):69–73.
20. Sastry AV, Abbadessa B, Wayne MG, Steele JG, Cooperman AM. What is the incidence of biliary carcinoma in choledochal cysts, when do they develop, and how should it affect management? World J Surg. 2015;39(2):487–92.
21. Ishibashi T, Kasahara K, Yasuda Y, Nagai H, Makino S, Kanazawa K. Malignant change in the biliary tract after excision of choledochal cyst. Br J Surg. 1997;84(12):1687–91.
22. Kobayashi S, Asano T, Yamasaki M, Kenmochi T, Nakagohri T, Ochiai T. Risk of bile duct carcinogenesis after excision of extrahepatic bile ducts in pancreaticobiliary maljunction. Surgery. 1999;126(5):939–44.
23. Tocchi A, Mazzoni G, Liotta G, Lepre L, Cassini D, Miccini M. Late development of bile duct cancer in patients who had biliary-enteric drainage for benign disease: a follow-up study of more than 1,000 patients. Ann Surg. 2001;234(2):210–4.
24. Atkinson HD, Fischer CP, de Jong CH, Madhavan KK, Parks RW, Garden OJ. Choledochal cysts in adults and their complications. HPB (Oxford). 2003;5(2):105–10.
25. Bettschart V, Clayton RA, Parks RW, Garden OJ, Bellamy CO. Cholangiocarcinoma arising after biliary-enteric drainage procedures for benign disease. Gut. 2002;51(1):128–9.
26. Xia HT, Dong JH, Yang T, Liang B, Zeng JP. Selection of the surgical approach for reoperation of adult choledochal cysts. J Gastrointest Surg. 2015;19(2):290–7.
27. Kobayashi S, Asano T, Yamasaki M, Kenmochi T, Saigo K, Ochiai T. Prophylactic excision of the gallbladder and bile duct for patients with pancreaticobiliary maljunction. Arch Surg. 2001;136(7):759–63.
28. Todani T, Watanabe Y, Urushihara N, Noda T, Morotomi Y. Biliary complications after excisional procedure for choledochal cyst. J Pediatr Surg. 1995;30(3):478–81.
29. Senthilnathan P, Patel ND, Nair AS, Nalankilli VP, Vijay A, Palanivelu C. Laparoscopic Management of Choledochal Cyst-Technical Modifications and Outcome Analysis. World J Surg. 2015;39(10):2550–6.
30. Xia HT, Dong JH, Yang T, Zeng JP, Liang B. Extrahepatic cyst excision and partial hepatectomy for Todani type IV-A cysts. Dig Liver Dis. 2014;46(11):1025–30.
31. Nakayama H, Masuda H, Ugajin W, Koshinaga T, Fukuzawa M. Left hepatic lobectomy for type IV-A choledochal cyst. Am Surg. 2000;66(11):1020–2.
32. Dong JH, Yang SZ, Xia HT, Duan WD, Ji WB, Gu WQ, et al. Aggressive hepatectomy for the curative treatment of bilobar involvement of type IV-A bile duct cyst. Ann Surg. 2013;258(1):122–8.
33. Chijiiwa K, Tanaka M. Late complications after excisional operation in patients with choledochal cyst. J Am Coll Surg. 1994;179(2):139–44.

34. Chijiiwa K, Komura M, Kameoka N. Postoperative follow-up of patients with type IVa choledochal cysts after excision of extrahepatic cyst. J Am Coll Surg. 1994;179(6):641–5.
35. Soares KC, Kim Y, Spolverato G, Maithel S, Bauer TW, Marques H, et al. Presentation and clinical outcomes of choledochal cysts in children and adults: a multi-institutional analysis. JAMA Surg. 2015;150(6):577–84.
36. Ohtsuka H, Fukase K, Yoshida H, Motoi F, Hayashi H, Morikawa T, et al. Long-term outcomes after extrahepatic excision of congenital choladocal cysts: 30 years of experience at a single center. Hepatogastroenterology. 2015;62(137):1–5.
37. Ronnekleiv-Kelly SM, Soares KC, Ejaz A, Pawlik TM. Management of choledochal cysts. Curr Opin Gastroenterol. 2016;32(3):225–31.

Bile Duct Injury at the Hepatic Confluence

17

Miguel-Angel Mercado, Mario Vilatoba and Bruno A. Gonzalez-Nolasco

Clinical Case

A 32-year-old female with history of biliary colic underwent a cholecystectomy with no incidents reported. During the third postoperative day, abdominal pain and distention were noted. An abdominal ultrasound showed free abdominal fluid. An exploratory laparoscopic procedure was performed, showing bile in the abdominal cavity, which was drained accordingly, and several surgical drains were left in the cavity.

An endoscopic retrograde cholangiopancreatography (ERCP) was performed, which showed complete transection of the common hepatic duct. The right upper abdominal drain showed continuous drainage between 500 and 750 ml a day.

The patient was referred to our center on the eighth postoperative week. Upon physical examination, the patient was in good general condition, without signs of peritoneal irritation or jaundice. The abdomen was flat with adequate peristalsis. A drain on the right upper quadrant continued to actively drain bile. A magnetic resonance cholangiopancreatography (MRCP) was performed (Fig. 17.1), showing a biliary injury classified as Strasberg E-4; therefore, no attempts to place a percutaneous drainage were done, and the patient was scheduled for surgical repair.

Surgical treatment of bile duct injury is indicated when loss of duct continuity is found and an endoscopic and/or radiological approach is ruled out [1]. Roux-en-Y hepaticojejunostomy has been proven to be the best treatment option by several groups [2–5]. A high-quality bilioenteric anastomosis, defined as a tension-free, wide, with adequate suture material, done in healthy, non-scarred non-ischemic

M.-A. Mercado (✉) · M. Vilatoba · B.A. Gonzalez-Nolasco
Department of General Surgery, National Institute of Medical Sciences and Nutrition "Salvador Zubiran", Vasco de Quiroga no. 15, Col. Seccion XVI, Tlalpan, Mexico City 14080, Mexico
e-mail: mercadiazma@yahoo.com

T.M. Pawlik et al. (eds.), *Case-Based Lessons in the Management of Complex Hepato-Pancreato-Biliary Surgery*, DOI 10.1007/978-3-319-50868-9_17

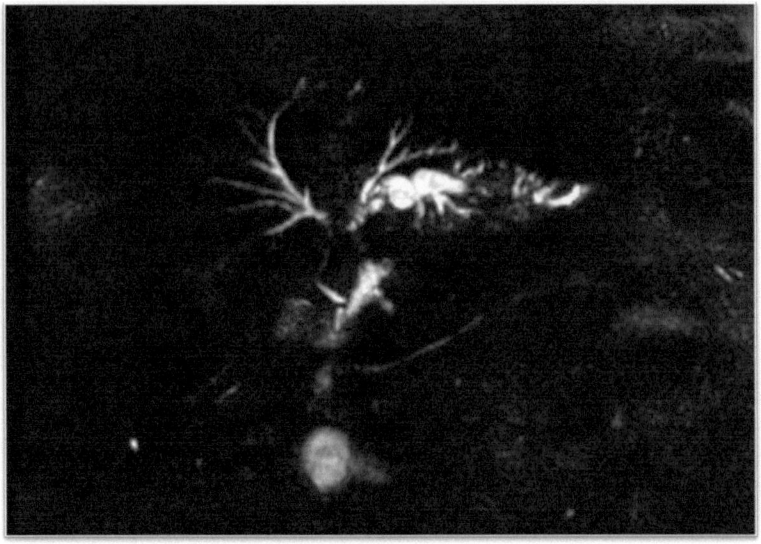

Fig. 17.1 MRI showing loss of confluence.

ducts that are anastomosed to a defunctionalized Roux-en-Y jejunal limb, offers the best results [6]. There are several technical maneuvers that can be done in order to reach this goal, including the anterior opening of the confluence and the left duct, as well as partial removal of hepatic segments IV and V [7].

Our group has shown that an anastomosis performed in a patient with preserved confluence offers the best results [8]. These results can also be optimized if the patient has no stones or biliary sludge, which are usually developed as a result of bacterial colonization.

Loss of confluence, classified as a Bismuth IV [9] or a Strasberg E-4, [3] is a technical challenge for the surgeon. This is also, in our experience, the most undesirable scenario for repair and long-term results are unpredictable. In some cases, the anatomical variation of a low confluence results in a higher rate of bile duct injury [10]. After section and ablation of the duct, two separated lumens can be observed.

In other situations, ischemic damage due to thermal energy may be the cause of the injury, secondary to the heuristic error in which the common bile duct is mistaken with the cystic duct. Also, the presence of a biloma (infected or not), as well as the anatomical deformity contribute to the ductal damage. The most common cause for biliary injury in our series is a technically deficient repair attempt, usually performed by the primary-care surgeon.

Intraoperative Technical Pearls

- Nearby organs should be methodically separated and, in patients who have previously undergone biliodigestive derivation, it is particularly important to free the small intestine in order to determine whether the anastomosed loop is not obstructed or defunctionalized, in case there is an enteral anastomotic variant (Omega loop with Braun anastomosis, Nakayama Beta-anastomosis), or if there is an abnormal positioning of the loop compromising its appropriate function.
- In our center's experience, longitudinally sectioning the anterior aspect of the duct (considering circulation is located on the lateral aspects) and directing this section toward the left duct without moving its posterior aspect makes creating the confluence a simpler task. Every section on the anterior aspect measures approximately 2–3 mm, having thoroughly verified and certified the direction of the ducts.
- In order to expose the hepatic hilum, the base of segment IV is removed with a 3 × 3 × 3 cm wedge. The small parenchymal vessels bleeding are controlled mainly through compression and, in some cases, using transfictive 5-0 sutures. This maneuver adequately exposes the left duct that follows an extrahepatic trajectory, from the confluence to the round ligament's end.

The loss of confluence can be easily diagnosed nowadays with the aid of MRCP. Endoscopic management can be a suitable therapeutic procedure by placing a percutaneous biliary drain or stents in order to maintain the function of the ducts. When endoscopic treatment is not an option, the surgical alternatives available for complex biliary injuries are: Portoenterostomy, double barrell anastomosis, construction of a neoconfluence, partial hepatectomy, and liver transplantation.

Portoenterostomy

This is the adult variant of the Kasai procedure [11]. It is the least desired option hence it has presented a high failure rate in our center [12]. We suggest its usage when very small, joined ducts are found and the construction of a high-quality bilioenteric anastomosis (wide, tension free, with appropriate epithelization of mucosae, done in healthy ducts using adequate suture material) is not feasible. In some cases, it is possible to place percutaneous stents during the preoperative or postoperative period in order to advance them to the intestinal lumen at the time of portoenterostomy. Along with periodical changes of the percutaneous stents, this option allows the patient to maintain an acceptable quality of life (without jaundice and cholangitis, with the evident disadvantage of having an indwelling catheter for a long period of time).

When the stents are removed, failure of the patency of the ducts is almost constant. In our hands, several of these cases are enrolled into the liver transplant waiting list.

Double Barrell Anastomosis

This variant can be performed when the ducts are widely separated (more than 1 cm). The right duct anastomosis is technically demanding and it anticipates a high chance of long-term dysfunction. Even after stenting, the final outcome after removal is unpredictable.

The anastomosis to the left duct can usually be done with a moderate level of difficulty by extending the incision to the anterior aspect of the duct. We have less than 10 cases repaired with this surgical approach. Complications such as secondary biliary cirrhosis may arise (with or without cholangitis, which in some conditions is severe). A couple of cases in our series have been treated by means of unilobar portal vein embolization with the objective of inducing atrophy of the affected liver lobe. Segmentary portal vein embolization does not offer good results.

Alternative Approaches and Controversies

- There are unfortunate isolated cases in which an appropriate anastomosis is impossible to perform. The anastomosis of the jejunal opening to the hepatic parenchyma and the need of stents in every duct included in the anastomosis technically leads to a portoenterostomy, similar to the one described by Kasai [13]. In our experience and that of others, these are very infrequent cases that often require prolonged stenting, and may also develop acute cholangitis episodes, and thus should be considered for liver transplant.
- Endoscopic access is not a simple procedure in these types of patients since it is challenging to insufflate the intestinal loop. If this is feasible, there is also the problem of identifying the anastomosis that oftentimes is punctiform and/or obstructed.
- There are numerous reports that have discussed the use of hepaticoduodenal derivation to successfully repair the biliary tract, such as Traverso's and Stewart–Way's groups; [14] it has been recommended for injuries in which the ductus choledochus is of acceptable length and there is no loss of tissue. From our viewpoint, it has the disadvantage of exposing the anastomosis to acidic content, and food and vegetable residues that hinder the anastomosis' function. Another disadvantage of this type of derivation is that if early dehiscence develops, aside from a biliary fistula, a duodenal fistula also appears with disastrous short- and long-term consequences.

Construction of a Neoconfluence

This has been our preferred approach for patients suitable for it [13]. Once more, on a case-to-case basis, in order to obtain a high-quality bilioenteric anastomosis, we remove the hepatic segments IV and V. Removal of liver parenchyma at this level allows us better visualization of the ducts. In some instances, a flap of bile duct is obtained (when the anterior aspect of the left duct is cut) in order to reach the right duct. An anastomosis is performed between the ducts with noninverted, fine sutures. Usually three to four stitches are enough. The result is a wide anterior opening of the left duct and an adequate diameter of the right duct, allowing a high-quality bilioenteric anastomosis. Our results with this approach are encouraging, similar to those obtained with a preserved confluence (Fig. 17.2).

Partial Hepatectomy

This approach is done in selected cases. In more than 800 patients treated, we have performed around 20 partial hepatectomies (2.5% of the cases). We suggest this approach in scenarios in which the lobar duct cannot be rehabilitated (small duct,

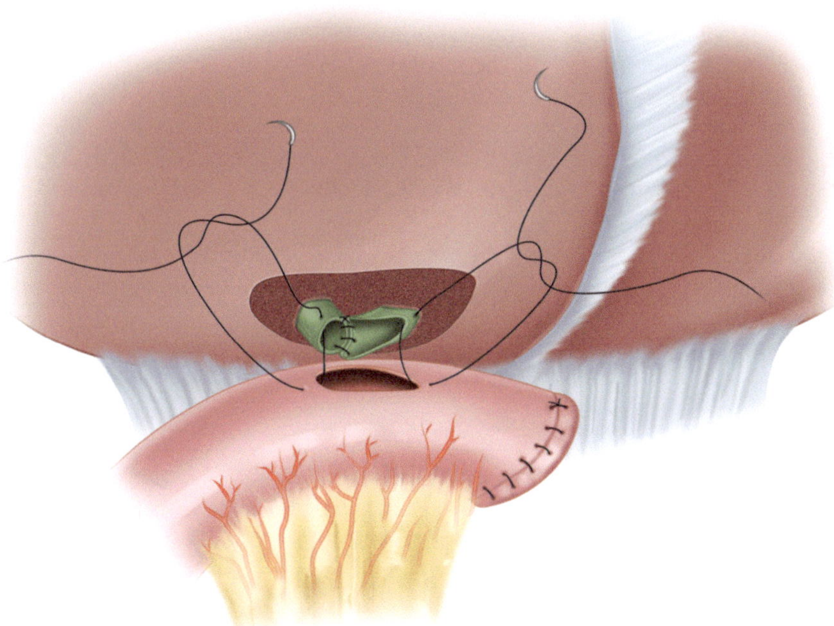

Fig. 17.2 Neoconfluence.

intralobar stricture with abscesses, refractory segmentary cholangitis). The right hepatic lobe is generally the one removed. In our series, only one case of left lobe removal was recorded.

Liver Transplantation

All patients with loss of confluence should be evaluated by a multidisciplinary team, including a transplant surgeon. There are cases in which, after arterial damage concomitant to the bile duct injury, ischemia of the intrahepatic ducts is observed, and a vanishing bile duct syndrome occurs.

Most of the injuries in our experience occur in healthy individuals. There are some cases in which a high-quality anastomosis is performed and even then, they develop obstruction of the anastomosis with intrahepatic strictures. In case of extreme damage to the ducts, liver transplantation should be considered as an option.

In patients with loss of confluence, bile duct repair after an injury is not always feasible and in some others the injury is so complex, involving a vascular component, that a poor prognosis is expected. This could lead to acute liver failure, recurrent cholangitis, and furthermore, secondary biliary cirrhosis.

In our series, 10 patients with recurrent cholangitis and end-stage liver disease secondary to bile duct injury were included in the liver transplant waiting list. So far, six patients have received an organ, including one man and five women, with a median age of 44 years old. The right hepatic artery was injured in one case; and, mean transoperative bleeding was 7,138 ml. All patients had received surgical treatment before liver transplant. The median time between bile duct injury and liver transplant was 96 months. The mean time on waiting list was 5.5 months. One patient died in the postoperative period secondary to hemorrhagic and septic shock; and, five patients are alive and have had minor complications, with a median follow-up of 30 months. Mean intensive care unit and hospital stay was two and seven days, respectively.

Any surgeon who attempts to do a liver transplant under these conditions should be aware of the high risk of bleeding, and technical difficulties due to surgical adhesions.

Conclusion

An injury that includes the confluence of the duct represents a surgical challenge. There are several treatment options to be considered (neoconfluence, double anastomosis, and portoenterostomy) and selected on a patient-to-patient basis.

Global Pearls

- Injuries leading to complete section of the duct have two associated components to consider: duct devascularization and tissue loss. This leads to high-tension, high-risk anastomoses in spite of performing broad maneuvers to avoid this scenario, such as an extensive Kocher maneuver that allows access to the duodenum or the distal duct.
- Silastic stents cause a minimal inflammatory reaction and oftentimes, upon removal, there may be bile accumulations, since an adequate trajectory is not formed. Therefore, if the postoperative plan includes repeated procedures, leaving a vulcanized rubber or latex stent is preferable, since they create an appropriate trajectory, ideal for radiological instrumentation.
- It is not unusual for a patient with a biliodigestive derivation, particularly high-risk anastomoses, to develop small calculi due to biliary sludge and bacterial colonization, or as a result of the shedding of sutures into the anastomosis' lumen. It is thus recommended to perform the anastomosis with disposable hydrolysable sutures that cannot act as a nest for calculi formation and accumulation.

References

1. de Santibanes E, Ardiles V, Pekolj J. Complex bile duct injuries: management. HPB. 2008;10(1):4–12.
2. Sicklick JK, Camp MS, Lillemoe KD, Melton GB, Yeo CJ, Campbell KA, et al. Surgical management of bile duct injuries sustained during laparoscopic cholecystectomy: perioperative results in 200 patients. Ann Surg. 2005;241(5):786–92; discussion 93–5.
3. Strasberg SM, Hertl M, Soper NJ. An analysis of the problem of biliary injury during laparoscopic cholecystectomy. J Am Coll Surg. 1995;180(1):101–25.
4. Winslow ER, Fialkowski EA, Linehan DC, Hawkins WG, Picus DD, Strasberg SM. "Sideways": results of repair of biliary injuries using a policy of side-to-side hepatico-jejunostomy. Ann Surg. 2009;249(3):426–34.
5. Kapoor VK. Bile duct injury repair: when? what? who? J Hepatobiliary Pancreat Surg. 2007;14(5):476–9.
6. Mercado MA, Vilatoba M, Chan C, Dominguez I, Leal RP, Olivera MA. Intrahepatic bilioenteric anastomosis after biliary complications of liver transplantation: operative rescue of surgical failures. World J Surg. 2009;33(3):534–8.
7. Mercado MA, Orozco H, de la Garza L, Lopez-Martinez LM, Contreras A, Guillen-Navarro E. Biliary duct injury: partial segment IV resection for intrahepatic reconstruction of biliary lesions. Arch Surg. 1999;134(9):1008–10.
8. Mercado MA, Chan C, Orozco H, Hinojosa CA, Podgaetz E, Ramos-Gallardo G, et al. Prognostic implications of preserved bile duct confluence after iatrogenic injury. Hepatogastroenterology. 2005;52(61):40–4.

9. Bismuth H, Majno PE. Biliary strictures: classification based on the principles of surgical treatment. World J Surg. 2001;25(10):1241–4.
10. Uysal F, Obuz F, Ucar A, Secil M, Igci E, Dicle O. Anatomic variations of the intrahepatic bile ducts: analysis of magnetic resonance cholangiopancreatography in 1011 consecutive patients. Digestion. 2014;89(3):194–200.
11. Garcia AV, Cowles RA, Kato T, Hardy MA. Morio Kasai: a remarkable impact beyond the Kasai procedure. J Pediatr Surg. 2012;47(5):1023–7.
12. Mercado MA, Franssen B, Dominguez I, Arriola-Cabrera JC, Ramírez-Del Val F, Elnecavé-Olaiz A, et al. Transition from a low: to a high-volume centre for bile duct repair: changes in technique and improved outcome. HPB (Oxford). 2011;13(11):767–73.
13. Mercado MA, Vilatoba M, Contreras A, Leal-Leyte P, Cervantes-Alvarez E, Arriola JC, et al. Iatrogenic bile duct injury with loss of confluence. World J Gastrointest Surg. 2015;7 (10):254–60.
14. Moraca RJ, Lee FT, Ryan JA, Jr., Traverso LW. Long-term biliary function after reconstruction of major bile duct injuries with hepaticoduodenostomy or hepaticojejunostomy. Arch Surg. 2002;137(8):889–93; discussion 93–4.

18 Posterior Right Disconnected Bile Duct

Umberto Cillo, Riccardo Boetto, Agostino Maria De Rose, Domenico Bassi, Francesco Ardito and Felice Giuliante

Case Presentation

A 50-year-old woman underwent a laparoscopic cholecystectomy for acute cholecystitis. Symptoms included right upper quadrant pain and fever without jaundice, and the patient was suspected to have Mirizzi Syndrome, based on pre-operative imaging.

A conversion to open cholecystectomy was required because of unclear anatomy due to local inflammation; a Mirizzi Type II Syndrome was identified. A retrograde cholecystectomy with T-Tube placement in the common bile duct was performed,

U. Cillo (✉) · R. Boetto · D. Bassi
UOC Chirurgia Epatobiliare e Trapianti Epatici, Università degli Studi di Padova,
Via Giustiniani no 2, 35128 Padua, Italy
e-mail: cillo@unipd.it

R. Boetto
e-mail: rboetto@hotmail.com

D. Bassi
e-mail: domenico.bassi@gmail.com

A.M. De Rose · F. Ardito · F. Giuliante
UOC Chirurgia Epatobiliare, Fondazione Policlinico Universitario A. Gemelli,
00168 Rome, Italy
e-mail: agostinomaria.derose@rm.unicatt.it

F. Ardito
e-mail: francesco.ardito@unicatt.it

F. Giuliante
e-mail: felice.giuliante@unicatt.it

T.M. Pawlik et al. (eds.), *Case-Based Lessons in the Management of Complex Hepato-Pancreato-Biliary Surgery*, DOI 10.1007/978-3-319-50868-9_18

and the patient was uneventfully discharged on postoperative day six. The T-Tube was removed four months later under fluoroscopic guidance, without biliary leakage or any other complication.

Two years later, the patient was referred to our tertiary Hepato-Pancreatic-Biliary (HPB) Surgery Center after an episode of mild cholangitis because of vague symptoms such as fatigue, mild upper right quadrant abdominal pain, and abdominal bloating; no weight loss was noted.

An abdominal ultrasound (US) revealed dilatation of the right posterior biliary ducts. A physical examination was normal; there was no jaundice or incisional hernias; there was mild pain on abdominal palpation. Blood tests were normal, revealing only a mild elevation in GGT levels (345 UI/L) with negative Ca 19-9 levels.

Management consisted of: (1) radiological assessment; (2) multidisciplinary evaluation and differential diagnosis analysis; (3) intraoperative cholangioscopy, and (4) liver resection.

Preoperative Assessment

The patient presented with a clinical suspicion of right posterior disconnected bile duct of unclear origin two years after a complex cholecystectomy. Focal intrahepatic strictures often present with vague symptoms such as fever, jaundice, or abdominal pain, the latter due to cholangitis. About 30% of patients with an incidentally identified lesion are asymptomatic at diagnosis [1].

A differential diagnosis based on the patient's clinical history and basic imaging data should be carried out and should included iatrogenic biliary injury and non-iatrogenic causes of segmental cholangiectasia.

Given the patient's surgical history, and in particular the intraoperative finding of Mirizzi Syndrome (with a fistula between the gallbladder wall and the common duct due to inflammation and erosion of the impacted stone), an unspecified biliary anomaly and T-tube positioning, the possibility of a surgical bile duct injury should be initially evaluated [2].

A bile duct injury is considered one of the most severe complications of laparoscopic cholecystectomy, with a reported incidence of 0.4–0.7%. Its incidence is 3.2–8.4 times higher in the presence of anomalies of the biliary anatomy. An aberrant right posterior sectoral hepatic duct (supraportal or infraportal type) represents the most dangerous biliary variant which may cause a bile duct injury, and accounts for about 5% of anomalies found in patients undergoing major hepatectomy with extrahepatic bile duct resection [3].

A segmental intrahepatic bile duct dilatation (cholangiectasia) could instead be sustained by several benign and malignant processes resulting in strictures. Benign causes include:

- Hepatic arterial ischaemia: such as TACE (0.3%) [4] and radiofrequency ablation [5]
- Chronic cholangitis: primary sclerosing cholangitis (PSC), immunoglobulin G4–associated sclerosing cholangitis, and infectious cholangitis [6]
- Hepatolithiasis [7]
- Portal biliopathy [6]

Malignant Causes

- Cholangiocarcinoma is the principal neoplastic cause of intrahepatic strictures (50–53%); periductal infiltrating and intraductal growth types can produce a stricture without a mass [1, 8].
- Neuroendocrine tumors can cause a sectoral bile duct dilatation [9].
- Intraductal papillary neoplasm is a preneoplastic condition that should be considered [10].

Technical Pearls

- Intra-operative cholangiography and/or cholangioscopy are crucial in better defining biliary anomalies. In the presence of extensive adhesions due to previous surgery, choledochotomy or cholangioscopy, via a longitudinal choledochotomy immediately above the duodenum, should be performed. It is possible to use a combined US and choledochoscopic approach as well.
- In particular, it is important to avoid excessive hilar dissection in the proximity of an intrahepatic biliary stricture and to resect the posterior section, if possible, using a "no touch" technique including the biliary confluence.
- Intraoperative pathology of the stricture after posterior section removal should be requested. If it is positive, extending the resection to improve radicality should be considered.

Diagnostic Tools

In settings other than primary sclerosing cholangitis, Ca 19-9 levels > 100 U/ml have a sensitivity of 53% and a specificity of 92% for malignancy prediction, but a negative result cannot exclude cholangiocarcinoma [11].

Although ultrasound (US) can detect intrahepatic dilated ducts >2 mm, it has only a limited ability to characterize strictures [12]. Computed tomography (CT) scan is better able to uncover the stricture's location, the presence of wall thickening (≥ 5 mm) or enhancement, and vascular or nodal (≥ 10 mm) invasion; but it is unable to clearly discriminate between benign and malignant causes [13, 14].

Magnetic resonance cholangiopancreatography (MRCP) presents high sensitivity and specificity, respectively 93.5 and 94.4%, for detecting strictures, and also allows vascular involvement assessment [15]. Endoscopic retrograde Cholangiopancreatography (ERCP) is usually attempted before percutaneous transhepatic cholangiography (PTC) is carried out.

Cholangiographic features of intrahepatic strictures include interruption of contrast medium, bile duct separation, tapering, shouldering, mucosal irregularity, a filling defect, or absence of opacification of the draining biliary tree segment. Sectoral bile duct dilatation due to an intrahepatic obstruction may be misdiagnosed because of insufficient contrast filling, or may be obscured by overlying opacified ducts.

Achieving a clear differentiation diagnosis between benign strictures and malignancy based on cholangiography is usually difficult [13].

Endoscopic Procedures

Endoscopic ultrasound (EUS) can be used when MRCP fails to lead to a diagnosis (10% of cases), but no data regarding sensitivity or specificity for intrahepatic strictures are available. Intraductal ultrasound (IDUS) may be useful in evaluating the extent and the longitudinal spread of bile duct carcinoma of the proximal system; in non-primary sclerosing cholangitis (PSC) patients, it has a high sensitivity (97%) and specificity (89%) rate for detection of malignancy detection; no specific data for intrahepatic strictures are available.

Cholangioscopy permits direct exploration of the bile duct lumen, making it possible to carry out targeted biopsies with a sensitivity rate ranging from 76 to 82% in malignancy detection. It can be performed endoscopically or percutaneously with a not-negligible complication rate (cholangitis 11.7% and haemobilia 5.8%) [16].

Tissue sampling can be performed using three techniques:

1. Aspiration cytology: via ERCP, PTC or nasobiliary drain aspiration with a malignancy detection sensitivity of 55%, specificity of 100% and accuracy of 56% [17].
2. Brush cytology: the sensitivity rate for malignancy detection ranges from 33 to 58% [18, 19].

3. Biopsy: during ERCP, PTC or EUS, it is associated to a 53 to 86% sensitivity rate for cholangiocarcinoma [19].

A triple modality approach including cytology, biopsy, and fluorescence in situ hybridization (FISH) has been reported to have an overall sensitivity of 0.82, a specificity of 1.00, a positive predictive value of 1.00, and negative predictive value of 0.87 [20].

The radiological assessment included:

- CT scan: liver parenchymal focal lesions were absent, in the presence of right posterior sector biliary dilatation were absent (Fig. 18.1).
- MRCP: intrahepatic biliary dilatation of the posterior sector (S6/S7), with a mild stenosis of the common duct above the bifurcation that was more extended and tighter on the right side (Fig. 18.2).

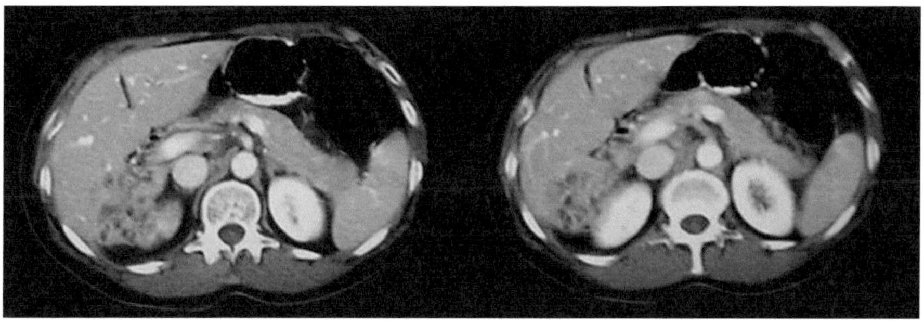

Fig. 18.1 Computed tomography (CT) scan with right posterior bile duct dilatation, no parenchymal focal lesions

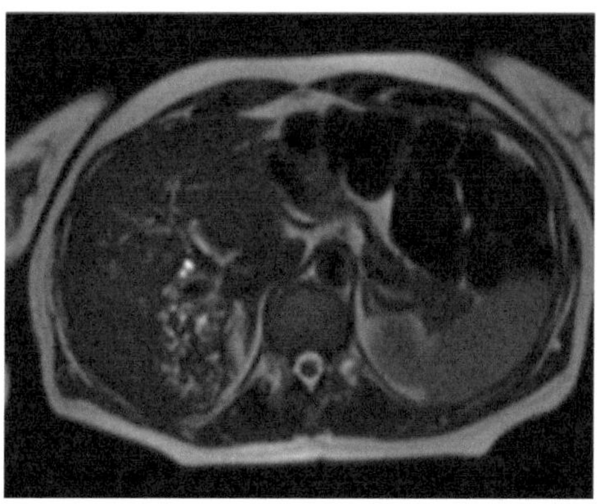

Fig. 18.2 Magnetic resonance cholangiopancreatography (MRCP) revealed intrahepatic biliary dilatation of S6/S7 with a mild stenosis of the common ducts above the confluence that was more extended and narrower on the *right* side

- ERCP confirmed a posterior right bile duct disconnection; brush cytology was negative.

Alternative Approaches and Management Controversies

- A conservative "wait and see" management, even though controversial, may be considered. However, in such a case, close follow-up with CT or MRCP should be adopted.
- If a conservative approach is chosen, posterior sector atrophy induction with either combined portal vein embolization alone or with percutaneous biliary drainage may be an option.

Multidisciplinary Evaluation and Operative Treatment

Several management options are available for the treatment of focal intrahepatic strictures in fit patients, and each should take into consideration the risk of malignancy and the presence of symptoms. The steps to be taken are as follows:

1. Observation
2. Endoscopic or Percutaneous dilatation/stenting
3. Surgical resection
4. Atrophy induction with combined portal vein embolization and percutaneous biliary drainage [21]

Given the difficulty in ruling out malignancy (which occurs in 50–70% of the cases), a liver resection should be considered, as it can provide the data necessary to establish a definitive diagnosis and to set up an oncologically correct treatment plan [16].

The case was discussed during our Hepato-Oncological Multidisciplinary meeting and on the basis of the imaging and preoperative data that was available, it was impossible to exclude the possibility of an underlying neoplasm causing sectoral dilatation in this young, symptomatic female patient. The low sensitivity of brush cytology and negative Ca 19-9 levels were likewise unable to rule out a malignant stricture.

An explorative laparotomy with hepatectomy, sectoral bile duct resection, and lymphadenectomy was planned. An atrophic right posterior liver sector in the absence of peritoneal or extrahepatic neoplastic diffusion was detected after a prolonged adhesiolysis at laparotomy (Fig. 18.3).

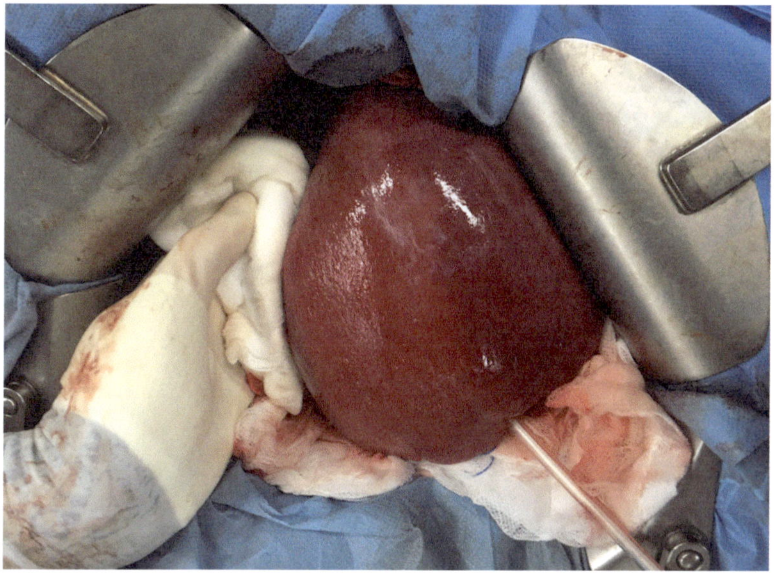

Fig. 18.3 Laparotomy with atrophic right posterior liver sector

An intraoperative US confirmed isolated right posterior bile duct dilatation with a small hyperechoic intraductal mass. An aberrant low confluence of right and left hepatic ducts was also evident.

A complex hilar dissection due to the previous biliary surgery was then performed, with palpatory evidence of a small mass apparently involving the right bile duct. The common bile duct was sectioned above the duodenum. Cholangioscopy, which was then performed, confirmed the anatomic variation, including a very low bile duct confluence and a completely obstructing stricture of the right posterior duct (Fig. 18.4).

The right periportal and common hepatic artery nodal sampling was negative for malignant cells. The right portal and arterial branches were selectively encircled and sectioned; the right hepatic vein was isolated and encircled.

A right posterior sectionectomy (S6-S7) with resection of the biliary aberrant confluence was performed, due to the close proximity with the pseudonodular obstruction of the right posterior duct. A bi-ductal Roux-en-Y hepatico-jejunostomy was performed. The patient was uneventfully discharged on postoperative day 7.

The final pathology revealed a sectoral chronic aspecific cholangitis with proximal duct inflammatory sclerotic stenosis that was negative for cancer cells. The picture was compatible with an iatrogenic biliary injury.

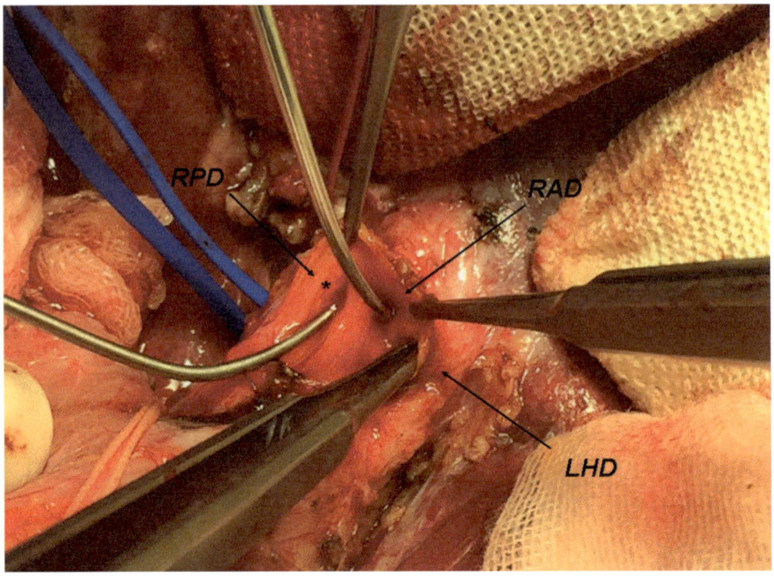

Fig. 18.4 Common bile duct section with evidence of anomalous low confluence. Right posterior duct (RPD) was disconnected at cholangioscopy as well as at surgical sampling; *RAD* right anterior duct; *LHD* left hepatic duct

Overall Management

- A crucial role in the management of technically demanding intraoperative scenarios involving the biliary tract is early referral to tertiary specialized hepatobiliary high-volume centers.
- Given the difficulty in ruling out malignancy in the context of a probable history of a iatrogenic lesion, an "oncologic" approach should always be taken.
- Adequate morphologic patient evaluation is mandatory including: CT scan, MRCP, ERCP with also specific endoscopic procedures (such as EUS, IDUS or Cholangioscopy) and tissue sampling.

References

1. Seo DW, Kim MH, Sk Lee, Myung SJ, Kang GH, Ha HK, et al. Usefulness of cholangioscopy in patients with focal stricture of the intrahepatic duct unrelated to intrahepatic stones. Gastrointest Endosc. 1999;49(2):204–9.

2. Erben Y, Benavente-Chenhalls LA, Donohue JM, Que FG, Kendrick ML, Reid-Lombardo KM, et al. Diagnosis and treatment of Mirizzi syndrome: 23-year Mayo Clinic experience. J Am Coll Surg. 2011;213(1):114–9. doi:10.1016/j.jamcollsurg.2011.03.008.
3. Kurata M, Honda G, Okuda Y, Kobayashi S, Sakamoto K, Iwasaki S, et al. Preoperative detection and handling of aberrant right posterior sectoral hepatic duct during laparoscopic cholecystectomy. J Hepatobiliary Pancreat Sci. 2015;22(7):558–62. doi:10.1002/jhbp.252.
4. Miyayama S, Yamashiro M, Okuda M, Yoshie Y, Nakashima Y, Ikeno H, et al. Main bile duct stricture occurring after transcatheter arterial chemoembolization for hepatocellular carcinoma. Cardiovasc Intervent Radiol. 2010;33(6):1168–79. doi:10.1007/s00270-009-9781-6.
5. Kim SH, Lim HK, Choi D, Lee WJ, Kim MJ, Lee SJ, et al. Changes in bile ducts after radiofrequency ablation of hepatocellular carcinoma: frequency and clinical significance. AJR Am J Roentgenol. 2004;183(6):1611–7.
6. Zhao L, Hosseini M, Wilcox R, Liu Q, Crook T, Taxy JB, et al. Segmental cholangiectasia clinically worrisome for cholangiocarcinoma: comparison with recurrent pyogenic cholangitis. Hum Pathol. 2015;46(3):426–33. doi:10.1016/j.humpath.2014.11.019.
7. Matsumoto Y, Fujii H, Yoshioka M, Sekikawa T, Wada T, Yamamoto M, et al. Biliary strictures as a cause of primary intrahepatic bile duct stones. World J Surg. 1986;10(5):867–75.
8. Blechacz B, Komuta M, Roskams T, Gores GJ. Clinical diagnosis and staging of cholangiocarcinoma. Nat Rev Gastroenterol Hepatol. 2011;8(9):512–22.
9. Zheng SL, Yip VS, Pedica F, Prachalias A, Quaglia A. Intrahepatic bile duct mixed adenoneuroendocrine carcinoma: a case report and review of the literature. Diagn Pathol. 2015;10:204. doi:10.1186/s13000-015-0439-1.
10. Hachiya H, Kita J, Shiraki T, Iso Y, Shimoda M, Kubota K. Intraductal papillary neoplasm of the bile duct developing in a patient with primary sclerosing cholangitis: a case report. World J Gastroenterol. 2014;20(42):15925–30. doi:10.3748/wjg.v20.i42.15925.
11. Patel AH, Harnois DM, Klee GG, LaRusso NF, Gores GJ. The utility of CA 19-9 in the diagnoses of cholangiocarcinoma in patients without primary sclerosing cholangitis. Am J Gastroenterol. 2000;95(1):204–7.
12. Foley WD, Quiroz FA. The role of sonography in imaging of the biliary tract. Ultrasound. 2007;23(2):123–35.
13. Kim HJ, Lee KT, Kim SH, Lee JK, Lim JH, Paik SW, et al. Differential diagnosis of intrahepatic bile duct dilatation without demonstrable mass on ultrasonography or CT: benign versus malignancy. J Gastroenterol Hepatol. 2003;18(11):1287–92.
14. Park HS, Lee JM, Kim SH, Jeong JY, Kim YJ, Lee KH, et al. CT Differentiation of cholangiocarcinoma from periductal fibrosis in patients with hepatolithiasis. Am J Roentgenol. 2006;187(2):445–53.
15. Pecchi A, De Santis M, Di Benedetto F, Gibertini M, Gerunda G, Torricelli P. Role of magnetic resonance cholangiography in biliary complications of orthotopic liver transplantation. Radiol Med. 2010;115(7):1065–79.
16. Yeo D, Perini MV, Muralidharan V, Chritophi C. Focal intrahepatic strictures: a review of diagnosis and management. HPB (Oxford). 2012;14(7):425–34. doi:10.1111/j.1477-2574.2012.00481.x.
17. Hattori M, Nagino M, Ebata T, Kato K, Okada K, Shimoyama Y. Prospective study of biliary cytology in suspected perihilar cholangiocarcinoma. Br J Surg. 2011;98(5):704–9.
18. Howell DA, Beveridge RP, Bosco J, Jones M. Endoscopic needle aspiration biopsy at ERCP in the diagnosis of biliary strictures. Gastrointest Endosc. 1992;38(5):531–5.
19. Ferrari Junior AP, Lichtenstein DR, Slivka A, Chang C, Carr-Locke DL. Brush cytology during ERCP for the diagnosis of biliary and pancreatic malignancies. Gastrointest Endosc. 1994;40(2 Pt 1):140–5.

20. Nanda A, Brown JM, Berger SH, Lewis MM, Barr Fritcher MG, Gores GJ, et al. Triple modality testing by endoscopic retrograde cholangiopancreatography for the diagnosis of cholangiocarcinoma. Therap Adv Gastroenterol. 2015;8(2):56–65.
21. Hwang S, Yoon SY, Jung SW, Namgoong JM, Park GC, Gwon DI, et al. Therapeutic induction of hepatic atrophy for isolated injury of the right anterior sectoral duct following laparoscopic cholecystectomy. Korean J Hepatobiliary Pancreat Surg. 2011;15(3):189–93.

19 Management of Contralateral Bile Duct Injury Following Liver Resection

Michael McCall, Jean-Michel Aubin and Elijah Dixon

Case 1

A 78-year-old gentleman, known for a coronary artery bypass graft (CABG) nine years prior, a right hemicolectomy for a large, benign polyp, and no known liver disease, initially presented with weakness and fatigue and was found to be anemic. He underwent upper and lower endoscopies, as well as cross-sectional imaging. Imaging (computed tomography and contrast-enhanced ultrasound) revealed a 7.9 × 4.0 × 4.7 cm hypodense lesion bridging segments 4b and 5 of the liver and abutting the fundus of the gallbladder, suggestive of an intrahepatic cholangiocarcinoma (Fig. 19.1). Given his exceptional functional status, excision was offered.

Intraoperatively, the lesion was found to encompass segment 4b and involve segment 5, abut the gallbladder, and encroach on the hepatic hilum. A meso-axial hepatectomy was carried out, with the use of the Aquamantys® (Medtronic; Minneapolis, MN, USA) device for parenchymal dissection. Hemostasis and absence of bile were confirmed at the end of the procedure. No drains were placed.

M. McCall
Department of Surgery, Division of General Surgery, Foothills Medical Centre, University of Calgary, 1403 29th Street NW, T2N 2T9 Calgary, AB, Canada
e-mail: mmccall@ualberta.ca

J.-M. Aubin
Department of Surgery, Foothills Medical Centre, University of Calgary, 1403 29th Street NW, T2N 2T9 Calgary, AB, Canada
e-mail: jmraubin@gmail.com

E. Dixon (✉)
Foothills Medical Centre, University of Calgary, EG - 26, 1403 29th Street NW, T2N 2T9 Calgary, AB, Canada
e-mail: Elijah.Dixon@albertahealthservices.ca

T.M. Pawlik et al. (eds.), *Case-Based Lessons in the Management of Complex Hepato-Pancreato-Biliary Surgery*, DOI 10.1007/978-3-319-50868-9_19

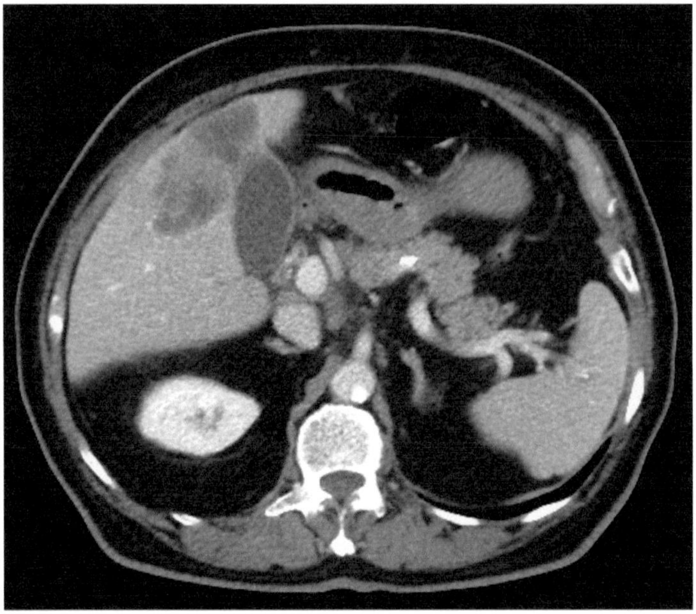

Fig. 19.1 Preoperative axial CT image showing concerning hypodense lesion bridging segments 4b/5

Pathologic assessment of the hepatic lesion revealed a poorly differentiated hepatocellular carcinoma, solid variant, with portal vein invasion. Resection margins were free of tumor.

Hyperbilirubinemia ensued early in the postoperative course (bilirubin POD 1: 125umol/L). The postoperative day 5 level was 44 and a nadir of 30 occurred on POD 7 (Fig. 19.2a). His international normalized ratio (INR) did not follow a similar trend (POD 1: 1.3; POD 5: 1.2; peak on POD 8: 1.5) (Fig. 19.2b). Following the development of fevers and a leukocytosis, cross-sectional imaging revealed a collection in the resection bed (Fig. 19.3). A percutaneous drain was placed and bilious fluid was noted.

Sequential imaging eventually revealed bile duct dilation. At this point, a percutaneous transhepatic cholangiogram (PTC) was obtained (Fig. 19.4a) to assess the biliary tree and characterize the suspected stricture. Once the cholangiogram was obtained, the stricture was traversed with a guidewire and an internal/external catheter was placed for biliary drainage and stenting of the stricture (Fig. 19.4b).

The bilirubin level gradually decreased, but never normalized (nadir post PTC insertion of 48). The PTC was sequentially upsized to a 14Fr caliber to optimize bilioenteric flow. Bilious drainage eventually ceased via the percutaneous drain in the surgical bed.

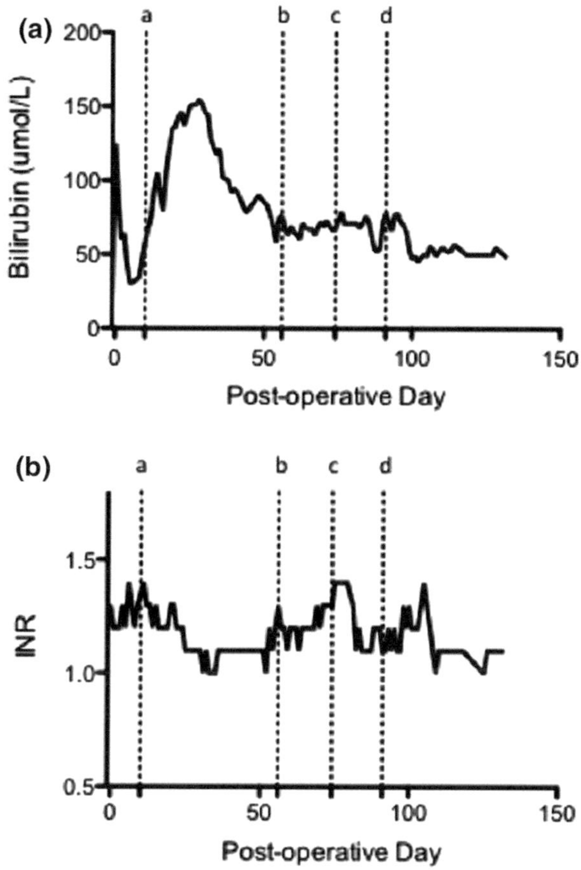

Fig. 19.2 Case 1 postoperative bilirubin (**a**) and INR (**b**) values. *Lines* denote (*a*) placement of percutaneous drain, (*b*) placement of *left* PTC, (*c*) upsizing of PTC to 12 Fr, and (*d*) upsizing of PTC to 14 Fr

Case 2

A 58-year-old gentleman initially presented with hematochezia and was found to have a large malignant polyp. Following completion of metastatic workup, he underwent a laparoscopic anterior resection. Cross-sectional imaging of the abdomen revealed a large cystic lesion centrally located in his liver (Fig. 19.5). A cystadenoma was suspected, and consequently surgical resection was recommended.

His colonic lesion proved to be a T2N0 low-grade adenocarcinoma. As no systemic therapy was planned, focus shifted to his hepatic lesion. Enucleation was pursued, due to intimate relation of the cystic lesion with the central Glissonian sheath and hilar plate. Though tedious, careful dissection was employed, without use of an energy device, in proximity of the central structures. Following resection,

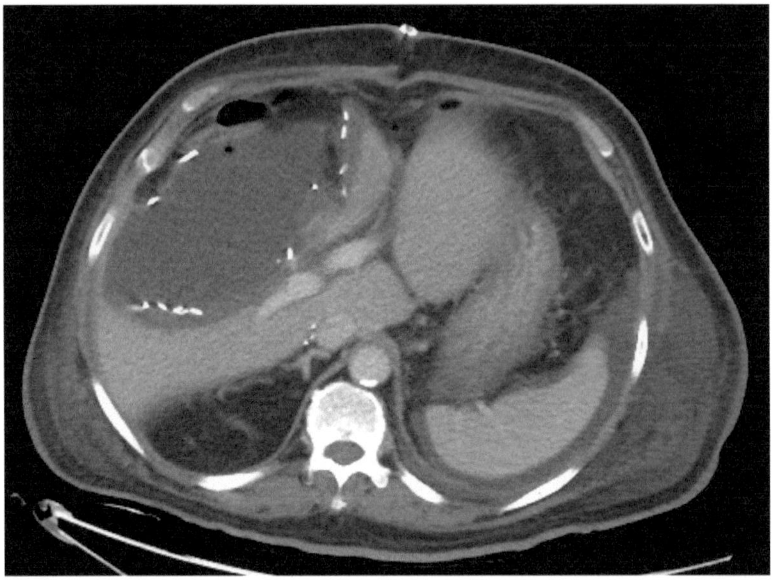

Fig. 19.3 Postoperative axial CT image demonstrating fluid collection in resection bed. A percutaneous drain was subsequently placed

hemostasis and absence of bile leaks was confirmed. No drains were placed. Pathologic assessment confirmed the diagnosis of cystadenoma, without dysplasia.

Unfortunately, this patient also developed fevers and leukocytosis, prompting cross-sectional imaging. A fluid collection was also identified and drained percutaneously (Fig. 19.6). Clinical improvement was then observed, and the patient was discharged home with drain in situ. He then presented to the Emergency Department eight weeks postoperatively with jaundice (bilirubin 152umol/L).

Given the delayed presentation, duct dilation was readily evident on imaging, and was amenable to percutaneous access. Both biliary systems were initially accessed and found to lead to inaccessible strictures at the proximal hepatic ducts (Figs. 19.7A, B). Bilateral external drains were placed.

The finding of bilateral occluded hepatic ducts resulted in a challenging scenario. Serial instrumentation of the bile ducts and attempts at traversing the stricture resulted in the transgression of the bile duct wall and free communication of both biliary systems with the central cavity initially drained postoperatively.

With technical expertise, a guidewire was eventually manipulated down the biliary tree, through to the cavity and back into the common hepatic duct. Bilateral PTCs were then placed well into the duodenum, to establish internal/external drainage (Fig. 19.7C). Multiple peri-procedural episodes of low-grade cholangitis were encountered and managed with antibiotics and external drainage.

(a)

(b)

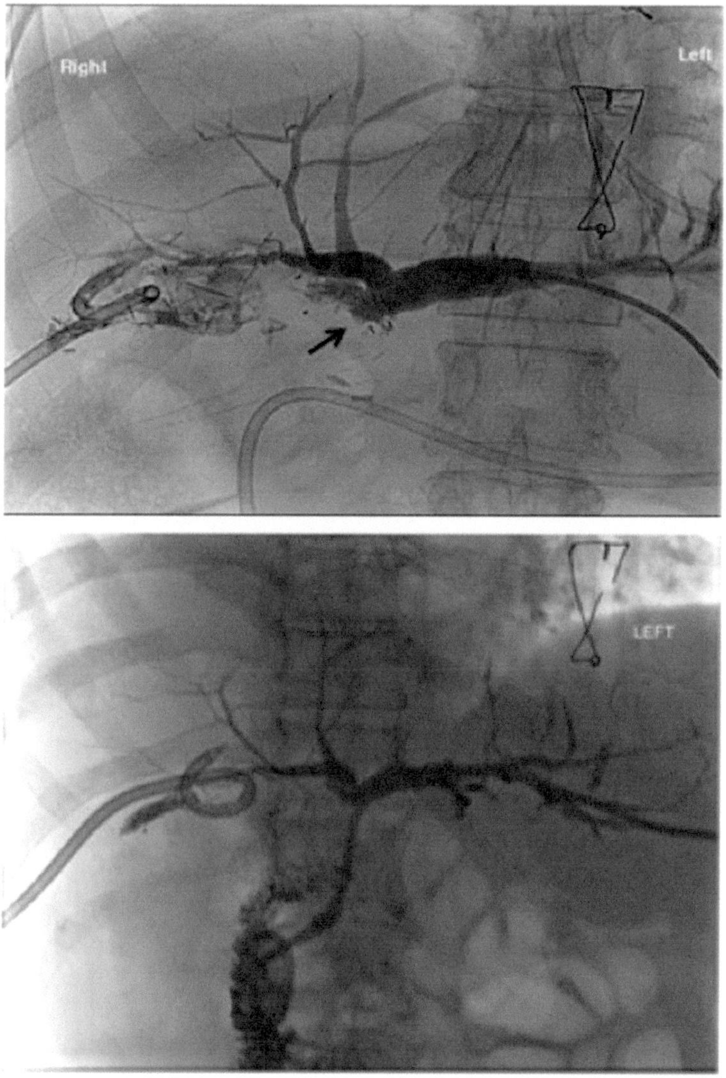

Fig. 19.4 Postoperative percutaneous transhepatic cholangiography demonstrating **a** complete biliary stricture (*arrow*), and **b** passage of wire across stricture with distal filling

Both PTCs remained in place for an extended duration of time until the percutaneous drain output decreased and became less bilious. Following this, the PTCs were sequentially closed, to allow internalized drainage. Cholangiograms and cross-sectional imaging eventually confirmed resolution of the central collection, as well as integrity of the bile ducts. The PTCs were then discontinued, at 7 and 8 months respectively. Follow-up is ongoing to monitor for further stricture development.

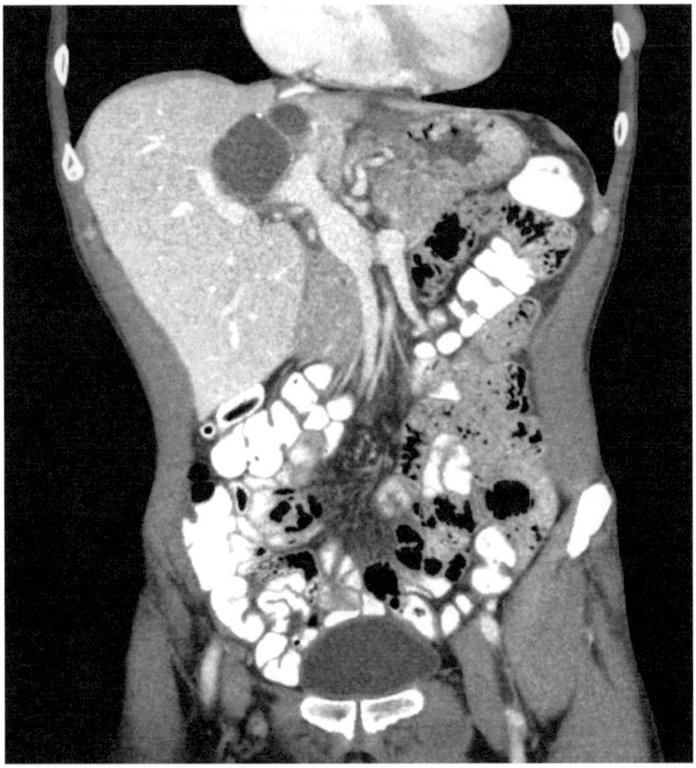

Fig. 19.5 Computed tomography coronal image showing central hepatic cystic lesion. Final pathology revealed a cystadenoma

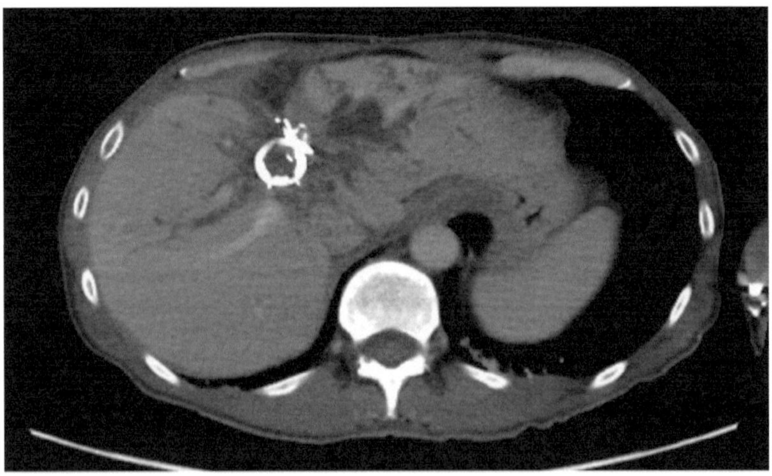

Fig. 19.6 Percutaneous drainage of a central hepatic fluid collection after liver resection

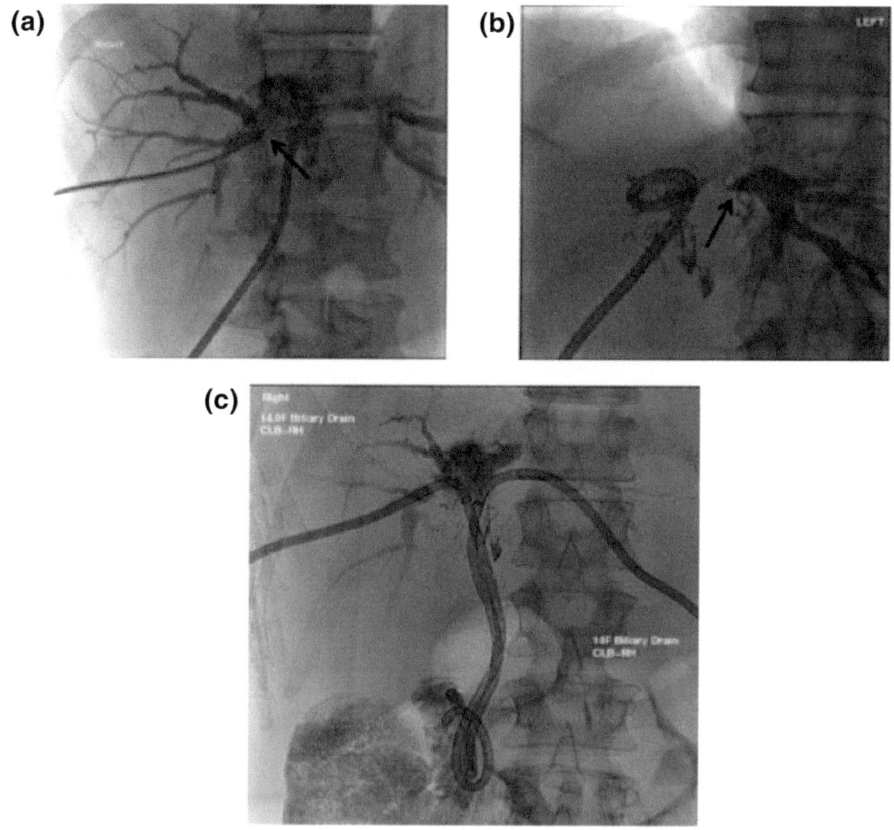

Fig. 19.7 Postoperative percutaneous transhepatic cholangiography showing both **a** *right* and **b** *left* biliary strictures (*arrow*). Eventual placement of bilateral percutaneous transhepatic internal/external biliary drains (**c**)

Intra-operative Pearls

1. Extra-parenchymal dissection of portal structures and lowering of the hilar plate can allow their displacement away from the transection margin, notably when there is foreshortening due to tumor.
2. Placing a tape around the opposite portal pedicle can help retract hilar structures away from staplers.
3. Passing a finger around the portal pedicle to be transected can help create more space around it.
4. Nonenergy device parenchymal transection methods should be employed in proximity to central structures or hilum.

5. As dissection approaches the hilum or the point of closest involvement, early transection of hepatic outflow (after extrahepatic inflow control) or cephalad transection can allow retrograde parenchymal dissection towards the hilum, and more careful dissection around central structures.

Discussion

These cases demonstrate one of the most devastating injuries after hepatic resection—that of a contralateral bile duct injury. While biliary complications occur in 3.6–10% of liver resections in the modern era, they account for nearly one-third of the mortality. [1–4] The majority of the current literature focuses on bile leakage and biloma formation (i.e., from the liver parenchyma) without considering bile duct injury as an independent entity. Boonstra et al. specifically studied this latter entity and determined that intraoperative blood loss, reoperative liver surgery, and the type of resection, especially extended left hepatectomy, were all associated with an increased risk of bile duct injury. [5] Other risk factors are anatomical variants, large central tumors, and tumors encroaching on the bile duct.

The short extrahepatic course of the right bile and its varied anatomy, especially in the setting of large central tumors, puts extended left resection at increased risk of ductal injury. Lesions with a central location in the liver can be resected via non-anatomical resection, anatomical hemi-hepatectomy, or via meso-axial hepatectomy (see Case 1, above). This is driven by the size of the lesion, proximity to vascular or biliary structures, and the quality and quantity of anticipated remnant liver. Oncologic outcomes are reportedly similar, [6] though anecdotal experience suggests a higher rate of bile leak. Meso-axial hepatectomy, or mesohepatectomy, can be considered when remnant volume is a concern, which is particularly true when operating on hepatocellular carcinomas, given the underlying fibrosis or cirrhosis. [6] Reoperative surgery and blood loss likely play similar roles to lesion location in bile duct injury—both can be linked to more difficult dissection and visualization.

Initial Presentation and Workup

The initial presentation is one of biliary leak, biliary stricture/obstruction or both. If a drain was left in situ at the initial operation, then a bile-stained effluent or a bilirubin level greater than three times the serum concentration will point to the diagnosis. In the early postoperative period, those with a bile leak will present with fevers, tachycardia, and a rising white blood cell count. A computed tomography (CT) scan is our initial investigation of choice (Fig. 19.8). In most cases, a perihepatic fluid collection will be discovered, leading to percutaneous placement of an image-guided catheter. Once again, a bilious effluent clinches the diagnosis. This, however, does not indicate a major biliary leak, as most postoperative bile leaks

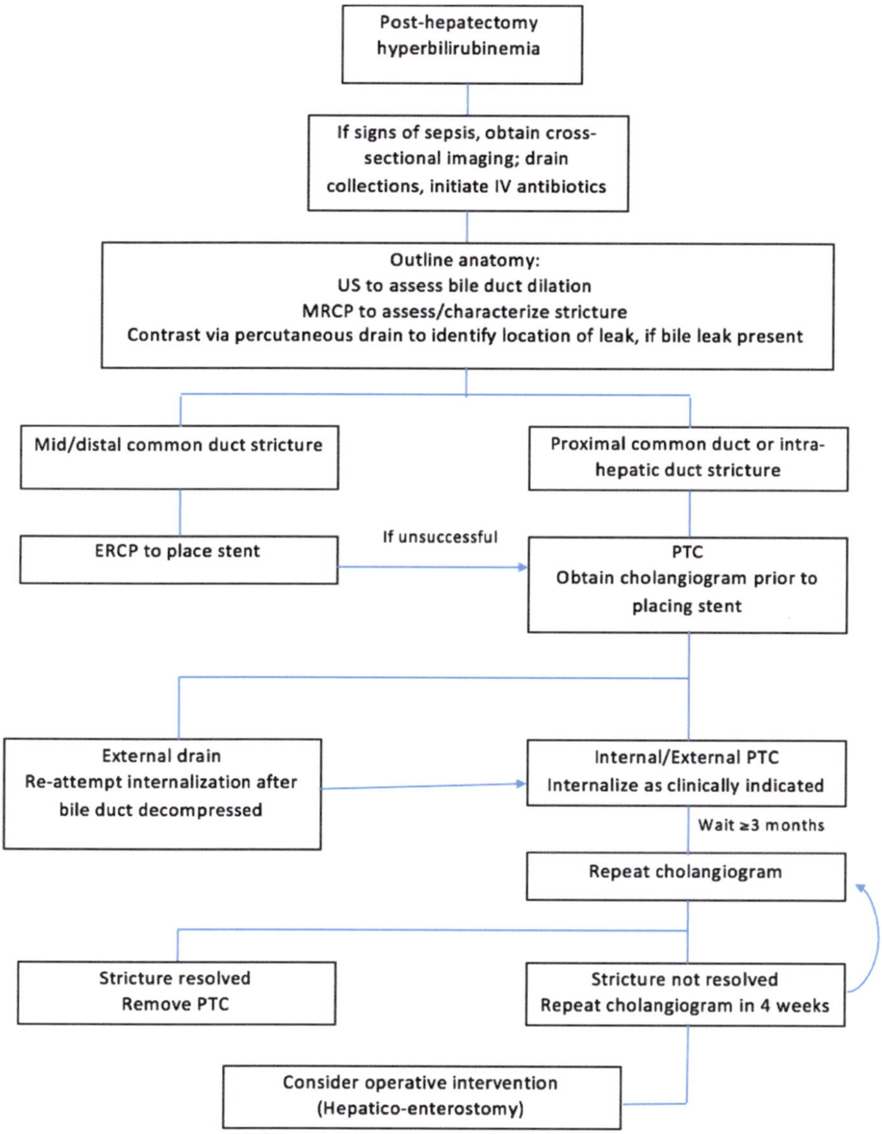

Fig. 19.8 Proposed algorithm for assessment and management of contralateral bile duct injury after liver resection

originate from the transected hepatic surface and cease spontaneously after drainage. [7]. In those with continued drainage, we have selectively employed sinogram analysis, injection of contrast via the drain under fluoroscopic guidance, in order to locate the origin of the leak. This is especially helpful when a bilioenteric anastomosis, such as in the case of a Klatskin tumor, is considered a possible source of the leak.

A rising bilirubin and alkaline phosphatase usually points to a biliary injury and resulting stricture. Our institution typically employs the 50/50 criteria to define liver failure. [8] This is defined by a 50% reduction in INR (INR > 1.7) as well as a bilirubin above 50 on POD 5. Neither of our patients met these criteria. Given the late rise in bilirubin and isolated hyperbilirubinemia for both patients, a pattern suggestive of an obstructive cause, a stricture from ischemia or inflammatory process was suspected. These could also present in a more protracted course once the patient has been discharged from their initial postoperative hospital stay (see Case 2, above). Once again cross-sectional imaging with CT or Magnetic Resonance Imaging (MRI) is appropriate as an initial investigation. A dilated biliary tree can be followed to the point of obstruction.

Initial Management

The initial management goals include resuscitation and treatment of sepsis. Our initial management strategy is nonoperative in nature. In those with a perihepatic collection, percutaneous drainage is employed. Continued drainage or a dilated biliary system on imaging usually points toward injury to a major ductal injury. In these, our preference is percutaneous transhepatic cholangiography and catheter (percurtaneous transhepatic catheter, PTC) placement. While an endoscopic route could be considered, our approach is weighted toward the percutaneous route. One advantage of the endoscopic (endoscopic retrograde cholagiopancreatography, ERCP) route is the ability to place an early stent and improve distal drainage. However, it goes without saying that this approach is unhelpful in the setting of a proximal obstruction.

If percutaneous biliary access is successful, we employ initial external drainage followed by drain internalization, and eventual clamping. For those with bile leaks, percutaneous drain output can be monitored as an outpatient. Once drainage ceases, cholangiography can be performed followed by PTC removal. This process may take months.

For those with strictures, balloon dilatation can be successful. Long-term effectiveness can be achieved after a single dilatation with a 59% patency rate at 25 years. [9] This increases to 80% if a second dilatation is performed. Overall success rate with a percutaneous approach is nearly 75%. [9, 10] Our local experience mirrors this; the majority of patients avoid reoperation and are managed percutaneously. In order to achieve this, serial upsizing of the drain is usually employed until normal biliary caliber is reached. As noted in Case 2, above, this approach is not without its possible complications—communication and collaboration with the interventional radiology team is of the utmost importance.

Operative Management

Fortunately, neither of our cases required operative management in order to repair contralateral biliary complications. However, this is the most definitive management option in those not controlled with the aforementioned maneuvers. Once sepsis has been controlled, and adequate drainage is achieved, an operative strategy is planned. Repeat cross-sectional imaging is usually employed and anatomy is defined. Ideally, these cases should be referred to high-volume hepatobiliary centers for definitive surgical management.

Re-operative surgery in any instance is difficult. In the setting of prior liver resection with postoperative biliary leak, this is even more challenging. Dissection is carried out in a methodical and cautious manner using anatomic landmarks for guidance. These can include the hepatoduodenal ligament, ligamentum teres, and the umbilical fissure. We clear the common bile duct distally and follow it proximally to the hilum. The injured bile duct is then defined. Tenets of repair include exposure of the injured segment, dissection back to healthy bile duct, and formation of a Roux-en-Y hepaticoenterostomy. Healthy bile duct is sewn to well-vascularized jejunal mucosa. We do not use external t-tubes or primary repair in these cases, as they have proven to have inferior outcomes.

Alternative Management Options

1. Avoid use of energy devices in proximity of the hilum.
2. Protect the portal structures with sponges and continuous suction.
3. Early placement of PTCs across strictures to avoid occlusion/near-occlusion.

Prevention of Contralateral Bile Duct Injury

Perhaps the best strategy to manage a contralateral biliary injury would be to avoid it entirely. One can likely predict the cases at risk for this devastating complication based on the preoperative imaging. Central tumors and those encroaching on the hilum make for difficult dissection and an increase in risk of contralateral biliary injury. With this in mind, there are a number of techniques to mitigate this risk. Although a Cochrane review showed no difference between liver transection techniques, those that involve energy must be used with caution near the contralateral bile ducts. [11] This is especially true with devices that couple energy with irrigation (such as the Aquamantys®); spread of the superheated irrigation outside of the transection plane to the hilum could lead to biliary injury. We recommend the use of nonenergy devices when in close approximation to the hilar structures. If this is impossible, then methods to decrease heat exposure are employed, including soaked sponges and carefully directed suctioning. When the portal pedicle is reached, many surgeons will use staplers to achieve control vascular structures. We find that passing a tape around the pedicle and using it apply counter-traction in the direction of the remaining liver parenchyma can serve to displace the contralateral bile duct. Similarly, lowering of the hilar plate and earlier transection of venous outflow can serve to displace the contralateral hilar structures. All of the techniques are selectively employed in our institution to decrease the chance of contralateral biliary injury.

Clinical Pearls

When facing a post-hepatectomy biliary stricture:

1. Define anatomy with cholangiography, either by percutaneous access or MRCP.
2. Gain control of the stricture with a PTC as soon as safely possible (dilated ducts ideal, but not necessary).
3. Consider peri-procedural antibiotic coverage when instrumenting obstructed bile ducts due to risk of cholangitis.
4. Drain perihepatic collections externally to control sepsis; allow time for inflammatory/ischemic process to resolve.
5. Plan for prolonged placement of PTC.

Conclusion

Although an uncommon occurrence, contralateral bile duct injuries are a recognized complication of liver resection. These can present as either bile leakage or stricture. Two cases show different elements of patient presentation and management. In both cases, the patient was successfully managed nonoperatively with percutaneous techniques, although certainly this is not definitive management in all cases.

References

1. Lo CM, Fan ST, Liu CL, Lai EC, Wong J. Biliary complications after hepatic resection: risk factors, management, and outcome. Arch Surg. 1998;133(2):156–61.
2. Yamashita Y, Hamatsu T, Rikimaru T, Tanaka S, Shirabe K, Shimada M, et al. Bile leakage after hepatic resection. Ann Surg. 2001;233(1):45–50.
3. Jarnagin WR, Gonen M, Fong Y, DeMatteo RP, Ben-Porat L, Little S, et al. Improvement in perioperative outcome after hepatic resection: analysis of 1,803 consecutive cases over the past decade. Ann Surg. 2002;236(4):397–406; discussion 407.
4. Imamura H, Seyama Y, Kokudo N, Maema A, Sugawara Y, Sano K, et al. One thousand fifty-six hepatectomies without mortality in 8 years. Arch Surg. 2003;138(11):1198–206; discussion 206.
5. Boonstra EA, de Boer MT, Sieders E, Peeters PM, de Jong KP, Slooff MJ, et al. Risk factors for central bile duct injury complicating partial liver resection. Br J Surg. 2012;99(2):256–62.
6. Yang LY, Chang RM, Lau WY, Ou DP, Wu W, Zeng ZJ. Mesohepatectomy for centrally located large hepatocellular carcinoma: indications, techniques, and outcomes. Surgery. 2014;156(5):1177–87.
7. Capussotti L, Ferrero A, Vigano L, Sgotto E, Muratore A, Polastri R. Bile leakage and liver resection: where is the risk? Arch Surg. 2006;141(7):690–4; discussion 695.
8. Balzan S, Belghiti J, Farges O, Ogata S, Sauvanet A, Delefosse D, et al. The 50-50 Criteria on Postoperative Day 5. Ann Surg. 2005;242(6):824–9.
9. Cantwell CP, Pena CS, Gervais DA, Hahn PF, Dawson SL, Mueller PR. Thirty years' experience with balloon dilation of benign postoperative biliary strictures: long-term outcomes. Radiology. 2008;249(3):1050–7.
10. Janssen JJ, van Delden OM, van Lienden KP, Rauws EA, Busch OR, van Gulik TM, et al. Percutaneous balloon dilatation and long-term drainage as treatment of anastomotic and nonanastomotic benign biliary strictures. Cardiovasc Intervent Radiol. 2014;37(6):1559–67.
11. Gurusamy KS, Pamecha V, Sharma D, Davidson BR. Techniques for liver parenchymal transection in liver resection. Cochrane Database Syst Rev. 2009(1):CD006880.

Transplantation for Hilar Cholangiocarcinoma

20

Caroline C. Jadlowiec and Charles B. Rosen

Introduction

Cholangiocarcinoma arises from epithelial cells of the intra- and extrahepatic bile ducts and is the second most common primary malignant tumor of the liver. Current understanding of cholangiocarcinoma has led to anatomic differentiation of these tumors based on the location (extrahepatic, hilar, and intrahepatic) and growth pattern (sclerotic, polypoid, and mass). The tumor node metastasis (TNM) staging system was updated in 2010 to reflect this current understanding, as treatment and outcomes are dependent on anatomy [1]. Hilar cholangiocarcinoma most often grows in a sclerotic pattern, and is notorious for infiltration of tissues adjacent to the duct. Potentially curative treatment options for hilar cholangiocarcinoma include resection and liver transplantation. Optimal surgical treatment for patients with resectable de novo hilar cholangiocarcinoma is en bloc resection of the extrahepatic bile duct and the involved ipsilateral liver, including the caudate with regional lymphadenectomy. Patients with hilar cholangiocarcinoma arising in the setting of primary sclerosing cholangitis (PSC) often have advanced liver disease and/or multifocal cholangiocarcinoma precluding resection.

C.C. Jadlowiec · C.B. Rosen (✉)
Division of Transplantation Surgery and Department of Surgery,
Mayo Clinic, 200 First Street SW, Rochester, MN 55905, USA
e-mail: rosen.charles@mayo.edu

C.C. Jadlowiec
e-mail: Jadlowiec.Caroline@Mayo.edu

T.M. Pawlik et al. (eds.), *Case-Based Lessons in the Management of Complex Hepato-Pancreato-Biliary Surgery*, DOI 10.1007/978-3-319-50868-9_20

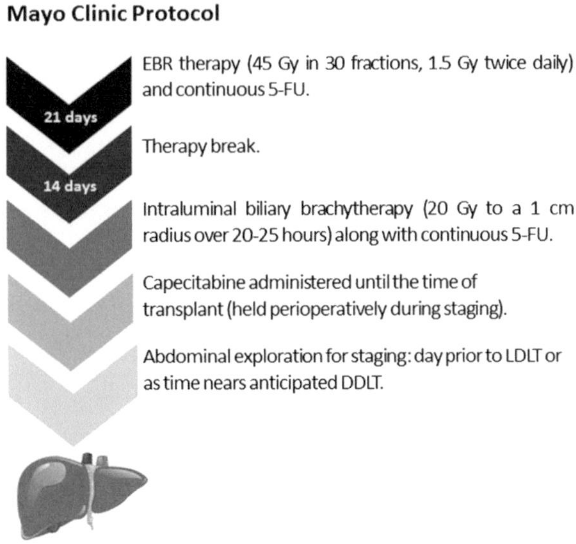

Fig. 20.1 Mayo Clinic Protocol. Neoadjuvant therapy is targeted to the primary tumor and regional lymph nodes. *EBR*, external beam radiation. Intraluminal brachytherapy with iridium is administered through an endoscopically placed biliary tube. *LDLT*, living donor liver transplant. *DDLT*, deceased donor liver transplant [8, 9]

Early experiences with liver transplantation for cholangiocarcinoma yielded poor results with 20–30% 3- to 5-year survival and greater than 50% recurrence rates [2–4]. Some patients with early stage disease, negative margins, and no regional lymph node involvement benefited from transplantation [5]. The University of Nebraska piloted an aggressive protocol for hilar cholangiocarcinoma patients using neoadjuvant high-dose brachytherapy (6 cGy) and 5-fluorouracil (5-FU) prior to liver transplantation [6, 7]. There was a high complication rate from the high-dose brachytherapy, but excellent tumor responses were observed in a small series of patients. The Mayo Clinic adopted that concept and initiated a similar protocol in 1993, combining neoadjuvant high-dose external beam therapy, lower dose brachytherapy, and chemosensitization with 5-FU in order to achieve the best possible results. The treatment protocol also included strict selection criteria and operative staging prior to transplantation (Fig. 20.1 and Table 20.1) [8–12]. Mayo

Table 20.1 Criteria for neoadjuvant therapy and liver transplantation

Criteria for neoadjuvant therapy and liver transplantation
1.Diagnosis of cholangiocarcinoma
• Transcatheter biopsy or brush cytology
• CA 19-9 > 100 U/mL or mass on cross-sectional imaging with a malignant-appearing stricture on cholangiography
• Biliary ploidy by FISH with a malignant-appearing stricture on cholangiography
2. Unresectable tumor above the cystic duct
• Pancreaticoduodenectomy for microscopic involvement of the CBD
• Resectable CCA arising in PSC
3. Radial tumor diameter $\leq$ 3 cm
4. Absence of intra- and extrahepatic metastases
5. Candidate for liver transplantation

Clinic has entered 283 patients in this treatment protocol, and 181 patients have undergone liver transplantation as of March 2016 (personal communication). The most current 5-year-survival rates after transplantation are 77% for 113 patients with cholangiocarcinoma arising in PSC, and 56% for 68 patients with de novo unresectable cholangiocarcinoma.

CASE 1

A 61-year-old male with no significant medical history other than hyperlipidemia presented with jaundice and a cholestatic liver profile (total bilirubin 3.3 mg/dL, alkaline phosphatase 350 U/L). Initial workup included a normal ultrasound that did not show any ductal dilatation or intrahepatic masses. His symptoms were attributed to drug-induced (atorvastatin) cholestatic hepatitis. Despite discontinuation of the medication, the patient had progression of his cholestatic profile, a 20-pound weight loss, and developed mild epigastric and back pain over the next 2 months. He also developed pruritus, acholic stools, and dark urine.

A malignant-appearing hilar bile duct stricture was finally detected by endoscopic retrograde cholangiography (ERC), and magnetic resonance imaging (MRI) subsequently demonstrated a type IIIB de novo hilar cholangiocarcinoma involving the midportion of the common hepatic duct with extension into the left duct. In addition to mild atrophy of the left liver with compensatory hypertrophy of the right liver, there was concern for encasement of the right hepatic artery. Given these findings, it was felt that resection was not an option, and the patient was referred for evaluation for neoadjuvant therapy and liver transplantation. He was found to be a candidate (see Table 20.1) and completed neoadjuvant radiotherapy with chemosensitization (see Fig. 20.1).

The patient did not have a suitable living donor and was placed on the deceased donor liver waiting list. As time neared for deceased donor organ availability, he underwent hand-assisted laparoscopic staging. The staging operation was negative, and the patient underwent liver transplantation with a liver from a 70-year-old deceased donor. Use of the extended criteria donor enabled him to undergo transplantation several months sooner than would have been possible with a standard criteria donor. Liver transplantation was performed with a standard caval-sparing hepatectomy and end-to-side caval implantation. The hepatic artery was reconstructed with an aortic jump graft using a younger donor iliac artery (Fig. 20.2). Biliary reconstruction was performed with Roux-en-Y choledochojejunostomy (Fig. 20.3).

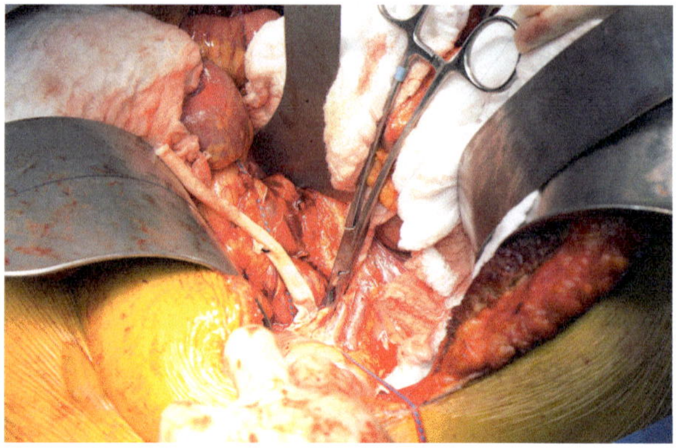

Fig. 20.2 Aortic jump graft. For deceased donors, an infrarenal aortic jump graft is created using donor iliac artery

Intraoperative Pearls

1. Avoidance of dissection in the liver hilus
2. Increased risk of early and late hepatic artery thrombosis
3. Biliary Roux limb reconstruction
   - Choledochojejunostomy in a deceased donor allograft
   - Hepaticojejunostomy in a living donor allograft
4. Increased risk of late portal vein stenosis
5. Pancreaticoduodenectomy for distal common bile duct involvement
   - En bloc pancreaticoduodenectomy without division of the common bile duct in patients with known common bile duct involvement detected by preoperative cytology or biopsy
   - Reconstruction with a double jejunal limb in living donors separating the biliary and pancreatic anastomoses
   - Non-pylorus-preserving distal gastrectomy secondary to radiation exposure.

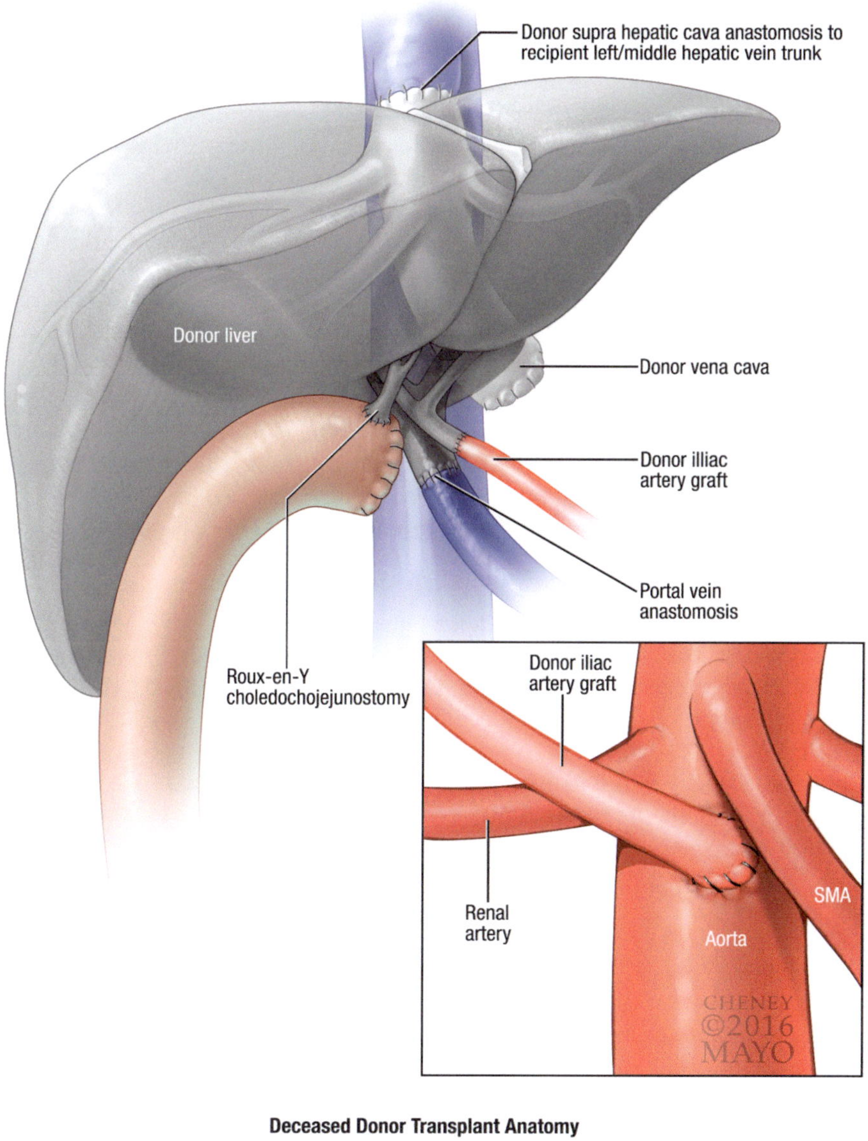

Fig. 20.3 Deceased donor liver transplant for cholangiocarcinoma. A Roux-en-Y choledochojejunostomy is created for biliary reconstruction, and an infrarenal aortic graft is created for hepatic artery inflow. Used with permission of Mayo Foundation for Medical Education and Research.

Discussion

The risk of cholangiocarcinoma in PSC patients ranges from 7 to 13%. Due to this risk, the majority of PSC patients undergo routine surveillance cholangiography [13]. In contrast, patients with cholangiocarcinoma arising de novo are frequently diagnosed when they develop jaundice later after the onset of nonspecific symptoms. De novo cholangiocarcinoma is often diagnosed at a more advanced stage of disease than cholangiocarcinoma arising in PSC. Indeed, in the Mayo Clinic experience, de novo patients are more likely to have a mass visible on cross-sectional imaging. Thus, it is not surprising that the results with neoadjuvant therapy and liver transplantation are better for patients with cholangiocarcinoma arising in PSC than those with de novo disease. Current 2-year-survival rates at Mayo Clinic are 60% for PSC patients and 30% for de novo patients after the start of neoadjuvant therapy, and 77 and 56% after liver transplantation. The differences in survival are likely due to earlier detection in PSC patients, since there were no significant differences in survival for de novo cholangiocarcinoma patients following adjustment for patient age, lymph node metastases, and tumor size [14]. Due to limited donor resources and equivocal results compared to resection, neoadjuvant therapy and liver transplantation is not the preferred treatment for de novo patients with resectable disease (Table 20.2) [15]. In contrast, patients with underlying PSC have a predisposition to multifocal cancer; they often have underlying parenchymal disease and/or cholangiopathy such that they are best treated by neoadjuvant therapy and liver transplantation regardless of tumor resectability.

In preparation for liver transplantation, all patients should undergo operative staging following completion of neoadjuvant therapy. Operative staging is best performed the day prior to living donor liver transplantation, such that it has minimal impact on technical difficulty and patient recovery. Patients awaiting deceased donor liver transplantation should undergo operative staging as the time nears for donor organ availability. Timing of the operation depends on ABO-specific MELD scores for patients undergoing deceased donor transplantation and will vary between transplant center willingness to accept extended criteria donors, donor service areas, and UNOS regions in the United States. MELD exception scores are granted by UNOS regional review boards for patients with cholangiocarcinoma which fulfill UNOS diagnosis guidelines and are enrolled in a neoadjuvant therapy protocol. MELD scores for cholangiocarcinoma begin at 22 and increase to a score representing a 10% increase in risk every 3 months, a score increase identical to that for hepatocellular carcinoma (22, 25, 27, 29, 31, 33, etc.).

Table 20.2 Criteria for unresectability of non-metastatic hilar cholangiocarcinoma

Criteria for unresectability of non-metastatic hilar cholangiocarcinoma
1. Bilateral segmental duct extension
2. Unilateral atrophy with either contralateral segmental ductal or vascular inflow involvement
3. Unilateral segmental ductal extension with contralateral vascular inflow involvement

Operative staging was done in an open fashion at our institution between 1993 and 2005. Since 2005, we have been able to accomplish most staging operations using hand-assisted laparoscopy. The hand port is placed through a right subcostal incision, which is later incorporated in the bilateral subcostal incision required for liver transplantation. Operative staging involves thorough intraperitoneal examination with biopsy of any suspicious peritoneal nodules or intrahepatic nodules, excision of the hepatic artery lymph node overlying the takeoff of the gastroduodenal artery, excision of a pericholedochal lymph node usually found posterior to the bile duct, and excision of any suspicious lymph nodes within the hepatoduodenal pedicle. If patients were to have had a cholecystectomy shortly before diagnosis of cholangiocarcinoma (which is not infrequent), the cystic duct stump should be excised for pathological examination. Clinical factors associated with a high likelihood of positive staging and/or patient dropout prior to transplantation include a CA 19-9 $\geq$ 500 U/L, mass $\geq$3 cm in radial diameter, and a biologic MELD $\geq$20 [16].

Although initially controversial, the use of deceased donors for treatment of cholangiocarcinoma has gained acceptance and is necessary for patients who do not have a suitable living donor. Despite being granted MELD exception points, cholangiocarcinoma patients remain disadvantaged and at risk for dropout while awaiting a deceased donor organ. As a result, marginal, high risk, and other extended criteria donor livers are often accepted for these patients to enable transplantation sooner than would otherwise be possible.

In the past, we used donor livers procured after circulatory arrest (donation after cardiac death, DCD). DCD livers have a high risk for cholangiopathy, which can lead to recurrent and severe cholangitis and require retransplantation in up to 30% of patients [17, 18]. We have been able to achieve a 5.9% risk of cholangiopathy by using experienced staff surgeons for DCD procurement and minimizing preservation time, but only for patients amenable to duct-to-duct or choledochoduodenostomy biliary reconstruction. Despite our efforts, we still have a 30% incidence of cholangiopathy with cholangiocarcinoma patients that require Roux-en-Y choledochojejunostomy (due to resection of the recipient duct and irradiation of the duodenum). We now avoid use of DCD donor livers for cholangiocarcinoma patients and reserve their use for patients much less likely to develop cholangiopathy. Older donor livers, however, are excellent grafts for cholangiocarcinoma patients. These donors often have significant iliac artery arteriosclerosis, so a graft from a younger donor should be available for use if necessary.

Technical modifications necessary during liver transplantation for cholangiocarcinoma are outlined below. In order to perform the best possible cancer operation, dissection in the liver hilus is avoided to prevent tumor seeding. Similarly, the hepatoduodenal ligament is dissected close to the duodenum and pancreas with proximal division of the proper hepatic artery and portal vein. Intraoperatively, it can be difficult to differentiate tumor from radiation-induced fibrosis and a generalized desmoplastic response. It can also be very difficult to separate the common bile duct from the portal vein. The portal vein wall can be very friable. Examination of explanted livers has shown that, in most instances, these findings are the result of

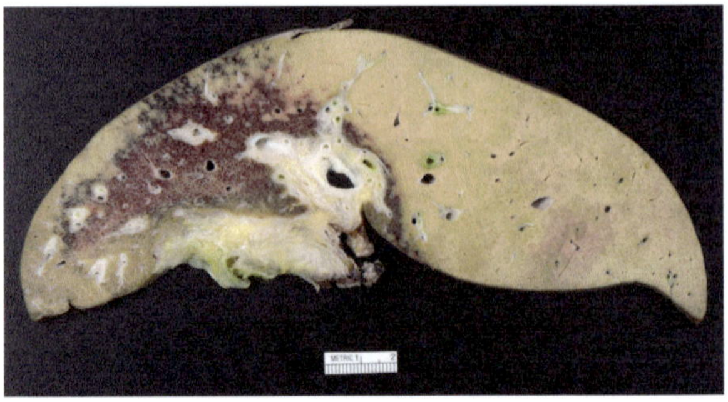

Fig. 20.4 Explant. Radiation-induced scarring involving the biliary tree

radiation injury and not tumor infiltration of the soft tissues surrounding the duct (Fig. 20.4).

Technical Modifications

1. Avoidance of the hilus during hepatectomy
2. Low division of the common bile duct (all patients) with intraoperative frozen section examination of the margin (PSC patients)
3. Isolation and division of the portal vein as close to the pancreas as possible
4. Avoidance of the irradiated recipient common hepatic artery during deceased donor transplantation
5. Use of a portal vein interposition graft during living donor liver transplantation
6. Separate jejunal limbs for biliary and pancreatic anastomoses after pancreaticoduodenectomy during living donor liver transplantation.

Neoadjuvant radiotherapy can have an adverse and unpredictable effect on the native hepatic artery. During our early experience, we observed higher incidences of hepatic artery thrombosis and late hepatic artery stenosis than with non-cholangiocarcinoma patients. As a result, we prefer using a donor iliac artery as a jump graft between the donor hepatic artery and the recipient infrarenal abdominal aorta during deceased donor transplantation, as shown in Figs. 20.2 and 20.3. We tried this approach when we began using living donors in 2000, and our results were poor due to the size mismatches between the living donor hepatic arteries and deceased donor iliac grafts. We switched back to using the recipient common hepatic artery for reconstruction during living donor transplantation. This approach is associated with a 20% incidence of arterial stenosis, [11, 19] and we rely on frequent Doppler ultrasound examinations to detect changes in arterial flow that prompt angiography with angioplasty and stent insertion.

Neoadjuvant radiotherapy also affects the recipient portal vein, and 20% of transplant recipients develop portal vein stenosis within four months of transplantation. Doppler ultrasound may detect a portal stenosis, but stenosis is best seen by CT, which is done at four months. Portal vein stenosis is treated with percutaneous transhepatic angioplasty with stent insertion. Biliary reconstruction requires a Roux-en-Y choledochojejunostomy for deceased donor recipients, as shown in Fig. 20.3, and a Roux-en-Y hepaticojejunostomy for living donor recipients.

CASE 2

A 15-year-old female with a history of ulcerative colitis presented with a 2-week history of jaundice, fatigue, and pruritus. Ultrasound revealed a hepatic hilar mass. Subsequent MRI imaging confirmed the presence of a hilar mass arising in the right hepatic duct with right and left intrahepatic duct obstruction. The greatest radial dimension was 3.0 cm (Fig. 20.5). An ERC and endoscopic ultrasound (EUS) demonstrated a malignant-appearing stricture with an obstructing mass. Intraluminal biopsy of the tumor confirmed adenocarcinoma, and EUS-guided aspirations of regional lymph nodes were negative for metastases. The patient completed neoadjuvant radiotherapy and chemosensitization (see Fig. 20.1). Her mother was found to be an excellent living donor. She underwent hand-assisted laparoscopic staging, which was negative, and living donor liver transplantation the following day. Hepatectomy included low isolation of the portal vein with division of the proper hepatic artery at its origin on the common hepatic artery. The common bile duct was divided as low as possible, just as it entered the head of the pancreas. Unfortunately, frozen section of the common bile duct margin demonstrated invasive adenocarcinoma. Pancreaticodudenectomy was performed prior to division of the portal vein. The head of the pancreas was removed along with the entire duodenum, gastric antrum, and a short segment of jejunum. The pancreatic neck

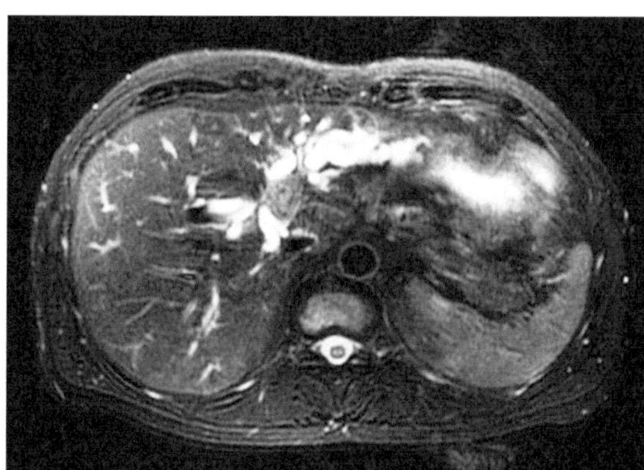

Fig. 20.5 Hilar mass on MRI imaging

was divided along the right lateral aspect of the superior mesenteric vein such that the neck of the pancreas would be as long as possible to facilitate pancreatojejunostomy. The gastroduodenal artery was divided as well. The liver was then removed by caval-sparing hepatectomy. The living donor right liver graft had been prepared for implantation by sewing a segment of deceased donor iliac vein to the segment V and VIII veins along the division interface, and sewing another segment to the right portal vein as an extension graft. The donor liver was implanted with and end-to-end right hepatic vein anastomosis, an end-to-side anastomosis between the segment V and VIII vein graft to the recipient inferior vena cava, and an end-to-end anastomosis between the portal vein extension graft and the recipient portal vein. After portal reperfusion, the donor right hepatic artery was sewn to the recipient common hepatic artery. Pancreaticoduodenectomy reconstruction was done with an end-to-side pancreatojejunostomy and a right hepaticojejunostomy to a separate Roux-en-Y jejunal limb in order to isolate the pancreatic and biliary anastomoses (Fig. 20.6). A gastrojejunostomy was done to restore enteric continuity.

Hilar Cholangiocarcinoma: Controversies

1. Utilization of liver transplantation
   - PSC patients with either resectable or unresectable CCA are best treated with neoadjuvant radiotherapy and chemosensitization followed by operative staging and transplantation
   - Patients with de novo resectable CCA should undergo liver resection
2. Exclusion of patients who have undergone percutaneous cholangiography
   - Although there have been cases of tube site recurrence, these patients are currently not excluded
   - Transperitoneal aspiration or biopsy of the primary tumor should be avoided because of high risk of tumor seeding; these patients are excluded from liver transplantation
3. Longitudinal extension of cancer along the bile duct
   - Not considered a contraindication to transplantation
4. Vascular encasement
   - Not considered a contraindication to transplantation.

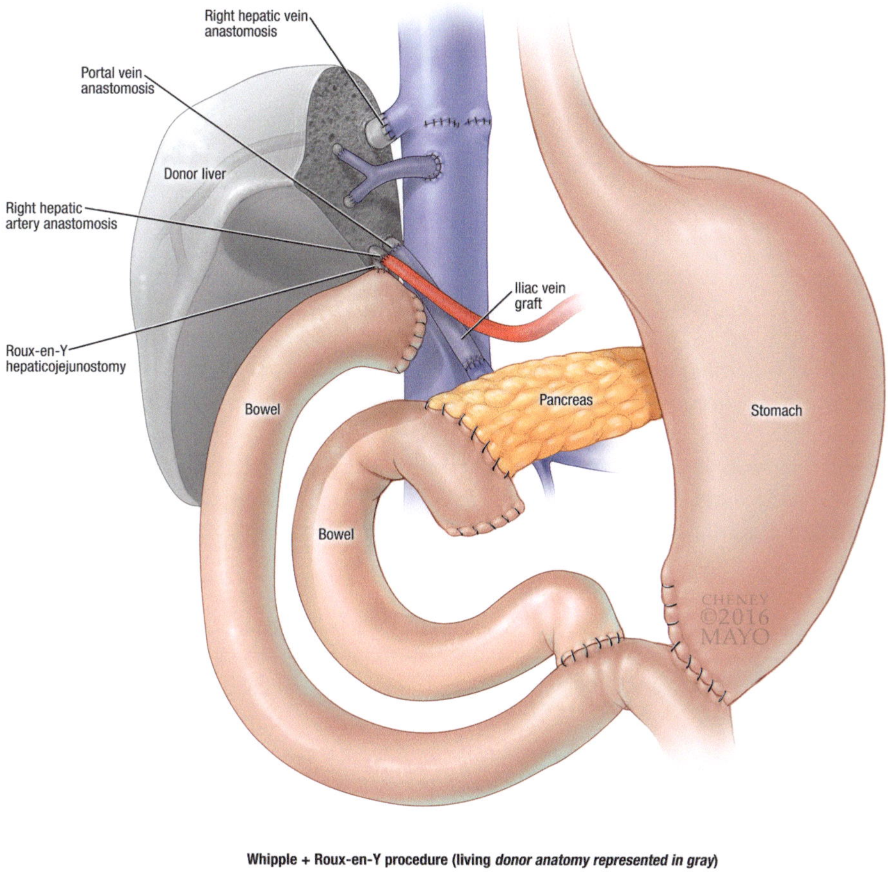

Fig. 20.6 Living donor liver transplant for cholangiocarcinoma. A right lobe allograft is depicted with venous outflow from the right hepatic vein. Outflow is further augmented by reconstructing draining veins from segments V and VIII. A double jejunal limb reconstruction is created in clinical scenarios necessitating a pancreaticoduodenectomy, thus separating the biliary and pancreatic anastomoses. Used with permission of Mayo Foundation for Medical Education and Research.

Discussion

Neoadjuvant therapy and liver transplantation is the preferred surgical treatment for patients with cholangiocarcinoma arising in the setting of PSC. Despite the obvious finding of a hilar mass, the pathological confirmation of cholangiocarcinoma in this setting remains challenging, with endoscopic biopsies and brushings frequently yielding falsely negative results. Fluorescence in situ hybridization (FISH), endoscopic cytology, and CA 19-9 are helpful in establishing a diagnosis of cholangiocarcinoma (Table 20.3) [20, 21].

Table 20.3 Accepted criteria for diagnosis of hilar cholangiocarcinoma

Accepted criteria for diagnosis of hilar cholangiocarcinoma
1. Transluminal biopsy or brush cytology with pathological confirmation of malignancy
or
2. Malignant-appearing stricture on cholangiography and at least one of the following:
• Elevated CA 19-9 (>100 U/mL)
• Polysomy by FISH
• Mass on cross-sectional imaging at the site of stricture

Microscopic extension of hilar cholangiocarcinoma to the common bile duct margin or a separate focus of microscopic tumor at the margin occurs in approximately 10% of patients with cholangiocarcinoma arising in the setting of PSC. Common bile duct involvement or multifocal disease is rare in patients with cholangiocarcinoma arising de novo. Thus, we routinely obtain a frozen section examination of the common bile duct margin in PSC patients, but not in those with de novo cholangiocarcinoma. When the margin is positive, pancreaticoduodenectomy provides the best chance for cure. We have reexcised the duct in three patients, and all three developed recurrent cancer. On occasion, we have planned an en bloc hepatectomy with pancreaticoduodenectomy for patients with known microscopic cancer within the pancreatic portion of the common bile duct, or for patients with prior choledochoduodenostomy, which precludes division of the common bile duct below the cancer. With a planned pancreaticoduodenectomy, the native liver, gastric antrum, pancreatic head, and associated duodenum are removed en bloc so as to avoid the potential for seeding by cutting through tumor or exposing tumor to the peritoneum. Since the risk of a biliary leak is very low with a deceased donor liver, we perform a standard pancreaticoduodenectomy reconstruction during deceased donor liver transplantation. The risk of a biliary leak is much higher with living donor liver transplantation, so it is our preference to isolate the pancreatic and biliary anastomoses to separate bowel limbs. An end-to-side pancreatojejunostomy is done using the proximal jejunum, and a separate Roux-en-Y jejunal limb is fashioned for the biliary anastomosis, as shown in Fig. 20.6. Pylorus preservation is avoided due to irradiation of the proximal jejunum from neoadjuvant therapy.

Conclusion

Liver transplantation in combination with neoadjuvant radiotherapy and chemosensitization is highly effective surgical treatment for selected patients with early stage hilar cholangiocarcinoma arising in the setting of PSC and early stage unresectable hilar cholangiocarcinoma arising de novo. Success requires modification of standard liver transplantation technique. Specific modifications include avoidance of the liver hilus with low division of the common bile duct; frozen section examination of the common bile duct margin in patients with PSC; use of an arterial graft between the donor artery and infrarenal aorta during deceased donor transplantation; use of a vein graft between the donor portal vein and recipient portal vein during living donor transplantation; and close postoperative monitoring by ultrasound and CT to detect late arterial stenosis following living donor transplantation, and late portal vein stenosis following transplantation regardless of donor type. Pancreaticoduodenectomy is indicated for patients with common bile duct margin involvement or known microscopic cancer in the intrapancreatic segment of the common bile duct. If pancreaticoduodenectomy is necessary during living donor transplantation, it is advisable to use a separate Roux-en-Y jejunal limb for the biliary anastomosis to isolate it from the pancreatojejunostomy.

Despite these technical challenges, excellent results are possible for patients with unresectable hilar cholangiocarcinoma or hilar cholangiocarcinoma arising in the setting of PSC.

Hilar Cholangiocarcinoma: Overall Management

1. Careful patient selection
   - Patients with CCA in the setting of PSC or unresectable patients with de novo cholangiocarcinoma fitting inclusion and exclusion criteria
2. Completion of neoadjuvant chemosensitization and radiotherapy
3. Pretransplant staging to exclude locoregional disease
   - The day prior to a living donor liver transplant
   - As MELD score increases and time nears for deceased donor organ availability
4. Liver transplantation
   - Living donor allograft with hepaticojejunostomy reconstruction
   - Deceased donor allograft with choledochojejunostomy and aortahepatic artery jump graft reconstruction
   - Pancreaticoduodenectomy for positive distal bile duct involvement
5. Careful postoperative allograft surveillance
   - Increased incidences of radiation-induced hepatic artery and portal vein stenoses.

References

1. American joint committee on cancer staging manual. 7th ed. New York: Springer; 2010. p. 201.
2. Meyer CG, Penn I, James L. Liver transplantation for cholangiocarcinoma: results in 207 patients. Transplantation. 2000;69(8):1633–7.
3. Robles R, Figueras J, Turrión VS, Margarit C, Moya A, Varo E, et al. Spanish experience in liver transplantation for hilar and peripheral cholangiocarcinoma. Ann Surg. 2004;39(2): 265–71.
4. Alessiani M, Tzakis A, Todo S, Demetris AJ, Fung JJ, Starzl TE. Assessment of five-year experience with abdominal organ cluster transplantation. J Am Coll Surg. 1995;180(1):1–9.
5. Shimoda M, Farmer DG, Colquhoun SD, Rosove M, Ghobrial RM, Yersiz H, et al. Liver transplantation for cholangiocellular carcinoma: analysis of a single-center experience and review of the literature. Liver Transpl. 2001;7(12):1023–33.
6. Foo ML, Gunderson LL, Bender CE, Buskirk SJ. External radiation therapy and transcatheter iridium in the treatment of extrahepatic bile duct carcinoma. Int J Radiat Oncol Biol Phys. 1997;39(4):929–35. Review.
7. Sudan D, DeRoover A, Chinnakotla S, Fox I, Shaw B Jr, McCashland T, et al. Radiochemotherapy and transplantation allow long-term survival for nonresectable hilar cholangiocarcinoma. Am J Transplant. 2002;2(8):774–9.
8. Rosen CB, Heimbach JK, Gores GJ. Liver transplantation for cholangiocarcinoma. Transpl Int. 2010;23(7):692–7.
9. Rea DJ, Rosen CB, Nagorney DM, Heimbach JK, Gores GJ. Transplantation for cholangiocarcinoma: when and for whom? Surg Oncol Clin N Am. 2009;18(2):325–37.
10. Rea DJ, Heimbach JK, Rosen CB, Haddock HG, Alberts SR, Kremers WK, et al. Liver transplantation with neoadjuvant chemoradiation is more effective than resection for hilar cholangiocarcinoma. Ann Surg. 2005;242(3):451–61.
11. Burns JM, Rosen CB, Heimbach JK, Gores GJ. Blumgart's surgery of the liver, biliary tract, and pancreas. 5th ed. Philadelphia: Elsevier; 2012. p. 1712–21.
12. Heimbach JK, Gores GJ, Nagorney DM, Rosen CB. Liver transplantation for perihilar cholangiocarcinoma after aggressive neoadjuvant therapy: a new paradigm for liver and biliary malignancies? Surgery. 2006;140(3):331–4.
13. Lazaridis KN, Gores GJ. Lazaridis KN. Gores GJ Semin Liver Dis. 2006;26(1):42–51.
14. Croome KP, Rosen CB, Heimbach JK, Nagorney DM. Is liver transplantation appropriate for patients with potentially resectable de novo hilar cholangiocarcinoma? J Am Coll Surg. 2015;221(1):130–9.
15. Mansour JC, Aloia TA, Crane CH, Heimbach JK, Nagino M, Vauthey JN. Hilar cholangiocarcinoma: expert consensus statement. HPB (Oxford). 2015;17(8):691–9.
16. Darwish Murad S, Kim WR, Therneau T, Gores GJ, Rosen CB, Martenson JA, et al. Predictors of pretransplant dropout and posttransplant recurrence in patients with perihilar cholangiocarcinoma. Hepatology. 2012;56(3):972–81.
17. Taner CB, Bulatao IG, Willingham DL, Perry DK, Sibulesky L, Pungpapong S, et al. Events in procurement as risk factors for ischemic cholangiopathy in liver transplantation using donation after cardiac death donors. Liver Transpl. 2012;18(1):100–11.
18. Mathur AK, Heimbach J, Steffick DE, Sonnenday CJ, Goodrich NP, Merion RM. Donation after cardiac death liver transplantation: predictors of outcome. Am J Transplant. 2010;10 (11):2512–9.
19. Mantel HT, Rosen CB, Heimbach JK, Nyberg SL, Ishitani MB, Andrews JC, et al. Vascular complications after orthotopic liver transplantation after neoadjuvant therapy for hilar cholangiocarcinoma. Liver Transpl. 2007;13(10):1372–81.

20. Kipp BR, Stadheim LM, Halling SA, Pochron NL, Harmsen S, Nagorney DM, et al. A comparison of routine cytology and fluorescence in situ hybridization for the detection of malignant bile duct strictures. Am J Gastroenterol. 2004;99(9):1675–81.
21. Nichols JC, Gores GJ, LaRusso NF, Wiesner RH, Nagorney DM, Ritts RE Jr. Diagnostic role of serum CA 19-9 for cholangiocarcinoma in patients with primary sclerosing cholangitis. Mayo Clin Proc. 1993;68(9):874–9.

Part III
Pancreas

Pancreatic Adenocarcinoma in the Head of the Pancreas with Portal Vein Involvement

21

Gyulnara G. Kasumova and Jennifer F. Tseng

Case Presentation

A 67-year-old male presented with new onset painless jaundice and hyperbilirubinemia. He underwent ERCP, where a biliary stricture was seen and a plastic biliary stent placed. At the time of ERCP, bile duct brushings were obtained and were negative. He underwent further evaluation with a CTA of the abdomen and pelvis, which revealed a 2.1 cm hypodense lesion within the pancreatic head with peri-portal and peri-pancreatic adenopathy.

Diagnosis and Workup

The patient demonstrated findings highly suspicious for pancreatic malignancy. His case was presented at pancreaticobiliary multidisciplinary conference (MDC), which includes surgical oncologists, medical oncologists, gastroenterologists, radiologists, pathologists, and radiation oncologists. MDC has been shown to resolve staging and treatment discrepancies, as well as to increase treatment rates, administration of multimodality and neoadjuvant therapy, and decrease time to initiation of treatment. Review of the scan demonstrated the mass to be in contact with the splenic/portal

G.G. Kasumova · J.F. Tseng (✉)
Department of Surgery, Beth Israel Deaconess Medical Center,
Harvard Medical School, 330 Brookline Avenue, Stoneman 9, Boston, MA 02215, USA
e-mail: jftseng@bidmc.harvard.edu

G.G. Kasumova
e-mail: gkasumov@bidmc.harvard.edu

T.M. Pawlik et al. (eds.), *Case-Based Lessons in the Management of Complex Hepato-Pancreato-Biliary Surgery*, DOI 10.1007/978-3-319-50868-9_21

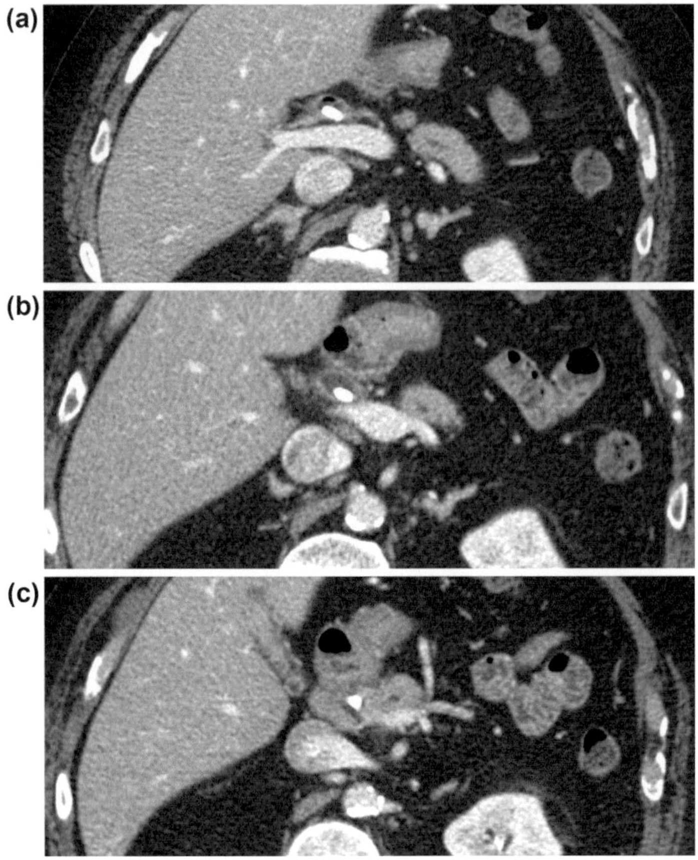

Fig. 21.1 Pre-operative imaging. Axial images of venous phase pancreatic protocol CT scan demonstrating hypodense lesion in pancreatic head: **a** portal vein free of tumor; **b** abutment of the portal vein with tumor; **c** tumor involvement of the splenic-portal vein confluence

vein confluence and adjacent superior mesenteric vein (Fig. 21.1). To obtain a tissue diagnosis, the patient underwent endoscopic ultrasound with fine needle aspiration (FNA) of the pancreatic mass and a porta hepatis lymph node. While the patient had an elevated CA 19-9 level of 939 U/mL (normal: <34 U/mL), both FNA samples were negative for malignant cells. The decision was made to proceed with open pancreatic biopsy and simultaneous port-a-cath placement, due to the high suspicion of malignancy. Open biopsy was performed using a Tru-Cut needle with three passes through a small palpable mass in the head of the pancreas. Frozen section confirmed pancreatic adenocarcinoma with duodenal invasion. The patient then underwent a chest CT, which was negative for metastatic disease.

Management

The patient presented with borderline resectable pancreatic adenocarcinoma. He received three cycles of neoadjuvant FOLFIRINOX (folinic acid, fluorouracil [5-FU], irinotecan and oxaliplatin) chemotherapy followed by stereotactic body radiotherapy (SBRT) with a cumulative dose of 2400 cGy. There was no progression of disease during treatment and, approximately 5 weeks after his last dose of chemotherapy and 3.5 weeks after his last radiation treatment, he proceeded to pancreaticoduodenectomy (PD) with venous resection and reconstruction with interposition of the internal jugular vein and splenic vein preservation. The patient is currently alive and well, undergoing workup for possible recurrence but presently biopsy-negative, more than 2 years after PD with venous reconstruction.

The above patient case demonstrates the application of neoadjuvant therapy for pancreatic adenocarcinoma, followed by restaging and pancreaticoduodenectomy with vascular reconstruction. The first extended pancreaticoduodenectomy with concomitant superior mesenteric vein (SMV) resection and reconstruction was performed in 1951 [4].

Pancreaticoduodenectomy with portal vein (PV) resection and reconstruction as part of an en bloc resection of the pancreas and surrounding structures to improve survival was first described in Japan[5]. Nearly a decade later, a similar “regional pancreatectomy” involving resection of the major peri-pancreatic vasculature with wide soft tissue clearance was described by Fortner in the United States [6]. However, contrary to early beliefs, no survival benefit had been demonstrated for patients undergoing radical or extended PD [7, 8]. It was not until recently that venous resection (VR) has demonstrated more favorable results, with comparable survival for patients with tumor involvement of major venous structures requiring venous resection and reconstruction compared to standard PD [9].

Subsequent studies within the last decade have found that patients with locally advanced disease requiring venous resection of the superior mesenteric and/or portal veins demonstrated similar survival [10] and postoperative morbidity and mortality [11] compared to patients who underwent standard PD. Findings were similar for those limited to tumors of the head [12–14]. Also, the results were not affected when PD was performed for other indications (ampullary and distal common bile duct cancers) [15]. One study [16] and several meta-analyses [17, 18] evaluating mesenteric-portal vein resection for all pancreatectomy types found similar results for survival, mortality, and morbidity. Multiple review articles have also concluded that portal vein and/or superior mesenteric vein resection is safe and confers a presumed survival advantage [19]. One study noted that patients who underwent SMV/PV resection had decreased survival relative to patients without resection; however, this study included a heterogeneous population of resectable and borderline resectable patients [20]. Another large database retrospective review found that patients undergoing pancreaticoduodenectomy with concomitant vascular resection had significantly increased rates of perioperative mortality and morbidity compared to those who did not [21]; although the interpretation of these results has been criticized, as large database work is limited by difficulty defining entry criteria and venous resection procedures resulting in mixing of cases of emergent versus planned reconstructions, as well as the inclusion of a potentially heterogeneous patient population not described in the context of multimodality cancer treatment [22]. Only one recent large meta-analysis demonstrated that patients undergoing PV-SMV resection had increased mortality, higher rates of R1/R2 resections, and worse survival [23]. Numerous studies have found that tumor-free margins [10, 16, 23–27], as well as the presence of tumor infiltration on venous resection [16, 17, 28, 29] were the most important prognostic factors. Only one study found no survival difference in the presence or absence of venous tumor infiltration [15] (Table 21.1).

Venous resection is often undertaken after neoadjuvant therapy. While neoadjuvant therapy for borderline resectable tumors has been subject to debate, the latest National Comprehensive Cancer Network (NCCN) guidelines recommend neoadjuvant therapy prior to attempted surgical resection [26, 30–32]. However, the International Study Group of Pancreatic Surgery (ISGPS) supports venous resection for borderline tumors without necessitating neoadjuvant treatment [33, 34].

Pre-operative Planning

Appropriate patient selection is crucial for successful venous resection. Radiographic imaging should be reviewed to ensure that (1) no metastatic disease is present; (2) there is no evidence of tumor involvement of the superior mesenteric artery (SMA) or celiac axis; and (3) the SMV and PV are patent without evidence of segmental or complete thrombosis [35].

The addition of vascular resection and reconstruction increases the complexity of PD and should be performed in the setting of (1) a multidisciplinary evaluation of the patient, with strong consideration of neoadjuvant treatment unless contraindicated; and (2) a high-volume surgical and perioperative team with extensive experience in vascular reconstruction and vascular surgical expertise available for preoperative and intraoperative consultation. Appropriate venous phase imaging must be obtained preoperatively to appreciate tumor abutment of the lateral or posterolateral wall of the SMV or superior mesenteric-portal vein (SMPV) confluence, the presence of which should indicate the need for venous resection [24]. Poor patient performance status and underlying organ system damage (especially hepatic or renal insufficiency) may serve as relative contraindications for vascular resection and consideration of other local therapies such as definitive SBRT may apply.

Table 21.1 Pancreaticoduodenectomy for pancreatic adenocarcinoma with venous resection reported in the literature since 2004

First author (year)	No. patients total (adeno)	No. patients (+VR)	No. patients (−VR)	% Operative mortality (+VR)	% Operative mortality (−VR)	Morbidity (+VR)	Morbidity (−VR)	Median survival (mo) (+VR)	Median survival (mo) (−VR)	No. positive margin (R1/2) (+VR) (%)	**No. positive margin (R1/2) (-VR) (%)**	**% vein infiltrate/ specimen examined**
Tseng (2004)	291	110	181	1 (0.9%)	2 (1.1%) ($p = 0.86$)	20 (18.2%)	39 (21.5%)	23.4	26.5	24/110 (21.8%)	21/181 (11.6%)	38/62 (61%)
Poon (2004)	50	12	38	0	1 (2.6%)	5 (41.7%)	16 (42.1)	19.5	20.7	8.3%	15.8%	6/12 (50%)
Riediger (2006)	125	40	85	2/53* (3.8%)	7/169* (4.1%)	22/53* (41.5%)	81/169* (47.9%)	22	15	13 (33%)	19 (24%)	16/29 (55%)
Carrere (2006)	133	45	88	2 (4.4%)	5 (5.7%)	25 (55.6%)	56 (63.6%)	15	19	8 (17.8%)	13 (14.8%)	29/45 (64%)
Ravikumar (2014)	1070	230	840	10 (4.6%)	26 (4.2%)	151/230 (65.6%)	432/840 (51.4%)	18.2	18.0	144/229 (62.9%)	423/820 (51.6%)	150 (65.2%) #
Cheung (2014)	78	32^	46	1/32 (3.1%)$^{+}$	2/46 (4.3%)$^{+}$	10/32 (31.5%)	20/46 (43.5%)	70.6%; 33.3% ***	71.1%; 23.6%***	7/32 (21.9%)	11/45 (24.4%)	–
Murakami (2015)	937**	435	502	–	–	–	–	18.5$^{\pm}$	25.8$^{\pm}$	–	–	–
Wang (2015)	208	42	166	1/42 (2.4%)	2/166 (1.2%)	16/42 (38.1%)	50/166 (30.0%)	20.0	26.0	8/42 (19.0%)	36/166 (21.7%)	100%
Kulemann (2015)	338	131	208	2/131 (1.5%)	8/208 (3.8%)	73/131 (55.7%)	104/208 (50%)	21.6	19.7	46/131 (35.4%)	49/208 (23.8%)	–

PubMed was used to search the terms pancreatic + adenocarcinoma + venous resection + portal vein. Review studies were not included. Inclusion criteria were tumors of the head, pancreatic adenocarcinoma, and PD. Studies that involved other pathologies were included if separate analyses were performed for head adenocarcinomas. A total of 18 full text articles were reviewed and 9 met inclusion criteria

+VR: venous resection; −VR: no venous resection; No.: number

*Includes pancreatic head cancer, ampullary cancer, bile duct cancer, and other

#Lymphovascular invasion

**Included patients who were resectable, borderline with venous involvement only, and borderline with arterial abutment

^Three pts also included resection of SMA

***1 and 3-yr survival rates

$^{+}$In-hospital mortality

$^{\pm}p < 0.05$

–Not reported

Clinical Pearls

- Review patient imaging both preoperatively and intraoperatively to help plan and direct dissection
- Obtain proximal and distal control of the splenic vein/SMV/PV early in the operation prior to removing the tumor specimen
- If planning to use an interposition graft, prepare conduit (internal jugular vein) early in the operation
- Make sure to correctly identify the specimen's retroperitoneal margin upon removal and determine R0/R1 *vs.* R2 resection status

Intra-operative Approach

In general, the need for vascular resection should be identified prior to operation with preoperative imaging and discussed with the patient and family, and the appropriate subspecialists, such as vascular surgery, should be alerted. Tumors of the pancreatic head and uncinate process are in close proximity to the portal and superior mesenteric veins and thereby place these vessels at risk of involvement and need for resection and reconstruction. However, it should be noted that resection of the SMV, PV, and SMPV confluence should only be performed when the vein segment cannot be separated from the pancreatic tumor and never to improve R0 margin distance or lymphatic clearance [9]. The SMV, which drains the midgut, runs posterior to the neck of the pancreas and joins the splenic vein to form the portal vein. The superior mesenteric artery (SMA) courses posterior to the pancreas and, in the majority of cases, will be located posteromedial to the SMV. The close relationship of the artery and vein makes involvement of the SMA without the SMV unlikely, only occurring if there is a posteriorly located tumor of the uncinate process; similarly, complete occlusion of the SMPV confluence often indicates tumor involvement of the SMA [35]. The SMA is surrounded by a perineural plexus that extends into pancreatic parenchyma and is a potential conduit for tumor extension [35]. While the clearance of the retroperitoneal margin and SMA dissection should be optimized, the surgeon must be wary of circumferential skeletonization of the vessel, which can result in denervation of the small bowel and increased transit time with increased risk of subsequent malnutrition [24].

If the PV and SMV are unable to be dissected free of tumor and grossly negative margins achieved, then venous resection and reconstruction is indicated. Segmental venous resection can be accomplished with or without division of the splenic vein. However, division of the splenic vein allows complete SMA exposure medial to the SMV and separation of the SMV and PV from the splenic vein, allowing for increased vein length for resection and primary anastomosis without the need for interposition grafting. To free the tumor from attachment at the SMPV confluence after division of the splenic vein, vascular clamps are placed 2–3 cm proximal (on the PV) and distal (on the SMV) to the involved segment and the vein is transected. A common practice for any anticipated lengthy (>30 min) occlusion of the portal vein is to perform SMA inflow occlusion after systemic heparinization and prior to SMV/PV occlusion to prevent small bowel edema impairing anastomosis.

Ideally, the splenic vein should be preserved when tumor involvement is limited to the PV and/or SMV. In cases of segmental involvement of the PV/SMV, splenic vein preservation limits mobilization of the PV and may require interposition grafting following SMV resection. Furthermore, preservation of the splenic vein can limit access to the proximal SMA [35]. For interposition grafting, we prefer to use internal jugular vein as the conduit. The conduit should be harvested early, prior to venous resection, and be prepared before vascular clamping for efficient anastomosis and minimal ischemia time.

As described in 2004, five general types of venous resection and reconstruction can be performed [35] (Fig. 21.2). When only a small portion of the SMPV confluence is involved by tumor, a tangential resection followed by vein patch repair (commonly from the greater saphenous vein) may be performed (Fig. 21.2, V1). If splenic vein ligation is necessary due to tumor involvement at the confluence, approximation of the superior mesenteric and portal veins may be either through a primary anastomosis without tension in an end-to-end fashion (Fig. 21.2, V2) or using an internal jugular vein interposition graft (Fig. 21.2, V3). If the splenic vein can be preserved in the setting of isolated tumor involvement of the PV or SMV, reconstruction may be similarly performed either as a tensionless primary end-to-end anastomosis (Fig. 21.2, V4) or with the use of an interposition graft (Fig. 21.2, V5).

After removal of the specimen, the surgeon must identify and ink the retroperitoneal margin for pathologic evaluation by permanent section [35]. Possible R1 versus R2 resection must also be determined by the surgeon at the time of operation; for clinically margin-negative resections as documented by the surgeon, microscopic pathological analysis will differentiate between R0 and R1 resection [35].

Controversies Around Management

- Whether or not to clamp the superior mesenteric artery prior to portal vein-superior mesenteric vein resection
- Whether the splenic vein can be ligated or reimplantation is necessary
- Whether or not to administer systemic heparin

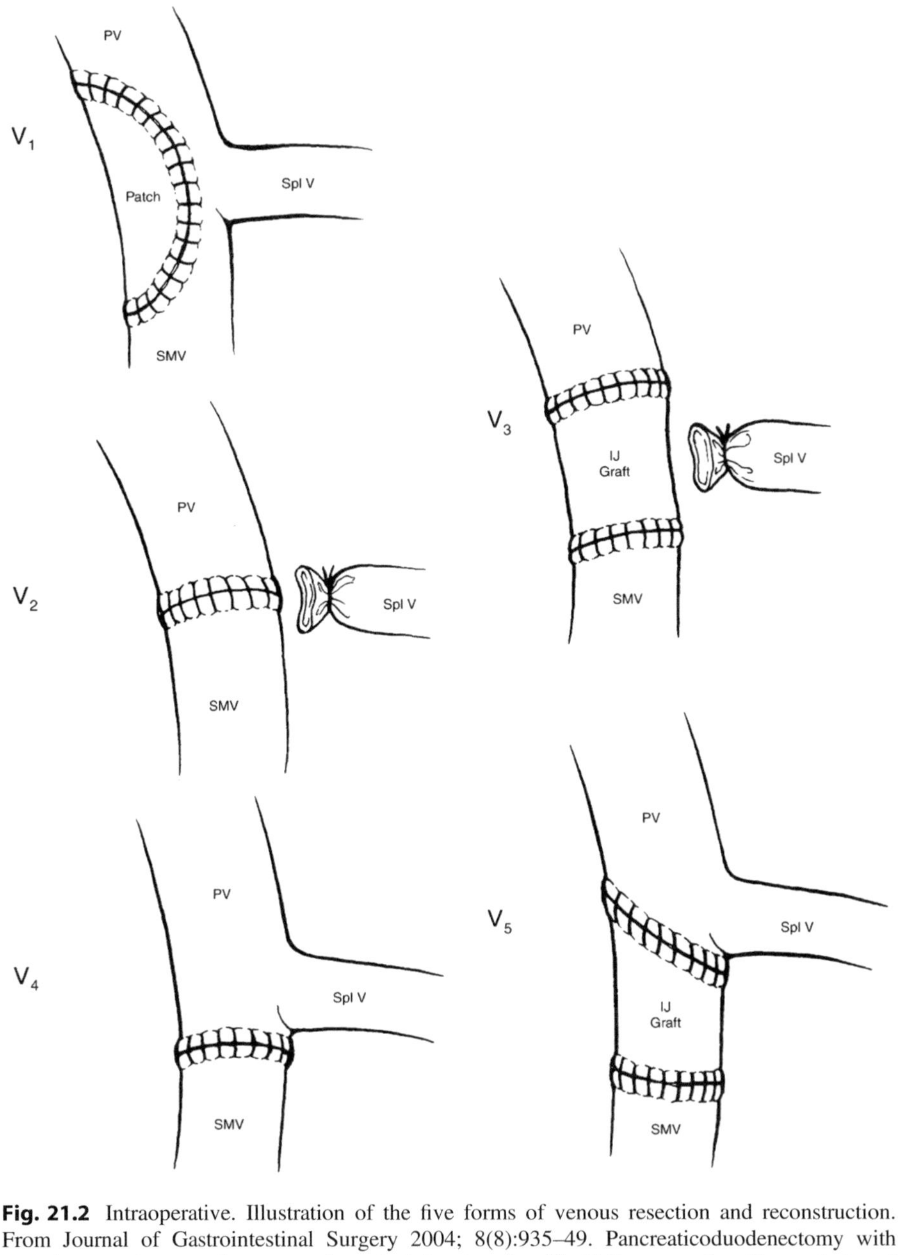

Fig. 21.2 Intraoperative. Illustration of the five forms of venous resection and reconstruction. From Journal of Gastrointestinal Surgery 2004; 8(8):935–49. Pancreaticoduodenectomy with vascular resection: margin status and survival duration; Jennifer F. Tseng *et al.*; with permission of Springer

Post-operative Course

Patients undergoing vascular reconstruction should follow the routine post-Whipple pathway per high-volume institutional standards. Some surgeons will obtain a duplex ultrasound to establish portal venous flow on postoperative day 2 or 3; otherwise, they will allow clinical examination and routine laboratory values to determine the need for imaging. Elevated liver function tests, new pressor/volume requirements, hepatic or renal dysfunction, and elevated lactate and ascites/drain output can suggest portal venous insufficiency or other related complication and warrant immediate investigation.

Patency rates for venous reconstruction are relatively high, although some variation between techniques has been noted [36], with significantly increased thrombosis rates with the use of prosthetic grafts [37]. Studies reporting occlusion rates suggest a venous occlusion range of 9–18% at median follow-up of 10.4–13 months [36, 38] and 7–13% at 1-year follow-up [9, 37]. However, no consensus regarding the use of prophylactic anticoagulation has been reached, and while some studies maintained all patients on aspirin post-operatively [38], others placed patients on prophylactic heparin at the discretion of the surgeon [37, 38]. No benefit of prophylactic aspirin administration alone has been found [36]. A recent systematic review evaluating various anticoagulation regimens following venous resection during pancreatectomy did not find an impact on the rates of early thrombosis or comorbidity [39].

In general, venous resection during PD has been deemed relatively safe when appropriate patient selection is utilized [19], but reports of postoperative complication rates have been mixed. Single-center studies have found no difference in the rates of perioperative 30-day [9, 10, 13, 15, 16, 20, 27] and in-hospital [13, 14] mortality in patients undergoing venous resection compared to standard procedure. These single-center studies have also demonstrated comparable rates of postoperative morbidity, including pancreatic fistulas, postoperative hemorrhage, delayed gastric emptying, intraabdominal abscesses, anastomotic leak, and wound infections [9–12, 14–16, 27]. Two meta-analyses found no differences in perioperative morbidity or mortality following pancreatectomy with or without venous resection [17, 18]. However, several larger studies noted significant differences between groups, with one retrospective database review finding increased overall morbidity and 30-day mortality for patients undergoing vascular resection [21]; but these results should be interpreted cautiously due to the study's retrospective nature and the heterogeneous patient population included, as discussed previously [9]. The most recent and largest meta-analysis also noted a slightly increased mortality rate (risk difference of 0.01) and increased overall morbidity for patients who underwent VR, as well as higher rates of reoperation and postoperative bleeding [23]. Appropriate selection criteria and careful operative planning are crucial for maximizing benefit to patients presenting with more advanced disease with venous involvement [24].

Global Pearls Related to Overall Management

- Patient selection: Review imaging of pancreas protocol CT at MDC to ensure no M1 or T4 disease (involvement of SMA or celiac axis)
- Direct attention to resection margins: Optimize SMA dissection and clearance of retroperitoneal margin
- Knowledge of venous anatomy: Understand strategies for resection of the SMV, PV, and SMPV confluence and use of interposition grafting

Conclusion

In the current era of pancreatic cancer surgery, venous resection and reconstruction is increasingly utilized at the time of pancreatectomy. Appropriately deployed, PD with VR can allow patients who would otherwise be considered unresectable to be rendered NED (no evidence of disease). However, given the complex nature of pancreatic surgery with vascular resection, a multidisciplinary team approach and the presence of an experienced pancreatic surgical and perioperative team is essential. Strong consideration should be given to administration of preoperative systemic therapy for pancreatic adenocarcinoma patients with venous involvement.

References

1. Schiffman SC, Abberbock S, Winters S, Valko C, Steve J, Zureikat AH, et al. A pancreatic cancer multidisciplinary clinic: insights and outcomes. J Surg Res. 2016;202(2):246–52.
2. Gardner TB, Barth RJ, Zaki BI, Boulay BR, McGowan MM, Sutton JE, et al. Effect of initiating a multidisciplinary care clinic on access and time to treatment in patients with pancreatic adenocarcinoma. J Oncol Pract. 2010;6(6):288–92.
3. Pawlik TM, Laheru D, Hruban RH, Coleman J, Wolfgang CL, Campbell K, et al. Evaluating the impact of a single-day multidisciplinary clinic on the management of pancreatic cancer. Ann Surg Oncol. 2008;15(8):2081–8.
4. Moore GE, Sako Y, Thomas LB. Radical pancreatoduodenectomy with resection and reanastomosis of the superior mesenteric vein. Surgery. 1951;30(3):550–3.
5. Asada S, Itaya H, Nakamura K, Isohashi T, Masuoka S. Radical pancreatoduodenectomy and portal vein resection. Report of two successful cases with transplantation of portal vein. Arch Surg. 1963;87:609–13.
6. Fortner JG. Regional resection of cancer of the pancreas: a new surgical approach. Surgery. 1973;73(2):307–20.
7. Yeo CJ, Cameron JL, Lillemoe KD, Sohn TA, Campbell KA, Sauter PK, et al. Pancreaticoduodenectomy with or without distal gastrectomy and extended retroperitoneal lymphadenectomy for periampullary adenocarcinoma, part 2: randomized controlled trial evaluating survival, morbidity, and mortality. Ann Surg. 2002;236(3):355–66; discussion 66–8.

8. Riall TS, Cameron JL, Lillemoe KD, Campbell KA, Sauter PK, Coleman J, et al. Pancreaticoduodenectomy with or without distal gastrectomy and extended retroperitoneal lymphadenectomy for periampullary adenocarcinoma–part 3: update on 5-year survival. J Gastrointest Surg. 2005;9(9):1191–204; discussion 204–6.
9. Tseng JF, Raut CP, Lee JE, Pisters PW, Vauthey JN, Abdalla EK, et al. Pancreaticoduodenectomy with vascular resection: margin status and survival duration. J Gastrointest Surg. 2004;8(8):935–49; discussion 49–50.
10. Carrere N, Sauvanet A, Goere D, Kianmanesh R, Vullierme MP, Couvelard A, et al. Pancreaticoduodenectomy with mesentericoportal vein resection for adenocarcinoma of the pancreatic head. World J Surg. 2006;30(8):1526–35.
11. Riediger H, Makowiec F, Fischer E, Adam U, Hopt UT. Postoperative morbidity and long-term survival after pancreaticoduodenectomy with superior mesenterico-portal vein resection. J Gastrointest Surg. 2006;10(8):1106–15.
12. Cheung TT, Poon RT, Chok KS, Chan AC, Tsang SH, Dai WC, et al. Pancreaticoduodenectomy with vascular reconstruction for adenocarcinoma of the pancreas with borderline resectability. World J Gastroenterol. 2014;20(46):17448–55.
13. Kulemann B, Hoeppner J, Wittel U, Glatz T, Keck T, Wellner UF, et al. Perioperative and long-term outcome after standard pancreaticoduodenectomy, additional portal vein and multivisceral resection for pancreatic head cancer. J Gastrointest Surg. 2015;19(3):438–44.
14. Ravikumar R, Sabin C, Abu Hilal M, Bramhall S, White S, Wigmore S, et al. Portal vein resection in borderline resectable pancreatic cancer: a United Kingdom multicenter study. J Am Coll Surg. 2014;218(3):401–11.
15. Yekebas EF, Bogoevski D, Cataldegirmen G, Kunze C, Marx A, Vashist YK, et al. En bloc vascular resection for locally advanced pancreatic malignancies infiltrating major blood vessels: perioperative outcome and long-term survival in 136 patients. Ann Surg. 2008;247 (2):300–9.
16. Beltrame V, Gruppo M, Pedrazzoli S, Merigliano S, Pastorelli D, Sperti C. Mesenteric-portal vein resection during pancreatectomy for pancreatic cancer. Gastroenterol Res Pract. 2015;2015:659730.
17. Yu XZ, Li J, Fu DL, Di Y, Yang F, Hao SJ, et al. Benefit from synchronous portal-superior mesenteric vein resection during pancreaticoduodenectomy for cancer: a meta-analysis. Eur J Surg Oncol. 2014;40(4):371–8.
18. Zhou Y, Zhang Z, Liu Y, Li B, Xu D. Pancreatectomy combined with superior mesenteric vein-portal vein resection for pancreatic cancer: a meta-analysis. World J Surg. 2012;36 (4):884–91.
19. Ramacciato G, Mercantini P, Petrucciani N, Giaccaglia V, Nigri G, Ravaioli M, et al. Does portal-superior mesenteric vein invasion still indicate irresectability for pancreatic carcinoma? Ann Surg Oncol. 2009;16(4):817–25.
20. Murakami Y, Satoi S, Motoi F, Sho M, Kawai M, Matsumoto I, et al. Portal or superior mesenteric vein resection in pancreatoduodenectomy for pancreatic head carcinoma. Br J Surg. 2015;102(7):837–46.
21. Castleberry AW, White RR, De La Fuente SG, Clary BM, Blazer DG 3rd, McCann RL, et al. The impact of vascular resection on early postoperative outcomes after pancreaticoduodenectomy: an analysis of the American College of Surgeons National Surgical Quality Improvement Program database. Ann Surg Oncol. 2012;19(13):4068–77.
22. Tseng JF. Proceed with caution: vascular resection at pancreaticoduodenectomy. Ann Surg Oncol. 2012;19(13):4001–2.
23. Giovinazzo F, Turri G, Katz MH, Heaton N, Ahmed I. Meta-analysis of benefits of portal-superior mesenteric vein resection in pancreatic resection for ductal adenocarcinoma. Br J Surg. 2016;103(3):179–91.
24. Christians K, Evans DB. Pancreaticoduodenectomy and vascular resection: persistent controversy and current recommendations. Ann Surg Oncol. 2009;16(4):789–91.

25. Selvaggi F, Mascetta G, Daskalaki D, dal Molin M, Salvia R, Butturini G, et al. Outcome of superior mesenteric-portal vein resection during pancreatectomy for borderline ductal adenocarcinoma: results of a prospective comparative study. Langenbecks Arch Surg. 2014;399(5):659–65.
26. Delpero JR, Boher JM, Sauvanet A, Le Treut YP, Sa-Cunha A, Mabrut JY, et al. Pancreatic adenocarcinoma with venous involvement: is up-front synchronous portal-superior mesenteric vein resection still justified? A survey of the Association Francaise de Chirurgie. Ann Surg Oncol. 2015;22(6):1874–83.
27. Wang WL, Ye S, Yan S, Shen Y, Zhang M, Wu J, et al. Pancreaticoduodenectomy with portal vein/superior mesenteric vein resection for patients with pancreatic cancer with venous invasion. Hepatobiliary Pancreat Dis Int. 2015;14(4):429–35.
28. Lapshyn H, Bronsert P, Bolm L, Werner M, Hopt UT, Makowiec F, et al. Prognostic factors after pancreatoduodenectomy with en bloc portal venous resection for pancreatic cancer. Langenbecks Arch Surg. 2016;401(1):63–9.
29. Ramacciato G, Nigri G, Petrucciani N, Pinna AD, Ravaioli M, Jovine E, et al. Pancreatectomy with mesenteric and portal vein resection for borderline resectable pancreatic cancer: multicenter study of 406 patients. Ann Surg Oncol. 2016;23(6):2028–37.
30. Tang K, Lu W, Qin W, Wu Y. Neoadjuvant therapy for patients with borderline resectable pancreatic cancer: a systematic review and meta-analysis of response and resection percentages. Pancreatology. 2016;16(1):28–37.
31. Hackert T, Ulrich A, Buchler MW. Borderline resectable pancreatic cancer. Cancer Lett. 2016;375(2):231–7.
32. National Comprehensive Cancer Network. NCCN clinical practice guidelines in oncology: pancreatic adenocarcinoma, version 1.2016. https://www.nccn.org/professionals/physician_gls/f_guidelines.asp.
33. Bockhorn M, Uzunoglu FG, Adham M, Imrie C, Milicevic M, Sandberg AA, et al. Borderline resectable pancreatic cancer: a consensus statement by the International Study Group of Pancreatic Surgery (ISGPS). Surgery. 2014;155(6):977–88.
34. Kelly KJ, Winslow E, Kooby D, Lad NL, Parikh AA, Scoggins CR, et al. Vein involvement during pancreaticoduodenectomy: is there a need for redefinition of “borderline resectable disease”? J Gastrointest Surg. 2013;17(7):1209–17; discussion 1217.
35. Tseng JF, Tamm EP, Lee JE, Pisters PW, Evans DB. Venous resection in pancreatic cancer surgery. Best Pract Res Clin Gastroenterol. 2006;20(2):349–64.
36. Dua MM, Tran TB, Klausner J, Hwa KJ, Poultsides GA, Norton JA, et al. Pancreatectomy with vein reconstruction: technique matters. HPB (Oxford). 2015;17(9):824–31.
37. Glebova NO, Hicks CW, Piazza KM, Abularrage CJ, Cameron AM, Schulick RD, et al. Technical risk factors for portal vein reconstruction thrombosis in pancreatic resection. J Vasc Surg. 2015;62(2):424–33.
38. Krepline AN, Christians KK, Duelge K, Mahmoud A, Ritch P, George B, et al. Patency rates of portal vein/superior mesenteric vein reconstruction after pancreatectomy for pancreatic cancer. J Gastrointest Surg: Off J Soc Surg Aliment Tract. 2014;18(11):2016–25.
39. Chandrasegaram MD, Eslick GD, Lee W, Brooke-Smith ME, Padbury R, Worthley CS, et al. Anticoagulation policy after venous resection with a pancreatectomy: a systematic review. HPB (Oxford). 2014;16(8):691–8.

Implications of a Completely Replaced Right Hepatic Artery and Pancreatoduodenectomy

22

Anubhav Mittal, Sanjay Pandanaboyana and John Albert Windsor

Introduction

Pancreatoduodenectomy is dissection of the head of pancreas and duodenum away from the major adjacent veins (portal-superior mesenteric vein and tributaries) and arteries (coeliac, common hepatic, superior mesenteric arteries, and their branches). Anomalies of these vessels can present significant technical and oncologic challenges to the surgeon.

Historically, the resectability of a ductal adenocarcinoma arising in the head of the pancreas has been determined by its relationship to the portal-superior mesenteric vein, with significant narrowing and/or invasion being a contraindication to resection [1]. This is no longer the case, with *en bloc* synchronous vein resection justified when it allows for a margin-negative resection [2, 3]. What remains contentious is the place of synchronous arterial resection during pancreatoduodenectomy. Two recent concepts are relevant to this discussion, whether or not there is anomalous arterial anatomy. The first concept is the defining of "borderline resectable" pancreatic ductal adenocarcinoma [4], which has probably contributed to an

A. Mittal
Royal North Shore Hospital, St Leonards, NSW 2065, Australia
e-mail: mittal.surgery@gmail.com

S. Pandanaboyana
Department of Hepatobiliary and Pancreatic Surgery, Auckland City Hospital, Park Road, Grafton, Auckland 1010, New Zealand
e-mail: Spandanaboyana@adhb.govt.nz

J.A. Windsor (✉)
HBP/Upper GI Unit, Department of General Surgery, Auckland City Hospital, Park Road, Grafton, Auckland 1142, New Zealand
e-mail: j.windsor@auckland.ac.nz

T.M. Pawlik et al. (eds.), *Case-Based Lessons in the Management of Complex Hepato-Pancreato-Biliary Surgery*, DOI 10.1007/978-3-319-50868-9_22

increased frequency of synchronous arterial resection following neoadjuvant chemotherapy [5]. The second concept is that of the "artery-first approach" to PD which aims to determine resectability, including arterial involvement, at an earlier stage and before the point of no return. Although the benefits of both the "borderline resectable" and the "artery-first" concepts are being more widely adopted, the evidence that these improve survival is sparse. Nevertheless, the artery-first approach is helpful in the early confirmation and safe dissection of arterial anomalies [6]. The aim of this chapter is to consider the significance and approach to the most common arterial anomalies encountered in patients undergoing PD.

Anatomical Considerations

Approximately six decades ago Michels published his detailed classification of the extrahepatic arterial anatomy based on 200 cadaveric dissections [7] and his findings were confirmed by Hiatt more recently [8] (Fig. 22.1). This classification system has formed the basis for more recent studies using modern imaging methods, including a study of 600 patients using digital subtraction angiography [9]. This study revealed that standard or normal arterial anatomy was found in only 61% of cases, and that anomalous RHA anatomy was present in approximately 17% of patients, with a completely replaced common hepatic artery (CHA) arising from the SMA in 2%. The most common variations of RHA anatomy are summarized in Table 22.1 [9]. These anomalies of the RHA can be further subdivided between those that are a complete replacement (RRHA) and accessory (ARHA) of the right hepatic arteries (Fig. 22.1). From these studies, anomalies of the right hepatic artery occur in between 17 [1] and 26% [2] of the general population.

The anatomical course of RRHA and ARHA are important because this determines both the vulnerability to inadvertent injury and whether intentional arterial resection will be required during the course of PD. There are three different variations to the course taken by the anomalous RHA [10]. In 87.5% of patients, after originating from the SMA, the RRHA courses posterior to the head of the pancreas (Type 1); in 10.7% it courses through the pancreatic parenchyma (Type 2); and in 3.7% it courses through the SMV groove deep to the pancreatic neck (Type 3).

Preoperative Considerations

Given the significance of these anomalies it is vital to identify them and to delineate the arterial course in relation to the pancreas, the tumor and expected dissection planes before embarking on the PD [11]. Dedicated visceral arterial angiography is no longer required prior to surgery [12]. Preoperative arterial phase computer-aided tomography (CT) is able to accurately detect anomalous RHA anatomy with a high degree of reliability [13], and the arterial phase should be a routine part of

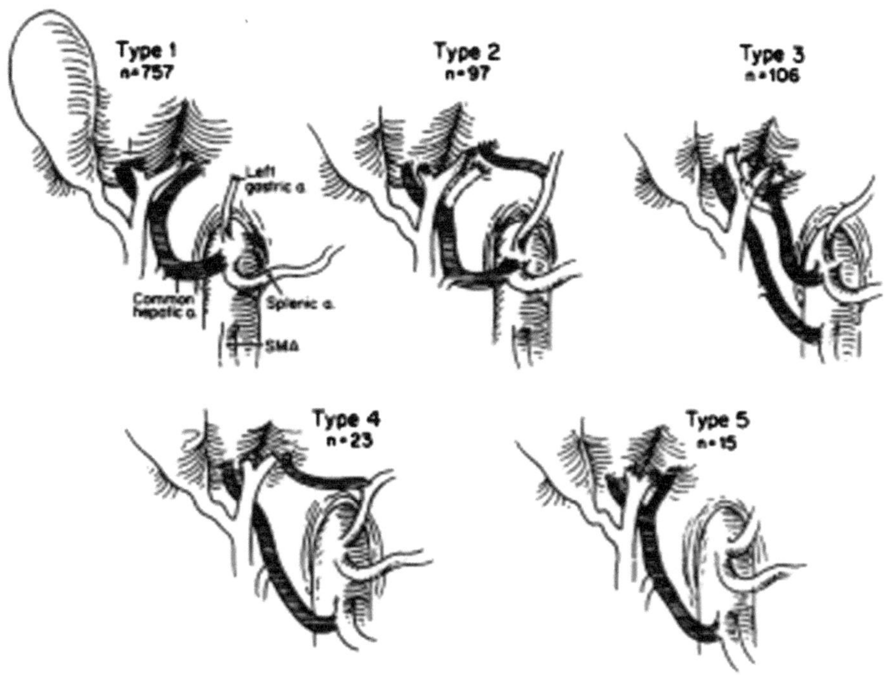

Fig. 22.1 Michel classification applied to a series of 1000 patients *Type 1* is normal; *Type 2* accessory left hepatic artery from the left gastric artery; *Type 3* accessory left hepatic artery from superior mesenteric artery; *Type 4* double accessory or replaced anomaly; *Type 5* common hepatic artery from the superior mesenteric artery. Not shown is the common hepatic artery arising from the aorta ($n = 2$). From Hiatt J, Gabbay J, and Busuttil R. Surgical Anatomy of the Hepatic Arteries in 1000 Cases. Annals of Surgery. 1994;220(1):50–2. With permission from Wolters Kluwer

Table 22.1 The most common anomalies of the RHA [9]

Type of RHA anomaly	Frequency (%)
RRHA from SMA	8.7
RRHA and RLHA	3.0
ARHA from SMA	1.5
ARHA and ALHA	1.0
ARHA and LHA and RRHA or RLHA	3.0

RRHA completely replaced right hipatic artery; *RLHA* completely replaced left hepatic artery; *ARHA* accessory right hepatic artery; *ALHA* accessory left hepatic artery; *SMA* superior mesenteric artery

preoperative CT imaging. It is uncertain whether 3D reconstruction of the arterial anatomy is helpful [14]. What is clear is that delineation of the course of the anomalous RHA is essential in preoperative planning of the intraoperative strategy for a PD.

Surgical Considerations

The key questions to be answered when an anomalous RHA is identified prior to a PD, is whether the artery can be preserved without compromising clearance of the cancer, whether it can be sacrificed, or whether it will require resection and reconstruction with either primary anastomosis or grafting.

Injury to a RRHA without reconstruction is likely to lead to hepatic ischaemia and necrosis. The bile duct is also at risk because the RHA becomes the primary arterial supply to the common bile duct after division of the gastroduodenal artery (GDA) during PD. The consequences of this include the early risk of a leak from the hepaticojejunostomy and later risk of anastomotic stricture. Injury to an ARHA is less of a concern. An ARHA can be safely resected without reconstruction if there is adequate flow in the main RHA. This can usually be evaluated by palpation with preservation of the vascular thrill with temporary clamping of the ARHA, or by intraoperative Doppler ultrasonography.

The Type 1 anomaly of the RHA [5] can usually be preserved because it runs posterior to the pancreatic head (Fig. 22.2). The exception is when it is directly invaded when all other resection margins are expected to be R0, which means that resection and reconstruction is indicated. Arterial resection is often required for Type 2 RHA anomalies, since the artery is usually encased by the cancer within the head of the pancreas. Arterial resection is occasionally required for a Type 3 RHA anomaly.

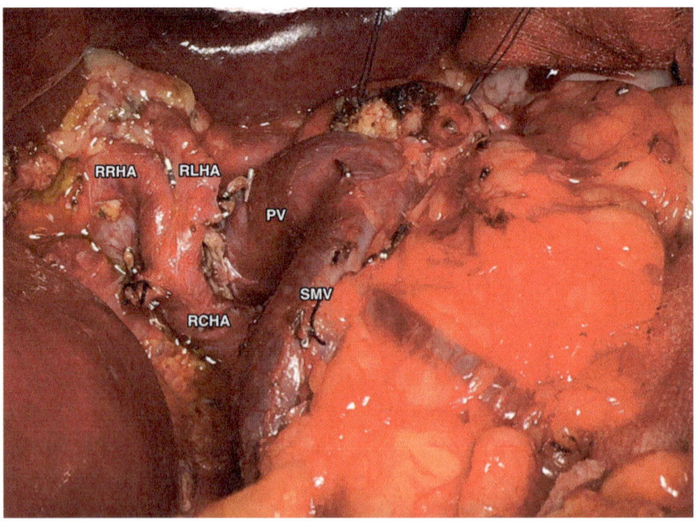

Fig. 22.2 Replaced common hepatic artery (*RCHA*) originating from the superior mesenteric artery with a *RRHA* and a *RLHA*. Portal vein (*PV*) and superior mesenteric vein (*SMV*) are displayed

It has been suggested that the distance between the margin of the pancreatic cancer to the origin of an anomalous RRHA is predictive of whether there will be an R0 or an R1 resection [15]. If the cancer margin is <10 mm from the origin of the RRHA on preoperative imaging, and PD is performed without arterial resection, the R1 rate with pancreatoduodectomy is 78% without arterial resection, which is more than 10 times the 6% risk of an R1 resection if the cancer margin is >10 mm from the origin of the RHA. On this basis, planned resection of a RRHA should be considered if the tumor is <10 mm from the origin of the RRHA in order to reduce the R1 rates.

A recent systematic review evaluated the management and impact of anomalous RHA on the outcomes of pancreatoduodenectomy [3]. This included 10 retrospective studies and 2278 patients [11]. The overall incidence of an anomalous RHA was 19% (n = 440). The majority of patients (n = 346, 87%) had the anomalous RHA coursing away from the tumor, and therefore did not require resection of the RHA. In 31 (7%) of the patients, the RHA was sacrificed without the need for reconstruction. In four of the studies, the authors performed a clamp test with intraoperative Doppler ultrasonography to confirm adequate arterial flow in the right hemi-liver from collateral circulation. Arterial reconstruction was only required in 17 (4%) patients. This was achieved by primary anastomosis of the divided arterial ends, vein or PTFE graft, or anastomosis of the divided RHA to the GDA stump. The outcome of patients undergoing arterial resection with or without reconstruction was compared in this systemic review [3]. There was no significant difference in short-term morbidity or mortality. There was also no difference in the positive (R1/R2) rates or overall survival.

Key Points

1. Anomalous right hepatic artery (RHA) is seen in 17–26% of the population.
2. The most common of the anamolies are a complete replacement of the RHA, followed by an accessory right hepatic artery, both arising from the superior mesenteric artery.
3. Preoperative arterial phase CT scan is able to accurately detect the type of anomaly and course the RHA anatomy with a high degree of reliability.
4. An artery-first approach to pancreatoduodenectomy will allow earlier identification and safe dissection of a replaced RHA, and should be considered if preoperative imaging suggests the presence of this anomaly.
5. Planned resection of an anomalous RHA should be considered if the tumor is <10 mm from the origin of the anomalous RHA in order to reduce the R1 rates.

Conclusion

Anomalous RHA anatomy is relatively common, and should be identified prior to pancreatoduodenectomy. Preoperative planning is important in deciding whether to preserve, sacrifice, or reconstruct an anomalous artery. The relationship of the tumor to the origin of the anomalous RHA is important to note. Pancreatoduodenecotmy with or without arterial resection can be safely performed in patients with anomalous RHA, although the evidence is derived from small retrospective case series. Artery-first approach may be adopted in patients with anomalous RHA anatomy to allow earlier identification and safer dissection during PD.

References

1. Barreto SG, Windsor JA. Justifying vein resection with pancreatoduodenectomy. Lancet Oncol. 2016;17(3):e118–24.
2. De Reuver PR, Mittal A, Neale M, Gill AJ, Samra JS. Extended pancreatoduodenectomy as defined by the International Study Group for Pancreatic Surgery is associated with worse survival but not with increased morbidity. Surgery. 2015;158(1):183–90.
3. Bockhorn M, Uzunoglu FG, Adham M, Imrie C, Milicevic M, Sandberg AA, et al. Borderline resectable pancreatic cancer: a consensus statement by the International Study Group of Pancreatic Surgery (ISGPS). Surgery. 2014;155(6):977–88.
4. Katz MHG, Pisters PWT, Evans DB, Sun CC, Lee JE, Fleming JB, et al. Borderline resectable pancreatic cancer: the importance of this emerging stage of disease. J Am Coll Surg. 2008;206 (5):833–46.
5. Amano R, Kimura K, Nakata B, Yamazoe S, Motomura H, Yamamoto A, et al. Pancreatectomy with major arterial resection after neoadjuvant chemoradiotherapy gemcitabine and S-1 and concurrent radiotherapy for locally advanced unresectable pancreatic cancer. Surgery. 2015;158(1):191–200.
6. Sanjay P, Takaori K, Govil S, Shrikhande SV, Windsor JA. "Artery-first" approaches to pancreatoduodenectomy. Br J Sur. 2012;99(8):1027–35.
7. Michels NA. The hepatic, cystic and retroduodenal arteries and their relations to the biliary ducts. Ann Surg. 1951;133(4):503–24.
8. Hiatt JR, Gabbay J, Busuttil RW. Surgical anatomy of the hepatic arteries in 1000 cases. Ann Surg. 1994;220(1):50–2.
9. Covey AM, Brody LA, Maluccio MA, Getrajdman GI, Brown KT. Variant hepatic arterial anatomy revisited: digital subtraction angiography performed in 600 patients. Radiology. 2002;224(2):542–7.
10. Jah A, Jamieson N, Huguet E, Praseedom R. The implications of the presence of an aberrant right hepatic artery in patients undergoing a pancreaticoduodenectomy. Surg Today. 2009;39 (8):669–74.
11. El Amrani M, Pruvot F-R, Truant S. Management of the right hepatic artery in pancreaticoduodenectomy: a systematic review. J Gastrointest Oncol. 2016;7(2):298–305.
12. Murugiah M, Windsor JA, Redhead DN, O'Neill JS, Suc B, Garden OJ, et al. The role of selective visceral angiography in the management of pancreatic and periampullary cancer. World J Surg. 1993;17(6):796–800.
13. Chong M, Freeny PC, Schmiedl UP. Pancreatic arterial anatomy: depiction with dual-phase helical CT. Radiology. 1998;208(2):537–42.

14. Tanikake M, Shimizu T, Narabayashi I, Matsuki M, Masuda K, Yamamoto K, et al. Three-dimensional CT angiography of the hepatic artery: use of multi-detector row helical CT and a contrast agent. Radiology. 2003;227(3):883–9.
15. Okada KI, Kawai M, Hirono S, Miyazawa M, Shimizu A, Kitahata Y, et al. The preservation of replaced right hepatic artery adjacent to pancreatic carcinoma correlates high resection rate in pancreaticoduodenectomy. Gastroenterology. 2015;148(4):S1145.

Pancreatic Adenocarcinoma in the Neck of the Pancreas Involving the Celiac Trunk (Appleby Procedure)

23

Richard A. Burkhart and Matthew J. Weiss

Introduction

Pancreatic ductal adenocarcinoma (PDA) is a devastating disease. Despite progress in other malignancies, the only chance for cure remains complete surgical extirpation of locally confined disease. PDA arising in the neck or body of the gland is insidious, often only becoming apparent after local or distant disease progression. Here we review our approach to patients who present with locally advanced PDA in the pancreatic neck involving the celiac axis. Our preoperative workup with laboratory and imaging analysis is detailed. Key considerations before entertaining surgical resection via a modified Appleby procedure are highlighted. Intra-operative decision-making and technical challenges are reviewed in detail. Peri-operative and postoperative care is reviewed in the context of a case recently encountered at our institution. Throughout, clinical pearls are offered to assist advanced pancreatic surgeons in the management of these complex patients.

R.A. Burkhart
Department of Surgery, The Johns Hopkins Hospital, 600 North Wolfe Street, Blalock 611, Baltimore, MD 21287, USA
e-mail: rburkha6@jhmi.edu

M.J. Weiss (✉)
Department of Surgery, The Johns Hopkins Hospital, 600 North Wolfe Street, Halsted 608, Baltimore, MD 21287, USA
e-mail: mweiss5@jhmi.edu

T.M. Pawlik et al. (eds.), *Case-Based Lessons in the Management of Complex Hepato-Pancreato-Biliary Surgery*, DOI 10.1007/978-3-319-50868-9_23

Case Presentation

A 48-year-old woman with mild hypertension presents to your surgical clinic with a chief complaint of vague upper abdominal discomfort for 9 months. Her pain is described as mild, 2 out of 10 in intensity, persistent, and located in the mid epigastrum. Associated symptoms include intermittent nausea and postprandial bloating. She cannot identify any aggravating or alleviating factors. Her primary care physician suspected gastritis and prescribed proton pump inhibitor therapy. This failed to improve her symptoms and an abdominal contrast-enhanced computed tomography (CT) scan was performed. This demonstrated a mass-like lesion appearing to arise from the neck pancreas and involving the common hepatic artery. This lesion was 5 cm in size and hypodense in relation to the surrounding pancreatic parenchyma. She arrives in your clinic with her husband and children to discuss surgical management of this disease.

Workup

Despite the improvements in survival seen in many types of gastrointestinal malignancies, pancreatic ductal adenocarcinoma (PDA) remains a highly lethal disease. The disease burden in the United States is increasing, with an incidence of nearly 50,000 cases annually [1]. With mortality rates approaching the incidence of the disease, a diagnosis of PDA can be devastating. Only 7% of patients will be alive at 5 years, with nearly all having disease surgically resected while still locally confined [1]. Despite being only the 12th most frequent cancer encountered in the U.S., it is currently the fourth leading cause of cancer-related death. Epidemiologic estimates suggest that PDA will surpass breast and prostate cancer to become the second-leading cause of cancer-related death in the U.S. by 2030 [2].

When considering a diagnosis of PDA, the initial clinic visit should include a review of the patient's medical history in detail and a thorough physical examination. Common presenting symptoms for patients with PDA can be vague, particularly when disease is located in the neck or body of the gland. Historical review of these patients finds abdominal pain to be present in nearly 90% of patients, with other symptoms including weight loss, nausea, vomiting, diarrhea, jaundice, and constipation occurring at a far less frequent rate [3]. A review of personal, family, and social history should focus on risk factors for pancreatic disease (including, at a minimum, a personal history of pancreatitis, cancer, or endocrine neoplasia; a family history of malignancy; or a social history of tobacco use). Physical examination should include an evaluation for jaundice, lymphadenopathy, abdominal mass, liver fullness or mass, pain in the back or abdomen, and presence or absence of ascites. An evaluation of blood work during this initial visit should also be completed and should include complete blood count, chemistry profile (including liver function testing), and pancreatic tumor markers (carbohydrate antigen 19-9 and carcinoembryonic antigen).

High-quality contrast-enhanced cross-sectional imaging is imperative when evaluating solid pancreatic masses. In many cases, the initial study obtained will be insufficient to provide an accurate characterization of the lesion. Clinicians entertaining a diagnosis of pancreatic malignancy should not hesitate to repeat abdominal imaging in these scenarios. Both CT and magnetic resonance imaging are good options, with a preference in our institution for CT due to physician experience and preference. Technical keys to CT performance are optimal timing of contrast administration (in both the arterial and portal venous phases) and highly selective use of oral contrast (in practice, oral contrast is rarely necessary and can sometimes prove detrimental when evaluating pancreatic pathology).

Unfortunately, as is the case in our patient (Fig. 23.1), tumors that arise in the body and tail of the pancreas are more often large (>2 cm) and less likely amenable to immediate surgical resection than those patients who have tumors in the head of the gland [4, 5]. When this is the case, further workup is required to obtain a tissue diagnosis and guide therapy. The most commonly used modality is endoscopy with ultrasound and needle biopsy. An experienced endoscopist should focus on the mass' location and tissue of origin, evaluate the locoregional lymphatic drainage basins, and evaluate for evidence of vascular encasement or invasion. Biopsy can be performed with either fine-needle aspiration or core needle sampling, based on the practitioner and institutional experience. After cross-sectional imaging in our patient, she underwent endoscopy with ultrasound and fine-needle aspirate biopsy to conclude her workup.

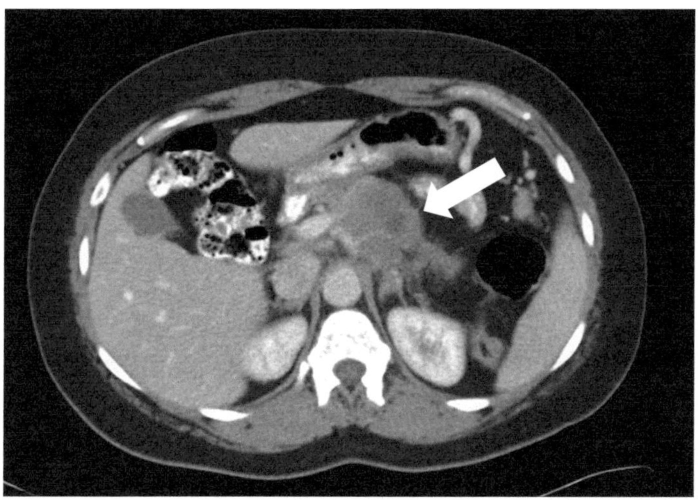

Fig. 23.1 Diagnostic imaging with contrast-enhanced computed tomography (CT) scan. Our diagnostic preference is to obtain a high-quality, intravenous contrast-enhanced CT scan. The scan should be completed with dual phase images, once during arterial enhancement and once during portal venous enhancement. Here we show our patient with a 5 cm mass in the neck/body of the pancreas (*white arrow*) that completely encases the celiac axis and its proximal branches

Diagnosis and Staging

A diagnosis of PDA can be made definitely based on histopathologic analysis of biopsy specimens. Typical findings include pleomorphic and hypercellular fragments of tissue with ductal features in a relative paucity of acinar epithelium. The nuclei are characteristically enlarged with irregular contours. Multinucleated cells and mitosis are often encountered. Cells are often found to be arranged haphazardly and with a lack of discernible polarity, often described as a "drunken honeycomb" arrangement [6]. Once the diagnosis has been confirmed, information gleaned from the patient's physical exam, imaging studies, endoscopy, and histology are combined to accurately stage the patient's disease.

The most common staging system used for PDA (Table 23.1) is derived from a consensus of experts in conjunction with the American Joint Committee on Cancer with a goal of facilitating treatment decisions and prognosis [7]. Currently in its seventh edition, the backbone relies on an evaluation of the primary tumor (T-stage), regional lymph nodes (N-stage), and presence or absence of metastasis (M-stage). Final anatomic or prognostic staging involves grouping of T, N, and M categories as can be seen in Table 23.1. The T and M-stage categories reflect the major determinant of survival in PDA: the capacity for complete surgical resection. When the primary tumor extends beyond the pancreas to involve the celiac axis or the superior mesenteric artery for greater than 180°, the term locally advanced PDA is used. This is generally regarded as unresectable disease (T4). In the absence of metastatic disease, a T4 tumor is considered stage III disease regardless of nodal status. When associated with evidence of metastasis a T4 tumor is considered stage IV.

It is worth a moment to discuss issues that arise in delivering a diagnosis of PDA in the clinic to our patient. As one of the most commonly encountered malignancies causing death, she may have preconceived notions regarding the meaning of the diagnosis. Certainly, there is a fair amount of nihilism that is associated with PDA in the general public. Practically, it can be helpful to deliver this news, when the patient allows, in the presence of family and her loved ones, as this support system may be an important part of the overall treatment plans. It can also be helpful to ask what they may know of the disease and use this as a starting point for counsel and guidance with medical decision-making (reinforcing accurate notions and correcting knowledge gaps). Ultimately, it is important to provide your patient with accurate clinical knowledge so she and her family can formulate clear and consistent goals of care throughout her treatment course.

At the time of diagnosis, only 20% of PDA are amenable to complete surgical resection [8, 9]. Of the remaining 80%, approximately one-third will have locally advanced disease without evidence of metastasis (stage III). Due to a high incidence of perioperative complications and a high rate of disease recurrence with poor response to adjuvant therapies, patients with stage III disease have rarely been offered attempts at surgical extirpation in the past. However, improvements in peri-operative outcomes and responses to systemic chemotherapeutics have led to more aggressive approaches in a highly selected group of patients. In the case

Table 23.1 Pancreatic cancer staging

Primary tumor (T)			
Tis	Carcinoma in situ		
T1	Tumor limited to the pancreas, <2 cm		
T2	Tumor limited to the pancreas, >2 cm		
T3	Tumor extends beyond the pancreas but without involvement of CA or SMA		
T4	Tumor involves CA or SMA		
Regional lymph nodes (N)			
N0	No regional lymph node metastasis		
N1	Regional lymph node metastasis		
Distant metastasis (M)			
M0	No distant metastasis		
M1	Distant metastasis		
Anatomic stage			
Stage 0	Tis	N0	M0
Stage IA	T1	N0	M0
Stage IB	T2	N0	M0
Stage IIA	T3	N0	M0
Stage IIB	T1	N1	M0
	T2	N1	M0
	T3	N1	M0
Stage III	T4	Any N	M0
Stage IV	Any T	Any N	M1

Adapted from the 7th edition of the AJCC cancer staging manual [7]
CA celiac axis; *SMA* superior mesenteric artery

presented here, we will discuss the management of a stage III PDA with tumor in the pancreatic neck and body with involvement of the celiac trunk and common hepatic artery.

Technical Pearls

- Diagnostic laparoscopy prior to laparotomy for planned curative resection can be used liberally in this patient cohort, as patients with unresectable or metastatic disease rarely require intestinal or biliary bypass.
- Prior to addressing the technically challenging hepatoduodenal ligament and superior pancreatic dissection, assessment of the retroperitoneal vasculature can be completed by mobilizing the duodenum and right colon with wide kocherization and a Cattell–Braasch maneuver.

- Liver perfusion is dependent upon retrograde flow through the gastroduodenal artery (GDA) to the proper hepatic artery. Double-check adequacy of flow with both palpation and Doppler before common hepatic artery transection. Protect the GDA by transecting the pancreas well away from its course over the pancreatic head and neck.

Preoperative Management

In a simplified model, patients such as ours with locally advanced PDA arising in the neck and body of the pancreas can be separated into two groups (Fig. 23.2). In the first group, patients are thought to have "poor" disease biology, with rapid local tumor growth and evidence of early disease metastasis. The second group is said to have "favorable" disease biology, with a long period of time during which the

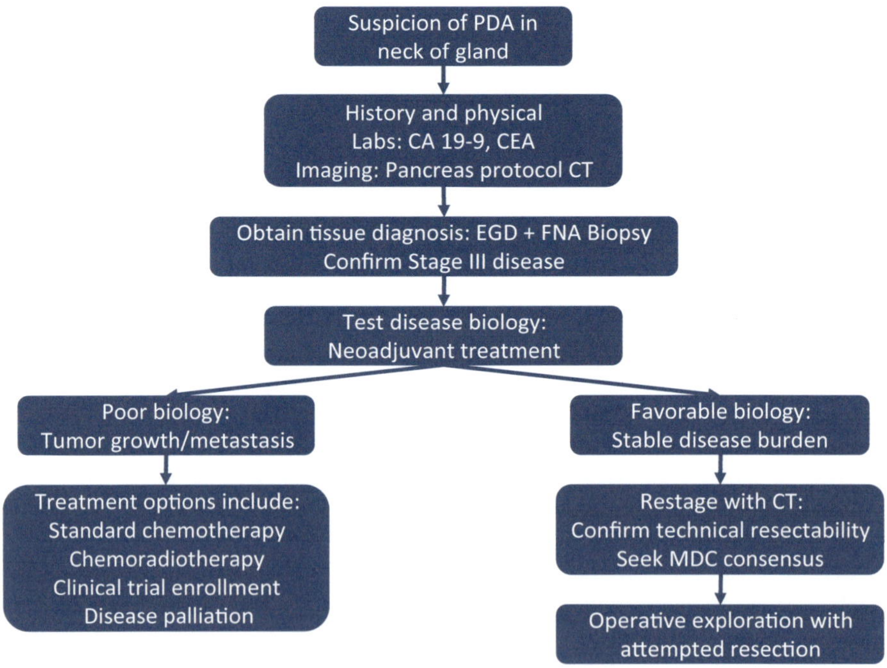

Fig. 23.2 Treatment diagram outlining the steps taken when pancreatic ductal adenocarcinoma is suspected in the neck of the gland. *PDA* pancreatic ductal adenocarcinoma; *CA 19-9* carbohydrate antigen 19-9; *CEA* carcinoembryonic antigen; *CT* computed tomography; *EGD* esophagogastroduodenoscopy; *FNA* fine-needle aspiration; *MDC* multidisciplinary conference

disease burden will remain relatively stable, without further local growth or evidence of metastasis. It is this second group that may benefit from more aggressive surgical therapies for local disease control. The rationale here is twofold: first, identification of a group of patients in whom disease is truly limited to the gland and surrounding structures where resection would therefore achieve cure (i.e., resect all disease prior to metastasis); and second, identification of a group of patients in whom survival will be driven primarily by local, rather than systemic, disease (i.e., systemic disease appears to be well controlled by chemotherapeutics).

Despite a plethora of research on the topic, there remains no prospective way to dichotomize patients into these two biologic groups based on the tissue sampling or clinical laboratory analysis at the time of diagnosis. As a result, our preferred method for patient selection based on disease biology is by treating first with non-surgical therapies and restaging at an interval. Experience with neoadjuvant approaches to stage III PDA is increasingly being reported in the literature [10–12]. Combination cytotoxic chemotherapeutics, particularly modified fluorouracil, leucovorin, irinotecan, and oxaliplatin (mFOLFIRINOX) with or without radiotherapy, is beginning to repeatedly demonstrate a capacity to downstage patients into a surgical paradigm of management. In data focused primarily on pancreatic head lesions, R0 resection in locally advanced disease can be achieved at rates exceeding 85% [10, 13, 14]. Experience with these regimens appears safe, with variable levels of toxicity based predominantly on the appearance of side effects from systemic chemotherapeutics.

Following neoadjuvant therapy, restaging of the patient should be performed as a surrogate indicator of disease biology. "Favorable" biology, as evident by disease stability or regression in combination with an absence of metastatic spread over time, should be a trigger to critically evaluate the patient's imaging for technical barriers to surgical extirpation. In those patients with elevated CA19-9 levels upon presentation, a decrease in that laboratory value may also be an indicator of favorable disease biology. The importance of surgical resection for the group of patients with favorable tumor biology and technically resectable disease should not be trivialized. Surgical resection, even in a locally advanced cohort of patients, remains the only chance for cure. Direct tumor invasion into adjacent locoregional structures does not always preclude an operation. Shoup et al., for example, demonstrated that patients requiring multivisceral resections for PDA of the body or tail have improved survival over locally advanced patients who do not undergo resection. Further, the long-term survival after multivisceral resection is similar to that following standard pancreatic resection [15].

PDA involving the celiac (CA) and common hepatic (CHA) arteries represents a unique surgical challenge. En-bloc resection of these arterial structures has been avoided in the past due to increased perioperative morbidity and questionable benefit. As the relative oncologic benefit improves (better chemotherapies, favorable tumor biology), the perioperative morbidity may become acceptable for select patients. Increased morbidity, as compared to standard distal pancreatectomy, is largely due to the potential for ischemia from devascularization of the liver, stomach, and spleen. In practice, ligation of the splenic artery is required for splenectomy, and carries little to no added morbidity. Similarly, ligation of the left gastric artery should have little effect on a stomach with intact collateralization. In stark contrast, however, devascularization of the liver remains a concern, as collateralization through the GDA is required to maintain adequate perfusion.

Resection of the distal pancreas and spleen, en-bloc with the CA, was first described by Appleby in 1953 as a surgical therapy for locally advanced gastric cancer [16]. Modification of this original operation, leaving the stomach intact, for use in resection of locally advanced PDA was first proposed in Japan and has been subsequently reported with increasing frequency in the literature [11, 12, 17–19]. With expanded experience, many high-volume pancreas centers have now demonstrated the safety of the modified Appleby procedure for PDA. Multidisciplinary management is a key to appropriate patient selection in this cohort. For example, if concern exists regarding the adequacy of collateral flow to the liver, preoperative angiography with coil embolization can be considered and, if needed, safely utilized [11, 14].

In our case, our female patient was seen in our multidisciplinary pancreas clinic by surgeons, oncologists, radiation oncologists, pathologists, and radiologists, where consensus supported initial combination cytotoxic chemotherapy (mFOLFIRINOX) followed by chemoradiotherapy (stereotactic body radiation therapy: 33 Gy). Her total course of therapy lasted 9 months, at which time she was restaged with cross-sectional imaging. She had disease, which remained confined to the pancreatic body and surrounding tissues without growth or metastasis, suggesting favorable disease biology. Her imaging continued to show circumferential involvement of the celiac trunk and common hepatic artery, while the portal vein and superior mesenteric artery remained free from involvement. The distal common hepatic artery at the GDA takeoff, as well as the entire length of the GDA, remained free from tumor involvement. She therefore was determined to have biologically favorable locally advanced (stage III) PDA of the pancreatic neck and body that was amenable to extended surgical resection (i.e., distal pancreatectomy and splenectomy with en-bloc celiac resection, a modified Appleby procedure).

Operative Management

Patients undergoing an Appleby procedure are evaluated in an anesthesia preoperative clinic at least 1 week prior to the planned operation. Additional consultation with cardiology or pulmonology staff is obtained based on patient comorbidities and risk factors for complications. On the day of operation, oral intake is prohibited after midnight. Preoperative placement of large-bore peripheral intravenous access and a radial arterial line is done after anesthetic induction and orotracheal intubation. Intravenous antibiotics and a prophylactic dose of subcutaneous heparin are administered within 1-hour prior to incision. A nasogastric tube is placed for gastric decompression. Placement of an epidural catheter and a central venous catheter is at the discretion of the operating team.

The technical performance of a modified Appleby procedure at our institution was first described by Makary et al. and has changed little since [20]. There are two main approaches to the aorta that are commonly utilized during the modified Appleby—an anterior approach and the "right-sided" approach [14]. We prefer, and describe, the approach to the celiac axis from an anterior direction.

In the operating room, laparoscopic exploration is routinely used to rule out occult disease metastasis. When satisfied, a midline incision is used to enter the abdomen. Any adhesive disease encountered is taken down sharply, and exposure is established using self-retaining retractors. The peritoneal cavity is then explored to rule out evidence of distant metastasis. A Cattell–Braasch maneuver is then performed and the duodenum is kocherized to assess the retroperitoneal vasculature. At this point, any involvement of tumor on the posterior aspect of the superior mesenteric artery, the inferior vena cava, or the aorta is a cause for concern, as this would preclude the ability to complete an R0 resection with a modified Appleby procedure.

The lesser sac is then entered by dividing the gastrocolic ligament, and the inferior border of the pancreatic neck is defined and mobilized out of the retroperitoneum. The superior mesenteric vein is identified and dissected along its course toward the pancreas. A tunnel is created in the avascular space between the neck of the pancreas anteriorly, and the mesenteric-portal vein confluence posteriorly. The splenic vein can often be identified here and looped for future transection.

Dissection then begins in the hepatoduodenal ligament to identify the proper hepatic artery. This vessel is dissected proximally to identify the GDA and CHA. The key at this point is to recall that the blood supply to the liver following successful Appleby is dependent upon collateral retrograde blood flow from the GDA into the proper hepatic artery. Therefore, any involvement of tumor at, or distal to, the GDA takeoff from the CHA will make CA resection without reconstruction impossible. If space allows at this point in the dissection, a clamp can be placed on the CHA and perfusion to the liver via retrograde GDA flow can be assessed with palpation or Doppler ultrasound evaluation. The portal vein is then identified posterior to the GDA and CHA, and the tunnel started at the inferior border of the pancreas is now completed at the superior border. A penrose drain is used to loop the gland, taking care to avoid the course of the GDA.

Subsequently, an anterior approach to the aorta is used to identify the CA. The surface of the aorta and trunk of the CA is cleaned and looped. The remainder of the aorta between the CA and SMA is palpated to ensure it is not involved by local tumor growth. If not done prior, atraumatic vascular clamps are placed on the trunk of the CA and across the CHA to assess flow to the liver. At this point, it is important to take great care to clamp the CA and not the SMA, as these two vessels branch from the aorta in close proximity. If the liver perfusion is poor after CA test clamp, the risks and benefits of an arterial reconstruction would be considered prior to continuing the extirpation. If perfusion to the liver is preserved, the operation is continued with division of the CA and distal CHA. The pancreas can then be divided at the neck, and the distal pancreas and spleen are mobilized from their retroperitoneal attachments in standard fashion. After specimen removal, the pancreas neck margin can be closed per surgeon preference, and perfusion to the liver is assessed once more by palpation and Doppler. Typically, a drain is left in the resection bed to facilitate drainage in the event of a pancreatic leak, and the nasogastric tube is left in place overnight.

Our patient underwent an uncomplicated modified Appleby procedure and was extubated at the conclusion of the case. One surgical drain was left in the pancreaticosplenic operative bed. Pathologic evaluation of the specimen revealed a 4.5 cm ductal adenocarcinoma with substantial treatment effect and without evidence of metastasis to locoregional lymph nodes. The margins were uninvolved with tumor.

Management Controversies and Alternative Approaches

- Despite case series demonstrating favorable oncologic outcomes, the decision to operate in the setting of locally advanced pancreatic ductal adenocarcinoma remains controversial and should only be entertained in high-volume centers with pancreatic expertise.
- In general, oncologic benefit is dependent more upon the biology of the disease than the technical performance of the operation. As such, using response to neoadjuvant chemotherapy or chemoradiotherapy as a surrogate marker for disease biology can help select those patients most likely to benefit from aggressive surgical therapy.
- The management of patients who have insufficient collateralization to support liver perfusion when the common hepatic artery is transected remains controversial. Specifically, the role of arterial reconstruction in these patients is unclear.

Peri-operative Care

Patients undergoing a modified Appleby can typically be extubated at the conclusion of the case, and transferred to an intensive care setting for serial physical examination and laboratory analysis over the first 24 h. Our standard post-distal pancreatectomy pathway has been generalized for use in this patient population, and this highlights the similarities in care that these patients require. There are two specific complications that are unique to Appleby that the care team must remain vigilant for: delayed gastric emptying (DGE) and hepatic ischemia. DGE is common in historical reports from Eastern literature, but appears to be relatively rare in more modern experience [13, 18, 21]. While mild transient transaminitis and hyperbilirubinemia occur often, significant hepatic ischemia is exceedingly rare when care is taken intraoperatively to assess adequacy of collateral flow; nevertheless, this complication can be devastating. Should concern for hepatic dysfunction arise in the immediate perioperative period, Doppler ultrasonography can be used liberally to assess adequacy of the hepatic arterial circulation. Optimal therapy for catastrophic liver ischemia is unknown, given the paucity of data in the literature, and our group has no experience in the management of this complication. Likely, this would require emergent bypass and arterial revascularization as a salvage approach. Other complications that occur after standard DP can be common after a modified Appleby procedure, including pancreatic fistula and wound infections. These are managed in identical fashion to those that occur after standard DP.

Postoperative Care and Considerations for Follow-Up

Routine postoperative office care for patients undergoing an uncomplicated modified Appleby procedure is similar to that for patients after standard distal pancreatectomy. Patients are asked to return to clinic for evaluation, at the discretion of the surgeon. A visit 2–4 weeks postoperatively is common in our practice. Initial recovery can take 2–4 weeks, with fatigue lasting up to 2 months at times. Clinically relevant pancreatic fistula can be effectively managed with prolonged peritoneal drainage. Though drains are typically removed during the patient's initial postoperative course, in the setting of a pancreatic leak, removal generally occurs around 1 month postoperatively. Triggers for drain removal in the setting of a pancreatic fistula are based on declining output in patients who otherwise appear clinically well.

The management of pain postoperatively can be unique in these patients. Some patients requiring opiods for pain control preoperatively may require appropriately tailored multimodal regimens in the initial postoperative period. Long-term pain control can be excellent, as many patients who have experienced severe pain preoperatively (presumably due to local tumor involvement) will have had the etiology of their pain removed with surgery [14].

Long-term complications from a modified Appleby procedure include risk of pancreatic endocrine and exocrine insufficiency. The percentage of patients who experience diabetes or diarrhea, for example, is likely similar to the cohort of patients undergoing standard distal pancreatectomy. New-onset diabetes can likely be expected in up to one-third of these patients [22, 23]. Though common in historical reports, exocrine insufficiency severe enough to cause diarrhea appears to be rare in modern experience [13, 14, 21].

A critical consideration in the postoperative management of these patients is the utilization of adjuvant therapies. These therapies can include cytotoxic chemotherapy or chemoradiotherapy, and vary based on the neoadjuvant treatment received. We strongly recommend shared decision-making in this setting, and commonly review these patients in a multidisciplinary tumor board. The use of adjuvant therapies following surgical extirpation is highly variable across different institutions, particularly when patients have been heavily pretreated [12, 13, 24]. The decision regarding the use of adjuvant therapies is also informed by peri-operative complications, and must be put into appropriate context. Generalizing from our experience with pancreaticoduodenectomy, we found that approximately 55% of patients receive adjuvant therapy, and that the presence of peri-operative complications decreases the likelihood of receiving adjuvant therapy [25].

Given the rarity of the procedure, a firm conclusion regarding the true oncologic benefit of this aggressive surgical approach has not been reached. Certainly, many centers have demonstrated that long-term local control and long-term survival (greater than 5 years) can be achieved in the setting of R0 resections [13, 21]. Similarly, Okada et al. demonstrated in their series that survival in margin-negative Appleby patients is similar to that after standard DP for PDA [18]. Again, it should be noted that these patients are highly selected and often heavily pretreated, making direct cohort comparisons difficult.

Our patient was successfully extubated at the conclusion of the case and transferred to the intensive care unit. She recovered well over the course of the first week, and was discharged home on postoperative day 7. An intraoperatively placed surgical drain was removed prior to discharge home. Her recovery over the first 2 months was notable for occasional nausea and constipation alternating with diarrhea. Her gastrointestinal symptoms were managed with dietary modification, continued protonix administration for a suspicion of gastritis, and judicious management of a bowel regimen. There were no concerning signs or symptoms of liver ischemia throughout her peri-operative course. Her incision healed well, and she

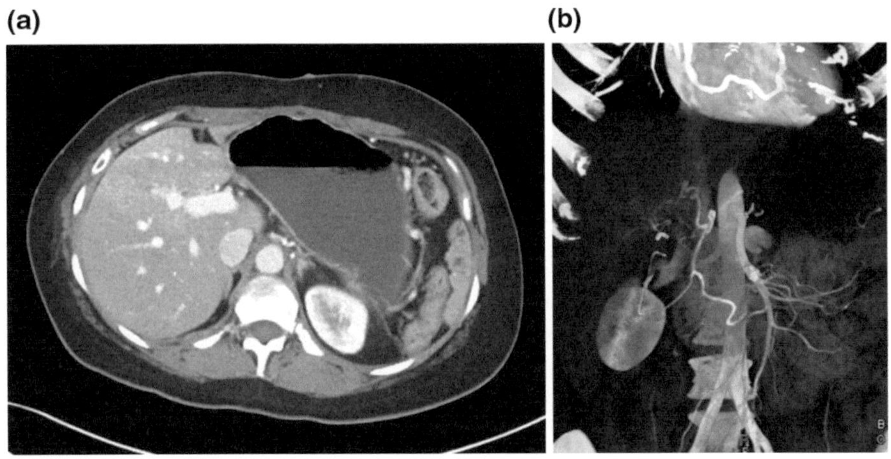

Fig. 23.3 Surveillance imaging 3 years following successful modified Appleby procedure. In addition to physical examination and laboratory analysis with tumor markers, we prefer to obtain high-quality imaging studies at an interval for surveillance. Here we show: **a** our patient's 3-year scan demonstrating no evidence of locoregional recurrence; **b** note the absence of the celiac takeoff from the aorta and reconstitution of the proper hepatic artery from retrograde flow supplied by the gastroduodenal artery

was seen in a multidisciplinary setting 3 months after operation. After much discussion, we declined to offer her further adjuvant therapy, given her heavily pretreated tumor and favorable pathology findings. We have followed her with sequential imaging for approximately 3 years without evidence of recurrent disease thus far (Fig. 23.3a, b).

Pearls for Overall Management of Pancreatic Adenocarcinoma in the Neck of the Gland

- High-quality cross-sectional imaging (commonly an intravenous contrast-enhanced pancreas-protocol computed tomography scan with virtual angiography) is imperative to accurately characterize the tumor's size, invasion into adjacent structures, and likelihood of successful extirpation.
- The use of neoadjuvant therapy, whether using cytotoxic chemotherapy alone or in combination with chemoradiotherapy, should be a standard approach for patients who present with pancreatic ductal adenocarcinoma in the neck of the gland with involvement of adjacent arterial structures.
- The decision to pursue operative management and consideration for continued adjuvant therapy should be made in a multidisciplinary setting on a case-by-case basis.

References

1. Siegel RL, Miller KD, Jemal A. Cancer statistics, 2016. CA Cancer J Clin. 2016;66(1):7–30.
2. Rahib L, Smith BD, Aizenberg R, Rosenzweig AB, Fleshman JM, Matrisian LM. Projecting cancer incidence and deaths to 2030: the unexpected burden of thyroid, liver, and pancreas cancers in the United States. Cancer Res. 2014;74(11):2913–21.
3. Nordback IH, Hruban RH, Boitnott JK, Pitt HA, Cameron JL. Carcinoma of the body and tail of the pancreas. Am J Surg. 1992;164(1):26–31.
4. Brennan MF, Moccia RD, Klimstra D. Management of adenocarcinoma of the body and tail of the pancreas. Ann Surg. 1996;223(5):506–11; discussion 511–2.
5. Sperti C, Pasquali C, Pedrazzoli S. Ductal adenocarcinoma of the body and tail of the pancreas. J Am Coll Surg. 1997;185(3):255–9.
6. Hruban RH, Ali SZ. Non-neoplastic and neoplastic pathology of the pancreas. In: Iacobuzio-Donahue CA, Montgomery E, editors. Gastrointestinal and liver pathology. Philadelphia: Churchill Livingstone Elsevier; 2005. p. 273.
7. Edge S, Byrd D, Compton C, Fritz A, Greene F, Trotti A. AJCC cancer staging manual. 7th ed. New York: Springer; 2010.
8. Bilimoria KY, Bentrem DJ, Ko CY, Stewart AK, Winchester DP, Talamonti MS. National failure to operate on early stage pancreatic cancer. Ann Surg. 2007;246(2):173–80.
9. Howlader N, Noone A, Krapcho M, Garshell J, Miller D, Altekruse S, et al. SEER Cancer statistics review, 1975–2012, National Cancer Institute. http://seer.cancer.gov/statfacts/html/pancreas.html. Accessed 1 March 2016.

10. Blazer M, Wu C, Goldberg RM, Phillips G, Schmidt C, Muscarella P, et al. Neoadjuvant modified (m) FOLFIRINOX for locally advanced unresectable (LAPC) and borderline resectable (BRPC) adenocarcinoma of the pancreas. Ann Surg Oncol. 2015;22(4):1153–9.
11. Cesaretti M, Abdel-Rehim M, Barbier L, Dokmak S, Hammel P, Sauvanet A. Modified Appleby procedure for borderline resectable/locally advanced distal pancreatic adenocarcinoma: a major procedure for selected patients. J Visc Surg. 2016;153(3):173–81.
12. Christians KK, Pilgrim CH, Tsai S, Ritch P, George B, Erickson B, et al. Arterial resection at the time of pancreatectomy for cancer. Surgery. 2014;155(5):919–26.
13. Baumgartner JM, Krasinskas A, Daouadi M, Zureikat A, Marsh W, Lee K, et al. Distal pancreatectomy with en bloc celiac axis resection for locally advanced pancreatic adenocarcinoma following neoadjuvant therapy. J Gastrointest Surg. 2012;16(6):1152–9.
14. Tanaka E, Hirano S, Tsuchikawa T, Kato K, Matsumoto J, Shichinohe T. Important technical remarks on distal pancreatectomy with en-bloc celiac axis resection for locally advanced pancreatic body cancer (with video). J Hepatobiliary Pancreat Sci. 2012;19(2):141–7.
15. Shoup M, Conlon KC, Klimstra D, Brennan MF. Is extended resection for adenocarcinoma of the body or tail of the pancreas justified? J Gastrointest Surg. 2003;7(8):946–52; discussion 952.
16. Appleby LH. The coeliac axis in the expansion of the operation for gastric carcinoma. Cancer. 1953;6(4):704–7.
17. Latona JA, Lamb KM, Pucci MJ, Maley WR, Yeo CJ. Modified Appleby procedure with arterial reconstruction for locally advanced pancreatic adenocarcinoma: a literature review and report of three unusual cases. J Gastrointest Surg. 2016;20(2):300–6.
18. Okada K, Kawai M, Tani M, Hirono S, Miyazawa M, Shimizu A, et al. Surgical strategy for patients with pancreatic body/tail carcinoma: who should undergo distal pancreatectomy with en-bloc celiac axis resection? Surgery. 2013;153(3):365–72.
19. Smoot RL, Donohue JH. Modified Appleby procedure for resection of tumors of the pancreatic body and tail with celiac axis involvement. J Gastrointest Surg. 2012;16(11):2167–9.
20. Makary MA, Fishman EK, Cameron JL. Resection of the celiac axis for invasive pancreatic cancer. J Gastrointest Surg. 2005;9(4):503–7.
21. Hirano S, Kondo S, Hara T, Ambo Y, Tanaka E, Shichinohe T, et al. Distal pancreatectomy with en bloc celiac axis resection for locally advanced pancreatic body cancer: long-term results. Ann Surg. 2007;246(1):46–51.
22. Burkhart RA, Gerber SM, Tholey RM, Lamb KM, Somasundaram A, McIntyre CA, et al. Incidence and severity of pancreatogenic diabetes after pancreatic resection. J Gastrointest Surg. 2015;19(2):217–25.
23. Shirakawa S, Matsumoto I, Toyama H, Shinzeki M, Ajiki T, Fukumoto T, et al. Pancreatic volumetric assessment as a predictor of new-onset diabetes following distal pancreatectomy. J Gastrointest Surg. 2012;16(12):2212–9.
24. Miura T, Hirano S, Nakamura T, Tanaka E, Shichinohe T, Tsuchikawa T, et al. A new preoperative prognostic scoring system to predict prognosis in patients with locally advanced pancreatic body cancer who undergo distal pancreatectomy with en bloc celiac axis resection: a retrospective cohort study. Surgery. 2014;155(3):457–67.
25. Wu W, He J, Cameron JL, Makary M, Soares K, Ahuja N, et al. The impact of postoperative complications on the administration of adjuvant therapy following pancreaticoduodenectomy for adenocarcinoma. Ann Surg Oncol. 2014;21(9):2873–81.

Laparoscopic Approaches to the Patient with Pancreatic Adenocarcinoma

24

Salila S. Hashmi and David A. Kooby

Case Presentation

We present a case of a 70-year-old Caucasian woman who presented with intermittent abdominal pain without any other associated symptoms. Physical examination and initial laboratory investigations were unremarkable. Due to persistent and focal nature of pain, she underwent an abdominal ultrasound, which revealed a mass in her pancreatic body. Magnetic resonance imaging (MRI) of abdomen and pelvis revealed a hypo-enhancing mass measuring 2 cm, located at the junction of the pancreatic body and tail, with progressive delayed enhancement, concerning for pancreatic adenocarcinoma (Fig. 24.1). There was no evidence of any vascular interface or any metastatic disease within the abdomen. An esophagogastroduodenoscopy (EGD) and endoscopic ultrasound (EUS) were performed, with multiple biopsies of the pancreatic mass that were consistent with pancreatic adenocarcinoma, and the serum CA19-9 level was 10 (normal range 0–37). A complete staging workup was performed and, given there were no signs of locally advanced or metastatic disease, the patient was taken to the operating room for surgical resection. The patient underwent a laparoscopic distal pancreatectomy (LDP) using radical antegrade modular pancreatosplenectomy (RAMPS) technique [1].

S.S. Hashmi (✉)
Emory University Hospital School of Medicine,
Atlanta, GA 303022, USA
e-mail: sshashm@emory.edu

D.A. Kooby
Emory University School of Medicine, 1365 C Clifton Road,
NE, 2nd Floor, Atlanta, GA 303022, USA
e-mail: dkooby@emory.edu

T.M. Pawlik et al. (eds.), *Case-Based Lessons in the Management of Complex Hepato-Pancreato-Biliary Surgery*, DOI 10.1007/978-3-319-50868-9_24

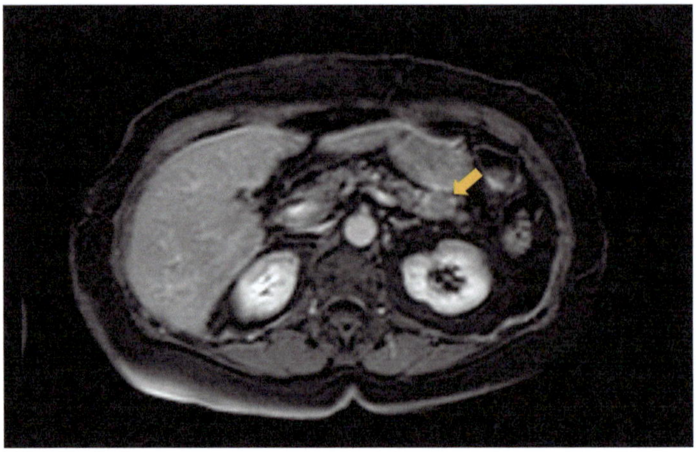

Fig. 24.1 Hypo-enhancing mass (marked by an *arrow*) along the caudal aspect of the pancreatic body/tail junction, suspicious for adenocarcinoma

Operative Technique for Laparoscopic Distal Pancreatectomy

The patient is positioned in a lazy right lateral decubitus position on a bean bag and secured well to the operating table with straps, tape, and appropriate padding. Usually the right arm is placed on an arm board with an axillary roll, and the left arm crosses the chest and is supported on another arm board. The left knee is flexed, with padding between the legs. This lateral positioning helps with visualization of the body and tail of pancreas, as the stomach and spleen are retracted inferiorly.

The abdominal cavity is accessed with a 5 mm port in the left upper quadrant using the optiview technique with a 5 mm 0° laparoscope. Alternatively, a 10-mm 30° laparoscope is placed above the umbilicus using the open Hasson technique. A diagnostic laparoscopy is then performed for two purposes—first for assessment of any inadvertent intra-abdominal injury during entry into the peritoneal cavity, and second to determine presence of any metastatic disease. If there is any suspicion for any metastatic disease, tissue biopsies are sent for frozen section. If positive for metastases, surgery is aborted, and the patient is referred for definitive chemotherapy.

In the absence of metastatic disease, additional ports are then placed for surgery (Fig. 24.2). These include a periumbilical 10–12 mm port (if a 5 mm port in the left upper quadrant was used initially) and two additional 5 mm ports in the left upper quadrant. These ports are placed in a transverse line along the left abdomen, with the lateral port being in the anterior axillary line. The ports are positioned about 5–8 cm apart in a craniocaudal manner, to permit bimanual operation without any restrictions.

Next the omentum is reflected superiorly, and a transverse incision is made in the gastrocolic ligament using harmonic scalpel or bipolar dissector to gain access to the lesser sac. Once in the lesser sac, short gastric vessels are sealed and divided

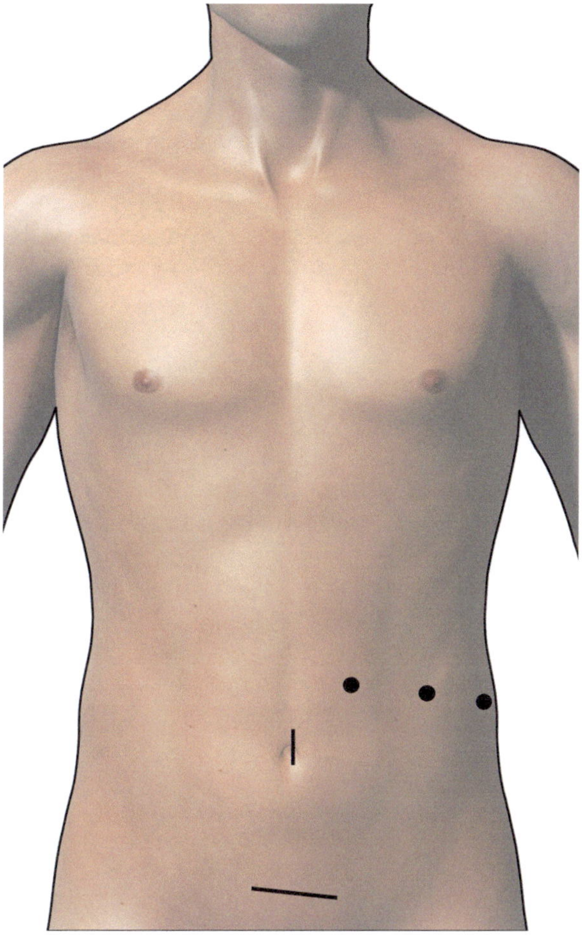

Fig. 24.2 Location of the port sites and Pfannestiel incision for specimen retrieval

along the greater curvature of the stomach all the way up to the hiatus, keeping the gastroepiploic intact. The patient can be placed in a reverse Trendelenburg position to assist in exposure and visualization of key structures. The transverse colon and splenic flexure are mobilized to gain access to the inferior border of the pancreas. The pancreas is inspected to identify the mass, and intraoperative ultrasound is typically used to assess both the tumor margins and relationship with vascular structures.

Dissection and vascular ligation is then carried out using a stepwise right-to-left or medial-to-lateral approach, recognizing the proximity of the junction of the fourth part of duodenum and jejunum in this area. The left gastric artery can be followed down to the celiac axis, defining the junction of splenic and hepatic arteries. If the patient is placed in Trendelenburg position, the splenic artery will be positioned more anteriorly and the hepatic artery will be angled away [2].

The splenic artery is then dissected at the upper border of the pancreas. Once dissected free, it is encircled using a right-angle clamp and a silicon loop which is secured with a clip, allowing for control in case of bleeding. The artery is then divided and the ends are either divided with a vascular stapler, tied and sutured, or tied and clipped. Ligation of the splenic artery allows for additional mobility of the junction of the pancreatic neck and body and helps to identify the splenic vein insertion into the portal vein. Peritoneum along the inferior margin of the pancreatic body and tail is divided. A retro-pancreatic tunnel can be created under direct visualization. The splenic vein can be transected alone or en-bloc with the pancreatic parenchyma, taking special caution that the main portal vein is away from the plane where en-bloc transection is being performed. Separate transection of these structures ensures safe ligation of the splenic vein without injuring portal or mesenteric veins, and is therefore preferred. Ligation is usually performed using a linear vascular stapler. Following this, the pancreatic parenchyma is transected with a stapler (Fig. 24.3). This is usually done with a vascular load and a slow close technique, closing the stapler over a few minutes followed by slow transection, in attempts to avoid a leak from the cut end of the pancreas [3]. If the pancreatic duct is obviously visible, it is clipped or suture ligated. Another option is cautery transection of gland, suture ligation of the pancreatic duct, followed by oversewing of the pancreatic stump.

The remainder of the mobilization is performed from right to left along the retroperitoneum, starting with the fascia over the adrenal and then Gerota's fascia. Attachments of the spleen to the diaphragm and kidney are taken down, and this tissue is swept with the specimen. Once the specimen is free, it is placed in a retrieval bag and is removed via a small Pfannestiel incision. The specimen should be examined to confirm that the mass has been completely removed. A frozen section at the margin can be obtained, at the discretion of the surgeon. A drain may be left in the pancreatic resection bed. Ports are removed under direct visualization.

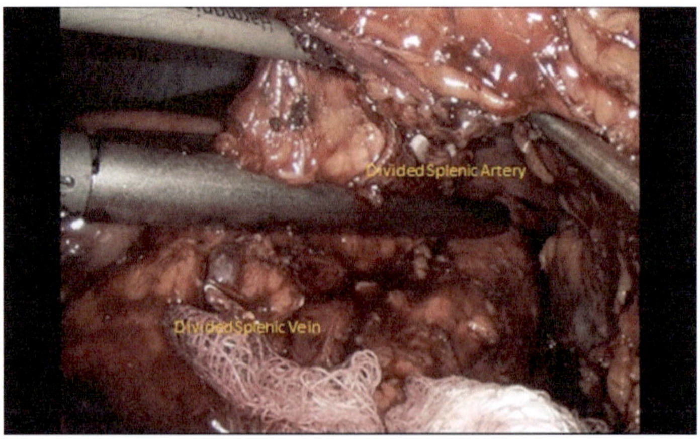

Fig. 24.3 Transection of the pancreas with a stapler, with the divided splenic artery and vein

Fascia for the 10–12 mm port site and Pfannestiel incision is closed. All incision sites are copiously irrigated, followed by skin closure.

Clinical Pearls

- Placing the patient in reverse Trendelenburg position after port placement aids in visualization of the key structures.
- Intraoperative ultrasound is a valuable tool to assess the tumor margins and its relationship with vascular structures.
- Caution must be taken when medial-to-lateral dissection is carried out, given the proximity of the junction of the 4th portion of the duodenum and early jejunum.
- Due to the patient positioning, the splenic artery may seem to be positioned more anteriorly (even though it is heading to the patient's left).
- A vascular cartridge for a laparoscopic stapler should be used for pancreatic parenchymal transection and the stapler should be fired using the slow close technique. If the pancreatic duct is seen it should be oversewn with a 3–0 silk suture on a tapered GI needle.

There remains debate regarding intraoperative drain placement after pancreatic resection. Multiple studies have shown that placement of closed suction drains during pancreaticoduodenectomy does not appear to decrease the rate of secondary drainage procedures or surgical exploration and, in fact, may be associated with increased pancreatic fistula (PF) formation and overall morbidity [4–7]. One randomized, controlled trial demonstrated that drains diminish the rate and severity of pancreatic fistula in patients with moderate/high risk for PF, but this could possibly be avoided in the roughly one-third of patients with negligible/low risk [8].

Alternative Techniques

RAMPS is an aggressive surgical approach designed to improve oncologic resection with a higher likelihood of negative (tangential) margins, increased rates of microscopically negative resections, and an improved lymph node dissection. It was originally described as an open technique in 2003 and then later adapted to laparoscopic and robotic surgery. Although it may be associated with improved disease-specific survival, it has similar 5-year overall survival compared to pancreaticoduodenectomy for adenocarcinoma [1, 9].

Alternative techniques include a laparoscopic hand-assist distal pancreatectomy [10, 11], or distal pancreatectomy with splenic preservation [11, 12]. Hand-assist involves a hand port that allows the surgeon's hand to access the peritoneal cavity during surgery. This assists the surgeon to palpate the tumor, allows for manual retraction and dissection, and application of direct pressure in case there is bleeding. This technique is usually employed in more difficult cases that involve resection of larger tumors, tumors with substantial inflammatory reaction around them, or in obese patients with thick abdominal walls [13].

Distal pancreatectomy with splenic preservation can be performed using what has been described as the Warshaw technique [11] or Kimura [12]. This involves either preservation of the splenic vasculature (Kimura) or preservation of the short gastrics to supply spleen (Warshaw). However, for malignant disease, splenic preservation at the expense of resection margins or thorough lymph node evaluation is not recommended.

Alternative Approaches

- RAMPS is an aggressive surgical approach designed to improve oncologic resection with a higher likelihood of negative (tangential) margins, increased rates of microscopically negative resections, and an improved lymph node dissection.
- Alternative techniques include a laparoscopic hand-assist distal pancreatectomy or distal pancreatectomy with splenic preservation. For malignant disease, splenic preservation at the expense of resection margins and adequate nodal harvest is not recommended.
- Intraoperative drain placement after pancreatic resection remains a great topic of debate. Closed suction drainage has not been shown to decrease the rate of secondary drainage procedures or surgical exploration, and may be associated with increased pancreatic fistula formation and overall morbidity.

Preoperative Evaluation for Pancreatic Adenocarcinoma

The two main goals of preoperative evaluation are to verify the histopathological diagnosis of pancreatic cancer and to determine resectability. This usually involves imaging with any preferred modality, EUS/EUS-guided biopsy, and serum tumor markers. Multiple imaging modalities are available for the evaluation of suspected pancreatic cancer, most common being multidetector computed tomography (MDCT) and magnetic resonance imaging (MRI). Usually the choice of either of these studies depends on available local expertise and the clinician's comfort with one or the other imaging technique, as there is not an evidence-based difference between the two techniques [14, 15]. In some cases, endoscopic decompression with biliary stent placement may be needed to manage obstructive jaundice (particularly for ampullary masses). EUS is a valuable tool for diagnosis. It has a negative predictive value as high as almost 100% in some series [16, 17]. EUS-guided biopsies help obtain a tissue diagnosis of primary tumor and any suspicious lymph nodes. These biopsies have been reported to have a high sensitivity (85%) and specificity (98%) for malignancy [18], although the utility may be limited in pancreatic body tumors. Serum CA 19-9 is a serum biomarker for pancreatic cancer, and has been shown to aid in diagnosis and can be used as a prognostic marker [19].

Postoperative Care

Postoperative care after LDP is not much different from management of any other postsurgical patient. Pain management is focused to avoid narcotics to help prevent ileus. Perioperative antibiotics are continued for 24 h after surgery. Fluid resuscitation is continued for at least 24–36 h, and sometimes longer, until the patient tolerates a diet. Urine output is used as an objective tool to guide fluid resuscitation. If the drain output is high, a drain amylase is measured and, if normal, the drain is removed prior to discharge. If amylase is high, patients are discharged with the drain and it is removed once the output is low.

Surveillance

The patient usually returns to see the surgeon 2–3 weeks after discharge. At this visit, the patient's clinical status is reviewed, their wounds are examined, their pathology is reviewed, and future care is arranged. Adjuvant chemotherapy with or without radiation therapy is typically recommended for fit patients following resection of pancreatic adenocarcinoma, and referral to an oncologist is ensured. Timing of follow-up visits are then individualized. MRI and serum CA 19-9 levels are obtained, usually at 1 month after surgery, and then per National Comprehensive Cancer Network guidelines [20].

Overall Management Pearls

- All patients need to undergo a complete staging workup and, only when no signs of locally advanced or metastatic disease, they are taken to the operating room for surgical resection.
- If there is any suspicion for metastatic disease at the start of the procedure, tissue biopsies must be sent for frozen section. If positive for metastases, surgery should be aborted and the patient should be referred for definitive chemotherapy.

- Postoperative care after LDP is not much different from management of any other postsurgical patient.
- Adjuvant chemotherapy, with or without radiation therapy, is typically recommended for fit patients following pancreatic resection.

Conclusion

About one-fourth of all pancreatic adenocarcinomas are located in the body or tail of the pancreas, and if they are detected at an early stage these are typically treated with distal (or left) pancreatectomy. The first reports of LDP were described by Cuschieri in 1994 [21]. With the recent advances in minimally invasive surgical techniques, there is an increasing trend in laparoscopic resection of pancreatic cancer. LDP can be a technically challenging operation, given the need of precise recognition of tissue planes and the proximity of critical vascular structures. There are only a few studies that compare open distal pancreatectomy (ODP) and minimally invasive distal pancreatectomy (MIDP) for resection of pancreatic adenocarcinoma. While there are multiple single-center studies [22–27] there is only one multicenter, case-controlled study focused on ductal adenocarcinoma published to date on this topic by the Central Pancreas Consortium (CPC) in the U.S. Results from this study showed that while open procedures were found to have higher estimated blood loss, increased wound infections, and increased need for drainage postoperatively, no difference was observed in the length of the operation, major complications, 30-day mortality, and pancreatic fistula development [28].

Although some single-center studies have reported lower positive margin (R1) rates [24–27], no difference was found in the study from CPC [28]. Based on single institution and SEER data, a minimum of 12 LNs should be harvested for resections of pancreatic adenocarcinoma. Only one single-center study shows a significantly greater node harvest in favor of a minimally invasive approach [23], while other studies found no significant difference [22–24]. Variable ranges with 5-year survival have been reported, but have not been found to be statistically different. No significant difference has been found in the use of adjuvant therapy between ODP and MIDP [22–25, 27, 28]. Table 24.1 shows cumulative results of these studies discussed above. Minimally invasive approach was used for smaller tumors and there was a higher incidence of positive margins when an open approach was used.

There is limited data to support that RAMPS approach to distal pancreatectomy potentially offers increased rates of R0 resections with negative tangential margins [29–31]. A recent Cochrane review concluded that existing studies investigating differences between open and laparoscopic approaches are not sufficient to eliminate bias, and randomized studies are needed [32].

Table 24.1 Cumulative results from studies comparing minimally invasive and open approach to distal pancreatectomy

Outcome	MIDP (minimally invasive distal pancreatectomy)	ODP (open distal pancreatectomy)
N	197	686
Tumor size (cm)	3.4	4
Positive Margin (%)	7	13
Total Nodes	15	12
Adjuvant therapy (%)	78	76
Overall survival	26 months	25 months

Cumulative results from studies comparing minimally invasive and open approach to distal pancreatectomy (presented at the 12th World Congress of the International Hepato-Pancreato-Biliary Association, April 2016, São Paulo 2016)

References

1. Strasberg SM, Linehan DC, Hawkins WG. Radical antegrade modular pancreatosplenectomy procedure for adenocarcinoma of the body and tail of the pancreas: ability to obtain negative tangential margins. J Am Coll Surg. 2007;204(2):244–9.
2. Kooby DA. Tips and tricks of laparoscopic distal pancreatectomy for ductal adenocarcinoma. J Hepatobiliary Pancreat Sci. 2016;23(6):E10–3.
3. Subhedar PD, Patel SH, Kneuertz PJ, Maithel SK, Staley CA, Sarmiento JM, et al. Risk factors for pancreatic fistula after stapled gland transection. Am Surg. 2011;77(8):965–70.
4. Conlon KC, Labow D, Leung D, Smith A, Jarnagin W, Coit DG, et al. Prospective randomized clinical trial of the value of intraperitoneal drainage after pancreatic resection. Ann Surg. 2001;234(4):487–94.
5. Mehta VV, Fisher SB, Maithel SK, Sarmiento JM, Staley CA, Kooby DA. Is it time to abandon routine operative drain use? A single institution assessment of 709 consecutive pancreaticoduodenectomies. J Am Coll Surg. 2013;216(4):635–42.
6. Van Buren G 2nd, Bloomston M, Hughes SJ, Winter J, Behrman SW, Zyromski NJ, et al. A randomized prospective multicenter trial of pancreaticoduodenectomy with and without routine intraperitoneal drainage. Ann Surg. 2014;259(4):605–12.
7. Behrman SW, Zarzaur BL, Parmar A, Riall TS, Hall BL, Pitt HA. Routine drainage of the operative bed following elective distal pancreatectomy does not reduce the occurrence of complications. J Gastrointest Surg. 2015;19(1):72–9.
8. McMillan MT, Fisher WE, Van Buren G 2nd, McElhany A, Bloomston M, Hughes SJ, et al. The value of drains as a fistula mitigation strategy for pancreatoduodenectomy: something for everyone? Results of a randomized prospective multi-institutional study. J Gastrointest Surg. 2015;19(1):21–31.
9. Mitchem JB, Hamilton N, Gao F, Hawkins WG, Linehan DC, Strasberg SM. Long-term results of resection of adenocarcinoma of the body and tail of the pancreas using radical antegrade modular pancreatosplenectomy procedure. J Am Coll Surg. 2012;214(1):46–52.
10. D'Angelica M, Are C, Jarnagin W, DeGregoris G, Coit D, Jaques D, et al. Initial experience with hand-assisted laparoscopic distal pancreatectomy. Surg Endosc. 2006;20(1):142–8.
11. Laxa BU, Carbonell AM, Cobb WS, Rosen MJ, Hardacre JM, Mekeel KL, et al. Laparoscopic and hand-assisted distal pancreatectomy. Am Surg. 2008;74(6):481–7.

12. Warshaw AL. Conservation of the spleen with distal pancreatectomy. Arch Surg. 1988; 123(5):550–3.
13. Kimura W, Inoue T, Futakawa N, Shinkai H, Han I, Muto T. Spleen-preserving distal pancreatectomy with conservation of the splenic artery and vein. Surgery. 1996;120(5): 885–90.
14. Postlewait LM, Kooby DA. Laparoscopic distal pancreatectomy for adenocarcinoma: safe and reasonable? J Gastrointest Oncol. 2015;6(4):406.
15. Tummala P, Junaidi O, Agarwal B. Imaging of pancreatic cancer: an overview. J Gastrointest Oncol. 2011;2(3):168–74.
16. Takakura K, Sumiyama K, Munakata K, Ashida H, Arihiro S, Kakutani H, et al. Clinical usefulness of diffusion-weighted MR imaging for detection of pancreatic cancer: comparison with enhanced multidetector-row CT. Abdom Imaging. 2011;36(4):457–62.
17. Klapman JB, Chang KJ, Lee JG, Nguyen P. Negative predictive value of endoscopic ultrasound in a large series of patients with a clinical suspicion of pancreatic cancer. Am J Gastroenterol. 2005;100(12):2658–61.
18. Agarwal B, Abu-Hamda E, Molke KL, Correa AM, Ho L. Endoscopic ultrasound-guided fine needle aspiration and multidetector spiral CT in the diagnosis of pancreatic cancer. Am J Gastroenterol. 2004;99(5):844–50.
19. Hewitt MJ, McPhail MJ, Possamai L, Dhar A, Vlavianos P, Monahan KJ. EUS-guided FNA for diagnosis of solid pancreatic neoplasms: a meta-analysis. Gastrointest Endosc. 2012; 75(2):319–31.
20. Goonetilleke KS, Siriwardena AK. Systematic review of carbohydrate antigen (CA 19-9) as a biochemical marker in the diagnosis of pancreatic cancer. Eur J Surg Oncol. 2007;33(3): 266–70.
21. NCCN Clinical Practice Guidelines in Oncology. Pancreatic Adenocarcinoma. Version 1.2016. https://www.nccn.org/professionals/physician_gls/f_guidelines.asp.
22. Cuschieri A. Laparoscopic surgery of the pancreas. J Royal Coll Surg Edinburgh. 1994; 39(3):178–84.
23. Magge D, Gooding W, Choudry H, Steve J, Steel J, Zureikat A, et al. Comparative effectiveness of minimally invasive and open distal pancreatectomy for ductal adenocarcinoma. JAMA Surg. 2013;148(6):525–31.
24. Hu M, Zhao G, Wang F, Zhao Z, Li C, Liu R. Laparoscopic versus open distal splenopancreatectomy for the treatment of pancreatic body and tail cancer: a retrospective, mid-term follow-up study at a single academic tertiary care institution. Surg Endosc. 2014; 28(9):2584–91.
25. Stauffer JA, Coppola A, Mody K, Asbun HJ. Laparoscopic versus open distal pancreatectomy for pancreatic adenocarcinoma. World J Surg. 2016;40(6):1477–84.
26. Shin S, Kim S, Song K, Hwang D, Lee J, Lee D, et al. A comparative study of laparoscopic vs open distal pancreatectomy for left-sided ductal adenocarcinoma: a propensity score-matched analysis. J Am Coll Surg. 2015;220(2):177–85.
27. Lee SY, Allen PJ, Sadot E, D'Angelica MI, DeMatteo RP, Fong Y, et al. Distal pancreatectomy: a single institution's experience in open, laparoscopic, and robotic approaches. J Am Coll Surg. 2015;220(1):18–27.
28. Zhang M, Fang R, Mou Y, Chen R, Xu X, Zhang R, et al. LDP vs ODP for pancreatic adenocarcinoma: a case matched study from a single-institution. BMC Gastroenterol. 2015; 15(1):1.
29. Kooby DA, Gillespie T, Bentrem D, Nakeeb A, Merchant NB, Parikh AA, et al. Left-sided pancreatectomy: a multicenter comparison of laparoscopic and open approaches. Ann Surg. 2008;248(3):438–46.
30. Choi SH, Kang CM, Lee WJ, Chi HS. Laparoscopic modified anterior RAMPS in well-selected left-sided pancreatic cancer: technical feasibility and interim results. Surg Endosc. 2011;25(7):2360–1.

31. Lee SH, Kang CM, Hwang HK, Choi SH, Lee WJ, Chi HS. Minimally invasive RAMPS in well-selected left-sided pancreatic cancer within Yonsei criteria: long-term (>median 3 years) oncologic outcomes. Surg Endosc. 2014;28(10):2848–55.
32. Riviere D, Gurusamy KS, Kooby DA, Vollmer CM, Besselink MG, Davidson BR, et al. Laparoscopic versus open distal pancreatectomy for pancreatic cancer. Cochrane Database Syst Rev. 2016;4:CD011391.

Robotic Approaches to the Patient with Pancreatic Adenocarcinoma

25

Jennifer L. Miller-Ocuin, Melissa E. Hogg, Amer H. Zureikat and Herbert J. Zeh III

Introduction

Pancreatic cancer is a systemic disease in a vast majority of the patients at the time of diagnosis; this mandates the clinician to carefully consider how to integrate local control of the tumor into the overall oncologic care of the patient. Current approaches of open surgery followed by adjuvant therapy have failed to significantly impact overall survival of this disease over the last 30 years. Re-sequencing of surgery and chemotherapy, integration of more effective chemotherapy regimens, and minimally invasive approaches to local control have the potential to improve current poor outcomes. In this chapter, we focus on how robotic pancreaticoduodenectomy is integrated into the multidisciplinary care of the patient with pancreatic

J.L. Miller-Ocuin
Department of Surgery, University of Pittsburgh Medical Center, 5112 Centre Avenue, Suite G.21, Pittsburgh, PA 15213, USA
e-mail: millerjl13@upmc.edu

M.E. Hogg · A.H. Zureikat
Department of Surgery, Division of Surgical Oncology, University of Pittsburgh Medical Center, 3550 Terrace Street, Scaife Hall, Suite 497, A-415, Pittsburgh, PA 15213, USA
e-mail: hoggme@upmc.edu

A.H. Zureikat
e-mail: zureikatah@upmc.edu

H.J. Zeh III (✉)
Department of Surgery, Division of Surgical Oncology, University of Pittsburgh Medical Center, 5150 Centre Avenue, Suite 414, Pittsburgh, PA 15232, USA
e-mail: zehxhx@upmc.edu

T.M. Pawlik et al. (eds.), *Case-Based Lessons in the Management of Complex Hepato-Pancreato-Biliary Surgery*, DOI 10.1007/978-3-319-50868-9_25

ductal adenocarcinoma. We will emphasize the diagnostic workup, technique, and outcomes of robotic-assisted pancreaticoduodenectomy in a patient with pancreatic adenocarcinoma.

Case Presentation

A 54-year-old male presented to the emergency department with a 3-month history of epigastric pain, early satiety, nausea and vomiting, and a 15-lb weight loss. His past medical history was significant for melanoma in situ, diverticulitis, gastroesophageal reflux disease, and hypertension. His family history was negative for pancreatic diseases and significant for multiple first-degree relatives with melanoma. CT scan without contrast enhancement demonstrated a dilated pancreatic duct in the setting of an elevated alkaline phosphatase on laboratory analysis. MRCP, performed to evaluate the pancreatic duct, was suspicious for an ampullary mass. EUS demonstrated a 2.4 cm mass that was biopsied. He underwent an endoscopic retrograde cholangiopancreatography (ERCP), demonstrating a distal common bile duct stricture; sphincterotomy was performed followed by placement of a 10 mm covered metal stent. He was referred to our multidisciplinary clinic for further evaluation.

Epidemiology

Pancreatic ductal adenocarcinoma (PDA) is the fourth leading cause of cancer deaths in the United States, and remains one of the few disease in which incidence and mortality remain nearly equal, despite improvements in medical technologies. Surgery remains the only potentially curative treatment for localized disease [1]. Although contemporary perioperative outcomes in patients undergoing resection for pancreatic cancer have improved significantly, long-term survival remains largely unchanged [2]. The poor prognosis of the disease is multifactorial secondary to biological factors [3], delayed presentation, complexity of surgery [4], and lack of effective therapy [5, 6]. Inherited pancreatic cancer syndromes, comprised of hereditary pancreatic cancer (identifiable gene mutation) and familial pancreatic cancer (at least one pair of first-degree relatives without an identifiable gene mutation), contribute to approximately 5–10% of all pancreatic adenocarcinoma cases [7]. Among these, Peutz–Jeghers Syndrome, BRCA2, Lynch Syndrome (hereditary non-polyposis colon cancer), and—in the case of our patient—familial atypical multiple mole melanoma syndrome (FAMMMS) should be considered.

Diagnostic Workup and Staging

All patients should undergo a comprehensive history and physical examination. Prior abdominal surgery or the presence of underlying comorbidities, such as chronic obstructive pulmonary disease, or congestive heart failure, should be kept in mind when choosing patients for minimally invasive pancreatectomy. At our institution, preoperative planning includes a triphasic (pancreatic protocol) CT scan of the abdomen and pelvis as well as endoscopic ultrasound (EUS). The combination of these two modalities has proven highly predictive of the ability to achieve an R0 resection in a validated model [8]. Contrast-enhanced MRI is also an acceptable imaging modality. These studies should be recent, ideally within 4–6 weeks of surgery [9].

Routine labs include complete blood count, coagulation panel, and hepatic function panel. We obtain a cancer antigen 19-9 (CA19-9) on all patients at the time of diagnosis (after serum bilirubin normalizes) and after completion of neoadjuvant chemotherapy. We have found that a serum CA19-9 response to neoadjuvant therapy of greater than 50% is predictive of improved overall survival, and is associated with higher R0 resection rate [10]. At our institution, preoperative chemotherapy is favored for a majority of patients, thus a short metal stent is placed.

Our patient had a triple-phase CT scan of the abdomen and pelvis that demonstrated a 2 cm hypodense mass in the pancreatic head (Fig. 25.1a) that was abutting the superior mesenteric vein at the splenoportal confluence (Fig. 25.1b). Endoscopic ultrasound demonstrated a 2.4 cm mass without vascular involvement, and cytology was consistent with pancreatic adenocarcinoma.

Following normalization of his serum bilirubin, tumor markers were significant for a cancer antigen 19-9 (CA19-9) of 149 U/ml (normal < 37 U/ml). Based on criteria from the NCCN, SSO, and AHPBA [11–13], the patient was classified as having resectable pancreatic cancer. The patient was discussed at multidisciplinary

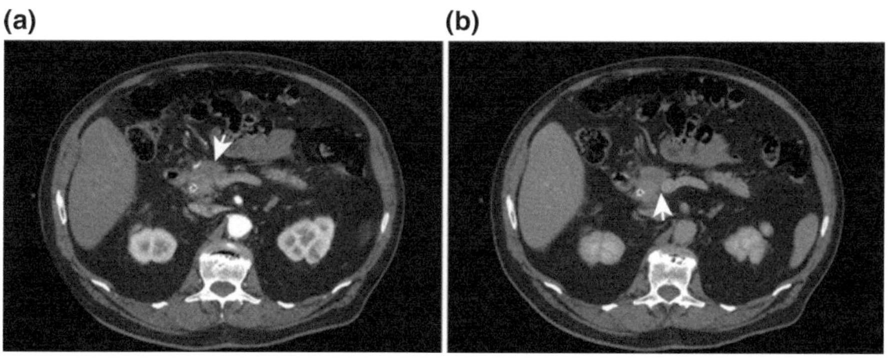

Fig. 25.1 Preoperative imaging demonstrating resectable pancreatic head mass. **a** Arterial phase shows hypoenhancing mass in the pancreatic head (*arrow*). **b** Portal venous phase demonstrates fat plane (*arrow*) between mass and SMV at the level of the splenic vein

tumor board. Curative intent treatment options offered to this patient included preoperative chemotherapy on or off protocol versus surgery upfront followed by adjuvant chemotherapy. Our patient chose to enroll in UPCI protocol 13-074 (two cycles of gemcitabine/nab-paclitaxel with or without the autophagy inhibitor hydroxychloroquine). He completed therapy and underwent repeat staging contrast-enhanced CT of the chest, abdomen, and pelvis, which demonstrated no distant disease and a stable primary. He had a favorable biochemical response, with CA19-9 decreasing to 28.1 [10]. Therefore, decision was made to proceed with robotic-assisted pancreaticoduodenectomy (PD).

Technical Pearls of Robotic-Assisted Pancreaticoduodenectomy

- Entry into lesser sac and mobilization of right colon
- Kocher maneuver and opening of ligament of Treitz
- Jejunal and gastric transection
- Portal dissection
  - Remove common hepatic artery node
  - Identify and ligate GDA
  - Identify suprapancreatic portal vein and begin tunnel
  - Portal lymphadenectomy and transection of bile duct
- Infrapancreatic SMV dissection and completion of the retropancreatic tunnel
- Division of the pancreas
- Uncinate dissection and specimen retrieval
- Cholecystectomy (if gallbladder present)
- Reconstruction.

Management

Pancreatic cancer is fundamentally a systemic disease in a majority of the patients at the time of diagnosis. This requires the clinician to integrate the timing of local control with the systemic management of this disease. The traditional sequencing of surgery followed by chemotherapy has proven inadequate despite dramatic improvements in mortality following the PD over the last 30 years, and morbidity of the open operation remains high. This high morbidity following the traditional open PD limits receipt of critical systemic chemotherapy that is required to improve survival. Several groups have demonstrated that postoperative complications affect ability to receive critical systemic chemotherapy with nearly 48% of subjects in one study never progressing to adjuvant therapy [4, 14]. There are several approaches to circumvent this clinical dilemma. First, it has been demonstrated that reversing the sequencing of surgery and chemotherapy results in more subjects receiving both modalities [15]. Second, we can reduce the morbidity of the surgery through the use of minimally invasive surgical (MIS) approaches. At our institution, we follow an innovative and aggressive algorithm in a majority of patients that favors administration of newer, more effective systemic chemotherapies preoperatively, followed by MIS PD and subsequent adjuvant chemotherapy. One additional potential benefit to this approach is that we are able to tailor the adjuvant chemotherapy based on the histopathologic response to the preoperative regimen.

Robotic Pancreaticoduodenectomy

Our institution utilizes seven ports for robotic-assisted pancreaticoduodenectomy, including a 10-mm camera port, three robotic arms, a 5-mm liver retractor, and two assistant ports. Port placement configuration is depicted in Fig. 25.2. Following abdominal access and insufflation, the abdomen is inspected for metastatic disease. Provided none is found, we proceed with mobilization, the first few steps of which can be performed laparoscopically or with robotic assistance. The patient is positioned in steep reverse Trendelenburg. We first enter the lesser sac through the gastrocolic ligament and continue dissection laterally to fully mobilize the right colon, exposing the duodenum. Next, a Kocher maneuver is performed to the level of the left renal vein, taking all the retroperitoneal attachments off of the pancreas and exposing the medial and inferior borders of the superior mesenteric artery (SMA). The ligament of Treitz is opened, allowing the proximal jejunum to be pulled underneath the SMA. The jejunum is transected with an endovascular stapler, and the mesentery is divided with a bipolar vessel sealer (LigaSure) at the border of the mesentery and serosa, completing the Kocher maneuver and linearizing the duodenum. We then divide the greater omentum at the level of the gastric antrum, and the right gastroepiploic artery is taken with the LigaSure. The lesser omentum is opened and the stomach is transected with an endovascular stapler. One unique aspect of the robotic PD is the inability of the surgeon to palpate the plain between the uncinate and SMA, as is classically described in the open approach. The decision of resectability and need for vascular resection must be appreciated before the operation based on adequate compute tomography. Thus the sequencing of the robotic PD is slightly different, and the jejeunum and stomach are divided early.

At this point, the robot is docked, if not already done. With the operating surgeon at the robotic console and the assisting surgeon positioned at the bedside between the patient's legs, the portal structures and retropancreatic tunnel are dissected. The common hepatic artery (CHA) is exposed by identification and removal of the CHA lymph node. CHA exposure is continued until the right gastric and gastroduodenal arteries (GDA) are exposed (Fig. 25.3a). CHA flow is confirmed on ultrasound by

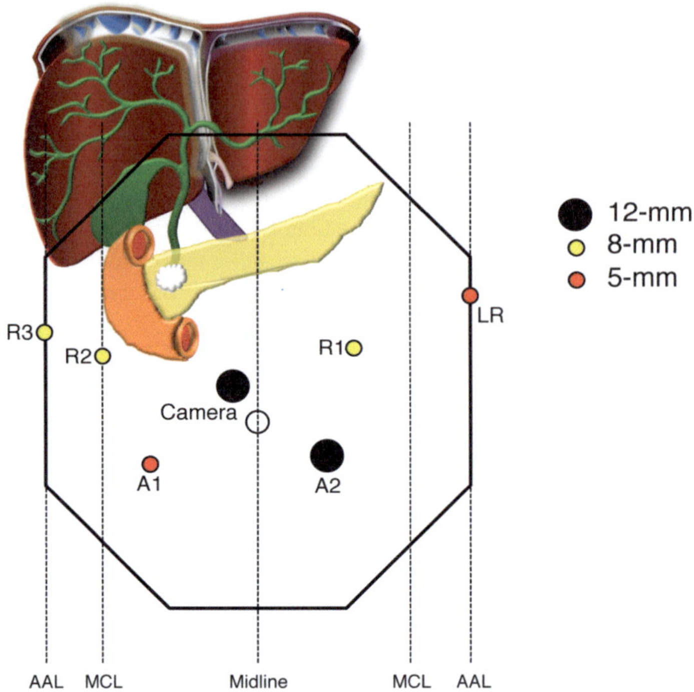

Fig. 25.2 Standard port placement for robotic-assisted pancreaticoduodenectomy. The peritoneum is accessed with a 5 mm optical viewing trochar using a 0° laparoscope in the left upper quadrant. This port is later exchanged for an 8 mm robotic port for Arm 1. The camera should be placed approximately 2 cm to the right and 2 cm above the umbilicus, to align with the SMV and optimize visualization of the uncinate dissection. Port placement can be moved up or down depending on the distance from the xiphoid process to the umbilicus (up for longer distance, down for shorter distance). The assistant ports should be placed approximately halfway between the camera and R2 (RLQ) and R1 (LLQ), respectively. The LLQ port site serves as the extraction site, and is converted to a GelPort following removal of the specimen

Doppler and color flow after vessel-loop facilitated occlusion of the GDA prior to GDA ligation. The suprapancreatic portal vein is identified at the apex of the triangle formed by the common hepatic artery, GDA, and superior border of the pancreas. The avascular plane is developed in a cephalad-to-caudad direction, thereby beginning the retropancreatic tunnel from above. We then identify the common bile duct (CBD), and all lymphatic tissue lateral and posterior to it is cleared inferiorly toward the specimen. An aberrant or replaced right hepatic artery, if present, will be identified posterior to the CBD, and should be dissected circumferentially and traced proximally toward the SMA. The CBD is transected with an endovascular stapler, as we have found that this minimizes bile spillage that is difficult to evacuate during the uncinate dissection (alternatively a bulldog clamp can be placed.) The peritoneum overlying the inferior border of the pancreas is opened, and dissection is carried down until the infrapancreatic SMV is identified. The retropancreatic tunnel is

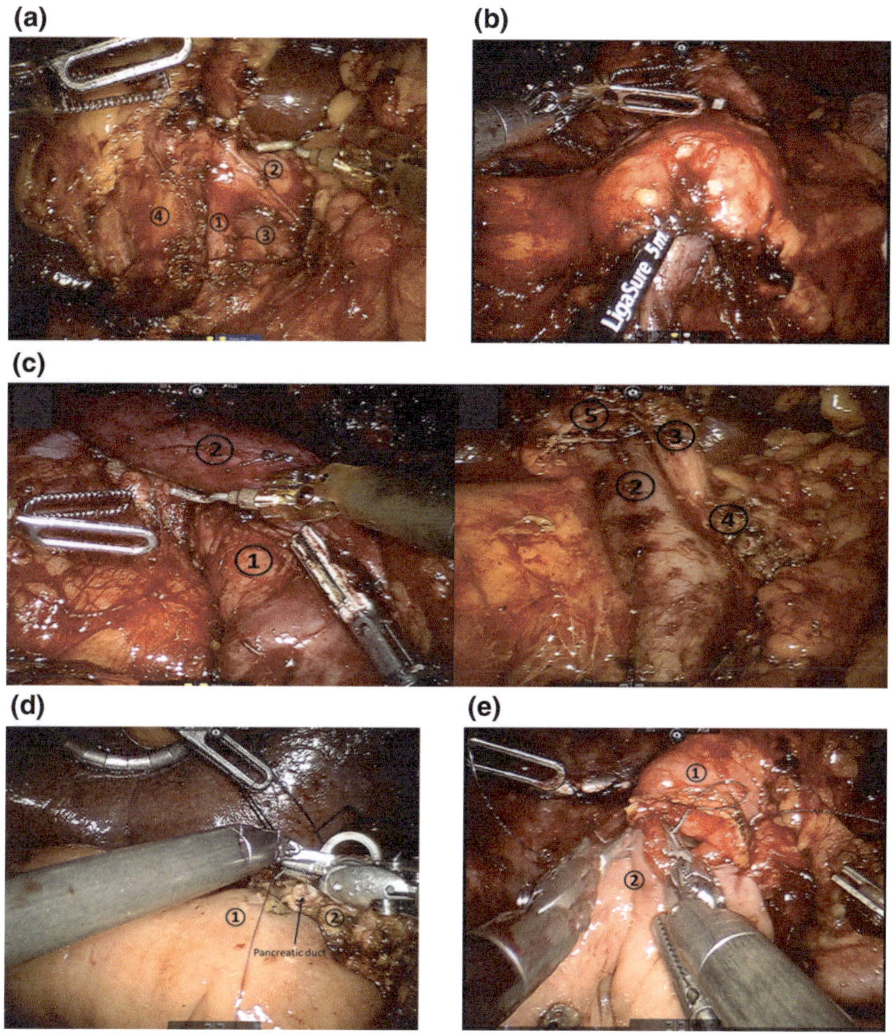

completed (Fig. 25.3b) and the pancreas is transected with electrocautery; "cold" transection is reserved for the duct.

After the pancreas is divided, attention is turned to dissecting the retroperitoneal margin and uncinate process. Special attention is given to the recurrent uncinated arterial and venous branches off of the SMA and SMV, as they are easily evulsed and can be a source of major intraoperative blood loss. Cephalad, we identify individually ligate the superior pancreaticoduodenal vein. The final resection bed is depicted in Fig. 25.3c. If the gallbladder is in situ, a cholecystectomy is performed at this point. The specimen is retrieved through the left lower quadrant assistant port, which must be enlarged. Pneumoperitoneum is reestablished with placement of a GelPort.

◀ **Fig. 25.3** Robotic-assisted pancreaticoduodenectomy. **a** Detailed view of portal dissection. The gastroduodenal artery (*1*) is isolated for ligation, typically via a vascular stapler and the stump is further reinforced with a clip. The common hepatic artery (*2*) and portal vein (*3*) can also be identified. The common bile duct (*4*) will also be transected using a stapler. **b** Creation of the retropancreatic tunnel. Dissection proceeds along the inferior and superior borders of the pancreas, at the level of the pancreatic neck, and allows for creation of a tunnel beneath the pancreas and above the mesenteric vasculature. **c** Completed pancreaticoduodenectomy resection view. *Left panel* with retraction of the superior mesenteric vein, shows careful dissection and removal of all the perivascular tissue along the plane of Leriche, clearing the superior mesenteric artery (*1*) and portal vein (*1*) margins. *Right panel* shows the dissected portal vein margin (*2*), the gastroduodenal artery stump (*3*), which is reinforced with a surgical clip, the cut edge of the pancreas (*4*), with a readily identifiable pancreatic duct, and the divided common bile duct (*5*). **d** Creation of pancreaticojejunostomy in modified Blumgart technique. The jejunum (*1*) is approximated to the pancreatic parenchyma (*2*) with 2-0 silk horizontal mattress sutures through the seromuscular layer of jejunum. Electrocautery is utilized to create a small enterotomy in the jejunum. Then, a duct-to-mucosa pancreaticojejunostomy is created using 5-0 PDS sutures over a Hobbs pancreatic stent (Hobbs Medical, Inc., Stafford Springs, CT, USA) to ensure duct patency. Finally, the anterior layer is created using 2-0 silk sutures to approximate the seromuscular layer of the jejunum to the pancreatic parenchyma. **e** Creation of the choledochojejunostomy. The common hepatic duct (*1*) is sutured to the jejunum (*2*) using interrupted absorbable 5-0 sutures for small ducts with or without a stent, or running 4-0 V-LOC suture (Covidien, New Haven, CT, USA) for larger, thicker ducts (shown here)

The enteric reconstruction is then carried out with meticulous attention, as most morbidity and mortality of PD is attributed to anastomotic leakage and failure. First a duct-to-mucosa modified-Blumgart pancreaticojejunostomy technique is performed (Fig. 25.3d), typically over a pancreatic duct stent [16]. We typically use 3 2-0 silk for the transpancreatic/seromuscular sutures, with the middle suture straddling the pancreatic duct. Once tied in place, an enterotomy is created, and we use 5-0 polydiaxanone for the duct-to-mucosa anastomosis. The anterior seromuscular layer is then placed. The bilio-enteric anastomosis is constructed, either by interrupted or continuous suture technique, depending on duct size; a running technique is employed for larger, thicker bile ducts, and an interrupted technique is used for smaller, softer ducts (Fig. 25.3e). Third, the gastrojejunostomy is performed by a stapled technique and sutured closure of the common enterotomy is done in two layers. Alternatively a "handsewn" gastrojejunostomy (or duodenojejunostomy) in a two-layered fashion can be formed. Following creation of the anastomoses, a 19 French closed suction, round, fluted surgical drain is placed anterior to the pancreaticojejunostomy and the hepaticojejunostomy, but posterior to the gastrojejunostomy. The falciform ligament is used to create a pedicled tissue flap to cover the GDA stump, which is marked with a 10 mm clip in case postoperative angiography is needed [17]. Unanticipated vascular involvement of the superior mesenteric vein or portal vein can be resected for an R0 resection due to the precision, control, and dexterity afforded by the robotic platform. We do not typically leave a nasogastric tube, as there is no evidence to support its routine use.

Postoperative care is focused on early diet advancement as tolerated, and conservative intravenous fluid management, titrated to hemodynamic parameters, and urine output through a modified enhanced recovery after surgery (ERAS) pathway.

The ICU is not routinely used. We use a modified Verona protocol [18] to manage the operative drain. Serum and drain amylase are measured on POD1 and POD3. If POD 1 amylase is less than 5000 and decreases by POD 3 in a clinically stable patient, the drain is removed on POD3.

Following robotic-assisted pancreaticoduodenectomy, our patient was discharged home on postoperative day 5 after an uneventful recovery. Final pathology demonstrated a poorly differentiated adenocarcinoma with Evans Grade IIB treatment [19] effect, positive for perineural invasion without definitive lymphovascular invasion, 0/65 lymph nodes positive for metastases, and negative (R0) resection margins.

Alternative Approaches and Controversies

- Open pancreaticoduodenectomy
  - Higher morbidity
- Fully laparoscopic pancreaticoduodenectomy
  - Steeper learning curve
  - Less easily disseminated.

Perioperative Outcomes Following Robotic PD

In 2006, one of the largest series of open PD to date was reported by Johns Hopkins, with 1,432 cases for pancreatic malignancies. Winter et al. reported a mean operative time of 380 min, a mean blood loss of 800 mL, mean length of stay of 9 days, 58% R0 resections, 5% pancreatic fistula rate (pre-ISPFG criteria), and a 2% mortality rate [20]. This impressive study provides a metric for comparison of outcomes when describing a new technical platform such as robotic-assisted PD.

Similar to the adoption of laparoscopic PD, early reports of robotic PD began with small case series; Giulianotti performed and reported the first series in 2003 [21]. Over time, experiences grew, leading to larger series. Data suggested similar oncologic outcomes, decreased blood loss, increased operative time, and increased cost (Table 25.1). A recent review of studies published before 2012 evaluated five series of robotic PD, including 131 patients; the (weighted) mean operative time was 510 min and complications occurred in 38.9% of patients, including 26% postoperative pancreatic fistula and 2.3% mortality [22].

The University of Pittsburgh reported the institution's first 250 consecutive robotic resections; 132 of these were RPD. With a conversion rate of 8% (4.5 in the last 112 cases), the review demonstrated a median estimated blood loss of 300 mL,

Table 25.1 Peri-operative outcomes of robotic-assisted pancreaticoduodenectomy

Author	Year published	Patients (n)	Time (min)	EBL (mL)	R0 resection (%)	Lymph nodes harvested (n)	POPF (%)	LOS (days)	30-day mortality (%)
Guilianotti [29]	2010	50	568	394	90	18	38	22	8
Buchs [30]	2011	44	444	387	90.9	16.8	18	13	4.5
Chan [31]	2011	8	478	200	.	.	33.3	12	0
Zureikat [23]	2011	24	512	320	.	.	21	9	4.2
Chalikonda [32]	2012	30	476	485	100	13.2	6.7	9.8	3.3
Lai [33]	2012	20	492	247	73	10	35	13.7	0
Zureikat [34]	2013	132	527	300	87.7	19	17	10	1.5
Bao [35]	2014	28	431	100	63	15	29	7.4	7
Baker [36]	2015	22	22	454	97.8	.	4.6	7	0
Chen [37]	2015	60	410	400	97.8	13.6	13.3	20	1.7

POPF Postoperative pancreatic fistula

mean length of stay of 10 days, 7.4% pancreatic leak (grade B and C) by ISGPF criteria, and a 1.5 and 3.8% 30- and 90-day mortality rate, respectively [23].

More recently, larger series of robotic PD are being reported. Additionally, some studies include matched comparisons to open PD. We have performed a contemporary cohort-matched multicenter comparison of perioperative outcomes of robotic PD and open PD that demonstrated reduced blood loss (mean difference = 181 mL, P = 0.04) and reduced major complications (OR = 0.64, P = 0.003) despite increased operative times (mean difference = 75.4 min, P = 0.01). Furthermore, the approaches were equivalent in terms of oncologic outcomes, with similar margin status and lymphadenectomy [24].

Our patient received 5 months, or five cycles, of adjuvant gemcitabine and nab-paclitaxel. He remains free of radiographic or biochemical evidence 24 months after surgery.

Adjuvant Therapy

As previously discussed, we believe that one of the principle impediments to improving survival in PDA over the last three decades is the significant morbidity of the pancreaticoduodenectomy, which often precludes administration of systemic chemotherapy [4]. Kendrick et al. have demonstrated that the minimally invasive approach can mitigate this morbidity and lead to more subjects receiving systemic chemotherapy. In this study 12% open patients undergoing open resection were delayed in receiving, or did not receive, adjuvant therapy versus 5% of totally laparoscopic pancreaticoduodectomy [25]. We see similar results in our own experience. A retrospective review of 463 patients at our institution demonstrates increased administration of adjuvant chemotherapy in the robotic approach versus open approach (82% vs. 70%; $p < 0.017$). Furthermore, robotic PD was an independent predictor of decreased complications (OR 0.47; $p = 0.011$) and increased adjuvant chemotherapy (OR 2.24; $p = 0.012$). Patients who received adjuvant chemotherapy had a longer OS compared to those who did not (31 vs. 13 months; $p < 0.0001$); patient receiving ≥ 6 cycles had a median OS of 39 months ($p < 0.0001$) (submitted for publication).

Posttreatment Surveillance and Interval Staging

Our current approach is to perform triple-phase CT scan, serum Ca 19-9, and physical exam every 6 months for 2 years and then yearly thereafter up to 10 years. Tzeng et al. compared five follow-up strategies—no scheduled follow-up as "baseline" and four increasing strategy groups with escalating utilization of CA 19-9, clinical examination, and imaging—and demonstrated that increased frequency and intensity of follow-up measures increases costs without any associated survival benefit [26].

Conclusion

We performed a review of quality metrics of all robotic PD cases performed at our institution, and determined that continuous assessment of quality metrics permitted safe and feasible implementation of the robotic approach [27]. This study identified benchmarks to optimize surgeons training in the approach. Subsequently, our institution has developed a mastery-based robotic simulation curriculum that combines virtual reality, inanimate object, and biotissue exercises to train surgeons on the robotic platform ex vivo. Training surgeons then develop skills at the patient bedside. Finally, trainees are gradually incorporated onto the robotic console in an increasing complexity of cases.

In order to safely implement minimally invasive pancreatic surgery, a structured training program is needed to allow new generations of surgeons to master skills of the approach while maintaining the tenets of open surgery. It is prudent to continuously analyze operative parameters, postoperative morbidity and mortality, and oncologic outcomes, as with any new surgical technology platform [28].

Box 25.3 General Pearls of Pancreaticoduodenectomy for Ductal Adenocarcinoma

- Good preoperative planning
  - Multidisciplinary strategy to maximize chances of receiving systemic chemotherapy
  - High-quality cross-sectional imaging and identification of anatomic variants (i.e., replaced/aberrant right hepatic artery) and vascular involvement
- Meticulous surgical technique—major steps should be performed the same way every time
- Careful attention to the recurrent uncinate vessels and the superior pancreaticoduodenal vein
- Leave an intraoperative drain
- Falciform ligament flap to cover the GDA stump.

References

1. Stojadinovic A, Brooks A, Hoos A, Jaques DP, Conlon KC, Brennan MF. An evidence-based approach to the surgical management of resectable pancreatic adenocarcinoma. J Am Coll Surg. 2003;196(6):954–64. doi:10.1016/S1072-7515(03)00010-3.
2. Winter JM, Brennan MF, Tang LH, D'Angelica MI, Dematteo RP, Fong Y, et al. Survival after resection of pancreatic adenocarcinoma: results from a single institution over three decades. Ann Surg Oncol. 2012;19(1):169–75. doi:10.1245/s10434-011-1900-3.

3. Poruk KE, Valero V 3rd, Saunders T, Blackford AL, Griffin JF, Poling J, et al. Circulating tumor cell phenotype predicts recurrence and survival in pancreatic adenocarcinoma. Ann Surg. 2016. [Epub ahead of print]. doi:10.1097/SLA.0000000000001600.
4. Wu W, He J, Cameron JL, Makary M, Soares K, Ahuja N, et al. The impact of postoperative complications on the administration of adjuvant therapy following pancreaticoduodenectomy for adenocarcinoma. Ann Surg Oncol. 2014;21(9):2873–81. doi:10.1245/s10434-014-3722-6.
5. Calvo F, Guillen Ponce C, Munoz Beltran M, Sanjuanbenito Dehesa A. Multidisciplinary management of locally advanced-borderline resectable adenocarcinoma of the head of the pancreas. Clin Transl Oncol. 2013;15(3):173–81. doi:10.1007/s12094-012-0962-4.
6. Kircher SM, Krantz SB, Nimeiri HS, Mulcahy MF, Munshi HG, Benson AB 3rd. Therapy of locally advanced pancreatic adenocarcinoma: unresectable and borderline patients. Expert Rev Anticancer Ther. 2011;11(10):1555–65. doi:10.1586/era.11.125.
7. Brand RE, Lerch MM, Rubinstein WS, Neoptolemos JP, Whitcomb DC, Hruban RH, et al. Advances in counselling and surveillance of patients at risk for pancreatic cancer. Gut. 2007;56(10):1460–9. doi:10.1136/gut.2006.108456.
8. Bao P, Potter D, Eisenberg DP, Lenzner D, Zeh HJ, Lee I, et al. Validation of a prediction rule to maximize curative (R0) resection of early-stage pancreatic adenocarcinoma. HPB (Oxford). 2009;11(7):606–11. doi:10.1111/j.1477-2574.2009.00110.x.
9. Dholakia AS, Hacker-Prietz A, Wild AT, Raman SP, Wood LD, Huang P, et al. Resection of borderline resectable pancreatic cancer after neoadjuvant chemoradiation does not depend on improved radiographic appearance of tumor-vessel relationships. J Radiat Oncol. 2013;2 (4):413–25. doi:10.1007/s13566-013-0115-6.
10. Boone BA, Steve J, Zenati MS, Hogg ME, Singhi AD, Bartlett DL, et al. Serum CA 19-9 response to neoadjuvant therapy is associated with outcome in pancreatic adenocarcinoma. Ann Surg Oncol. 2014;21(13):4351–8. doi:10.1245/s10434-014-3842-z.
11. Tempero MA, Malafa MP, Behrman SW, Benson AB 3rd, Casper ES, Chiorean EG, et al. Pancreatic adenocarcinoma, version 2.2014: featured updates to the NCCN guidelines. J Natl Compr Canc Netw. 2014;12(8):1083–93.
12. Varadhachary GR, Tamm EP, Abbruzzese JL, Xiong HQ, Crane CH, Wang H, et al. Borderline resectable pancreatic cancer: definitions, management, and role of preoperative therapy. Ann Surg Oncol. 2006;13(8):1035–46. doi:10.1245/ASO.2006.08.011.
13. Callery MP, Chang KJ, Fishman EK, Talamonti MS, William Traverso L, Linehan D.C. Pretreatment assessment of resectable and borderline resectable pancreatic cancer: expert consensus statement. Ann Surg Oncol. 2009;16(7):1727–33. doi:10.1245/s10434-009-0408-6.
14. Raut CP, Tseng JF, Sun CC, Wang H, Wolff RA, Crane CH, et al. Impact of resection status on pattern of failure and survival after pancreaticoduodenectomy for pancreatic adenocarcinoma. Ann Surg. 2007;246(1):52–60. doi:10.1097/01.sla.0000259391.84304.2b.
15. Wayne JD, Abdalla EK, Wolff RA, Crane CH, Pisters PW, Evans DB. Localized adenocarcinoma of the pancreas: the rationale for preoperative chemoradiation. Oncologist. 2002;7(1):34–45.
16. Grobmyer SR, Kooby D, Blumgart LH, Hochwald SN. Novel pancreaticojejunostomy with a low rate of anastomotic failure-related complications. J Am Coll Surg. 2010;210(1):54–9. doi:10.1016/j.jamcollsurg.2009.09.020.
17. Ching KC, Santos E, McCluskey KM, Orons PD, Bandi R, Friend CJ, et al. Covered stents and coil embolization for treatment of postpancreatectomy arterial hemorrhage. J Vasc Interv Radiol. 2016;27(1):73–9. doi:10.1016/j.jvir.2015.09.024.
18. Bassi C, Molinari E, Malleo G, Crippa S, Butturini G, Salvia R, et al. Early versus late drain removal after standard pancreatic resections: results of a prospective randomized trial. Ann Surg. 2010;252(2):207–14. doi:10.1097/SLA.0b013e3181e61e88.
19. Chatterjee D, Katz MH, Rashid A, Varadhachary GR, Wolff RA, Wang H, et al. Histologic grading of the extent of residual carcinoma following neoadjuvant chemoradiation in pancreatic ductal adenocarcinoma: a predictor for patient outcome. Cancer. 2012;118 (12):3182–90. doi:10.1002/cncr.26651.

20. Winter JM, Cameron JL, Campbell KA, Arnold MA, Chang DC, Coleman J, et al. 1423 pancreaticoduodenectomies for pancreatic cancer: a single-institution experience. J Gastrointest Surg. 2006;10(9):1199–210; discussion 1210–1. doi:10.1016/j.gassur.2006.08.018.
21. Giulianotti PC, Coratti A, Angelini M, Sbrana F, Cecconi S, Balestracci T, et al. Robotics in general surgery: personal experience in a large community hospital. Arch Surg. 2003;138(7):777–84. doi:10.1001/archsurg.138.7.777.
22. Strijker M, van Santvoort HC, Besselink MG, van Hillegersberg R, Borel Rinkes IH, Vriens MR, et al. Robot-assisted pancreatic surgery: a systematic review of the literature. HPB (Oxford). 2013;15(1):1–10. doi:10.1111/j.1477-2574.2012.00589.x.
23. Nguyen KT, Zureikat AH, Chalikonda S, Bartlet, DL. Moser AJ, Zeh HJ. Technical aspects of robotic-assisted pancreaticoduodenectomy (RAPD). J Gastrointest Surg. 2011;15(5):870–5. doi:10.1007/s11605-010-1362-0.
24. Zureikat AH, Postlewait LM, Liu Y, Gillespie TW, Weber SM, Abbott DE, et al. A multi-institutional comparison of perioperative outcomes of robotic and open pancreaticoduodenectomy. Ann Surg. 2016;264(4):640–9. doi:10.1097/SLA.0000000000001869.
25. Croome KP, Farnell MB, Que FG, Reid-Lombardo KM, Truty MJ, Nagorney DM, et al. Total laparoscopic pancreaticoduodenectomy for pancreatic ductal adenocarcinoma: oncologic advantages over open approaches? Ann Surg. 2014;260(4):633–8; discussion 638–40. doi:10.1097/SLA.0000000000000937.
26. Tzeng CW, Abbott DE, Cantor SB, Fleming JB, Lee JE, Pisters PW, et al. Frequency and intensity of postoperative surveillance after curative treatment of pancreatic cancer: a cost-effectiveness analysis. Ann Surg Oncol. 2013;20(7):2197–203. doi:10.1245/s10434-013-2889-6.
27. Boone BA, Zenati M, Hogg ME, Steve J, Moser AJ, Bartlett DL, et al. Assessment of quality outcomes for robotic pancreaticoduodenectomy: identification of the learning curve. JAMA Surg. 2015;150(5):416–22. doi:10.1001/jamasurg.2015.17.
28. Hogg ME, Zenati M, Novak S, Chen Y, Jun Y, Steve J, et al. Grading of surgeon technical performance predicts postoperative pancreatic fistula for pancreaticoduodenectomy independent of patient-related variables. Ann Surg. 2016;264(3):482–91. doi:10.1097/SLA.0000000000001862.
29. Giulianotti PC, Sbrana F, Bianco FM, Elli EF, Shah G, Addeo P, et al. Robot-assisted laparoscopic pancreatic surgery: single-surgeon experience. Surg Endosc. 2010;24(7):1646–57. doi:10.1007/s00464-009-0825-4.
30. Buchs NC, Addeo P, Bianco FM, Ayloo S, Benedetti E, Giulianotti PC. Robotic versus open pancreaticoduodenectomy: a comparative study at a single institution. World J Surg. 2011;35(12):2739–46. doi:10.1007/s00268-011-1276-3.
31. Chan OC, Tang CN, Lai EC, Yang GP, Li MK. Robotic hepatobiliary and pancreatic surgery: a cohort study. J Hepatobiliary Pancreat Sci. 2011;18(4):471–80. doi:10.1007/s00534-011-0389-2.
32. Chalikonda S, Aguilar-Saavedra JR, Walsh RM. Laparoscopic robotic-assisted pancreaticoduodenectomy: a case-matched comparison with open resection. Surg Endosc. 2012;26(9):2397–402. doi:10.1007/s00464-012-2207-6.
33. Lai EC, Yang GP, Tang CN. Robot-assisted laparoscopic pancreaticoduodenectomy versus open pancreaticoduodenectomy—a comparative study. Int J Surg. 2012;10(9):475–9. doi:10.1016/j.ijsu.2012.06.003.
34. Zureikat AH, Moser AJ, Boone BA, Bartlett DL, Zenati M, Zeh HJ, 3rd. 250 robotic pancreatic resections: safety and feasibility. Ann Surg. 2013;258(4):554–9; discussion 559–62. doi:10.1097/SLA.0b013e3182a4e87c.
35. Bao PQ, Mazirka PO, Watkins KT. Retrospective comparison of robot-assisted minimally invasive versus open pancreaticoduodenectomy for periampullary neoplasms. J Gastrointest Surg. 2014;18(4):682–9. doi:10.1007/s11605-013-2410-3.

36. Baker EH, Ross SW, Seshadri R, Swan RZ, Iannitti DA, Vrochides D, et al. Robotic pancreaticoduodenectomy: comparison of complications and cost to the open approach. Int J Med Robot. 2015;12(3):554–60. doi:10.1002/rcs.1688.
37. Chen S, Chen JZ, Zhan Q, Deng XX, Shen BY, Peng CH, et al. Robot-assisted laparoscopic versus open pancreaticoduodenectomy: a prospective, matched, mid-term follow-up study. Surg Endosc. 2015;29(12):3698–711. doi:10.1007/s00464-015-4140-y.

Pancreatic Neuroendocrine with Superior Mesenteric Vein–Portal Vein Thrombus

26

Jeffrey A. Norton, E. John Harris and Robert T. Jensen

Introduction

Recent studies suggest that pancreatic neuroendocrine tumors (PNET) account for 10% of all pancreatic tumors [1]. Nonfunctional tumors are the most common type of PNET. They can present as an incidentally identified pancreatic mass on a CT done for another reason, or as a large invasive tumor with or without distant metastases. Approximately 25% will have liver metastases [2]. In large nonfunctional PNETs, tumor thrombi may exist when the primary tumor invades through the wall of one or more adjacent venous structures [3]. Tumor venous thrombi are more frequently seen in renal cell cancer and hepatocellular cancer, and the treatment of this condition is well described. The incidence of venous thrombi with PNETS, the clinical impact of these thrombi, and the optimal surgical treatment of them, is unclear [4]. In patients with PNET that extend into the portal vein from either the superior mesenteric vein (SMV) or the splenic vein (SV), we have resected tumor from within these structures during the concomitant pancreatic resection. This chapter gives an in-depth review of the surgical procedures

J.A. Norton (✉)
Department of Sugery, Stanford University Medical Center,
300 Pasteur Drive, Room H3591, 94305-5641 Stanford, CA, USA
e-mail: janorton@stanford.edu

E. John Harris
Division of Vascular Surgery, Stanford University Medical Center,
300 Pasteur Drive, H-3641, 94305 Stanford, CA, USA
e-mail: edjohn@stanford.edu

R.T. Jensen
Digestive Diseases Branch, National Institutes of Health, Bdg. 10,
Rm 9C103, 20892 Bethesda, MD, USA
e-mail: robertj@bdg10.niddk.nih.gov

T.M. Pawlik et al. (eds.), *Case-Based Lessons in the Management of Complex Hepato-Pancreato-Biliary Surgery*, DOI 10.1007/978-3-319-50868-9_26

necessary to remove tumor thrombus from these structures, and the long-term outcome of patients with these findings.

Case Studies

Case #1

A 54-year-old truck driver from Oregon presents with hematemesis. He has had two episodes in which he was vomiting up large amounts of blood and he has had six units of pRBCs during the intitial episode and three units during the second episode. CT shows large gastric varices secondary to splenic vein occlusion by a large pNET that involves the body and tail of the pancreas, with extension into the portal vein (Fig. 26.1). There is tumor thrombus in the portal vein, without any evidence of distant metastases.

The splenic artery was embolized with coils on the night before surgery by interventional radiology. PNET resection required subtotal pancreatectomy with

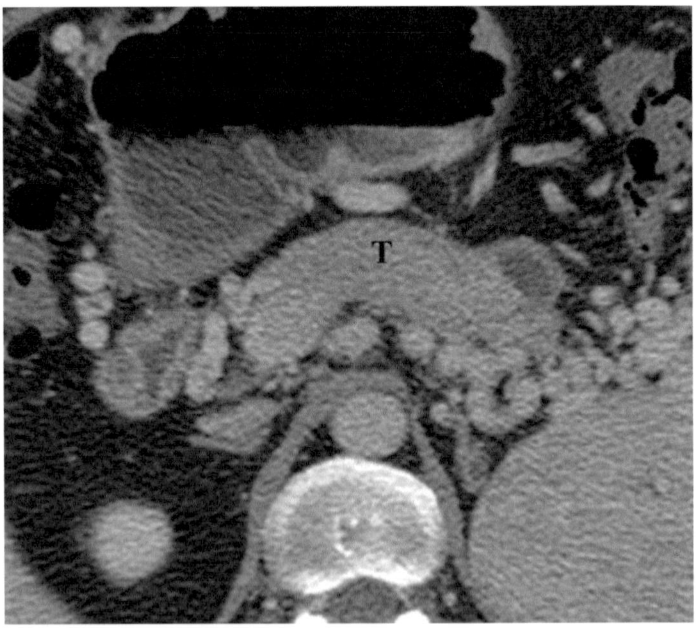

Fig. 26.1 Computed tomography (CT) of a pancreatic neuroendocrine tumor (T) in the body of the pancreas that obstructs the splenic vein with extensive short gastric collaterals and extends into the lumen of the portal vein

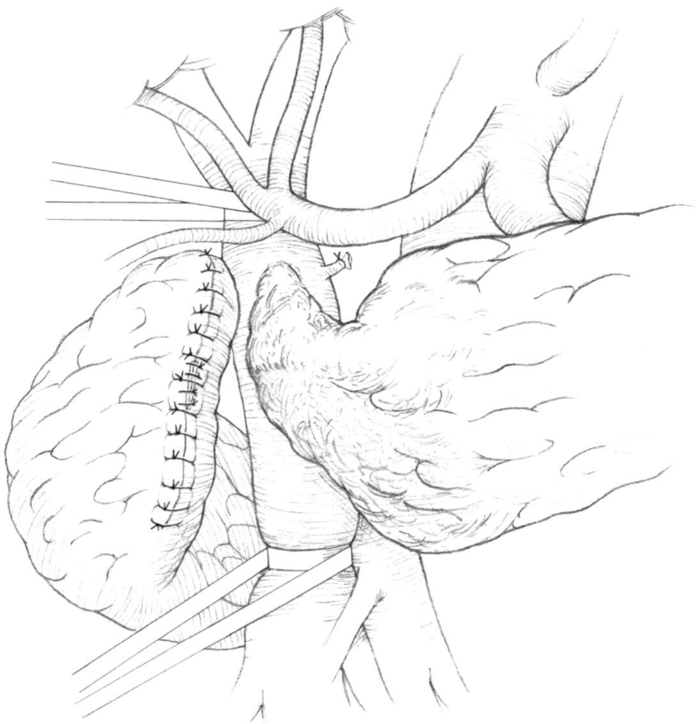

Fig. 26.2 Drawing of the tumor in Fig. 26.1 at surgery just prior to resection. One can see that the pancreas is transected and oversewn to the right of the superior mesenteric vein (SMV)/portal vein confluence. The coronary vein is ligated and divided. Vascular control of the portal vein and SMV proximal and distal to where the tumor extends through the splenic vein into the portal vein is obtained prior to resection of the tumor within the portal vein and splenic vein

splenectomy, obtaining proximal and distal control of the portal vein, and extraction of tumor thrombi from portal vein (Fig. 26.2) with patch closure of portal vein (Fig. 26.3).

Case #2

A 67-year-old man who presents with pain after eating, and weight loss. CT demonstrates a 3 cm pancreatic mass in the uncinate portion of the head abutting the SMV (Fig. 26.4), with subsequent evidence of invasion into the lumen (Fig. 26.5). EUS was performed and FNA of the pancreatic head tumor shows NET. At surgery he had a Whipple pancreaticoduodenectomy with obtaining proximal and distal control of the SMV, portal vein and splenic vein; given heparin; and removing the tumor thrombus from the portal vein and using a venous patch to reconstruct the SMV at the venotomy (Fig. 26.6).

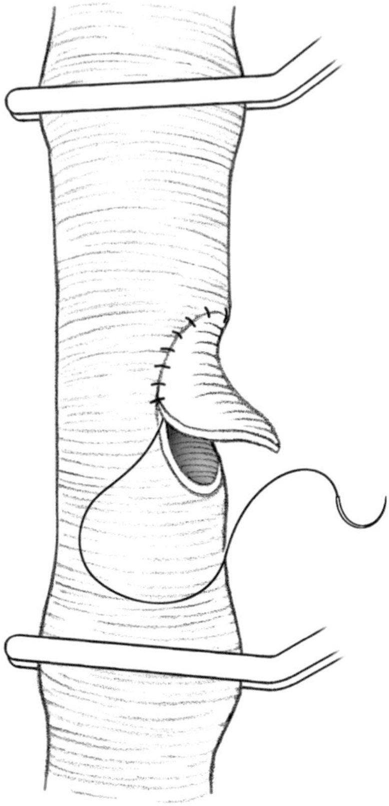

Fig. 26.3 Drawing of closure of a portal vein venotomy with a bovine patch. Proximal and distal control of the vein is obtained with vascular clamps. A venotomy is made and the tumor within the portal vein is excised. Following the excision of tumor a pericardial patch is used to reconstruct the vessel and not narrow the lumen

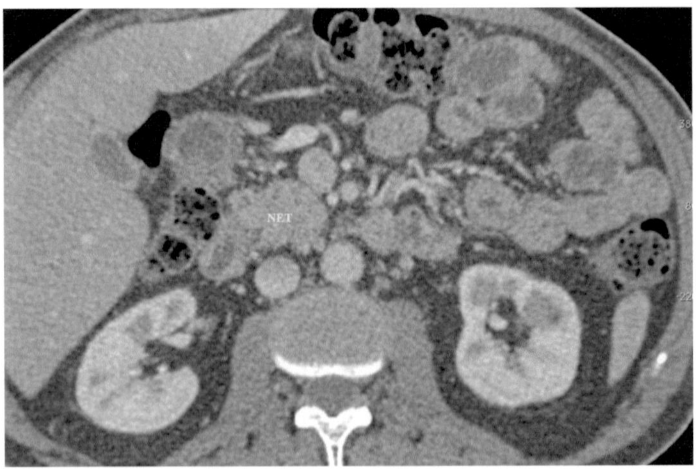

Fig. 26.4 Computed tomography (CT) of a neuroendocrine tumor (NET) in the uncinate portion of the head of the pancreas

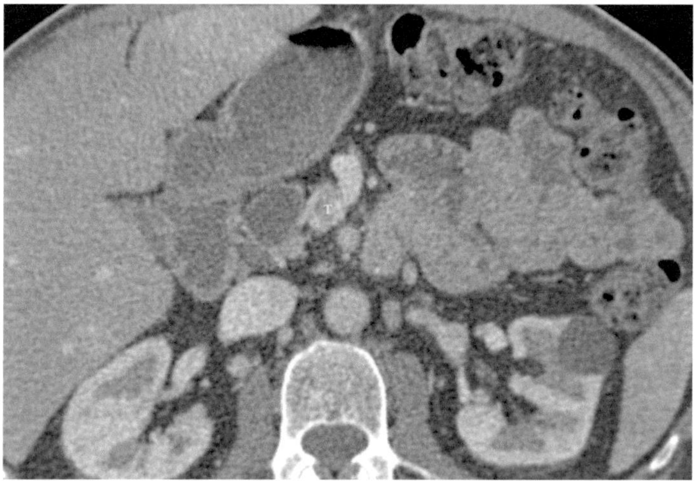

Fig. 26.5 The same PNET as seen in Fig. 26.4 extends through the wall of the superior mesenteric vein into the lumen of the portal vein (T) on superior CT cuts

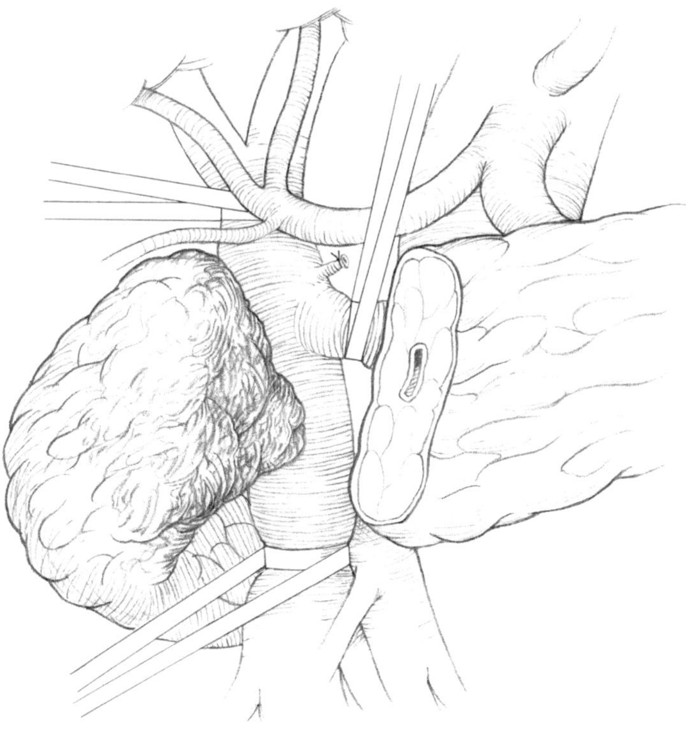

Fig. 26.6 Drawing of the PNET in Fig. 26.5 that extends into the SMV and is in the process of being removed surgically. Note vascular control of the SMV, portal vein, and coronary vein is obtained prior to excision

Proximal and distal control of the portal vein, splenic vein, inferior mesenteric vein, and the superior mesenteric vein is done with vessel loops and vascular clamps, as seen in Fig. 26.2. Any other smaller branches are ligated and divided. Systemic heparin is given at a dose of 100 Units per Kg IV prior to clamping. We incise the vein and use a spatula to mobilize the thrombus. It may require excision and reconstruction of the vein wall. This can be done with a pericardial patch venoplasty, shown in Fig. 26.3, a superficial femoral vein patch, or interposition graft. After closure of the vein, the heparin is revered with protamine at a dose of 1 mg per 100 units of heparin infused. We start 81 mg per day of aspirin on postoperative day 1. We do not use any other type of anticoagulation. Portal vein thrombectomy is either done with concomitant Whipple pancreaticoduodenectomy or subtotal pancreatectomy with splenectomy.

Clinical Pearls

- Proximal and distal control is necessary
- Ligate small posterior branches. Make sure that vein is free without any branches
- Draw a line on interposition vein to maintain proper orientation

Results

We have published a series of 46 patients with major vascular abutment, involvement, or encasement who underwent surgery to remove all gross neuroendocrine tumor [2]. Our series is contrasted to a more recent series from MD Anderson [1]. They reported on nine patients with PNETs who underwent portal venous tumor thrombectomy. The mean age was 42 and 51, respectively. There were approximately 50% men in both studies. Our study had a much higher percentage of MEN-1 (i.e., 26% compared to 0%). The mean tumor size was similar, approximately 5 cm. Most of their tumors were in the body and tail, while most of ours were in the head. Although not all of the head tumors in our experience required a Whipple pancreaticoduodenectomy, the rate was 23%. Whipple was performed in one-third of patients with pancreatic head tumors. The Ki67 rate was between 1 and 2% for all our tumors because we selected them based on a low malignant potential, which is defined as a positive SRS scan or a Ki67 $< 2\%$, while theirs had a high rate in several patients, and all except one was treated with preoperative chemotherapy. Each of their patients had blood vessel involvement while only 34% of ours had it. Since our patients had less blood vessel involvement; we performed fewer venotomies and vascular reconstructions (Table 26.1 and 26.2).

Table 26.1 Demographics of patients with PNETs and vascular involvement from two series

Study	# patients with pNET + vascular involvement	% Men	Mean age (range)	% functional NET	% MEN1	NET Size (cm)	% head of pancreas	% vessel involvement
MD Anderson	9	33	51 (38-67)	0	0	5.4	11	100
Stanford NIH	46	46	42 (24-76)	70	26	5.8	59	34

Table 26.2 Extent of surgery, complications, disease status, and survival

Study	% Up front chemotherapy	% Whipple procedures	% Vascular resection and reconstruction	% complications (deaths)	% Disease-free	Survival
MD Anderson	67	11	89	Not listed	33%	78% at 3 years
Stanford NIH	0	23	20	27 and no deaths	30%	60% at 10 years

However, the two illustrative cases presented here had tumor thrombus within the vessel that can be excised with a spatula, except where it entered the vessel. We used heparin for our venous procedures, and reversed it with protamine after the procedure on the vessel was completed; however, it is controversial, and some do not use it. We reconstructed the portal or superior mesenteric vein with a vein patch from the femoral vein, or a bovine pericardial patch, while some others use the internal jugular vein, but that is used more for complete replacement of these vessels. We had no cases developing thrombosis of the portal vein, as we have followed the flow through this vessel with Doppler ultrasound. These procedures are done with acceptable morbidity and no operative mortality. The disease-free survival was approximately 30% in both studies, and the long-term survival is between 60 and 70%, suggesting that it is worthwhile to perform this more aggressive surgery [1, 2].

Alternative Approaches

- Alternative systemic treatment
- Manage bleeding gastric varies with either sclerotherapy or embolization of splenic artery

Discussion

Malignant pancreatic neuroendocrine tumors have a good prognosis [5–9]. Unfortunately, a significant proportion present late, with large tumors that encase or invade adjacent blood vessels [3]. A number of studies have demonstrated that vascular invasion with PNETs is associated with decreased survival [5, 10, 11]. The surgical approach to this group of patients is controversial. Based on analogies to pancreatic adenocarcinoma and limited experience with attempted surgical resection of patients with advanced PETs, for many, involvement of the superior mesenteric vein (SMV), and portal vein (PV) is a contraindication to surgical resection [10, 12]. However, recent studies in standard pancreas cancer surgery question this approach. The operability of pancreatic tumors is usually defined by the results of thin-slice computed tomography with special protocols to enhance visualization of the pancreas and its blood vessels [12–16]. However, these studies may falsely determine operability. For example, in patients with adenocarcinoma of the pancreas, when preoperative imaging studies suggest that the tumor involves the SMV or PV, many surgeons suggest that the tumor is inoperable [10, 12, 13]. However, recent studies dispute this thinking, and suggest that these locally advanced tumors may be resectable for benefit [17–19]. Sarcomas involving blood vessels that were previously thought to be inoperable have been recently excised, with acceptable morbidity and good overall survival [20, 21]. Because PNETs are rare, there have only been two studies of the ability to surgically resect malignant PNETs that invade or involve the major mesenteric veins [1, 2]. Most reports have only a few patients [4, 22–26]. In this review we report the long-term results with PNETs that abut or involve major mesenteric vascular structures, including the PV and SMV. The findings suggest that major vascular involvement on preoperative imaging studies may not be a contraindication to resection of PNET.

This chapter focuses on the method and role of surgery in removing PNETs abutting the PV, or invading into the PV with tumor thrombi. This method is important for the following reasons:

1. A significant proportion of PNETs demonstrate aggressive behavior that is associated with decreased survival, and medical chemotherapy treatment of these large, advanced tumors is generally ineffective [10, 27, 28].
2. There are a number of studies in patients with metastatic PNETs to the liver that aggressive resection of liver metastases is associated with improved survival, [5, 6, 11–13] and the question is whether or not this more advanced surgery applies to patients whose tumor invades into the mesenteric veins.
3. Recent studies in series of patients with adenocarcinoma of the pancreas invading into these veins show that resection of these veins—even in patients with more aggressive and poorer prognosis types of cancer—can be done with acceptable morbidity and mortality, and is associated with improved survival [10, 13–16, 29].
4. Resection of other tumors like HCC and RCC that invade into large veins can be done safely with improved survival.
5. A locally aggressive, nonfunctional PNET that invades into the splenic vein and continues to grow into the portal vein can cause dramatic life-threatening complications like massive upper gastrointestinal bleeding from short gastric varices [30, 31]. Successful resection of these tumors may significantly delay or prevent the occurrence of such complications.

In a recent study we have shown resections were feasible, safe, and associated with long survival, even though tumors were large (5 cm), with distant metastatic disease [2]. One important concept is that in some, or even many, cases the tumor is not as involved with the vasculature as thought on the imaging study. In a recent study of patients with advanced large PNETs, 50% of patients thought to have vascular involvement from preoperative imaging studies were found at the time of surgery not to have vascular involvement or encasement [8, 10, 12, 29].

Computed tomography (CT) and magnetic resonance imaging (MRI) are thought to have similar excellent sensitivity for detecting vascular involvement, and are the standard imaging studies used to determine vascular involvement in patients with either pancreas cancer or PNET [6, 10, 12]. Our current preference is CT over MRI. CT with thin slices, intravenous contrast, arterial and venous phases, and 3-D reconstruction allows the surgeon to see the tumor and plan the resection effectively. Studies show that with PNETs, radiological abutment or even vascular involvement is frequently not synonymous with vascular involvement during surgery. In some studies, it has been reported that a small percentage of patients with PNETs who have CTs reporting vascular involvement are found not to have it at surgery [32]. In most patients, the PNET can be removed without vascular reconstruction. It requires careful dissection, but not vascular reconstruction. This is different than what is found in pancreatic adenocarcinoma, which usually requires vascular resection and reconstruction when the preoperative imaging studies suggest that is the case.

In our study, despite the extensive tumor and venous involvement, patients who underwent resection had an impressive actuarial and disease-free survival rates of 60 and 30% at 5 years [2]. The most important negative prognostic factor associated with decreased long-term survival is the presence of liver metastases [33]. In contrast, disease-free survival was not affected by either the extent or type of vascular involvement, or by any of the other factors that have been found to have prognostic significance in other studies of PNET patients [1, 2, 8, 9]. In our study, patients with nonfunctional PNETs and possible vascular involvement had a significantly decreased survival compared to the survival of similar patients with functional tumors [2]. Others have reported that patients with nonfunctional tumors have a poorer survival than those with functional tumors [1, 9, 34]. The decreased survival of patients with nonfunctional tumors is likely to be due to the presence of greater tumor burdens at diagnosis, and a more aggressive tumor nature [5]. In our study, the extent of tumor was similar for nonfunctional and functional tumors, suggesting that the aggressive nature of the nonfunctional tumors is the reason for decreased survival [2].

Factors that Negatively Influenced Subsequent Survival

- Liver resection
- Liver tumors
- Postoperative anti-tumor treatment
- Nonfunctional tumors affected disease-free survival negatively, but not overall survival

Unfortunately, these studies do not clearly establish the value of aggressive surgery to remove PNETs from within mesenteric blood vessels [35]. The studies do indicate and demonstrate that with proper planning, and possibly vascular consultation preoperatively, the surgery can be done safely. However, a number of findings in our study are suggestive of a benefit of this more aggressive surgery. First, despite the expected decreased survival of patients with malignant PNETs with vascular involvement or liver metastases, the overall survival rate was 60% at 5 years, and 30% of patients remained free of tumor [2]. These data are encouraging, because historical data show that patients with similar findings who did not undergo surgery have a 5-year survival rate of 30–40%.

Second, in our study the results were obtained in the setting of pancreatic resection (80%), liver resection (41%) and vascular reconstruction, (20%) and in that complex setting there were no deaths, and the operative morbidity was 27%, which is well within the rates of even lesser pancreatic surgical procedures [2].

Third, in our study five patients specifically presented with severe upper gastrointestinal hemorrhage from gastric varices secondary to splenic vein obstruction by tumor that was totally ameliorated by surgery to resect the tumor and reconstruct the portal vein. Others have described similar results in a series of case reports [30]. These findings indicate that resection of PNET is of great benefit to those who have splenic vein involvement and gastric varices, as the bleeding is life-threatening and difficult to control by other means [2].

Fourth, medical therapies for advanced PNETs have provided only modest benefits, with series showing only disease stabilization and a few partial responses [28]. Therefore, it is seldom possible to downsize malignant PNETs, as has been reported for other tumors, to make them surgically resectable. Our study and the results of others suggest that major vascular involvement is not a contraindication to surgery [1, 2]. Because radiographic evidence of vascular involvement exists in 20% of patients with malignant PNETs, these results apply to a significant number of patients with PNETs seen in the community, and such patients should be referred to specialized tertiary care centers where multidisciplinary expertise is readily available. In fact, Adams has written an editorial to support this strategy [36].

Overall Management

- With splenic vein occlusion and gastric hemorrhage, manage gastric varies with either sclerotherapy or splenic artery embolism
- Ascites from SMV or portal vein occlusion can be managed with lassie, aldactone, and albumin infusion

References

1. Prakash L, Lee JE, Yao J, Bhosale P, Balachandran A, Wang HM, et al. Role and operative technique of portal venous tumor thrombectomy in patients with pancreatic neuroendocrine tumors. J Gastrointest Surg. 2015;19(11):2011–8.
2. Norton JA, Harris EJ, Chen Y, Visser BC, Poultsides GA, Kunz PC, et al. Pancreatic endocrine tumors with major vascular abutment, involvement, or encasement and indication for resection. Arch Surg. 2011;146(6):724–32.
3. Bok EJ, Cho KJ, Williams DM, Brady TM, Weiss CA, Forrest ME. Venous involvement in islet cell tumors of the pancreas. Am J Roentgenol. 1984;142(2):319–22.
4. Bedirli A, Patiroglu TE, Sakrak O, Aritas Y. Portal vein resection for a portal vein thrombus caused by nonfunctioning islet cell carcinoma: report of a case. Surg Today. 2004;34(9):802–4.
5. Hochwald SN, Zee S, Conlon KC, Colleoni R, Louie O, Brennan MF, et al. Prognostic factors in pancreatic endocrine neoplasms: sn analysis of 136 cases with a proposal for low-grade and intermediate-grade groups. J Clin Oncol. 2002;20(11):2633–42.
6. Norton JA, Jensen RT. Resolved and unresolved controversies in the surgical management of patients with Zollinger-Ellison syndrome. Ann Surg. 2004;240(5):757–73.
7. Madeira I, Terris B, Voss M, Denys A, Sauvanet A, Flejou JF, et al. Prognostic factors in patients with endocrine tumours of the duodenopancreatic area. Gut. 1998;43(3):422–7.
8. Panzuto F, Nasoni S, Falconi M, Corleto VD, Capurso G, Cassetta S, et al. Prognostic factors and survival in endocrine tumor patients: comparison between gastrointestinal and pancreatic localization. Endocr-Relat Cancer. 2005;12(4):1083–92.
9. Ekeblad S, Skogseid B, Dunder K, Oberg K, Eriksson B. Prognostic factors and survival in 324 patients with pancreatic endocrine tumor treated at a single institution. Clin Cancer Res. 2008;14(23):7798–803.
10. Wray CJ, Ahmad SA, Matthews JB, Lowy AM. Surgery for pancreatic cancer: recent controversies and current practice. Gastroenterology. 2005;128(6):1626–41.
11. Ballian N, Loeffler AG, Rajamanickam V, Norstedt PA, Weber SM, Cho CS. A simplified prognostic system for resected pancreatic neuroendocrine neoplasms. HPB (Oxford). 2009;11 (5):422–8.
12. Buchs NC, Chilcott M, Poletti PA, Buhler LH, Morel P. Vascular invasion in pancreatic cancer: imaging modalities, preoperative diagnosis and surgical management. World J Gastroenterol. 2010;16(7):818–31.
13. Martin RCG, Scoggins CR, Egnatashvili V, Staley CA, McMasters KM, Kooby DA. Arterial and venous resection for pancreatic adenocarcinoma operative and long-term outcomes. Arch Surg. 2009;144(2):154–9.
14. Glanemann M, Shi BM, Liang F, Sun XG, Bahra M, Jacob D, et al. Surgical strategies for treatment of malignant pancreatic tumors: extended, standard or local surgery? World J Surg Oncol. 2008;6:123.
15. Tucker O, Rela M. Letter 2. Systematic review of outcome of synchronous portal-superior mesenteric vein resection during pancreatectomy for cancer. Brit J Surg. 2006;93(10):1303–4.
16. Siriwardana HP, Siriwardena AK. Systematic review of outcome of synchronous portal-superior mesenteric vein resection during pancreatectomy for cancer. Brit J Surg. 2006;93(6):662–73.
17. Harrison LE, Klimstra DS, Brennan MF. Isolated portal vein involvement in pancreatic adenocarcinoma—a contraindication for resection? Ann Surg. 1996;224(3):342–7.
18. Tseng JF, Tamm ER, Lee JE, Pisters PWT, Evans DB. Venous resection in pancreatic cancer surgery. Best Pract Res Clin Gastroenterol. 2006;20(2):349–64.
19. Ramacciato G, Mercantini P, Petrucciani N, Giaccaglia V, Nigri G, Ravaioli M, et al. Does portal-superior mesenteric vein invasion still indicate irresectability for pancreatic carcinoma? Ann Surg Oncol. 2009;16(4):817–25.
20. Song TK, Harris EJ, Raghavan S, Norton JA. Major blood vessel reconstruction during sarcoma surgery. Arch Surg. 2009;144(9):817–22.

21. Poultsides GA, Tran TB, Zambrano E, Janson L, Mohler DG, Mell MW, et al. Sarcoma resection with and without vascular reconstruction: a matched case-control study. Ann Surg. 2015;262(4):632–40.
22. Obuz F, Bora S, Sarioglu S. Malignant islet cell tumor of the pancreas associated with portal venous thrombus. Eur Radiol. 2001;11(9):1642–4.
23. Sakamoto E, Hasegawa H, Ogiso S, Igami T, Mori T, Mizuno T, et al. Curative resection for a pancreatic endocrine carcinoma involving the portal vein. Hepatogastroenterology. 2004;51 (60):1849–51.
24. Kawakami H, Kuwatani M, Hirano S, Kondo S, Nakanishi Y, Itoh T, et al. Pancreatic endocrine tumors with intraductal growth into the main pancreatic duct and tumor thrombus within the portal vein: a case report and review of the literature. Intern Med. 2007;46(6):273–7.
25. Akatsu T, Aiura K, Shimazu M, Ueda M, Wakabayashi G, Tanabe M, et al. Successful pancreatectomy with en-bloc resection of the celiac artery and portal vein for pancreatic endocrine carcinoma. Hepatogastroenterology. 2007;54(76):1269–71.
26. Yamato H, Kawakami H, Kuwatani M, Shinada K, Kondo S, Kubota K, et al. Pancreatic carcinoma associated with portal vein tumor thrombus: three case reports. Intern Med. 2009;48(3):143–50.
27. Yu F, Venzon DJ, Serrano J, Goebel SU, Doppman JL, Gibril F, et al. Prospective study of the clinical course, prognostic factors, causes of death, and survival in patients with long-standing Zollinger-Ellison syndrome. J Clin Oncol. 1999;17(2):615–30.
28. Strosberg JR, Kvols LK. Oncologic—a review of the current clinical trials for gastroenteropancreatic neuroendocrine tumours. Expert Opin Inv Drug. 2007;16(2):219–24.
29. Deshpande V, Fernandez-del Castillo C, Muzikansky A, Deshpande A, Zukerberg L, Warshaw AL, et al. Cytokeratin 19 is a powerful predictor of survival in pancreatic endocrine tumors. Am J Surg Pathol. 2004;28(9):1145–53.
30. Metz DC, Benjamin SB. Islet cell-carcinoma of the pancreas presenting as bleeding from isolated gastric varices—report of a case and review of the literature. Digest Dis Sci. 1991;36 (2):241–4.
31. Yamaguchi T, Takahashi H, Kagawa R, Takeda R, Sakata S, Yamamoto M, et al. Nonfunctioning pancreatic endocrine tumor presenting with hemorrhage from isolated gastric varices. Am Surg. 2005;71(12):1027–30.
32. Hellman P, Andersson M, Rastad J, Juhlin C, Karacagil S, Eriksson B, et al. Surgical strategy for large or malignant endocrine pancreatic tumors. World J Surg. 2000;24(11):1353–60.
33. Weber HC, Venzon DJ, Lin JT, Fishbein VA, Orbuch M, Strader DB, et al. Determinants of metastatic rate and survival in patients with Zollinger-Ellison syndrome—a prospective long-term study. Gastroenterology. 1995;108(6):1637–49.
34. Phan GO, Yeo CJ, Hruban RH, Lillemoe KD, Pitt HA, Cameron JL. Surgical experience with pancreatic and peripancreatic neuroendocrine tumors: 125 patients. Gastroenterology. 1997;112(4):A1465.
35. Gurusamy KS, Ramamoorthy R, Sharma D, Davidson BR. Liver resection versus other treatments for neuroendocrine tumours in patients with resectable liver metastases. Cochrane Database Syst Rev. 2009(2):CD007060.
36. Adams DB. Especially dangerous and therefore anxious operations. Arch Surg. 2011;146 (6):732–3.

Pancreatic Neuroendocrine Tumor in Tail of Pancreas with Splenic Vein Thrombus and Sinistral Portal Hypertension

27

Christina L. Costantino and Cristina R. Ferrone

Case Presentation

R.D. is a 53-year-old male in previously excellent health who presented with shortness of breath and a cough. He initially underwent a pulmonary workup, which was negative. He was found to have melanotic stool and anemia with a HCT of 28. He underwent upper endoscopy, which demonstrated multiple gastric varices with red wale marks consistent with recent bleeding. He had no esophageal varices. CT scan demonstrated a 3×2.8 cm pancreatic tail mass (Fig. 27.1), splenic vein thrombosis (Fig. 27.2), splenomegaly (16×6 cm), and multiple varices suggestive of sinistral hypertension (Fig. 27.3). He also had a 3 cm suspicious lesion in the right lobe of his liver. His chest CT was negative.

R.D. underwent a distal pancreatectomy and splenectomy for oncologic resection and decompression of his varices. Pathology demonstrated a well-differentiated neuroendocrine tumor with metastasis in 1/27 lymph nodes.

Pancreatic neuroendocrine tumors (PNETs) are rare and account for approximately 2–4% of pancreatic neoplasms. These tumors originate from the pancreatic islet cells and are classified according to the functional syndrome they produce [1]. Insulinoma and gastrinomas account for 70–90% of functional PNETs. Approximately 10–25% of PNETs are nonfunctional, in that they do not cause a syndrome related to hormonal hypersecretion [1]. These tend to be diagnosed at a more

C.L. Costantino
Department of Surgery, Massachusetts General Hospital, 55 Fruit Street, GRB-425, 02114 Boston, MA, USA
e-mail: clcostantino@partners.org

C.R. Ferrone (✉)
Massachusetts General Hospital, 15 Parkman St., WAC 460, 02114 Boston, MA, USA
e-mail: cferrone@mgh.harvard.edu

T.M. Pawlik et al. (eds.), *Case-Based Lessons in the Management of Complex Hepato-Pancreato-Biliary Surgery*, DOI 10.1007/978-3-319-50868-9_27

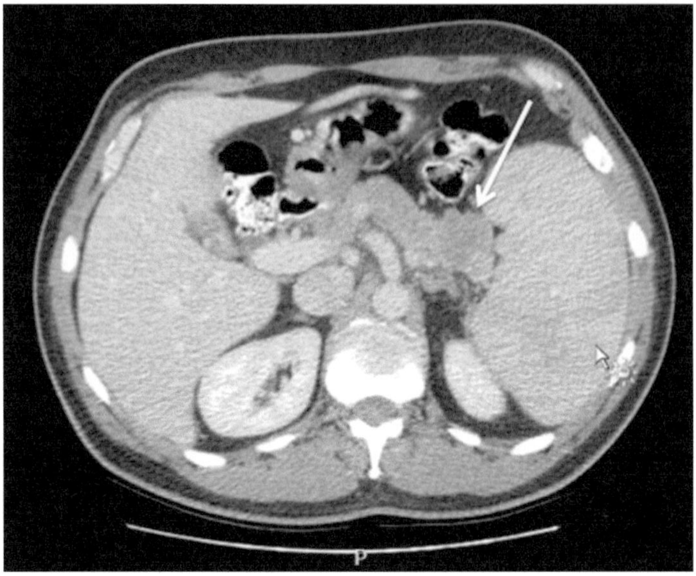

Fig. 27.1 CT scan demonstrating pancreatic tail mass

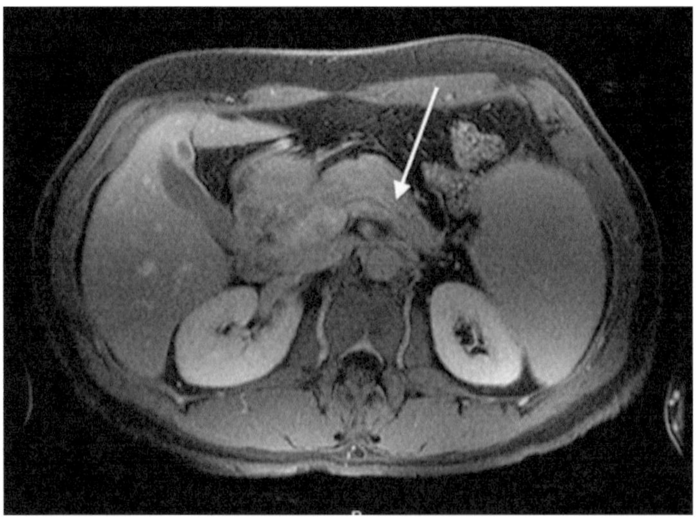

Fig. 27.2 MRI demonstrating splenic vein thrombosis

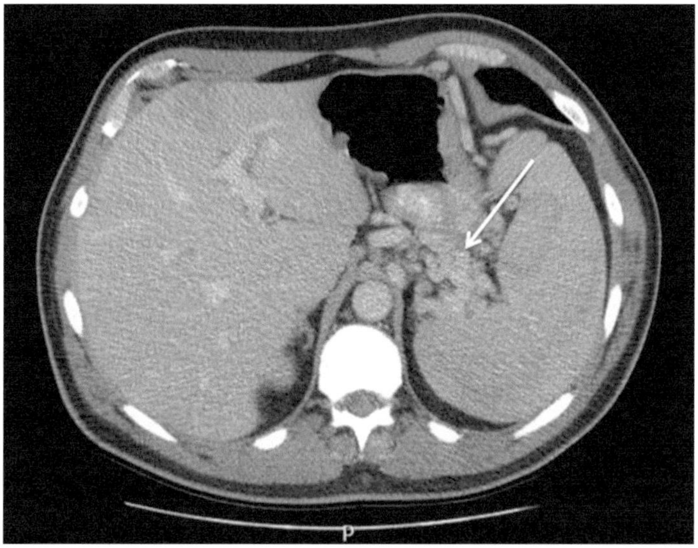

Fig. 27.3 CT scan demonstrating gastric varices secondary to sinistral hypertension

advanced stage, given patients do not present until tumors are commonly causing symptoms, such as abdominal pain, from mass effect.

Presentation

Patients with neuroendocrine tumors may present in a variety of ways, and may be subdivided into those producing hormonal syndromes (functioning) and those with nonfunctioning tumors. Functioning tumors tend to present when they are smaller in size, due to hormone hypersecretion resulting in hypoglycemia, peptic ulcer disease, or diarrhea [1]. Nonfunctioning tumors, however, tend to be larger and present later in their course, given they are often only symptomatic once they cause compression or, most commonly, abdominal pain [2]. Patients may also commonly experience symptoms of weight loss and nausea. Those patients who present with symptoms of anemia or GI hemorrhage must be considered for bleeding form gastric varices secondary to sinistral hypertension [3].

Intraoperative Technical Pearls

- Ligation of the splenic artery early before manipulation of the splenic vein or venous collaterals is critical, in order to decrease left-sided portal pressure in the venous system.

- The splenic vein is divided close to the junction of the mesenteric vein, or 1 cm from the most proximal edge of the lesion.
- Ideally, the inferior mesenteric vein is preserved.

Imaging

Given neuroendocrine tumors are hypervascular in comparison to the surrounding pancreatic parenchyma, thin-cut pancreatic protocol CT with IV contrast is the gold standard for preoperative planning. The majority of PNETs will "light up" on the arterial phase of the scan. MRI imaging sensitivity increases with tumor size, and is an alternate mode of imaging that may be used as an adjunct. Additionally, endoscopic ultrasound imaging is utilized to evaluate the extent of disease and perform preoperative biopsies. Immunohistochemical staining with chromogranin A can distinguish neuroendocrine tumors from pancreatic adenocarcinomas [1].

Staging studies include a Chest CT for evaluation of metastatic thoracic disease. Patients may also undergo an octreotide scan, or somatostatin receptor scintigraphy, to localize both primary and metastastic lesions. Octreotide, a synthetic analogue of somatostatin, is radiolabeled and injected into the venous system. A radioactive signal is produced when bound to somatostatin receptors, which are found on primary and metastatic neuroendocrine tumor cells [1].

Operative Planning: Splenic Preservation?

The indication for spleen conserving surgery must be carefully evaluated with each patient. Splenic preservation importantly decreases the risk of overwhelming infection related to encapsulated organisms, as well as provides other immunoprotective capacity. The Warshaw technique, first described in 1988, proposed preservation of the spleen during distal pancreatectomy for tail of the pancreas pathology [4]. This technique divides the splenic artery and vein with the body and tail of the pancreas. The spleen relies on the collateral vasculature via the short gastric and left gastroepiploic vessels to survive. Given the increased flow via these collaterals, patients may develop gastric varices, which theoretically may lead to hemorrhage. After a 23-year experience at MGH, only one-quarter of patients demonstrated asymptomatic perigastric varices on routine imaging, with no resultant clinical consequences [5].

Splenic vein thrombosis complicates pancreatic neoplasms in 7–10% of patients [6]. Splenic vein thrombosis (SVT) can occur secondary to direct tumor invasion or compression of the splenic vein by mass effect. Occlusion of the splenic vein results in sinistral portal hypertension. Greenwald et al. first described the pathophysiology of left-sided portal hypertension in 1939 [7]. Engorgement of the short gastrics and gastroepiploic veins result in gastric varices secondary to back pressure of the left portal venous system [1]. The incidence of gastric bleeding in sinistral portal hypertension varies from 4 to 72% [6].

Case study R.D. presented with symptomatic anemia and stigmata of recent bleeding. His gastric varices arose in the setting of a distal pancreatic neuroendocrine tumor with associated splenic vein thrombosis, leading to sinistral hypertension and gastric varices. Distal pancreatectomy and splenectomy is the procedure of choice for this patient, not simply for oncologic resection and regional lymphadenectomy, but for control of gastrointestinal hemorrhage by decompressing the left portal venous system.

Operative bleeding risk is substantial due to perigastric varices and inflammation. Coupling this bleeding risk is that many patients are at risk for thrombocytopenia from platelet sequestration in the splenic sinusoids [1]. There is a significantly higher rate of pancreas specific complications with splenic vein thrombosis (33% vs. 7%), in addition to bleeding [6]. Splenic artery embolization can be utilized to help mitigate this risk preoperatively, however, this is not widely utilized.

Operative Technique: Distal Pancreatectomy and Splenectomy

Exposure for distal pancreatectomy and splenectomy can be achieved laparoscopically, or utilizing an open technique with a subcostal or vertical midline incision that extends from the xyphoid process to the umbilicus. The abdomen is explored initially to evaluate for obvious metastasis requiring biopsy. Excellent visualization and retraction are keys to achieving appropriate exposure. First the gastrocolic ligament omentum is opened, allowing entry into the lesser sac. The lesser sac is entered by elevating the greater omentum off of the transverse colon. Dividing the splenocolic ligament will allow for mobilization of the colon caudally. The superior and inferior borders of the pancreas are incised, and a retropancreatic plane is developed to better visualize the dimensions of the mass and vasculature (Fig. 27.4). The splenic artery should be identified close to its origin close at the celiac trunk, where it can be clamped, transected, and suture ligated with 2-0 silk. Taking the arterial supply before attempting any manipulation of the splenic vein or venous collaterals is critical. This step decreases pressure within the venous system.

Next, the splenic vein is divided close to the junction of the mesenteric vein, or 1 cm from the most proximal edge of the lesion. Ideally, the inferior mesenteric vein is preserved. The greater curvature of the stomach is then taken down, paying

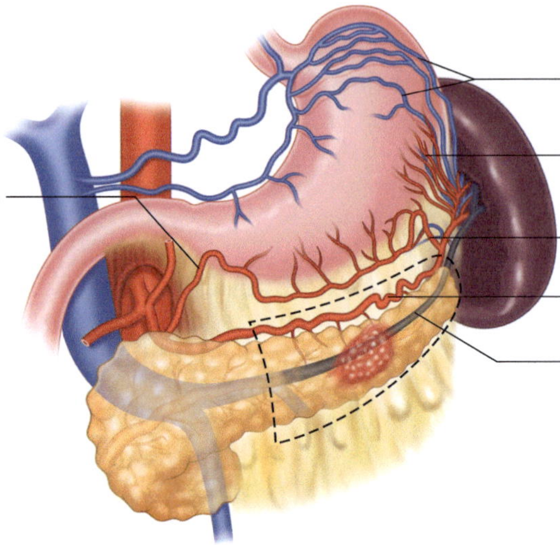

Fig. 27.4 Anatomic landmarks

close attention to preserve the gastroepiploic arcade, and clamping and tying the short gastric vessels with 2-0 silk or utilizing clips and the ligasure or the tri-stapler with the vascular staple load. We then reflect the stomach to the patient's right, exposing the pancreas. After the artery and vein have been divided, either the remaining lateral and inferior splenic attachments can be mobilized, or the pancreas can be divided. Division of the pancreatic body can be performed with a scalpel, stapler ± vicryl sheath, or harmonic/tissue link. Unfortunately, the rate of pancreatic fistula is equivalent no matter what transaction technique is utilized [5]. The spleen, with the pancreas, is delivered through the incision, carefully dividing any final retroperitoneal attachments. The surgical bed is inspected for good hemostasis. A surgical drain is left in place near the pancreatic stump.

Controversies and Alternative Approaches

- Splenic artery embolization can be utilized to help mitigate risk of gastrointestinal hemorrhage, however, this is not widely utilized.
- En bloc splenic resection is indicated for splenic vein thrombosis and sinistral hypertension.
- The drain in the surgical bed may be removed once the fluid amylase level is less than 600 cc or with an output less than 30 cc for 24 h.

Postoperative Management

Postoperatively, patients generally stay in the hospital for three days after a laparoscopic operation, and 5 days after an open operation. On postoperative day one or when the patient begins taking in fatty foods, an amylase level is sent of the drain fluid. This value is checked daily. If the fluid amylase level is less than 600 cc or the drain output is less than 30 cc for 24 h, then the drain is removed [8]. Patients should also undergo splenectomy vaccinations if they were not administered prior to resection, which include: pneumococcal, haemophilus influenzae, and meningococcal vaccines.

Overall Management

- Decreasing left-sided portal pressure in the venous system is important prior to manipulation, given risk of gastrointestinal hemorrhage.
- Distal pancreatectomy and splenectomy is the procedure of choice for oncologic resection and regional lymphadenectomy, and control of gastrointestinal hemorrhage by decompressing the left portal venous system.

Conclusion

Pancreatic neuroendocrine tumor of the pancreas is a rare disease, even more rare is associated splenic vein thrombosis with resultant sinistral hypertension. In the setting of bleeding, these PNETs should be excised en bloc with the spleen for both oncologic resection and decompression of gastric varices (Fig. 27.5).

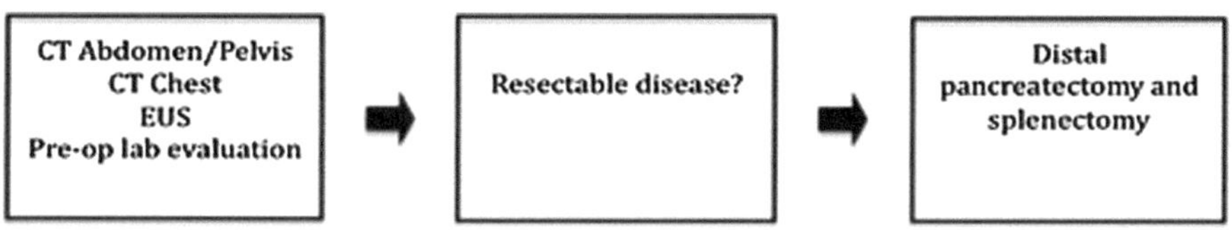

Fig. 27.5 Workflow diagram

References

1. Yeo CJ et al. Shackelford's surgery of the alimentary tract. Philadelphia, PA: Elsevier/Saunders;2013.
2. Nissen NN, Kim AS, Yu R, Wolin EM, Friedman ML, Lo SK, Wachsman AM, Colquhoun SD. Pancreatic neuroendocrine tumors: presentation, management, and outcomes. Am Surg. 2009;75(10):1025–9.
3. Evans GR, Yellin AE, Weaver FA, Stain SC. Sinistral (left-sided) portal hypertension. Am Surg. 1990;56:758–63.
4. Warshaw AL. Conservation of the Spleen With Distal Pancreatectomy. Arch Surg. 1988;123 (5):550–3.
5. Ferrone CR, Konstantinidis IT, Sahani DV, Wargo JA, Fernandez-del Castillo C, Warshaw AL. Twenty-three years of the Warshaw operation for distal pancreatectomy with preservation of the spleen. Ann Surg. 2011;253(6):1136–9.
6. Dedania N, Agrawal N, Winter JM, Koniaris LG, Rosato EL, Sauter PK, et al. Splenic vein thrombosis is associated with an increase in pancreas-specific complications and reduced survival in patients undergoing distal pancreatectomy for pancreatic exocrine cancer. J Gastrointest Surg. 2013;17(8):1392–8.
7. Greenwald HM, Wasch MG. The roentgenologic demonstration of esophageal varices as a diagnostic aid in chronic thrombosis of the splenic vein. J Pediatr. 1939;14:57–65.
8. Rodríguez JR, Madanat MG, Healy BC, Thayer SP, Warshaw AL. Castillo CF-D. Distal pancreatectomy with splenic preservation revisited. Surgery. 2007;141(5):619–25.

Multifocal Branch-Duct Intraductal Papillary Mucinous Neoplasm

28

Alexander P. Stark and O. Joe Hines

Case Presentation

A 68-year-old female in good health was noted to have numerous small pancreatic cysts during the work-up and subsequent operation for an abdominal liposarcoma. She had no personal history of pancreatic disease, nor any pertinent family history. In addition to the aforementioned liposarcoma, a preoperative CT scan of the abdomen demonstrated innumerable small cysts throughout the pancreatic parenchyma with apparent communication with the pancreatic duct, the greatest of which measured 0.9 cm in diameter. The pancreatic duct was noted to be 4 mm in maximum diameter. Postoperatively, the patient recovered uneventfully and received a dedicated work-up of these pancreatic cysts, including endoscopic ultrasound and fine needle aspiration (EUS-FNA). Definitive communication with the pancreatic duct was not identified. However, the largest cyst measuring 1.3×0.9 cm was found to have a mural nodule; cyst fluid aspirate was consistent with a mucinous lesion. A presumptive diagnosis of multifocal branch-duct type intraductal papillary mucinous neoplasm (BD-IPMN) was made, and a total pancreatectomy was recommended, given the extent of parenchymal involvement. The patient was referred for a second opinion regarding the management of these cysts.

A.P. Stark
Department of Surgery, David Geffen School of Medicine at UCLA,
10833 Le Conte Ave, 72-227, 90095 Los Angeles, CA, USA
e-mail: astark@mednet.ulca.edu

O.J. Hines (✉)
Department of Surgery, David Geffen School of Medicine at UCLA,
10833 Le Conte Ave, CHS 72-180, 90095-6904 Los Angeles, CA, USA
e-mail: joehines@mednet.ucla.edu

T.M. Pawlik et al. (eds.), *Case-Based Lessons in the Management of Complex Hepato-Pancreato-Biliary Surgery*, DOI 10.1007/978-3-319-50868-9_28

Overview of Multifocal Bd-IPMN

Pancreatic cysts are increasingly identified on cross-sectional imaging, occurring in approximately 2.4–19.6% percent of CT and MRI examinations [1, 2]. Of these, lesions with malignant potential—in particular mucinous cystic neoplasm, main-duct intraductal papillary neoplasm (MD-IPMN), and BD-IPMN—require prompt identification. BD-IPMN is generally believed to have the lowest malignant potential of the three. Invasive carcinoma *or* high-grade dysplasia (referred to as "malignant" disease) is reportedly found in 12–47% of resected BD-IPMN specimens [3–7]. This range narrows to 16.1–29.5% when looking only at series with $n > 100$ [8]. In contrast, the reported risk of malignant disease in patients with MD-IPMN ranges between 38 and 68% [4, 6, 8–13]. It should be noted that these numbers rely heavily on retrospective data subject to selection bias, particularly as they represent the risk of malignancy in series of resected specimens. Data regarding the true risk of malignancy in BD-IPMN remains elusive, as increasing numbers of patients with presumed BD-IPMN are observed rather than offered resection.

Guidelines have been issued to aid the clinician in identifying patients with presumed BD-IPMN at risk for malignancy. The 2012 International Association of Pancreatology Consensus Guidelines (ICG) identify *high-risk stigmata* (obstructive jaundice, enhancing solid component, main pancreatic duct >10 mm) and *worrisome features* (pancreatitis, cyst size ≥ 3 cm, main pancreatic duct 5–9 mm, non-enhancing mural nodule, and abrupt change in pancreatic duct diameter with distal pancreatic atrophy) of and for malignant BD-IPMN [8]. Cysts with high-risk stigmata should be considered for resection straight away; those with worrisome features require further investigation with EUS-FNA to better characterize the lesion. In 2015, the American Gastroenterological Association (AGA) issued evidence-based guidelines for the management of incidentally discovered pancreatic cysts [14, 15]. Neither the 2012 ICG nor the 2015 AGA guidelines directly address multifocal disease.

However, multifocal disease is common in patients with BD-IPMN, many of whom have innumerable lesions (Fig. 28.1). The reported incidence of multifocality varies widely from 0 to 83%, but a more conservative estimate of 25–41% is generally accepted [6, 16–18]. The pronounced incidence of multifocal disease has given rise to the notion that IPMN is a manifestation of a field defect of genetic susceptibility for the entire gland. Data demonstrating the risk of recurrence and malignancy in the remnant pancreas despite margin-negative resection of IPMN gives credence to such a theory [19, 20]. On the other hand, tissue analyses performed on patients with multifocal BD-IPMN have revealed striking genetic heterogeneity between synchronous lesions, indicating that each may result from an independent genetic event, even in the setting of diffuse disease [16].

The management of patients with suspected multifocal BD-IPMN presents the clinician with a number of additional challenges in addition to those inherent in the management of solitary BD-IPMN (see box below). Among these include the ability to confidently confirm the diagnosis of multifocal BD-IPMN. Disturbingly, in one series a significant percentage of multifocal lesions preoperatively classified as

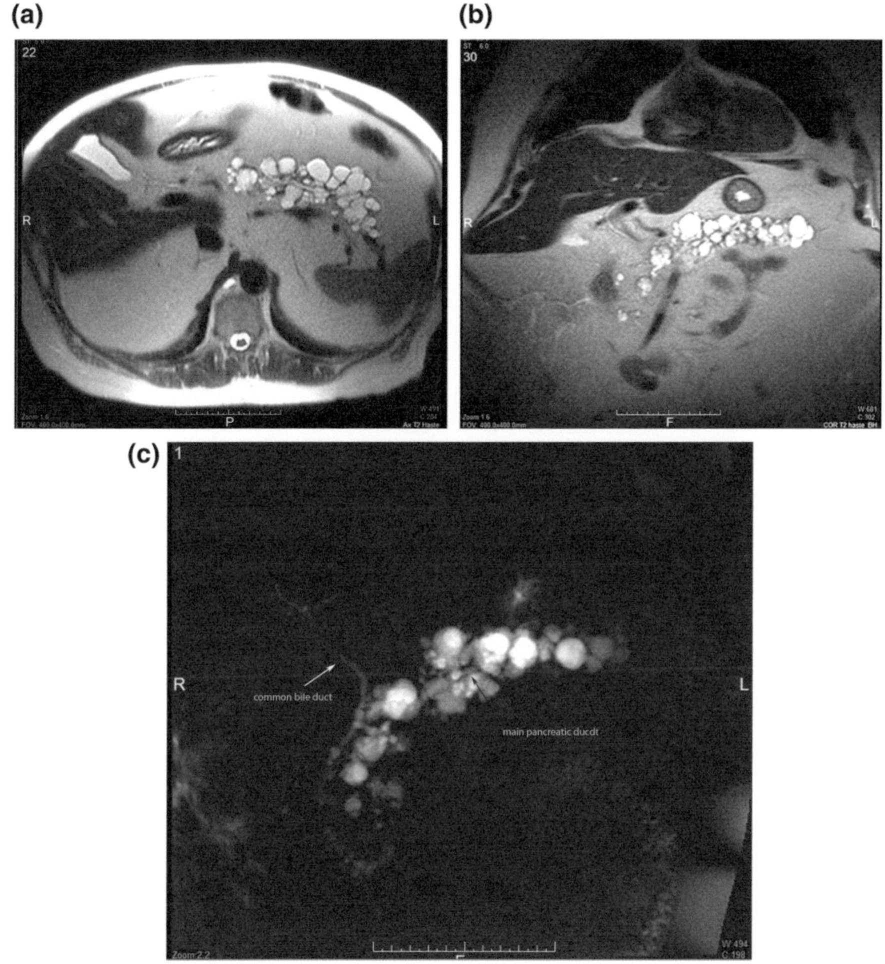

Fig.s 28.1 **a**, **b**, **c**—**a** Axial and **b** coronal T2 weighted magnetic resonance imaging of the abdomen in a patient with multifocal BD-IPMN demonstrating innumerable pancreatic cysts. No mural nodules or solid masses are appreciated; no cyst measures >3 cm in diameter. **c** Coronal magnetic resonance cholangiopancreatography (MRCP) image of the same patient. The common bile duct is normal in caliber (*white arrow*). The main pancreatic duct is incompletely visualized; the visible portion is normal in caliber (*black arrow*). In this patient, EUS was subsequently performed to confirm communication between these cysts and the main pancreatic duct. EUS was also performed to fully evaluate the diameter of the main pancreatic duct throughout the entire gland

BD-IPMN were found to have main pancreatic duct involvement, indicating a true diagnosis of mixed-IPMN [9]. Estimating the risk of malignancy is another challenge; even if no individual lesion displays high risk or worrisome features, is there reason to believe that multifocal disease itself is a marker of increased risk of malignancy? [21]. Fortunately, most series have not found an intrinsically higher rate of malignancy in patients with multifocal disease relative to unifocal disease (Table 28.1). In patients

Table 28.1 Comparison of rate of invasive or malignant disease in multifocal BD-IPMN versus unifocal BD-IPMN

Author	Year	*n*	Rate of multifocal disease, %	Rate of malignancy[a], unifocal %	Rate of malignancy[a], multifocal %	Rate of invasive disease, unifocal%	Rate of invasive disease, multifocal	*p*-value
Schmidt et al. [6]	2007	103	40.7 (42/103)	n/a	n/a	18.0 (11/61)	7.1 (3/42)	0.06
Rodriguez et al. [18]	2007	145	25.5 (37/145)	21.3 (23/108)	24.3 (9/37)	n/a	n/a	ns
Mori et al. [50]	2012	211	19.9 (42/211)	27.7 (15/54)[b]	33.3 (5/15) [b]	20.4 (11/54)	13.3 (2/15)	ns
Fritz et al. [51]	2014	233	19.3 (45/233)	25.5 (48/188)	20.0% (9/45)	n/a	n/a	ns

n/a = data unavailable; ns = not statistically significant
[a] the term malignant encompasses lesions with invasive carcinoma and/or carcinoma in situ/high-grade dysplasia
[b] rate of malignancy reported only for resected lesions with pathologic confirmation

with intermediate-risk solitary lesions, further characterization relies heavily on EUS-FNA. This is logistically problematic in patients with innumerable lesions, all of which cannot be reasonably sampled. Finally, if surgery is to be recommended, the extent of resection is often difficult to determine on an anatomic basis. Between 17 and 52% of patients with multifocal BD-IPMN have disease that is either diffuse in nature or extends beyond the boundaries of segmental resections such as pancreaticoduodenectomy, extended pancreaticoduodenectomy, central pancreatectomy, and distal pancreatectomy [6, 22]. The surgeon therefore must often choose to perform a total pancreatectomy or choose to leave gross disease behind.

Challenges in the management of multifocal BD-IPMN

- Confirmation of the diagnosis of multifocal BD-IPMN and excluding main pancreatic duct involvement.
- Assessment of malignancy risk in patients with innumerable cysts.
- Total pancreatectomy versus segmental resection of dominant cyst(s) with postoperative surveillance of residual disease.
- Determination of surveillance method, interval, and duration in patients undergoing observation.

Clinical Management of Multifocal BD-IPMN

The management of patients with multifocal BD-IPMN ranges from complete surgical clearance of all disease via total pancreatectomy, to segmental resection of the dominant cyst with subsequent surveillance of the remnant pancreas (with or without residual disease present), to prolonged surveillance of the entire gland without surgical resection. As is the case for all patients with pancreatic cysts, surgery is recommended for those with symptomatic disease on the basis of a well-established relationship between the presence of symptoms and the risk of high-grade dysplasia and invasive disease [23].

Similarly, surgery is recommended for patients suffering from recurrent episodes of pancreatitis in association with multifocal BD-IPMN—believed to result from obstruction of the main pancreatic duct by viscous mucin. Pancreatitis is typically mild when associated with IPMN but frequently recurrent and sometimes refractory in absence of surgical intervention. The majority of the literature does not indicate an increased risk of malignancy for IPMN-associated with pancreatitis, but this is an association that has been poorly studied [24, 25]. In patients with asymptomatic disease, selection of the appropriate course of management will depend on the characteristics of the dominant cyst(s) and the location of lesions with high-risk stigmata or worrisome features. Clinicians will also have to weigh the patient's fitness to undergo a major pancreatectomy, discuss the relative risks and benefits of surgery against the risks of prolonged surveillance, and take patient preference into account.

Total Pancreatectomy

Total pancreatectomy is the most definitive treatment for multifocal BD-IPMN, and the only curative procedure for patients with diffuse gland involvement. Total pancreatectomy has historically been avoided secondary to prohibitive perioperative morbidity and mortality, obligate pancreatic endocrine and exocrine insufficiency, and attendant poor quality of life. However, elective total pancreatectomy is being increasingly performed, and IPMN is an increasingly common indication [26–28]. A recent single-center review of 100 patients undergoing total pancreatectomy for pancreatic adenocarcinoma demonstrated a significant decrease in perioperative morbidity and mortality over the past four decades [27]. Perioperative morbidity remains common (between 19 and 66%) but is typically minor; perioperative mortality is now reported to be 2% [27, 29]. Once considered "brittle diabetes," it has been demonstrated that postoperative glycemic control after total pancreatectomy for IPMN can be managed with similar success as in patients with type 1 diabetes mellitus. Diabetes-related quality of life is also similar between type 1 diabetics and patients post-total pancreatectomy [30, 31]. Finally, patient-reported overall quality of life after total pancreatectomy approximates or is similar to patients undergoing partial pancreatic resection [32, 33]. Nonetheless, the postoperative management of these patients remains a challenge requiring diligent management; as many as one-half of patients may require readmission within 12 months of total pancreatectomy [34].

Data regarding the outcomes of total pancreatectomy for IPMN—let alone multifocal BD-IPMN—are extremely limited. Two small cohort studies describe individual patient outcomes after total pancreatectomy for IPMN ($n = 5$) [35, 36]. One series of 39 patients with IPMN who underwent elective total pancreatectomy demonstrated an overall five-year survival rate of 43%; five-year survival for noninvasive and invasive disease was 90 and 22%, respectively [34]. Unfortunately, these results were not stratified based on IPMN type (main-duct versus branch-duct). For patients with noninvasive IPMN (multifocality not specified), another series demonstrated a recurrence rate of 0% (0/13) after total pancreatectomy compared to 8% (5/60) after partial pancreatectomy [37].

Which patients with multifocal BD-IPMN should be considered for total pancreatectomy? Those patients with multiple high-risk lesions meeting ICG criteria for resection who are not amenable to segmental resection on an anatomic basis may require total pancreatectomy. An argument for total pancreatectomy can also be made for those with multifocal BD-IPMN and a strong family history of pancreatic cancer. When compared to patients without a family history of pancreatic cancer, those with familial pancreatic cancer are more likely to develop an

IPMN-associated malignancy in the setting of multifocal disease. These patients are also more likely to harbor high-grade dysplasia in sub-centimeter lesions [38].

Partial Pancreatectomy and Postoperative Surveillance

For the majority of patients with multifocal disease and one or more cysts that meet ICG criteria for resection, strong consideration should be given for partial pancreatectomy with postoperative surveillance. The argument for this management strategy is predicated on two facts which are supported by the literature: [1] leaving behind gross residual BD-IPMN does not increase the risk of developing subsequent *malignancy* in the remnant pancreas (provided no lesion with high-risk stigmata or worrisome features is missed), and [2] leaving gross residual disease does create a need for extended postoperative surveillance of the remnant pancreas, as such is required even after R0 resection of unifocal BD-IPMN. Unfortunately, supportive data is limited by the fact that the majority of series compile MD-, mixed-, and BD-IPMN together. However, it is known that the risk of recurrence and subsequent malignancy is higher after resection of MD- and mixed-IPMN compared to BD-IPMN [39]. In interpreting these studies for the purpose of managing patients with multifocal BD-IPMN, it is likely that the risk of recurrence and malignancy in the remnant pancreas is even lower than will be discussed.

Neither the presence of microscopic nor macroscopic disease in the remnant pancreas appears to increase the risk of developing IPMN-associated malignancy. In a study of 191 patients who underwent segmental resection for noninvasive IPMN (subtype not specified), 38 patients were left with disease in the remnant. One patient (1/38, 2.6%) developed invasive disease in the remnant during a mean follow-up of 41 months. Of the 153 patients with complete operative clearance of IPMN, 31 recurred in the remnant, and three developed invasive disease (3/153, 2.0%, mean follow-up 73 months). The authors therefore concluded that in comparison to those with complete operative clearance of IPMN, those with residual disease were not at increased risk for the development of malignancy [40]. Additional evidence is derived from numerous small studies demonstrating a benign course for residual BD-IPMN without high-risk stigmata or worrisome features. In a review of 37 patients with multifocal BD-IPMN, 22 patients had gross disease in the remnant that was observed with serial CT scans. Over a mean follow-up of 40 months, no clinically significant disease progression was identified [41]. Another small study demonstrated similar results, with no morphologic changes in ICG-negative BD-IPMN left in the remnant pancreas after 84 months mean follow-up (n = 16) [19]. Most recently, 33 patients with gross residual BD-IPMN after partial pancreatectomy were observed for a mean of 61 months; mean cyst size increased from 10 mm to 13 mm, and no lesion developed high-risk stigmata or worrisome features [42].

Furthermore, performing a partial pancreatectomy to remove a dominant cyst in a patient with multifocal BD-IPMN does not alter the need for postoperative surveillance. That is to say, nearly all patients undergoing partial pancreatectomy—

even those with complete operative clearance of BD-IPMN—require extended surveillance. It is known that the risk of recurrence is related to the type of IPMN, presence of invasive disease, and status of the surgical margin. The largest study to date demonstrates a 17% overall recurrence rate after resection, inclusive of all subtypes of IPMN [37, 39, 42, 43]. A positive surgical margin impacts the timing and risk of recurrence, but even in the setting of negative margins the reported recurrence rate for all IPMN subtypes is 13–14% [20, 42]. One series of 210 confirmed BD-IPMNs found the overall recurrence risk to be 15%; 85% of recurrences occurred in the remnant pancreas, and 32% were invasive [42]. Thus while segmental resection is not contraindicated in patients with multifocal BD-IPMN, many authors strongly recommend postoperative surveillance of the remnant pancreas. This recommendation applies to patients in whom there is complete operative clearance of BD-IPMN as well as those with residual BD-IPMN in the remnant pancreas [19, 20, 39, 44].

The ideal duration of surveillance is unclear. Some authors have identified recurrence up to 8 years after resection, and therefore recommend indefinite surveillance[43, 44]. As our understanding of the natural history of benign-appearing BD-IPMN evolves, the recommendations for surveillance may change. One study found that in the subset of patients that underwent resection for noninvasive BD-IPMN, recurrence was almost uniformly benign (95%), prompting the authors to suggest that surveillance in that population may be unnecessary [42]. Indeed, the AGA guidelines recommend MRI surveillance of the remnant pancreas every 2 years only if the resection specimen contained high-grade dysplasia or invasive disease; the guidelines recommend against routine surveillance of the remnant when no high-grade dysplasia or invasive disease was identified in the specimen. This is justified by the low risk of malignant recurrence after resection of noninvasive BD-IPMN [15].

Case Continued

Review of the patient's prior work-up revealed discordant findings between the CT and EUS performed at the outside institution. EUS did not confirm the communication between the main pancreatic duct and the many pancreatic cysts identified on CT. More importantly, however, was the EUS-identified mural nodule in the dominant cyst that was not seen on CT. Both findings—but in particular the latter—influence management; therefore a repeat EUS-FNA was performed out our institution.

Repeat EUS identified numerous small pancreatic cysts with clear communication with the main pancreatic duct. A dominant cyst measuring 1.5 × 0.8 cm was identified in the body of the pancreas. No mural nodule was identified in any cyst. The diameter of the main pancreatic duct was measured at 4 mm in the neck, tapering to 2–3 mm in the head and 1–2 mm in the tail. Cyst aspirate was consistent with a mucinous lesion. The results of the repeat EUS-FNA thus confirmed the diagnosis of multifocal BD-IPMN without main pancreatic ductal involvement.

Surveillance Alone

The ICG recommend treatment for patients with multifocal BD-IPMN based on the characteristics of the cyst with the highest risk of malignancy; if no lesion demonstrates high-risk stigmata or worrisome features, then a period of observation may be pursued [8]. This recommendation hinges on the presumption that multifocality is not itself an indicator of high risk. A detailed clinicopathologic review found a majority of multifocal BD-IPMN to be of gastric-foveolar epithelial subtype (less aggressive) with low to intermediate dysplasia, indicating multifocality itself is unlikely to be a manifestation of underlying aggressive tumor biology [16]. Observational data has demonstrated that multifocal disease is found in the same percentage of patients with and without invasive disease; additionally the percentage of patients who develop invasive disease during follow-up does not differ between patients with multifocal versus unifocal BD-IPMN [5]. In a retrospective review of a large cohort of 131 patients with a radiologic and/or pathologic diagnosis of multifocal BD-IPMN, 121 were managed conservatively and 10 underwent surgery. Of the 121 managed conservatively, all were alive and asymptomatic and none required surgery during a mean follow-up of 40 months (range 12–127 months) [22]. Another study directly compared a cohort of multifocal IPMN undergoing surveillance to a similar cohort of unifocal IPMN; cysts meeting ICG high-risk stigmata or worrisome features were excluded (n = 77 vs. n = 54). During follow-up, there was no difference in the progression—cyst growth, development of high-risk stigmata or worrisome features—of the dominant cyst in patients with multifocal disease as compared to the index lesion in patients with unifocal disease [45].

The true risk of developing malignancy while undergoing surveillance for multifocal BD-IPMN remains unknown; few studies address this question directly. However, extrapolating from data regarding unifocal BD-IPMN gives reason to believe this risk is low. A recent large meta-analysis and systematic review of patients with solitary BD-IPMN (20 studies included, n = 2177) found the risk of developing pancreatic malignancy to be 3.7% during follow-up (mean follow-up range 29.3–76.7 months). The rate of death related to pancreatic malignancy was 0.9% [46]. Another study of 211 patients with "low-risk" BD-IPMN found the cumulative risk of cancer at 7 years by Kaplan–Meier estimate to be 1.2% [47].

Prior to beginning a period of observation for what is thought to be low-risk multifocal BD-IPMN, one caveat requires careful consideration by the patient and clinician. Successful nonoperative management of low-risk BD-IPMN is contingent upon the accuracy with which this diagnosis can be clinically made. It has been recently demonstrated that main pancreatic duct involvement is frequently missed by preoperative imaging alone; in 233 patients with suspected isolated BD-IPMN, final pathologic diagnosis revealed main pancreatic duct involvement in 29% of patients [9]. Another study demonstrated that the diagnosis was confirmed in only 64% of suspected patients, and main pancreatic duct involvement was identified in 20% of patients [48]. Confidence in the diagnosis and a thorough investigation of the main pancreatic duct—with EUS if necessary—is therefore a critical component in the successful nonoperative management of these patients.

Finally, the duration of surveillance for low-risk multifocal BD-IPMN also remains unknown. As slow growth in cyst size and steady increase in the number of cysts have been documented over time, some clinicians recommend extended surveillance [49]. One study demonstrated a low but persistent risk of malignancy in low-risk BD-IPMN after 1 year of surveillance [47]. Although the evidence backing any decision regarding duration of surveillance is limited, the AGA guidelines recommend discontinuing surveillance of pancreatic cysts if no change has been noticed over 5 years [15].

Case Conclusion

As the patient's disease was confirmed to be multifocal BD-IPMN without any lesion demonstrating high-risk stigmata or worrisome features for malignancy, surveillance was recommended over resection as a primary management strategy. If the patient develops symptoms, suffers from recurrent pancreatitis, or develops a lesion meeting ICG criteria for resection during follow-up, a discussion of the relative risks and benefits of partial pancreatectomy versus total pancreatectomy will inform further management.

Conclusion

Multifocal disease is common in patients with BD-IPMN. Appropriate management hinges on a patient-by-patient appraisal of the risk of malignancy in the dominant lesion (if present) as well as the remainder of the gland. Currently, data upon which the clinician can make this appraisal is limited; understanding these limitations is of critical importance. As in the management of any patient with suspected BD-IPMN, the first step in management is the identification of the presence or absence of lesions containing high-risk stigmata or worrisome features for malignancy. ICG and AGA guidelines inform the decision of whether or not to operate. Patients with multifocal disease may be at increased risk for occult main pancreatic duct involvement entailing a higher risk of malignancy; observation may be safely pursued in patients with low-risk multifocal disease after a thorough investigation of the main pancreatic duct with MRCP and/or EUS. If an operation is required, then total pancreatectomy or partial pancreatectomy with postoperative surveillance is required.

Take-away Points for the Successful Management of Multifocal BD-IPMN

- Careful evaluation of the main pancreatic duct is necessary to rule out mixed-IPMN. Concordant MRCP and EUS findings are sought.

- The risk of malignancy is related to the features of the highest risk cyst.
- Total pancreatectomy no longer carries prohibitive morbidity and unacceptable quality of life in patients for whom it is indicated or preferred.
- Segmental pancreatectomy is acceptable even if gross residual disease is left behind, but only if none of the remaining lesions have high-risk stigmata or worrisome features for malignancy.
- Observation is a safe management strategy for patients confirmed to have multifocal BD-IPMN without any lesion meeting ICG criteria for resection.

References

1. Zhang XM, Mitchell DG, Dohke M, Holland GA, Parker L. Pancreatic cysts: depiction on single-shot fast spin-echo MR images. Radiology. 2002;223(2):547–53.
2. de Jong K, Nio CY, Hermans JJ, Dijkgraaf MG, Gouma DJ, van Eijck CH, et al. High prevalence of pancreatic cysts detected by screening magnetic resonance imaging examinations. Clin Gastroenterol Hepatol. 2010;8(9):806–11.
3. Correa-Gallego C, Do R, Lafemina J, Gonen M, D'Angelica MI, DeMatteo RP, et al. Predicting dysplasia and invasive carcinoma in intraductal papillary mucinous neoplasms of the pancreas: development of a preoperative nomogram. Ann Surg Oncol. 2013;20(13):4348–55.
4. Shimizu Y, Yamaue H, Maguchi H, Yamao K, Hirono S, Osanai M, et al. Predictors of malignancy in intraductal papillary mucinous neoplasm of the pancreas: analysis of 310 pancreatic resection patients at multiple high-volume centers. Pancreas. 2013;42(5):883–8.
5. Pelaez-Luna M, Chari ST, Smyrk TC, Takahashi N, Clain JE, Levy MJ, et al. Do consensus indications for resection in branch duct intraductal papillary mucinous neoplasm predict malignancy? a study of 147 patients. Am J Gastroenterol. 2007;102(8):1759–64.
6. Schmidt CM, White PB, Waters JA, Yiannoutsos CT, Cummings OW, Baker M, et al. Intraductal papillary mucinous neoplasms: predictors of malignant and invasive pathology. Ann Surg. 2007;246(4):644–51; discussion 51–4.
7. Fritz S, Klauss M, Bergmann F, Hackert T, Hartwig W, Strobel O, et al. Small (Sendai negative) branch-duct IPMNs: not harmless. Ann Surg. 2012;256(2):313–20.
8. Tanaka M, Fernandez-del Castillo C, Adsay V, Chari S, Falconi M, Jang JY, et al. International consensus guidelines 2012 for the management of IPMN and MCN of the pancreas. Pancreatology. 2012;12(3):183–97.
9. Fritz S, Schirren M, Klauss M, Bergmann F, Hackert T, Hartwig W, et al. Clinicopathologic characteristics of patients with resected multifocal intraductal papillary mucinous neoplasm of the pancreas. Surgery. 2012;152(3 Suppl 1):S74–80.
10. Salvia R, Fernandez-del Castillo C, Bassi C, Thayer SP, Falconi M, Mantovani W, et al. Main-duct intraductal papillary mucinous neoplasms of the pancreas: clinical predictors of malignancy and long-term survival following resection. Ann Surg. 2004;239(5):678–85; discussion 85–7.
11. Moriya T, Hashimoto Y, Traverso LW. The duration of symptoms predicts the presence of malignancy in 210 resected cases of pancreatic intraductal papillary mucinous neoplasms. J Gastrointest Surg. 2011;15(5):762–70; discussion 70–1.

12. Ferrone CR, Correa-Gallego C, Warshaw AL, Brugge WR, Forcione DG, Thayer SP, et al. Current trends in pancreatic cystic neoplasms. Arch Surg. 2009;144(5):448–54.
13. Hackert T, Fritz S, Klauss M, Bergmann F, Hinz U, Strobel O, et al. Main-duct intraductal papillary mucinous neoplasm: high cancer risk in duct diameter of 5 to 9 mm. Ann Surg. 2015;262(5):875–80; discussion 80–1.
14. Scheiman JM, Hwang JH, Moayyedi P. American gastroenterological association technical review on the diagnosis and management of asymptomatic neoplastic pancreatic cysts. Gastroenterology. 2015;148(4):824–48, e22.
15. Vege SS, Ziring B, Jain R, Moayyedi P. Clinical Guidelines C. American gastroenterological association institute guideline on the diagnosis and management of asymptomatic neoplastic pancreatic cysts. Gastroenterology. 2015;148(4):819–22.
16. Matthaei H, Norris AL, Tsiatis AC, Olino K, Hong SM, dal Molin M, et al. Clinicopathological characteristics and molecular analyses of multifocal intraductal papillary mucinous neoplasms of the pancreas. Ann Surg. 2012;255(2):326–33.
17. Waters JA, Schmidt CM, Pinchot JW, White PB, Cummings OW, Pitt HA, et al. CT vs MRCP: optimal classification of IPMN type and extent. J Gastrointest Surg. 2008;12 (1):101–9.
18. Rodriguez JR, Salvia R, Crippa S, Warshaw AL, Bassi C, Falconi M, et al. Branch-duct intraductal papillary mucinous neoplasms: observations in 145 patients who underwent resection. Gastroenterology. 2007;133(1):72–9; quiz 309–10.
19. Ohtsuka T, Kono H, Tanabe R, Nagayoshi Y, Mori Y, Sadakari Y, et al. Follow-up study after resection of intraductal papillary mucinous neoplasm of the pancreas; special references to the multifocal lesions and development of ductal carcinoma in the remnant pancreas. Am J Surg. 2012;204(1):44–8.
20. Winner M, Epelboym I, Remotti H, Lee JL, Schrope BA, Chabot JA, et al. Predictors of recurrence in intraductal papillary mucinous neoplasm: experience with 183 pancreatic resections. J Gastrointest Surg. 2013;17(9):1618–26.
21. Raman SP, Kawamoto S, Blackford A, Hruban RH, Lennon AM, Wolfgang CL, et al. Histopathologic findings of multifocal pancreatic intraductal papillary mucinous neoplasms on CT. Am J Roentgenol. 2013;200(3):563–9.
22. Salvia R, Partelli S, Crippa S, Landoni L, Capelli P, Manfredi R, et al. Intraductal papillary mucinous neoplasms of the pancreas with multifocal involvement of branch ducts. Am J Surg. 2009;198(5):709–14.
23. Stark A, Donahue TR, Reber HA, Hines OJ. Pancreatic cyst disease: a review. JAMA. 2016;315(17):1882–93.
24. Morales-Oyarvide V, Mino-Kenudson M, Ferrone CR, Gonzalez-Gonzalez LA, Warshaw AL, Lillemoe KD, et al. Acute pancreatitis in intraductal papillary mucinous neoplasms: a common predictor of malignant intestinal subtype. Surgery. 2015;158(5):1219–25.
25. Venkatesh PG, Navaneethan U, Vege SS. Intraductal papillary mucinous neoplasm and acute pancreatitis. J Clin Gastroenterol. 2011;45(9):755–8.
26. Almond M, Roberts KJ, Hodson J, Sutcliffe R, Marudanayagam R, Isaac J, et al. Changing indications for a total pancreatectomy: perspectives over a quarter of a century. HPB (Oxford). 2015;17(5):416–21.
27. Reddy S, Wolfgang CL, Cameron JL, Eckhauser F, Choti MA, Schulick RD, et al. Total pancreatectomy for pancreatic adenocarcinoma: evaluation of morbidity and long-term survival. Ann Surg. 2009;250(2):282–7.
28. Murphy MM, Knaus WJ 2nd, Ng SC, Hill JS, McPhee JT, Shah SA, et al. Total pancreatectomy: a national study. HPB (Oxford). 2009;11(6):476–82.
29. Stauffer JA, Nguyen JH, Heckman MG, Grewal MS, Dougherty M, Gill KR, et al. Patient outcomes after total pancreatectomy: a single centre contemporary experience. HPB (Oxford). 2009;11(6):483–92.

30. Jamil LH, Chindris AM, Gill KR, Scimeca D, Stauffer JA, Heckman MG, et al. Glycemic control after total pancreatectomy for intraductal papillary mucinous neoplasm: an exploratory study. HPB Surg. 2012;2012:381328.
31. Billings BJ, Christein JD, Harmsen WS, Harrington JR, Chari ST, Que FG, et al. Quality-of-life after total pancreatectomy: is it really that bad on long-term follow-up? J Gastrointest Surg. 2005;9(8):1059–66; discussion 66–7.
32. Epelboym I, Winner M, DiNorcia J, Lee MK, Lee JA, Schrope B, et al. Quality of life in patients after total pancreatectomy is comparable with quality of life in patients who undergo a partial pancreatic resection. J Surg Res. 2014;187(1):189–96.
33. Muller MW, Friess H, Kleeff J, Dahmen R, Wagner M, Hinz U, et al. Is there still a role for total pancreatectomy? Ann Surg. 2007;246(6):966–74; discussion 74–5.
34. Barbier L, Jamal W, Dokmak S, Aussilhou B, Corcos O, Ruszniewski P, et al. Impact of total pancreatectomy: short- and long-term assessment. HPB (Oxford). 2013;15(11):882–92.
35. Inagaki M, Obara M, Kino S, Goto J, Suzuki S, Ishizaki A, et al. Pylorus-preserving total pancreatectomy for an intraductal papillary-mucinous neoplasm of the pancreas. J Hepatobiliarypancreat Surg. 2007;14(3):264–9.
36. Yamaguchi K, Konomi H, Kobayashi K, Ogura Y, Sonoda Y, Kawamoto M, et al. Total pancreatectomy for intraductal papillary-mucinous tumor of the pancreas: reappraisal of total pancreatectomy. Hepatogastroenterology. 2005;52(65):1585–90.
37. Chari ST, Yadav D, Smyrk TC, DiMagno EP, Miller LJ, Raimondo M, et al. Study of recurrence after surgical resection of intraductal papillary mucinous neoplasm of the pancreas. Gastroenterology. 2002;123(5):1500–7.
38. Shi C, Klein AP, Goggins M, Maitra A, Canto M, Ali S, et al. Increased prevalence of precursor lesions in familial pancreatic cancer patients. Clin Cancer Res. 2009;15 (24):7737–43.
39. Passot G, Lebeau R, Hervieu V, Ponchon T, Pilleul F, Adham M. Recurrences after surgical resection of intraductal papillary mucinous neoplasm of the pancreas: a single-center study of recurrence predictive factors. Pancreas. 2012;41(1):137–41.
40. Miller JR, Meyer JE, Waters JA, Al-Haddad M, Dewitt J, Sherman S, et al. Outcome of the pancreatic remnant following segmental pancreatectomy for non-invasive intraductal papillary mucinous neoplasm. HPB (Oxford). 2011;13(11):759–66.
41. Kwon JH, Kim SC, Song KB, Lee JH, Hwang DW, Park KM, et al. Surgical outcomes of multifocal branch duct intraductal papillary mucinous neoplasms of pancreas. Korean J Hepatobiliary Pancreat Surg. 2014;18(4):152–8.
42. Marchegiani G, Mino-Kenudson M, Ferrone CR, Morales-Oyarvide V, Warshaw AL, Lillemoe KD, et al. Patterns of recurrence after resection of IPMN: who, when, and how? Ann Surg. 2015;262(6):1108–14.
43. Ridtitid W, DeWitt JM, Schmidt CM, Roch A, Stuart JS, Sherman S, et al. Management of branch-duct intraductal papillary mucinous neoplasms: a large single-center study to assess predictors of malignancy and long-term outcomes. Gastrointest Endosc. 2016;84(3):436–45.
44. White R, D'Angelica M, Katabi N, Tang L, Klimstra D, Fong Y, et al. Fate of the remnant pancreas after resection of noninvasive intraductal papillary mucinous neoplasm. J Am Coll Surg. 2007;204(5):987–93; discussion 993–5.
45. Rosenblatt R, Dorfman V, Epelboym I, Poneros JM, Sethi A, Lightdale C, et al. Demographic features and natural history of intermediate-risk multifocal versus unifocal intraductal papillary mucinous neoplasms. Pancreas. 2015;44(3):478–83.
46. Crippa S, Capurso G, Camma C, Delle Fave G, Castillo CF, Falconi M. Risk of pancreatic malignancy and mortality in branch-duct IPMNs undergoing surveillance: a systematic review and meta-analysis. Digest Liver Dis. 2016;48(5):473–9.
47. Lawson RD, Hunt GC, Giap AQ, Krinsky ML, Slezak J, Tang RS, et al. Pancreatic cysts suspected to be branch duct intraductal papillary mucinous neoplasm without concerning features have low risk for development of pancreatic cancer. Ann Gastroenterol. 2015;28 (4):487–94.

48. Correa-Gallego C, Ferrone CR, Thayer SP, Wargo JA, Warshaw AL. Fernandez-Del Castillo C. Incidental pancreatic cysts: do we really know what we are watching? Pancreatology. 2010;10(2–3):144–50.
49. Castelli F, Bosetti D, Negrelli R, Di Paola V, Zantedeschi L, Ventriglia A, et al. Multifocal branch-duct intraductal papillary mucinous neoplasms (IPMNs) of the pancreas: magnetic resonance (MR) imaging pattern and evolution over time. Radiol Med. 2013;118(6):917–29.
50. Mori Y, Ohtsuka T, Kono H, Ideno N, Aso T, Nagayoshi Y, et al. Management strategy for multifocal branch duct intraductal papillary mucinous neoplasms of the pancreas. Pancreas. 2012;41(7):1008–12.
51. Fritz S, Klauss M, Bergmann F, Strobel O, Schneider L, Werner J, et al. Pancreatic main-duct involvement in branch-duct IPMNs: an underestimated risk. Ann Surg. 2014;260(5):848–55; discussion 855–6.

Cavernous Transformation of the Portal Vein Requiring Temporary Mesocaval Shunt and Internal Jugular Vein Interposition Graft

29

George Younan, Douglas B. Evans and Kathleen K. Christians

Case Presentation

A 61-year-old woman was referred to our Pancreatic Cancer Program for a second opinion regarding surgical resection of her pancreatic cancer. She originally presented 10 months prior to our consultation with acute on chronic abdominal pain that radiated to the back. A pancreas protocol computed tomography (CT) scan demonstrated a hypoenhancing pancreatic neck mass that caused abutment of the celiac artery (CA) at its bifurcation into the splenic artery (SA) and the common hepatic artery (CHA) (Fig. 29.1a, b). The superior mesenteric vein–portal vein–splenic vein confluence (SMV-PV-SVV) was occluded, with resultant cavernous transformation of the PV (Fig. 29.1c) The bile duct was not obstructed. Serum level of carbohydrate antigen 19-9 (CA 19-9) at the time of diagnosis was 216 units/mL in the setting of a normal bilirubin. An endoscopic ultrasound (EUS) and fine-needle aspiration (FNA) of the tumor mass was positive for pancreatic adenocarcinoma. The patient sought care locally and the tumor was deemed unresectable. She subsequently received six cycles of Gemcitabine/nab-paclitaxel with minor treatment-associated side effects, followed by 50.4 Gy of Gemcitabine-based

G. Younan · K.K. Christians (✉)
Department of Surgery, Medical College of Wisconsin/Froedtert Hospital,
9200 W Wisconsin Ave, 53226 Milwaukee, WI, USA
e-mail: kchristi@mcw.edu

G. Younan
e-mail: grg.younan@gmail.com

D.B. Evans
Department of Surgery, Medical College of Wisconsin/Froedtert Hospital,
9200 W Wisconsin Ave, Suite 3510, 53226 Milwaukee, WI, USA

T.M. Pawlik et al. (eds.), *Case-Based Lessons in the Management of Complex Hepato-Pancreato-Biliary Surgery*, DOI 10.1007/978-3-319-50868-9_29

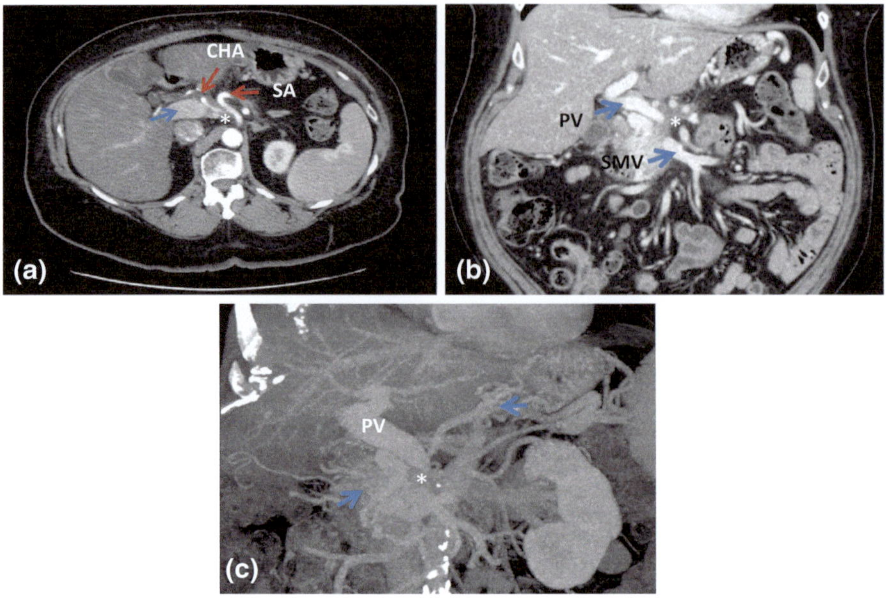

Fig. 29.1 **a–c**—**a** demonstrates a CT axial image of a hypoechoic tumor (*) at the bifurcation of the celiac artery into the splenic artery (SA) and common hepatic artery (CHA; *red arrows*). The *blue arrow marks* the portal vein. **b** is a computed tomography coronal image showing the portal vein (cephalad *blue arrow*) occluded by the tumor (*) and reconstituting into the superior mesenteric vein (*lower blue arrow*) and its branches caudal to the region of tumor involvement. **c** is a coronal CT venous reconstruction image showing cavernous transformation of the portal vein with associated venous collaterals (*blue arrows*). The *asterisk marks* the tumor location

chemoradiation. Restaging imaging showed stable disease and CA 19-9 level dropped to 33 units/mL. The tumor was still deemed unresectable, and thus she was referred to our program for a second opinion 8 weeks post-chemoradiation.

Diagnosis and Preoperative Management

Patients with newly diagnosed pancreatic cancer are treated by a multidisciplinary team with a combination of chemotherapy, radiation, and surgical resection (when possible) [1–3]. Venous resection and reconstruction during pancreatectomy are now considered standard of care for pancreatic cancer, as supported by the consensus statement published by the American Hepato-Pancreato-Biliary Association/Society of Surgical Oncology in 2009 [4]. Venous resection during pancreatectomy is done when the only obstacle for a complete R0 resection of the tumor is the inability to separate the tumor from the attached venous segment, presuming there is an adequate proximal and distal target available for reconstruction [5]. Although consensus statements such as the one referenced above imply that venous resection and reconstruction (at the time of pancreaticoduodenectomy or total pancreatectomy) has become somewhat routine, we would argue that such operations are of significant complexity, and require years of experience to both be performed safely and to result in a complete gross resection of the tumor.

The multimodality management of pancreatic cancer is founded on the initial staging of the tumor, which is based on anatomic tumor–vessel relationships. We have developed a CT-based staging algorithm for pancreatic cancer whereby we classify tumors as resectable, borderline resectable, locally advanced, or metastatic [2, 6, 7]. Tumors with more than 50% abutment of the SMV-PV are considered borderline resectable. Therefore, patients who require mesocaval shunting and segmental venous resection with interposition grafting have, by definition, borderline resectable disease at a minimum.

Experienced interventional endoscopists are a key part of the multidisciplinary team, as a tissue diagnosis is required prior to initiation of neoadjuvant therapy. EUS/FNA of the tumor is performed with an on-site cytopathologist specializing in pancreatic cytopathology. This facilitates a prompt, usually same setting, tissue diagnosis. Durable metallic endobiliary stents are inserted in patients with biliary obstruction prior to the initiation of neoadjuvant therapy [11].

After diagnosis and accurate staging, patients with borderline resectable pancreatic cancer receive neoadjuvant therapy. National guidelines support the use of neoadjuvant chemotherapy with/without chemoradiation in patients with borderline resectable disease [1, 8, 9]. Neoadjuvant therapy has been shown to increase the rate of R0 resections and reduce the number of patients with positive lymph nodes, both of which positively impact survival [8]. Neoadjuvant therapy also allows clinicians a window of time to assess tumor biology; thus, only patients with stable or responding disease at restaging are offered surgical resection directed at the primary tumor [1, 10].

Stage-specific treatment plans are assigned to every patient treated in our pancreatic cancer program. Serial restaging and assessment of treatment response are done at regular intervals following completion of each modality of therapy and again prior to surgery. Restaging includes assessment of three parameters: clinical, biochemical, and radiographic response to neoadjuvant treatment [2, 9]. Clinical response is based on performance status and symptoms (ECOG $\leq$ 1, improvement in pain). The biochemical response is based on serum tumor markers; we usually obtain a serum level of CA 19-9 at diagnosis once the bilirubin level has normalized, and then obtain serial levels at every restaging evaluation. Disease progression should be suspected when the CA 19-9 increases even in the absence of clinical or radiographic signs of disease progression. Our group and others have published the positive prognostic impact of a decline in Ca 19-9 to normal levels following neoadjuvant therapy [12, 13]. The radiographic response is also assessed at the end of every phase of the neoadjuvant therapy. This assessment is made accurate by the inclusion of experienced diagnostic radiologists and a weekly multidisciplinary pancreas tumor conference. Preoperative restaging scans are obtained no greater than 30 days prior to surgery, and normally within 2 weeks of the date of operation. Tumor–vessel relationships and the plan for vascular resection, if needed, are assessed and discussed one final time before surgery. It is important to note that the tumor–vessel relationship usually remains unchanged even when the primary tumor responds to therapy (gets smaller). Based on these clinical, biochemical, and radiographic assessments, patients are classified as having had a response to treatment, stable disease, or progressive disease [2, 7].

All patients with cavernous transformation of the PV or partial/complete occlusion of the PV or SMV are placed on a prophylactic dose of low-molecular-weight heparin at the time of diagnosis. Patients are medically supported (hydration, growth factor support, antiemetics, nutrition) throughout their neoadjuvant therapy by our multidisciplinary team. A surgical clinic visit is usually scheduled within 2 weeks of surgery to review restaging studies, to obtain medical clearance, and to develop a detailed operative plan. A consent form is signed for diagnostic laparoscopy, pancreatectomy, and possible internal jugular and saphenous vein harvest.

The patient reported herein was seen as a second opinion after completing preoperative systemic chemotherapy and chemoradiation for what was believed to be an unresectable tumor. When referred to our program, initial imaging and all restaging scans were reviewed. The tumor–vessel relationships were stable (unchanged) and there was total occlusion of the SMV-PV confluence with cavernous transformation of the PV forming collaterals around the head and neck of the pancreas. Venous reconstruction was possible due to the presence of proximal (PV) and distal (SMV) targets for segmental venous reconstruction. The pancreatic neck tumor was abutting the celiac axis bifurcation at the level of the SA and the CHA and the SA was encased. Her performance status was adequate (ECOG 0/1), and she was not requiring pain medication.

CA 19-9 had dropped from 216 to 33 units/mL. Consensus review was a favorable clinical and biochemical response and stable imaging findings. She was therefore consented for total pancreatectomy, en bloc splenectomy, and mesocaval shunting utilizing internal jugular vein.

Surgical Management

Patients receive prophylactic antibiotics on induction. Their power port is accessed and we do not usually utilize additional central venous access, in order to preserve the internal jugular veins if a mesocaval shunt/interposition graft is required. The abdomen, left neck, and the groin are widely prepped and a detailed procedure "time out" is completed. A diagnostic laparoscopy is routinely performed to rule out radiologically occult metastatic disease [14]. Pancreatectomy is completed as we have previously published [15]. Cavernous transformation of the PV is caused by gradual occlusion of the PV. This occlusion results in the development of multiple large venous collaterals, allowing for mesenteric venous return to the liver by bypassing the obstruction. This poses a significant risk of hemorrhage if the portal dissection were to be attempted without decompression of the venous collaterals [16]. We have used mesocaval shunting during pancreatectomy to safely address the

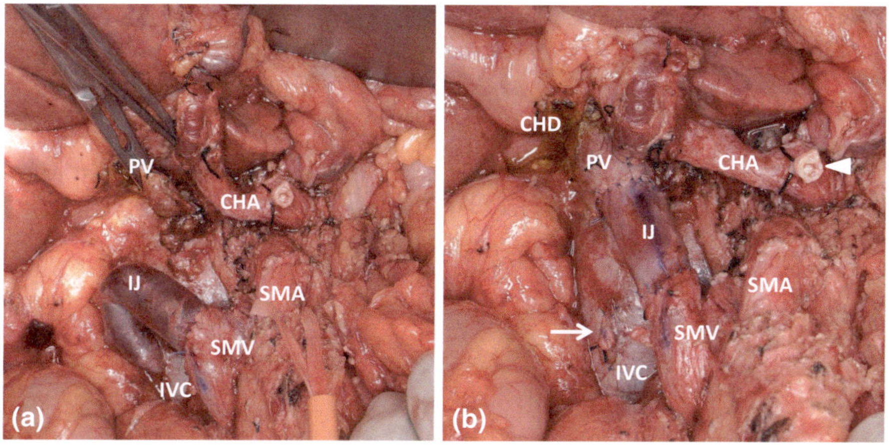

Fig. 29.2 **a, b—a** is an intraoperative photograph illustrating the internal jugular vein graft functioning as a mesocaval shunt between the superior mesenteric vein and inferior vena cava. **b** is an intraoperative photograph illustrating the anatomy once the cephalad end of the IJ interposition graft has been disconnected from the IVC, shortened, and sewn end-to-end to the PV restoring mesenteric venous flow to the liver. The *white arrow points* to the site of the temporary IJ-IVC anastomosis and the *arrowhead marks* the splenic artery stump. *SMA* superior mesenteric artery, *SMV* superior mesenteric vein, *PV* portal vein, *IVC* inferior vena cava, *CHA* common hepatic artery, *CHD* common hepatic duct

issue of large portal venous collaterals in the setting of an occluded PV [16, 17]. The SMV is exposed early in the operation, inferior to the neck of the pancreas or caudal to the area of tumor encasement; an area usually free of venous collaterals (Fig. 29.2a) The middle colic vein is usually divided to allow adequate exposure of the SMV. The anterior surface of the IVC is cleared caudal to the renal veins when performing a generous Kocher maneuver. Additional dissection at the root of the mesentery allows identification of the superior mesenteric artery (SMA) as well as the jejunal and ileal branches of the SMV (if the SMV is being approached cephalad to its bifurcation). Exposure of the SMA and SMV caudal to the tumor is critically important. An artery (SMA)-first approach, which involves separation of the pancreatic head and uncinate process from the SMA (before the SMV-PV), is often performed, even if not complete, as it will facilitate exposure of the IVC from the root of mesentery and allow for a bit more room to perform the SMV and the IVC anastomoses [18, 19]. The jejunal branch of the SMV usually courses posterior to the SMA [20]. An anterior jejunal branch allows easier access to the SMV, however it is associated with multiple venous anomalies [5]. When needed for oncologic and/or technical reasons, one of the first-order branches of the SMV may often be ligated without the need for reconstruction. This is acceptable if the caliber of the remaining ileal branch is suitable for reconstruction (at least 1.5 times the diameter of the SMA on the axial images of the CT scan). While anastomosis to the ileal branch of the SMV is quite reliable (as compared to the common trunk of the SMV), anastomosis to the jejunal branch is quite difficult, and should only be attempted in very rare situations by the most experienced surgeons [20]. Bowel ischemia and necrosis will occur if both the ileal and the jejunal branches of the SMV are divided [15].

After the distal target on the SMV is dissected and prepared and the IVC is exposed, one is then ready to divert venous outflow from the mid-gut with a mesocaval shunt. If total pancreatectomy is to be performed, we would also include early splenic artery ligation (or splenic artery embolization preoperatively if access to the splenic artery was anticipated to be difficult) and take down of short gastric vessels to eliminate all arterial blood flow to the pancreas and spleen. Eliminating splenic artery and short gastric arterial inflow, combined with a mesocaval shunt to decompress outflow, will result in optimal decompression of the large collaterals comprising the cavernous transformation of the PV. The left internal jugular (IJ) vein is harvested and an end SMV-to-side anterior IVC anastomosis is completed utilizing 5-0 or 6-0 prolene suture. This is usually done with a side-biting Satinsky clamp on the IVC. The SMV is then divided caudal to the site of tumor encasement, and an anastomosis is completed from the IJ graft to the SMV (Fig. 29.2b) This shunt effectively allows complete diversion of all venous return from the mid-gut into the IVC, and allows for a safe portal dissection, which is the next step to be performed in the operation. The remainder of the pancreatectomy is completed as we have previously described [15]. After a modest antrectomy and division of the bile duct and pancreas, the suprapancreatic PV is divided and the specimen is removed. Systemic heparinization and inflow occlusion of the SMA with a Rommel tourniquet is used for the final step in venous reconstruction. The IJ graft is then disconnected from the IVC, shortened to an adequate length, and an anastomosis is created between the end of the IJ and the PV, reestablishing forward flow from the SMV to the PV. Appropriate contour and size match of the interposition graft is the aim of this reconstruction, which decreases the risk of turbulent blood flow and graft thrombosis [21]. The PV anastomosis is performed with interrupted 6-0 prolene suture [15]. In this particular patient, a total pancreatectomy was done due to the complexity of arterial abutment/encasement and concomitant cavernous transformation of the PV.

Postoperative Care

The postoperative management of pancreatectomy patients in our institution is standardized. Most pancreaticoduodenectomy patients are admitted to the surgical floor (barring prohibitive comorbid conditions which increase risk for an early cardiovascular complication), whereas total pancreatectomy patients are admitted overnight to the surgical intensive care unit for close glucose monitoring. A multimodal pain regimen is used, which consists of patient-controlled analgesia, scheduled intravenous Tylenol, Toradol, and Gabapentin. Nasogastric tubes are removed two or three days postoperatively and diet is advanced thereafter as tolerated. Promotility agents are used as needed for delayed gastric emptying, most often in a prophylactic fashion. Many of our patients receive a feeding jejunostomy tube for enteral feeding support, which is started two days postoperatively and continued until adequate oral intake is met. Using this pathway we have achieved an average length of stay of seven to eight days.

Venous graft thrombosis remains a very rare occurrence in the acute postoperative period. In fact, we have not had a single patient experience this acute early complication in our cumulative experience at the Medical College of Wisconsin. Narrowing of the conduit can, however, be seen over time. Our 1-year patency rate for such segmental interposition grafts is 90% [21]. With the absence of guidelines on pharmacological management of venous conduits, we have developed our own standard protocol. which includes 300 mg of aspirin per rectum in the post-anesthesia care unit as well as prophylactic dose heparin. Patients are then switched to 325 mg of oral enteric-coated aspirin once they tolerate oral intake, and are discharged on that regimen. We selectively use once-a-day low-molecular-weight heparin injections on discharge for 2–4 weeks postoperatively.

Clinical Pearls and Pitfalls

- High-quality, triple-phase CT imaging followed by multidisciplinary review accurately determines the patient's stage and treatment course (hopefully as part of a clinical trial) including whether surgical resection will be possible; tumor–vessel relationships in pancreatic surgery usually do not change with treatment.
- In the setting of cavernous transformation of the portal vein, every attempt should be made to divert mesenteric flow from portal venous collaterals prior to portal dissection; diversion includes splenic and short gastric artery ligation, as well as mesocaval shunting. One should not attempt the portal dissection in this setting in the absence of maximal mesenteric venous diversion.
- An SMA first approach when possible, and in experienced hands, facilitates the more complex venous resection/reconstruction.
- Postoperative care is standardized across inpatient services, helping to facilitate patient care and minimize instances of failure to rescue.

References

1. Christians KK, Heimler JW, George B, Ritch PS, Erickson BA, Johnston F, et al. Survival of patients with resectable pancreatic cancer who received neoadjuvant therapy. Surgery. 2016;159(3):893–900. PubMed PMID: 26602840.
2. Evans DB, George B, Tsai S. Non-metastatic Pancreatic Cancer: Resectable, borderline resectable, and locally advanced-definitions of tncreasing importance for the optimal delivery of multimodality therapy. Ann Surg Oncol. 2015;22(11):3409–13. PubMed PMID: 26122369.

3. Evans DB, Crane CH, Charnsangavej C, Wolff RA. The added value of multidisciplinary care for patients with pancreatic cancer. Ann Surg Oncol. 2008;15(8):2078–80. PubMed PMID: 18546044. Pubmed Central PMCID: 2491408.
4. Evans DB, Farnell MB, Lillemoe KD, Vollmer C Jr, Strasberg SM, Schulick RD. Surgical treatment of resectable and borderline resectable pancreas cancer: expert consensus statement. Ann Surg Oncol. 2009;16(7):1736–44. PubMed PMID: 19387741.
5. Christians KK, Lal A, Pappas S, Quebbeman E, Evans DB. Portal vein resection. Surg Clin North Am. 2010;90(2):309–22. PubMed PMID: 20362788.
6. Appel BL, Tolat P, Evans DB, Tsai S. Current staging systems for pancreatic cancer. Cancer journal. 2012;18(6):539-49. PubMed PMID: 23187840.
7. Fathi A, Christians KK, George B, Ritch PS, Erickson BA, Tolat P, et al. Neoadjuvant therapy for localized pancreatic cancer: guiding principles. Journal of gastrointestinal oncology. 2015;6(4):418–29. PubMed PMID: 26261728. Pubmed Central PMCID: 4502155.
8. Christians KK, Tsai S, Mahmoud A, Ritch P, Thomas JP, Wiebe L, et al. Neoadjuvant FOLFIRINOX for borderline resectable pancreas cancer: a new treatment paradigm? Oncologist. 2014;19(3):266–74. PubMed PMID: 24569947. Pubmed Central PMCID: 3958454.
9. Evans DB, Ritch PS, Erickson BA. Neoadjuvant therapy for localized pancreatic cancer: support is growing? Ann Surg. 2015;261(1):18–20. PubMed PMID: 25599323.
10. Miura JT, Krepline AN, George B, Ritch PS, Erickson BA, Johnston FM, et al. Use of neoadjuvant therapy in patients 75 years of age and older with pancreatic cancer. Surgery. 2015;158(6):1545–55. PubMed PMID: 26243342.
11. Aadam AA, Evans DB, Khan A, Oh Y, Dua K. Efficacy and safety of self-expandable metal stents for biliary decompression in patients receiving neoadjuvant therapy for pancreatic cancer: a prospective study. Gastrointest Endosc. 2012;76(1):67–75. PubMed PMID: 22483859.
12. Katz MH, Varadhachary GR, Fleming JB, Wolff RA, Lee JE, Pisters PW, et al. Serum CA 19-9 as a marker of resectability and survival in patients with potentially resectable pancreatic cancer treated with neoadjuvant chemoradiation. Ann Surg oncology. 2010;17(7):1794-801. PubMed PMID: 20162463. Pubmed Central PMCID: 2889288.
13. Aldakkak M, Christians KK, Krepline AN, George B, Ritch PS, Erickson BA, et al. Pre-treatment carbohydrate antigen 19-9 does not predict the response to neoadjuvant therapy in patients with localized pancreatic cancer. HPB (Oxford). 2015;17(10):942–52. PubMed PMID: 26255895. Pubmed Central PMCID: 4571763.
14. Jayakrishnan TT, Nadeem H, Groeschl RT, George B, Thomas JP, Ritch PS, et al. Diagnostic laparoscopy should be performed before definitive resection for pancreatic cancer: a financial argument. HPB (Oxford). 2015;17(2):131–9. PubMed PMID: 25123702. Pubmed Central PMCID: 4299387.
15. Christians KK, Tsai S, Tolat PP, Evans DB. Critical steps for pancreaticoduodenectomy in the setting of pancreatic adenocarcinoma. J Surg Oncol. 2013;107(1):33–8. PubMed PMID: 22711619.
16. Christians KK, Riggle K, Keim R, Pappas S, Tsai S, Ritch P, et al. Distal splenorenal and temporary mesocaval shunting at the time of pancreatectomy for cancer: initial experience from the Medical College of Wisconsin. Surgery. 2013;154(1):123–31. PubMed PMID: 23305596.
17. Pilgrim CH, Tsai S, Evans DB, Christians KK. Mesocaval shunting: a novel technique to facilitate venous resection and reconstruction and enhance exposure of the superior mesenteric and celiac arteries during pancreaticoduodenectomy. J Am Coll Surg. 2013;217(3):e17–20. PubMed PMID: 23816382.
18. Leach SD, Davidson BS, Ames FC, Evans DB. Alternative method for exposure of the retropancreatic mesenteric vasculature during total pancreatectomy. J Surg Oncol. 1996;61(2):163–5. PubMed PMID: 8606551.

19. Younan G, Chimukangara M, Tsai S, Evans DB, Christians KK. Replaced gastroduodenal artery: Added benefit of the "artery first" approach during pancreaticoduodenectomy-A case report. Int J Surg Case Rep. 2016;13(23):93–7. PubMed PMID: 27124718.
20. Katz MH, Fleming JB, Pisters PW, Lee JE, Evans DB. Anatomy of the superior mesenteric vein with special reference to the surgical management of first-order branch involvement at pancreaticoduodenectomy. Ann Surg. 2008;248(6):1098–102. PubMed PMID: 19092356.
21. Krepline AN, Christians KK, Duelge K, Mahmoud A, Ritch P, George B, et al. Patency rates of portal vein/superior mesenteric vein reconstruction after pancreatectomy for pancreatic cancer. J Gastrointest Surg. 2014;18(11):2016–25. PubMed PMID: 25227638.

Chronic Pancreatitis: Puestow and Frey Procedures

30

Alex Chang and Daniel Abbott

Introduction

Chronic pancreatitis (CP) leads to inflammation and irreversible fibrotic obliteration of pancreatic parenchyma associated with progressive loss of endocrine function, exocrine function, and pain [1]. It can be difficult to diagnose early, as there is no diagnostic test with reliable predictive value. Thus, there are multiple diagnostic criteria and classifications of chronic pancreatitis, which make epidemiological comparisons for clinical and research purposes difficult [2]. In Western nations, the prevalence of chronic pancreatitis is reported to be between 28 per 100,000 with an incidence of 7 per 100,000; a much higher incidence of up to 14 per 100,000 has been reported in Asian nations. The mean age at diagnosis of CP is 46 years, with subsequent lower survival than in the background population—a standardized mortality ratio of 3.6 [3]. Additionally, the socioeconomic impact of chronic pancreatitis is great, due to the degree of disability as a result of recurring hospital admissions and loss of productivity [4]. A small risk of malignant transformation is also possible, although this increased risk is age- and duration-dependent and varies considerably between studies [2].

A. Chang
Department of Surgery, University of Cincinnati, 231 Albert Sabin Way, ML0558, Cincinnati, OH 45267, USA
e-mail: changax@ucmail.uc.edu

D. Abbott (✉)
University of Wisconsin School of Medicine and Public Health, 600 Highland Ave, K4/742, Madison, WI 53792, USA
e-mail: abbott@surgery.wisc.edu

T.M. Pawlik et al. (eds.), *Case-Based Lessons in the Management of Complex Hepato-Pancreato-Biliary Surgery*, DOI 10.1007/978-3-319-50868-9_30

Etiology

Chronic pancreatitis is attributed to a number of etiologic factors commonly described using the TIGAR-O acronym: Toxic-metabolic (including alcohol and tobacco), Idiopathic, Genetic (including PSS1, CFTR, and SPINK1 mutations), Autoimmune, Recurrent severe acute pancreatitis, and Obstruction (including pancreas divisum, strictures, neoplasms, and sphincter of Oddi dysfunction; see Table 30.1). In Western nations, long-standing alcohol abuse accounts for 65–85% of cases.

Table 30.1 TIGAR-O classification of chronic pancreatitis risk factors and etiology

Toxic-metabolic
• Alcohol consumption
• Tobacco smoking
• Hypercalcemia
• Hyperlipidemia
• Chronic renal failure
• Medication and toxins (organotin compounds)
Idiopathic
• Tropical calcific pancreatitis
• Fibrocalculous pancreatitis
• Other
Genetic
• Cationic trypsinogen (R122H)
• CFTR mutation
• SPINK1 mutation
• α1-antitrypsinogen mutation
Autoimmune
• Autoimmune pancreatitis
• Sjogren's syndrome
• Inflammatory bowel disease
• Primary biliary cirrhosis
Recurrent severe acute pancreatitis
• Postcomplicated severe acute pancreatitis
• Postradiation pancreatitis
• Ischemic pancreatitis
Obstructive
• Pancreatic divisum
• Sphincter of Oddi dysfunction
• Duct obstruction
• Periamullary and periductal tumors
• Pancreatic duct structures

Pathophysiology

Initiation of pancreatic injury differs between patients, however most follow common pathways, which include occlusion of ducts by external compression or protein plugs, leading to ductal and parenchymal hypertension, with resultant inflammation and fibrosis [5]. Often the onset of chronic pancreatitis is attributed to residual morphological pancreatic changes in the pancreas following an episode of acute pancreatitis, leading to alterations in the normal flow of pancreatic secretions [6]. Pancreatic duct pressures can rise from 7–15 mm Hg in healthy individuals to 80 mm Hg in severe cases. Ductal obstruction can occur in side branches of the pancreatic duct or at any point along the main duct. Ductal hypertension is attributed to ongoing exocrine secretion from pancreatic acini in conjunction with surrounding inelastic pancreatic parenchyma and capsule [7].

It has been long believed that relief of ductal hypertension by decompression of a dilated duct will relieve chronic pancreatitis-related pain [8]. However, the pathogenesis of pain, the major feature of chronic pancreatitis, is incompletely understood. Lack of any single successful therapeutic modality for CP pain suggests multifactorial and collusive mechanisms. Pancreatic sensation is derived from retroperitoneal autonomic nerves synapsing at the celiac ganglia, forming a neural network embedded in the periaortic fatty areolar tissue near the celiac and superior mesenteric arteries. Chronic pain levels correlate with perineural fibrosis and inflammatory cell infiltrates [9]. Increases in neural tissue, as well as hypertrophy from inflammatory infiltration, leave focal disruptions in the perineural sheath (which protects the nerves from inflammatory injury). Chronic stimulation of nociceptors with a concomitant decreased nerve stimulation threshold enhances responsiveness of nerves to stimuli and thus, increased pain.

Other mechanisms of pancreas injury include pancreatic ischemia, duct disruption, autodigestion by pancreatic enzymes, reactive oxygen species and oxidative injury, and activation of pancreatic stellate cells leading to fibrosis. Progressive loss of exocrine and endocrine function is often accompanied by unrelenting or recurrent pain requiring medical and/or surgical intervention. It is often observed that progressive cases of chronic pancreatitis may "burn out" after many decades, however this phenomenon is unpredictable and pain often persists despite loss of function.

Marseille, Cambridge, and Rosemont Classification Systems

An international consensus classification for inflammatory disease of the pancreas in use since 1963, termed the Marseille classification [10], groups pancreatitis patients into four main groups: (1) acute; (2) relapsing acute with no residual glandular injury; (3) chronic relapsing, characterized by pain and acute exacerbations; and (4) chronic, with progressive functional damage to the gland. Since that time, new technology has made anatomical and radiological determinations available to provide more sophisticated classification schemes [11].

While pancreatogram findings do not always correlate to disease pathology or patient symptoms, the popular Cambridge classification, first introduced in 1984, employs ERCP, ultrasound, or CT imaging to classify the severity of disease. Changes in MPD caliber and parenchymal changes (summarized in Table 30.2) stratify patients from normal to severe (Cambridge class III) pancreatitis [12].

Since the 1980s, endoscopic ultrasound has become an increasingly valuable tool to visualize changes in pancreatic parenchyma and duct, however the interobserver agreement for the diagnosis of chronic pancreatitis was highly variable. Previous diagnostic criteria typically required the presence of three to five features out of nine, and equally weighted endoscopic findings consistent with chronic pancreatitis [13]. Three or more endoscopic features have 83% sensitivity and 80% specificity for the diagnosis of chronic pancreatitis, with predictably higher specificity with more stringent requirements [14, 15]. A consensus statement introduced in 2009 termed the "Rosemont criteria" proposed standardized definitions and criteria for the diagnosis of chronic pancreatitis by endoscopic ultrasound (summarized in Table 30.3) [16].

Table 30.2 Cambridge classification for chronic pancreatitis

Cambridge class 0	
Severity	Equivocal
ERCP	Less than three abnormal side branches
Imaging	MPD 2–4 mm, gland 1–2 × normal size
Cambridge class I	
Severity	Mild
ERCP	3 or more abnormal side branches
Imaging	Cavities < 10 mm, MPD irregularity, focal acute necrosis, parenchymal heterogeneity, hyperechoic duct wall, contour irregularity of the gland
Cambridge class II	
Severity	Moderate
ERCP	More than 3 abnormal side branches and abnomal MPD
Imaging	Cavities < 10 mm, MPD irregularity, focal acute necrosis, parenchymal heterogeneity, hyperechoic duct wall, contour irregularity of the gland
Cambridge class III	
Severity	Severe
ERCP	>3 abnormal side branches + abnomal MPD + at least one additional finding (large cavity > 10 mm, intraductal filling defect, duct obstruction, or ductal dilation)
Imaging	Cavities < 10 mm, MPD irregularity, focal acute necrosis, parenchymal heterogeneity, hyperechoic duct wall, contour irregularity of the gland + at least one additional finding (large cavity > 10 mm, intraductal filling defect, duct obstruction, or ductal dilation, calcifications, organ invasion)

Table 30.3 Rosemont criteria for diagnosis of chronic pancreatitis

Rosemont endoscopic features of CP		
Major A features	Hyperechoic foci ($\geq$2 mm)	
	MPD calculi	
Major B features	Lobularity or honeycombing of parenchyma	
Minor features	Anechoic Cysts	
	Hyperechoic stranding ($\geq$3 mm)	
	Hyperechoic foci ($\geq$2 mm)	
	Dilated duct ($\geq$3.5 mm in body, $\geq$1.5 in tail)	
	Irregular MPD contour	
	$\geq$3 dilated side branches ($\geq$1 mm)	
	Hyperechoic MPD wall	
Rosemont criteria for diagnosis of CP		
Consistent with CP	1 major A feature	AND $\geq$ 3 minor features
	1 major A feature	AND 1 major B feature
	2 major A features alone	
Suggestive of CP	1 major A feature	AND < 3 minor features
	1 major B feature	AND $\geq$ 3 minor features
	$\geq$5 minor features	
Indeterminate for CP	3–4 minor features alone	
	major B feature alone	AND < 3 minor features
Normal	1 or 2 minor features	

Case Presentation: Surgical Treatment of Chronic Pancreatitis

A 42-year-old gentleman with a history of long-standing alcohol abuse and gallstone pancreatitis 2 years prior presents to the emergency department with complaints of abdominal pain. He reports his symptoms were provoked by alcohol consumption 1 day prior, and radiates bilaterally from the epigastric region to the spine. He also endorses nausea and anorexia. Review of his medical history reveals two prior episodes of self-limited abdominal pain in the current year, with no other contributing medical, surgical, or social comorbidities.

Differential Diagnosis

A broad differential diagnosis for the case of acute or recurrent epigastric abdominal pain includes, but is not limited to, the following:

- Pancreatitis
- Peptic ulcer disease

- Gastritis
- Intestinal obstruction
- Mesenteric ischemia
- Cardiac and pleural sources

In the United States, alcohol abuse continues to be the prominent risk factor for chronic pancreatitis, responsible for 45% of cases [17]. Chronic pancreatitis attributed to alcohol consumption usually presents in the fourth to sixth decades of life, and correlates with cumulative alcohol intake. While the patient in this case presented with a history of heavy alcohol intake, there is no safe level of alcohol consumption with regard to risk of chronic pancreatitis [18, 19]. A minority of alcoholics will develop alcoholic chronic pancreatitis, suggesting a genetic predisposition or other susceptibility in some patients [20].

A majority of cases of chronic pancreatitis not related to alcohol use are idiopathic. The presentation of idiopathic chronic pancreatitis has a bimodal age distribution, with an early onset group presenting during adolescence, and another late-onset group occurring at a mean age of 56 years. Pain is almost uniformly the first symptom in early onset chronic pancreatitis. Some cases can be attributed to an initial episode of severe acute pancreatitis, sometimes called the sentinel acute pancreatitis event, or SAPE. Late-onset disease is commonly associated with pain, however episodes of severe pain are less frequently reported [21].

The natural history of pain in all types of pancreatitis improves in severity and frequency in approximately two-thirds of cases. In a minority of cases, pain becomes worse over time. The course of progression in alcoholic chronic pancreatitis is reciprocal to the degree of alcohol abstinence. The pattern of recurrent pain also appears to follow two distinct patterns. In its early course, symptoms are akin to recurrent episodes of acute pancreatitis, with prolonged periods of absence between episodes. In later stages, many develop a "smoldering" pancreatitis, with episodes of exacerbation and associated endocrine dysfunction [22]. A sizable number of cases reach a terminal "burn out" of chronic pancreatitis, in which pain is improved or absent, and exocrine/endocrine deterioration comes to a halt [23, 24].

Long-standing chronic pancreatitis often leads to local complications responsible for significant additional morbidity. Intraductal calculi (pancreatolithiasis) and ductal stenosis are common and lead to duct dilation. Splenic vein thrombosis can occur due to its close proximity to the inflammatory process, and leads to hypersplenism and gastric varices. Pancreatic pseudocysts are common and frequently cause pain, portal vein compression, and sometimes even intestinal obstruction. Rarely, erosion into major vascular structures can lead to life-threatening hemorrhage. The risk of malignancy arising from a background of chronic pancreatitis is elevated four to six times that of the general population; however, the absolute risk is still low and may not warrant additional screening. In some cases, ductal dilation is accompanied by fibrosis and phlegmon of the pancreatic head. This can be concerning not only due to mass effect on surrounding structures, but also in shrouding the diagnosis of pancreatic head malignancies.

Technical Pearls

- Identifying a dilated pancreatic duct with a small-gauge needle and syringe, with or without ultrasound guidance, can help minimize blind attempts in finding the duct, and minimizing chances of unnecessary trauma to the pancreas.
- Ensure the Roux limb is at least 40 to 60 cm in length, to minimize the risk of gastrointestinal content reflux into the pancreaticojejunostomy.
- When performing a Frey procedure, ensure that the SMV and portal vein are clearly identified so as to minimize the risk of inadvertent injury.
- When performing a Frey procedure, perform a full Kocher maneuver to appreciate the thickness of the pancreatic head, and minimize the chance of full-thickness debridement.

Workup

Eliciting a history of recurrent abdominal pain, anorexia, and nausea which is exacerbated by food intake should provoke an investigation toward pancreatitis as a possible diagnosis. Patients may also exhibit hyperglycemia, jaundice, steatorrhea, weight loss, and endorse a history of heavy alcohol use. Symptoms are variable, and up to 20% of patients with pancreatitis will present with "painless pancreatitis." Initial laboratory testing should include serum amylase and lipase levels, however these markers may lose sensitivity after extensive glandular injury has impaired exocrine enzyme production. Extensive fibrosis and edema may lead to elevation of serum bilirubin and alkaline phosphatase in a minority of patients. Additionally, fecal fat excretion can be detected (alternatively Sudan staining of the feces can be utilized), although it is neither sensitive nor specific. Fecal chymotrypsin, trypsin, and elastase testing are now widely available, but suffer from low sensitivity in all but very late-stage disease. Enhanced pancreatic function tests have been studied, including MRCP and endoscopic-assisted secretin stimulation testing, but these techniques have yet to be widely adopted [25].

Endoscopic retrograde pancreatography (ERCP) was classically the reference imaging modality for the diagnosis of chronic pancreatitis, however, increasing consensus is developing around the use of endoscopic ultrasound (EUS) criteria. Studies comparing EUS to ERCP in the diagnosis of chronic pancreatitis have found good correlation between morphologic abnormalities seen on EUS with a sensitivity of 85–97% [26, 27]. However, in practice, computed tomography is almost always included as a powerful adjunct; modern CT scanning has 60–90% sensitivity, as well as 85–95% specificity in the diagnosis of chronic pancreatitis, with increasing sensitivity in more advanced disease [27, 28]. CT findings in chronic pancreatitis include parenchymal atrophy, inflammatory changes, calcifications, pseudocysts, and pancreatic and bile duct dilation. Irregular ductal contour, strictures, and side-branch abnormalities may be more prominent on ERCP and assist in classification and treatment planning. Transabdominal ultrasonography and plain films may detect large cysts, ductal dilation, and calcification, but are rarely used in guidance of treatment algorithms. Magnetic resonance imaging, while promising, is not clearly superior to ERCP and CT [5, 29].

Preoperative Evaluation for CP and a Dilated MPD

Preoperative laboratory evaluation revealed mildly elevated serum amylase and lipase, normal serum trypsin, glucose, calcium, and triglycerides. Nutrition status was normal. CT scan revealed multiple 8–10 mm dilations of the MPD in the body and tail of the pancreas, with a prominence of the pancreatic head. EUS confirms dilation of the MPD, lobularity in the remaining parenchyma, and multiple minor features of chronic pancreatitis.

Multidisciplinary approaches to the patient with chronic pancreatitis are recommended to achieve optimal results. Surgical therapy is reserved for patients in whom there is a high likelihood of symptomatic relief and preservation of exocrine and endocrine function. Resection may be required if pancreatic carcinoma cannot be excluded, or if there is concern for ineffective gland preservation. In the patient presented, classic endoscopic and laboratory findings combined with a history of recurrent episodes of abdominal pain, as well as a history of heavy alcohol use, confirmed a diagnosis of chronic pancreatitis. A dilated MPD with multiple strictures as well as an inflammatory mass in the pancreatic head is amenable to surgical therapy.

Levels of endocrine and exocrine function should be carefully documented prior to proceeding. In the case of alcohol-related pancreatitis, evidence of abstinence should be demonstrated. The goal of surgery is not to reverse the parenchymal injury, but to relieve pain, prevent future complications of chronic pancreatitis, and preserve remaining pancreatic function [30]. If delayed, chronic pain may become intractable and opioid-resistant, while endocrine and exocrine function continue to deteriorate. If operative therapy is undertaken with too much haste, patients with self-limited or stable chronic pancreatitis will be subjected to significant unnecessary operative risk.

The choice of operation is determined by the anatomic classification and severity of disease, degree of pancreatic insufficiency, MPD and side-branch anatomy, and therapeutic effect of previous interventions. Here, we detail two decompressive techniques commonly utilized for patients with dilated main pancreatic ducts, without (Puestow) or with (Frey) strictures, inflammatory masses, or stones in the head of the gland.

Operative Techniques

Puestow

The longitudinal pancreaticojejunostomy, first proposed by Puestow and Gillesby in 1958 [31], was the first most common pancreatic drainage procedure. A "chain-of-lakes" appearance of the MPD due to multiple strictures and dilations, or a MPD with diameter $\geq$ 7 mm, is effectively treated by longitudinal drainage (Figs. 30.1 and 30.2) [32]. The Puestow-Gillesby procedure was modified quickly by Partington and Rochelle, and this version of the procedure continues in surgical practice with high rates of success [33, 34].

The abdomen is entered either via upper midline laparotomy or a subcostal incision. Division of the gastrocolic ligament allows entrance to the lesser sac, and a Thompson retractor (or similar device) is used to expose the entire anterior surface of the pancreas. Lysis of adhesions to the posterior gastric wall is often required due to chronic inflammation of the pancreas and associated viscera. Care is taken to identify the infrapancreatic SMV, celiac trunk, hepatic artery, and gastroduodenal artery just cephalad and medial to the pancreatic head, so as not to inadvertently injure critical vasculature. Identification of the dilated pancreatic duct is accomplished by aspirating pancreatic fluid using a 21-gauge needle, with or without the assistance of intraoperative ultrasound. The length of the diseased MPD is opened, and adequate drainage is ensured by passing a blunt surgical probe through residual normal caliber duct.

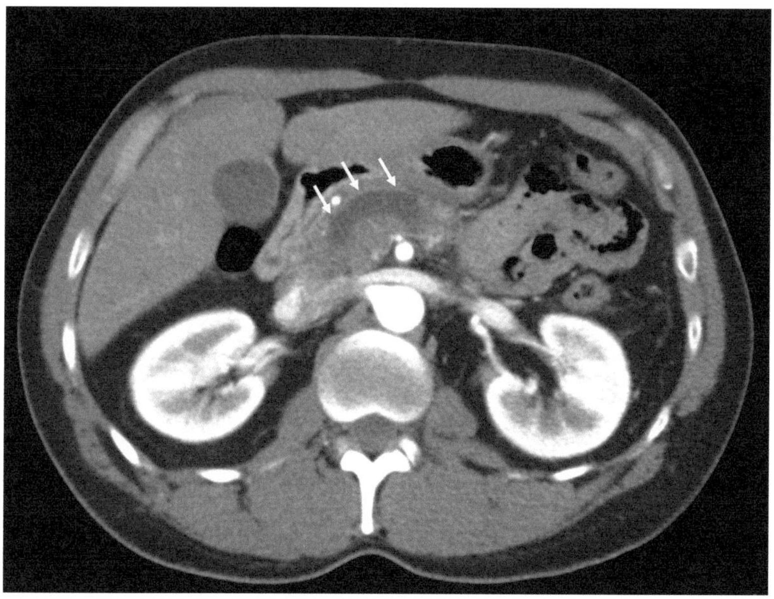

Fig. 30.1 Computed tomography of a 10-mm dilated main pancreatic duct in chronic pancreatitis (*white arrows*)

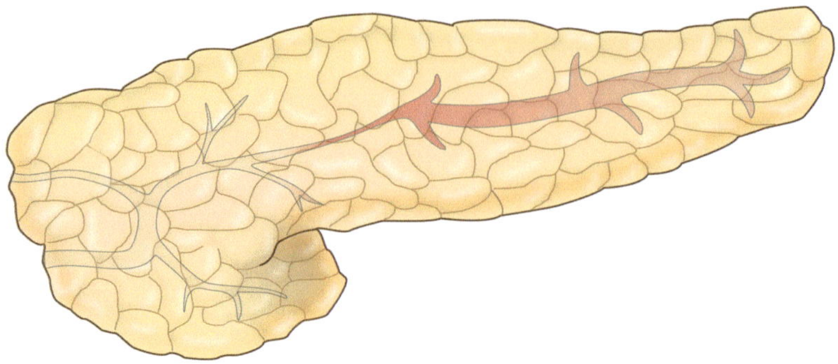

Fig. 30.2 Chronic pancreatitis with dilated main duct in the body and tail of the pancreas

The small bowel is divided using a linear cutting GIA stapler 10 to 20 cm distal to the ligament of Treitz. A 40 to 60 cm Roux limb is created and brought up, in a retrocolic fashion, to the pancreatic ductotomy. The Roux-en-Y reconstruction can be performed in a variety of ways. Some advocate a single, interrupted layer of monofilament suture between the edges of the ductotomy and full-thickness intestinal wall, while others perform the anastomosis with a single running layer of monofilament suture (absorbable and nonabsorbable are both used at the surgeon's discretion). A two-layer anastomosis can be performed by adding an outer layer of interrupted 3-0 silk sutures between the seromuscular layer of the jejunum and the pancreatic capsule. A drain is typically placed in the lesser sac to capture any clinically meaningful pancreatic leak.

Frey Modification of Beger's Procedure

In 1987 Frey introduced a technique to address commonly encountered pancreatic head-dominant disease (fibrosis, stones, or strictures), with a concomitant dilated MPD [35]. Traditional resectional therapy for pancreatic head-dominant disease includes pancreaticoduodenectomy and duodenum-sparing resection of the pancreatic head (Beger's procedure), though these operations are complicated by technical difficulty and increased operative risk due to scarring and neovascularization of the gland [36]. This modification avoids the dangerous dissection in the posterior neck of the pancreas, and includes only a single pancreatic anastomosis. Just as with a longitudinal pancreaticojejunostomy, the ductotomy is completed and then extended into the uncinated process. The pancreatic head tissue overlying the ducts of Wirsung and Santorini is removed, taking care to leave a posterior wall of pancreatic parenchyma intact. The Roux-en-Y reconstruction is then completed with interrupted suture to the pancreatic capsule and a running layer of monofilament suture to the pancreatic duct edge (Fig. 30.3).

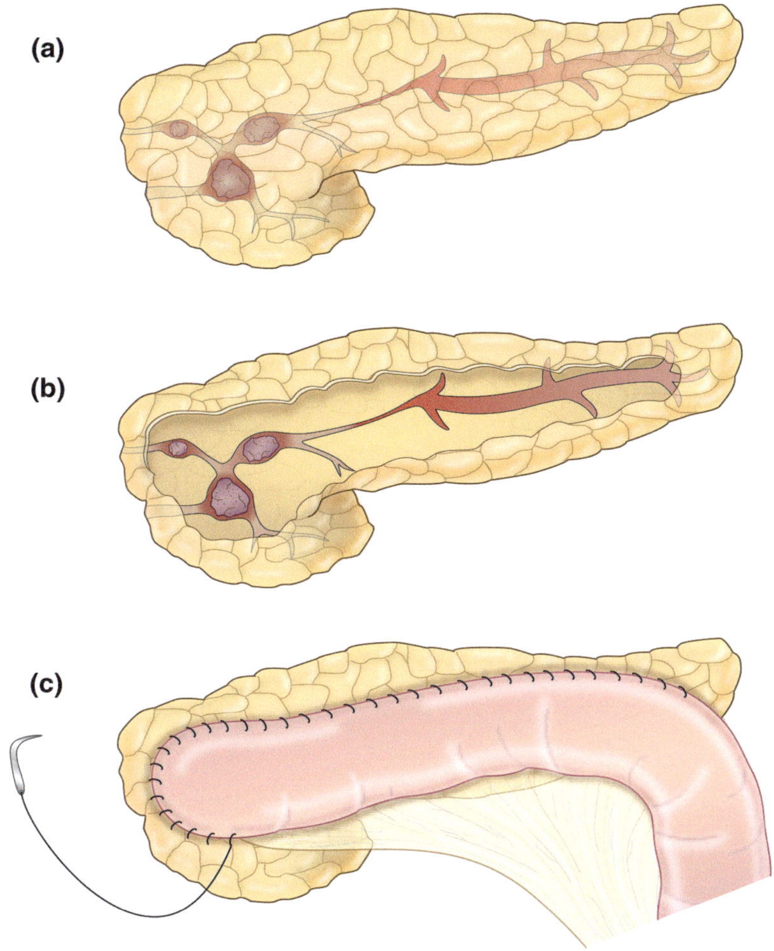

Fig. 30.3 Chronic pancreatitis with **a** multiple stones, strictures, and dilated duct in the body and tail of the pancreas; **b** coring out of diseased pancreatic parenchyma; **c** longitudinal ductotomy with Roux-en-Y pancreatojejunal anastomosis

Outcomes and Pitfalls

Overall operative mortality for a Frey or Puestow procedure is generally 1–3%, most often related to sepsis following pancreaticojejunal anastomotic dehiscence or cholangitis [37]. Postoperative morbidity of up to 19–22% is reported, with the most common complications including delayed gastric emptying, pancreatic fistula, abdominal abscesses, wound infection, and respiratory complications [38–40].

Studies show short-term pain relief, demonstrated by reduction in analgesia requirement and reduced admissions for pain following drainage procedures, to be 75–90% [41, 42], with no significant difference between Frey and Puestow procedures when patients are selected appropriately [43]. Compared to other resectional therapies, the Frey procedure is equally effective in achieving pain relief and preserving pancreas function, with the advantage of being a somewhat safer procedure [44]. Direct comparisons between longitudinal pancreatojejunostomy and Frey procedures are not forthcoming, as the resectional component of the Frey procedure addresses a heterogeneous patient population of patients with dilated MPD (those with head-dominant strictures and/or pancreatic duct stones).

Long-term pain control is a challenge in this patient population, with up to 14–35% of patients undergoing longitudinal pancreatojejunostomy requiring narcotic use [40, 45–47]. Compared to endoscopic drainage, surgical drainage procedures have a greater likelihood of complete or partial pain relief (80% vs. 38%) and require fewer additional interventions in a 5-year longitudinal study [48]. Pain relief following surgical drainage is more rapid, effective, and sustained compared to endoscopic drainage alone [48, 49]. Preoperative narcotic dependence, prior surgical interventions, and continued alcohol consumption are predictors of poor long-term success, and a lack of commonly accepted staging systems for chronic pancreatitis makes comparison across studies difficult. While no single intervention is greatly superior in all cases, surgical intervention should be tailored to each patient's anatomical and physiological disease.

Alternatives and Controversies

- Small-duct chronic pancreatitis is not amenable to pancreaticojejunostomy. While large-duct disease is relieved in the short term by surgical decompression, up to 50% of patients have recurrent pain within 5 years.
- Theoretical suppression of pancreatic exocrine excretion with digestive enzymes, cholecystokinin receptor antagonists, or somatostatin has shown some benefit in early trials, but have not gained wide acceptance.
- Endoscopic drainage and pancreatic duct stenting shows promising short-term results in select patients, however, direct comparison to surgical drainage is forthcoming.

Conclusion

Chronic pancreatitis is a difficult disease process that is best suited for a multidisciplinary approach. Treatment strategies based on patient anatomy and functional status should be tailored with the goal of preserving pancreatic function, relieving pain, and preventing complications of chronic pancreatitis. Longitudinal pancreatojejunostomy with or without resection of pancreatic head tissue should be considered in symptomatic patients if a diagnosis of chronic pancreatitis with main pancreatic duct dilation is clear. Prolonged delays in decompression should be avoided, to prevent loss of pancreatic function and chronic narcotic dependence.

Summary

- Chronic pancreatitis is characterized by a progressive loss of pancreatic parenchymal tissue leading to endocrine and exocrine insufficiency, often with a substantial subclinical phase.
- In general, chronic pancreatitis is caused by relative ductal obstruction leading to intraductal hypertension, although stones and intraductal plugs are rare. Relief of the intraductal hypertension can halt progression of parenchyma changes.
- Symptomatic chronic pancreatitis and those patients with progressive endocrine or exocrine insufficiency warrant invasive treatment including endoscopic and surgical decompression.
- Chronic pancreatitis with a dilated pancreatic duct should be treated with surgical decompression, while small ducts can be given a trial of medical or endoscopic treatment.
- Dilated pancreatic duct with multiple strictures are best addressed by lateral pancreaticojejunostomy, while head-dominant disease is best addressed by Beger or Frey procedures.

References

1. Strobel O, Büchler MW, Werner J. Surgical therapy of chronic pancreatitis: indications, techniques and results. Int J Surg. 2009;7(4):305–12.
2. Spanier BM, Dijkgraaf MG, Bruno MJ. Epidemiology, aetiology and outcome of acute and chronic pancreatitis: an update. Best Pract Res Clin Gastroenterol. 2008;22(1):45–63.
3. Lowenfels AB, Maisonneuve P, Cavallini G, Ammann RW, Lankisch PG, Andersen JR, et al. Prognosis of chronic pancreatitis: an international multicenter study. Am J Gastroenterol. 1994;89(9):1467–71.
4. Jupp J, Fine D, Johnson CD. The epidemiology and socioeconomic impact of chronic pancreatitis. Best Pract Res Clin Gastroenterol. 2010;24(3):219–31.
5. Steer ML, Waxman I, Freedman S. Chronic pancreatitis. N Engl J Med. 1995;332(22):1482–90.
6. Klöppel G, Maillet B. The morphologic basis for the evolution of acute pancreatitis into chronic pancreatitis. In: Beger HG, Buchler M, Malfertheiner P, editors. Standards in pancreatic surgery. Berlin: Springer; 1993. p. 290–6.
7. Karanjia ND, Singh SM, Widdison AL, Lutrin FJ, Reber HA. Pancreatic ductal and interstitial pressures in cats with chronic pancreatitis. Dig Dis Sci. 1992;37(2):268–73.
8. Bradley EL. Pancreatic duct pressure in chronic pancreatitis. Am J Surg. 1982;144(3):313–6.
9. Sakorafas GH, Tsiotou AG, Peros G. Mechanisms and natural history of pain in chronic pancreatitis: a surgical perspective. J Clin Gastroenterol. 2007;41(7):689–99.

10. Singer MV, Gyr K, Sarles H. Revised classification of pancreatitis. Report of the Second International Symposium on the Classification of Pancreatitis in Marseille, France, March 28–0, 1984. Gastroenterology. 1985;89(3):683–5.
11. Sarner M, Cotton PB. Classification of pancreatitis. Gut. 1984;25(7):756–9.
12. Axon AT, Classen M, Cotton PB, Cremer M, Freeny PC, Lees WR. Pancreatography in chronic pancreatitis: international definitions. Gut. 1984;25(10):1107–12.
13. Gardner TB, Taylor DJ, Gordon SR. Reported findings on endoscopic ultrasound examinations for chronic pancreatitis: toward establishing an endoscopic ultrasound quality benchmark. Pancreas. 2014;43(1):37–40.
14. Stevens T. Update on the role of endoscopic ultrasound in chronic pancreatitis. Curr Gastroenterol Rep. 2011;13(2):117–22.
15. Wiersema MJ, Hawes RH, Lehman GA, Kochman ML, Sherman S, Kopecky KK. Prospective evaluation of endoscopic ultrasonography and endoscopic retrograde cholangiopancreatography in patients with chronic abdominal pain of suspected pancreatic origin. Endoscopy. 1993;25(9):555–64.
16. Catalano MF, Sahai A, Levy M, Romagnuolo J, Wiersema M, Brugge W, et al. EUS-based criteria for the diagnosis of chronic pancreatitis: the Rosemont classification. Gastrointest Endosc. 2009;69(7):1251–61.
17. Coté GA, Yadav D, Slivka A, Hawes RH, Anderson MA, Burton FR, et al. Alcohol and smoking as risk factors in an epidemiology study of patients with chronic pancreatitis. Clin Gastroenterol Hepatol. 2011;9(3):266–73.
18. Bisceglie AM, Segal I. Cirrhosis and chronic pancreatitis in alcoholics. J Clin Gastroenterol. 1984;6(3):199–200.
19. Durbec J, Sarles H. Multicenter survey of the etiology of pancreatic diseases. Digestion. 1978;18(5–6):337–50.
20. Whitcomb DC. Genetic predisposition to alcoholic chronic pancreatitis. Pancreas. 2003;27(4):321–6.
21. Layer P, Yamamoto H, Kalthoff L, Clain JE, Bakken LJ, DiMagno EP. The different courses of early-and late-onset idiopathic and alcoholic chronic pancreatitis. Gastroenterology. 1994;107(5):1481–7.
22. Ammann RW, Muellhaupt B. Zurich Pancreatitis Study Group. The natural history of pain in alcoholic chronic pancreatitis. Gastroenterology. 1999;116(5):1132–40.
23. Lankisch P, Löhr-Happe A, Otto J, Creutzfeldt W. Natural course in chronic pancreatitis. Digestion. 1993;54(3):148–55.
24. Witt H, Apte MV, Keim V, Wilson JS. Chronic pancreatitis: challenges and advances in pathogenesis, genetics, diagnosis, and therapy. Gastroenterology. 2007;132(4):1557–73.
25. Lieb J 2nd, Draganov PV. Pancreatic function testing: here to stay for the 21st century. World J Gastroenterol. 2008;14(20):3149–58.
26. Hollerbach S, Klamann A, Topalidis T, Schmiegel WH. Endoscopic ultrasonography (EUS) and fine-needle aspiration (FNA) cytology for diagnosis of chronic pancreatitis. Endoscopy. 2001;33(10):824–31.
27. Choueiri NE, Balci NC, Alkaade S, Burton FR. Advanced imaging of chronic pancreatitis. Curr Gastroenterol Rep. 2010;12(2):114–20.
28. Buscail L, Escourrou J, Moreau J, Delvaux M, Louvel D, Lapeyre F, et al. Endoscopic ultrasonography in chronic pancreatitis: a comparative prospective study with conventional ultrasonography, computed tomography, and ERCP. Pancreas. 1995;10(3):251–7.
29. Miller FH, Keppke AL, Wadhwa A, Ly JN, Dalal K, Kamler V. MRI of pancreatitis and its complications: part 2, chronic pancreatitis. Am J Roentgenol. 2004;183(6):1645–52.
30. Potts JR, Moody FG. Surgical therapy for chronic pancreatitis: selecting the appropriate approach. Am J Surg. 1981;142(6):654–9.
31. Puestow CB, Gillesby WJ. Retrograde surgical drainage of pancreas for chronic relapsing pancreatitis. AMA Arch Surg. 1958;76(6):898–907.

32. Gaines RD. Current surgical management of chronic pancreatitis. J Natl Med Assoc. 1975;67 (1):50–4.
33. Partington PF, Rochelle RE. Modified Puestow procedure for retrograde drainage of the pancreatic duct. Ann Surg. 1960;152:1037–43.
34. Greenlee HB, Prinz RA, Aranha GV. Long-term results of side-to-side pancreaticojejunostomy. World J Surg. 1990;14(1):70–6.
35. Frey CF, Smith GJ. Description and rationale of a new operation for chronic pancreatitis. Pancreas. 1987;2(6):701–7.
36. Bell RH. Current surgical management of chronic pancreatitis. J Gastrointest Surg. 2005;9 (1):144–54.
37. Schnelldorfer T, Lewin DN, Adams DB. Operative management of chronic pancreatitis: longterm results in 372 patients. J Am Coll Surg. 2007;204(5):1039–45.
38. Izbicki JR, Bloechle C, Broering DC, Knoefel WT, Kuechler T, Broelsch CE. Extended drainage versus resection in surgery for chronic pancreatitis: a prospective randomized trial comparing the longitudinal pancreaticojejunostomy combined with local pancreatic head excision with the pylorus-preserving pancreatoduodenectomy. Ann Surg. 1998;228(6):771–9.
39. Prinz RA, Greenlee HB. Pancreatic duct drainage in 100 patients with chronic pancreatitis. Ann Surg. 1981;194(3):313–20.
40. Adams DB, Ford MC, Anderson MC. Outcome after lateral pancreaticojejunostomy for chronic pancreatitis. Ann Surg. 1994;219(5):481–7; discussion 487–9.
41. D'Haese JG, Ceyhan GO, Demir IE, Tieftrunk E, Friess H. Treatment options in painful chronic pancreatitis: a systematic review. HPB (Oxford). 2014;16(6):512–21.
42. Frey CF, Amikura K. Local resection of the head of the pancreas combined with longitudinal pancreaticojejunostomy in the management of patients with chronic pancreatitis. Ann Surg. 1994;220(4):492–504; discussion 504–7.
43. Terrace J, Paterson H, Garden O, Parks R, Madhavan K. Results of decompression surgery for pain in chronic pancreatitis. HPB (Oxford). 2007;9(4):308–11.
44. Frey CF, Mayer KL. Comparison of local resection of the head of the pancreas combined with longitudinal pancreaticojejunostomy (Frey procedure) and duodenum-preserving resection of the pancreatic head (Beger procedure). World J Surg. 2003;27(11):1217–30.
45. Bradley EL. Long-term results of pancreatojejunostomy in patients with chronic pancreatitis. Am J Surg. 1987;153(2):207–13.
46. Dite P, Ruzicka M, Zboril V, Novotny I. A prospective, randomized trial comparing endoscopic and surgical therapy for chronic pancreatitis. Endoscopy. 2003;35(7):553–8.
47. Thuluvath PJ, Imperio D, Nair S, Cameron JL. Chronic pancreatitis: long-term pain relief with or without surgery, cancer risk, and mortality. J Clin Gastroenterol. 2003;36(2):159–65.
48. Cahen DL, Gouma DJ, Laramée P, Nio Y, Rauws EA, Boermeester MA, et al. Long-term outcomes of endoscopic vs surgical drainage of the pancreatic duct in patients with chronic pancreatitis. Gastroenterology. 2011;141(5):1690–5.
49. Cahen DL, Gouma DJ, Nio Y, Rauws EA, Boermeester MA, Busch OR, et al. Endoscopic versus surgical drainage of the pancreatic duct in chronic pancreatitis. N Engl J Med. 2007;356(7):676–84.

Chronic Pancreatitis: Frey Procedure

31

Tyler S. Wahl and John D. Christein

Case Presentation

A 57-year-old white male with chronic obstructive pulmonary disease (COPD) and chronic pancreatitis from alcohol abuse of 40 years presents to your clinic with chronic abdominal pain. Patient notes having significant post-prandial abdominal bloating and boring epigastric pain radiating to his back in a band-like fashion, intermittently associated with diarrhea. His pain, nausea, and steatorrhea have progressed over several years, resulting in a 15-lb weight loss this past year, requiring initiation of pancreatic enzyme replacement with some improvement. First episode of pancreatitis occurred in 2008, followed by episodes in August 2014 and March 2015, requiring hospitalizations with a serum lipase of 1,544 units/L and normal liver function tests during his latest admission. Notable past medical history is significant for COPD, osteoarthritis, and pancreatitis, without evidence of choledocholithiasis, jaundice, abnormal liver function tests, or cirrhosis during prior hospitalizations. Your patient has no surgical history and has abstained from alcohol for 14 months; however, he continues to smoke half a pack of tobacco per day. Physical exam reveals stable vital signs and a non-tender epigastrum without guarding or rebound tenderness.

The patient received an abdominal computed tomography (CT) scan with intravenous and oral contrast (Fig. 31.1a–d) showing extensive dystrophic calcifications throughout the pancreatic head, with diffuse dilation of the proximal

T.S. Wahl · J.D. Christein (✉)
Department of Surgery, University of Alabama at Birmingham (UAB),
1922 7th Avenue South, Kracke Building 428, Birmingham, AL 35249, USA
e-mail: jchristein@uabmc.edu

T.S. Wahl
e-mail: twahl@uabmc.edu

T.M. Pawlik et al. (eds.), *Case-Based Lessons in the Management of Complex Hepato-Pancreato-Biliary Surgery*, DOI 10.1007/978-3-319-50868-9_31

main-pancreatic duct from an intra-pancreatic duct calculus. The pancreatic duct was dilated to the level of the pancreatic tail. The patient also underwent an endoscopic retrograde cholangiopancreatography (ERCP) with scout imaging showing numerous calcifications in the pancreatic gland and large mass of calcium in the pancreatic head. Cholangiogram was deferred given normal preoperative liver function tests. The pancreatogram revealed a pancreatic duct stricture in the head with some filling into a large mass of calcification.

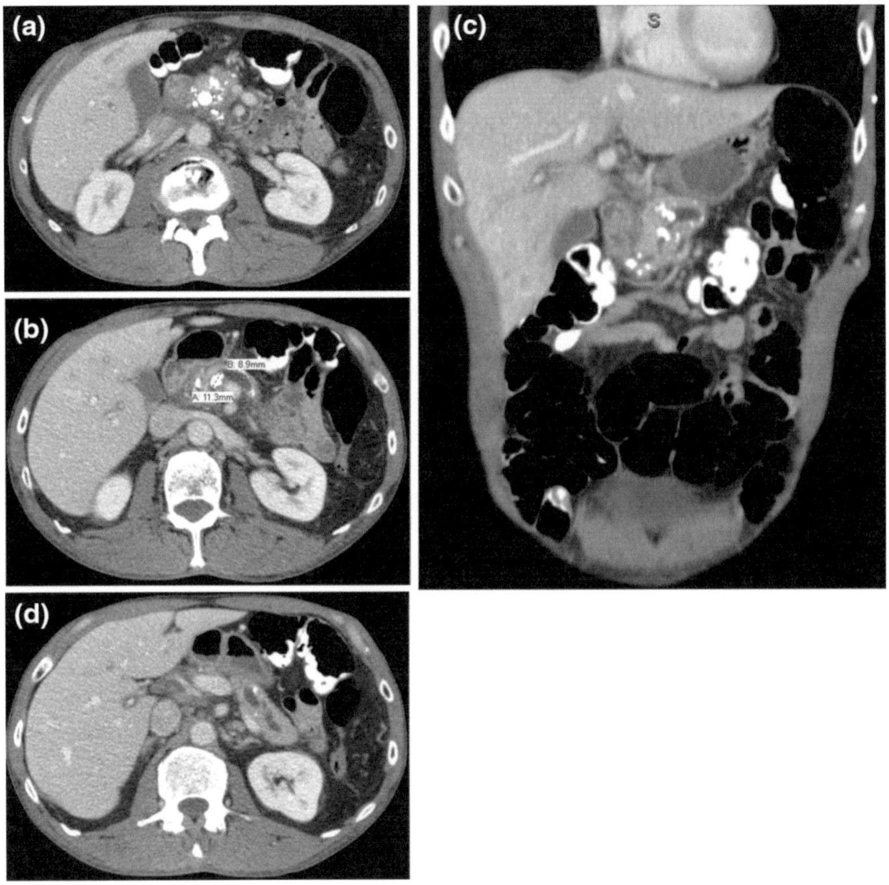

Fig. 31.1 CT abdomen with IV/PO contrast showing **a** extensive dystrophic calcifications throughout the pancreatic head with diffuse dilation of **b** the proximal main-pancreatic duct (9 mm), with an intra-pancreatic duct calculus associated with mild edema and peri-pancreatic stranding suggestive of acute on chronic pancreatitis. **c** coronal image of the pancreatic head with calculi and dilated duct. **d** pancreatic duct dilation extends to the body and tail

Diagnosis and Assessment

Chronic pancreatitis is a fibro-inflammatory syndrome of the pancreas provoked by inflammatory or stress conditions incited through genetic and/or environmental risk factors, leading to morphologic (parenchymal injury, irregular fibrosis) and physiologic (exocrine and endocrine) changes with acinar and islet cell loss [1–5]. The pathophysiology of chronic pancreatitis is multifactorial and complex. The TIGAR-O (toxic/metabolic, idiopathic, genetic, autoimmune, recurrent pancreatitis, obstructive) classification system identifies risk-factor categories associated with chronic pancreatitis [1].

Our patient demonstrates a common presentation of chronic pancreatitis with chronic alcohol and tobacco abuse, recurrent acute pancreatitis, post-prandial abdominal pain, malabsorption (exocrine insufficiency), and weight loss. His exposure to long-term use of alcohol and tobacco places him at an elevated risk for pancreatic disease development and progression [6–9]. The correlation between alcohol use and pancreatic disease is common worldwide, including the United States [10]. Recurrent acute pancreatitis attacks destroy parenchymal tissue over time through chronic inflammatory changes, including fibrosis and calcification, leading to impaired exocrine and endocrine functions [11]. Chronic pancreatitis in the advanced phases is associated with an increased risk for pancreatic cancer [12–14]. Exocrine insufficiency largely takes place when more than 90% of acinar cell function is lost leading to malabsorption [15]. Steatorrhea (fat malabsorption) precedes azotorrhea (protein malabsorption), leading to weight loss over months to years, as seen in our patient. Patients commonly present with boring epigastric pain radiating to the back in a band-like fashion. Pancreatic pseudocyst formation (not found in our patient) may also cause pain, early satiety, weight loss, and inability to eat, resulting in weight loss in the more acute setting.

Initial workup should include well-validated radiologic imaging, typically with CT, ERCP, endoscopic ultrasound (EUS) with biopsy, or magnetic resonance cholangiopancreatography (MRCP). CT imaging with a pancreas protocol (with and without IV contrast, IV contrast in arterial and portal venous phases, and water as oral contrast) is the first-line noninvasive imaging modality of choice, and our initial gold standard. Studies using this protocol are able to diagnose chronic pancreatitis and its complications with 90% confidence [1]. Endoscopic methods of imaging with ERCP and EUS can provide imaging and tissue for diagnosis with therapeutic intervention using ERCP technique. The risks of bleeding, bowel or duct perforation, and acute pancreatitis must be taken into account with perceived benefits on a case-by-case basis. It is essential to assess the pancreatic and biliary duct anatomy for evidence of obstruction preoperatively to optimize intraoperative intervention.

In terms of pancreatic exocrine dysfunction, functional testing is invasive and not necessarily diagnostic, and should have a limited role in chronic pancreatitis workup. Instead, history and clinical evidence of steatorrhea/azotorrhea with or without weight loss may be a signal of malabsorption and a malnourished, catabolic state. It is critical to evaluate the patient's nutritional status preoperatively through a metabolic and nutritional panel not limited to fat-soluble vitamins, liver function tests, pre-albumin, and albumin. Malnourished patients need nasojejunal enteral feedings for 2–4 weeks to reestablish an anabolic state to prepare for surgery.

Patients with chronic pancreatitis often present with glucose intolerance from endocrine insufficiency, as up to 60% of patients will require insulin replacement [16]. Further, chronic pancreatitis patients are at an increased risk for spontaneous or treatment-related hypoglycemia, likely attributed to glucagon insufficiency, malnutrition, and alcohol consumption [16]. Our patient did not have endocrine insufficiency.

Management

Whenever feasible, lifestyle modifications should be implemented for chronic pancreatitis patients prior to surgical intervention. In addition to multimodal pain therapies, alcohol and smoking cessation can further decrease pain and complications in chronic pancreatitis, with further risk mitigation of pancreatic calcification through smoking cessation [17–19]. Reductions in dietary fats for patients with severe refractory steatorrhea offer some benefit, yet medium-chain triglyceride supplementation are not indicated and require additional enzyme supplementation for proper digestion and absorption [11, 20]. Parenteral vitamin supplementation of fat-soluble vitamins and enteral pancreatic enzyme replacement is beneficial for patients with exocrine insufficiency and malabsorption [11]. Pancreatic enzyme supplementation normalizes fat-soluble vitamin, pre-albumin, and ferritin levels in chronic pancreatitis patients without steatorrhea [21]. Enzyme supplementation can be given in the absence of fecal-fat testing in patients with clinical malabsorption (loose, foul-smelling stool; weight loss; muscle wasting; osteopenia) [22]. A 72-h fecal-fat study is the gold standard to detect steatorrhea; however, this test may not be convenient or feasible given the sensitivity and specificity (100 and 95%, respectively) and positive predictive value (90%) of the acid steatocrit random-spot test [23].

Surgical intervention is warranted in our patient presenting with progressive frequency of pancreatitis episodes, severe and recurrent pain, signs of malabsorption, and evidence of pancreatic duct obstruction and dilation. Our patient warrants a duodenal-preserving partial resection of the pancreatic head, longitudinal ductotomy, and lateral pancreaticojejunostomy (Frey Procedure).

Indications for Frey Procedure

- Disabling or severe pain with ductal dilation $\geq$ 7 mm or dilated with multiple strictures
- Asymptomatic with ductal dilation $\geq$ 7 mm or dilated with multiple stricture

- Symptomatic inflammatory mass/calcification in pancreatic head causing ductal dilation
- Consideration: dilated with multiple strictures has a "chain of lakes" appearance

Intraoperative Technique

Positioning and Preparation

The patient is placed on the operating room table in the supine position. Intravenous access with two large-bore intravenous cannulas or one central venous line is established, along with arterial wave monitoring via a radial arterial line. Appropriate prophylactic antibiotics, urinary catheter, and compression hose-stockings with a sequential compression device are administered or placed prior to incision.

Exposure of the Pancreas

We begin with a bilateral subcostal incision with thorough exploration of the abdomen prior to exposing the pancreas (Fig. 31.2). The greater omentum is elevated off the transverse mesocolon to its origin on the stomach, and the gastrocolic ligament is divided to provide access into the lesser sac exposing the anterior pancreas body and tail (Fig. 31.3a, b). Exposure of the pancreas is challenging in the setting of chronic inflammation, as the posterior wall of the stomach is frequently densely adherent to the pancreas.

Longitudinal Pancreatic Ductotomy

First, identify the gastroduodenal artery (GDA) near the head. If the GDA can be palpated, ligate at the superior and inferior border of the pancreas for proximal and distal control, respectively, with interrupted figure-of-eight 4-0 Prolene sutures. If the GDA is not palpable due to extensive fibrosis, carefully dissect until the GDA is encountered, and control with manual compression until ligated. Once dissection approaches the neck, formal control of the GDA is performed superiorly and inferiorly to the pancreas as described. The pancreatic duct is identified within the pancreatic head with a needle and opened using cautery with a high setting (75–85) on fulgurate mode. We insert an appropriately sized probe into the duct upstream

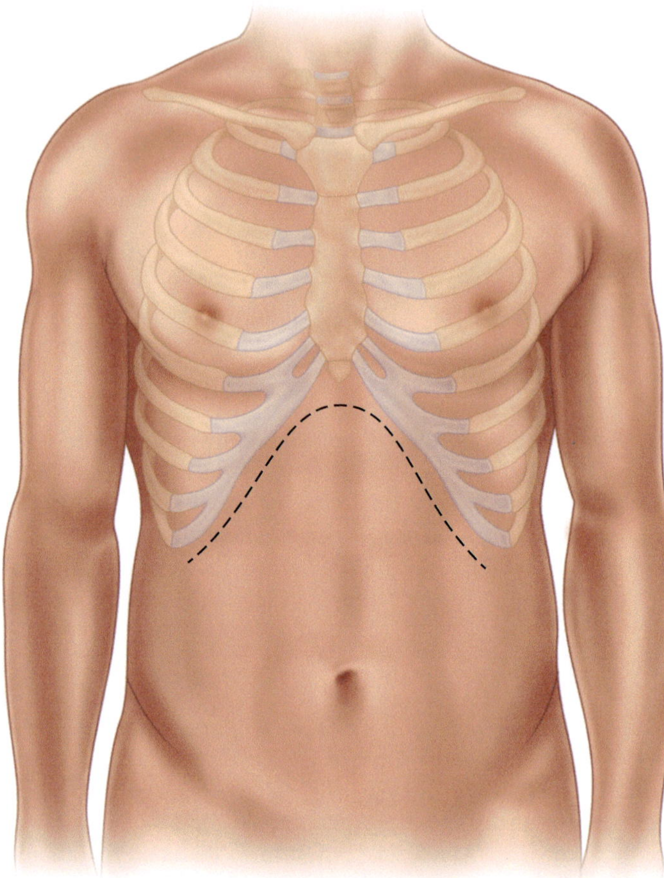

Fig. 31.2 Sub-costal incision or an upper midline incision may be utilized

toward the tail and cut down along the probe with high cautery. The ductotomy is then directed downstream toward the head to expose the entire main-pancreatic duct up to 1 cm from the papilla of Vater. All pancreatic stones and debris are removed.

Pancreatic Head Resection

The portal vein above the pancreas and superior mesenteric vein (SMV) below are visualized to ensure safe dissection of the anterior pancreatic head and uncinate process. With the GDA ligated, use high cautery to partially resect the pancreatic head, leaving only a thin rim of pancreatic tissue along the medial duodenal wall

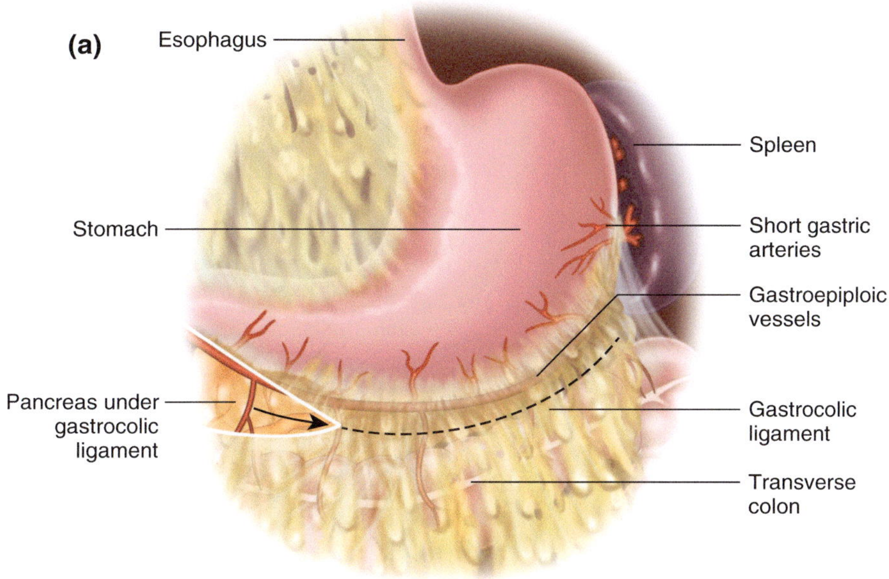

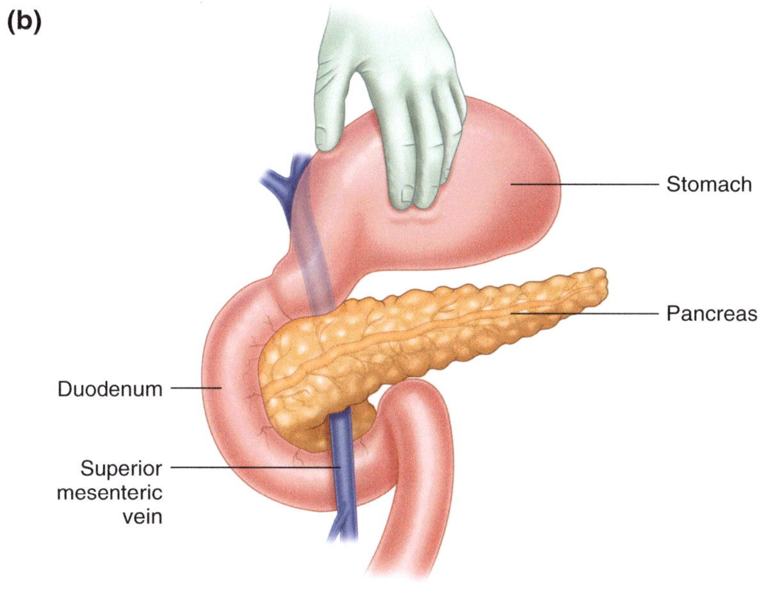

Fig. 31.3 **a** Divide the gastrocolic ligament to gain access into the lesser sac. **b** Reflect the stomach cephalad to expose the anterior pancreas

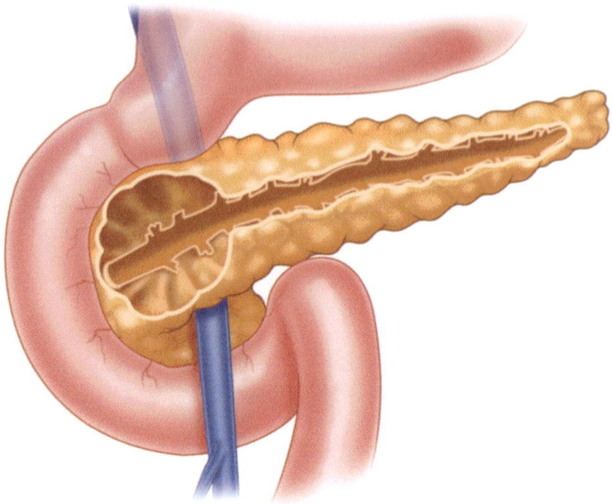

Fig. 31.4 The longitudinal ductotomy should expose the entire main duct from the tail to approximately 1 cm from the papilla of Vater. The partial pancreatic head resection is shown (note the dissection does not extend past the posterior border of the main duct). Remove all stones and debris from main and side-branch ducts

(Fig. 31.4). Once lateral to the neck, dissection can continue down to the uncinate process in a circular fashion with piece-meal resection of tissue, if necessary. Resection should not extend beyond the posterior border of the main duct, as deeper resections increase the risk of pancreatic division, compromising vascular structures, and promoting a pancreatic leak into the retroperitoneal space. We do not perform a Kocher maneuver as to avoid posterior capsule penetration. Meticulous care is taken to remove stones and debris from the main duct and side branches. Utilize suture ligation of brisk bleeding (5-0 Prolene sutures), as cautery temporarily seals arterial vessels. If the bile duct is encountered and opened unintentionally, the bile will ultimately drain into the pancreaticojejunostomy.

Roux-en-Y Pancreaticojejunostomy

A segment of jejunum is identified and divided 15 to 30 cm distal to the ligament of Treitz. The common enterotomy is closed with 3-0 Prolene as the mesentery is divided with ligation of bridging vessels toward the mesenteric origin to the right of the middle colic vasculature. The distal jejunum segment is pulled through the transverse mesocolon to deliver the Roux limb to the pancreas in a retrocolic position, or according to the patient's anatomy. Excess mesenteric defects are closed with interrupted 3-0 silk suture. The transected end of the Roux limb is oriented with the pancreatic tail to start a one-layer side-to-side pancreaticojejunostomy using multiple running 3-0 Prolene sutures, and secured to the transverse mesocolon with interrupted 3-0 silk suture once complete. The pancreaticojejunostomy continues toward the pancreatic head to allow complete drainage of the main duct, with progressive opening of the jejunum to avoid an excessively long jejunotomy (Fig. 31.5).

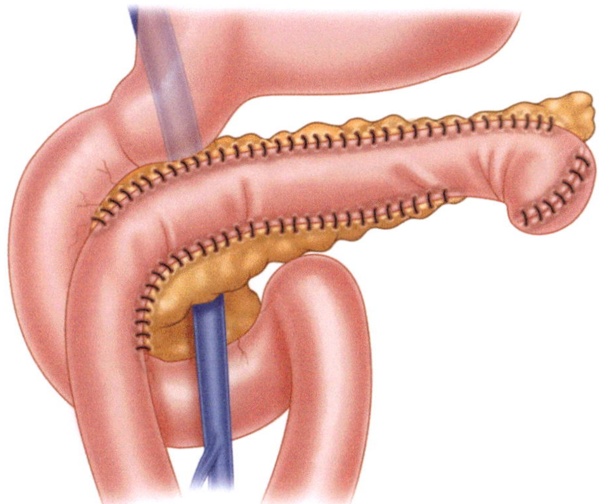

Fig. 31.5 Lateral pancreaticojejunostomy, anterior view. Remember to perform incremental opening of the Roux jejunal limb while performing the anastomosis from the tail toward the head, to avoid an overly long jejunotomy

Following completion of the pancreaticojejunostomy, an end-to-side jejunojejunostomy is created to complete the Roux-en-Y, approximately 40–50 cm distal to the pancreaticojejunostomy to reestablish intestinal continuity. One small, round drain is placed in the lesser sac, and fascia is closed in two layers with 1-0 Prolene sutures prior to skin irrigation and approximation with staples.

Technical Pearls

Exposure

- Enter the lesser scar through the gastrocolic ligament to expose the anterior pancreas

Ductotomy

- Ligate the gastroduodenal artery
- Ensure ductotomy extends the entire length of the gland using high-setting cautery (75–85) on fulgurate mode

Partial pancreatic head resection

- Pancreatic head tissue resection should leave only a thin rim of tissue around the duodenum and not extend past the posterior border of the main-pancreatic duct

Pancreaticojejunostomy

- Orient the Roux jejunal limb according to patient's anatomy with anastomoses starting from the tail with incremental openings to avoid an overly long jejunotomy

Postoperative Management

A monitored setting may be required for 24–48 h postoperatively in patients with high blood loss, given risk of further bleeding postoperatively. High fluid requirements may be needed if active inflammation is present or extensive adhesiolysis performed. Monitor urine output closely with a urinary catheter initially until patient is adequately resuscitated.

Early enteral nutrition initiation (feeding jejunostomy among malnourished patients) with enteral liquids by postoperative day (POD) 1. Check a drain amylase on POD 2 or 3 once diet is advanced with drain removal according to the International Study Group on Pancreatic Fistula (ISGPF) criteria. Projected goal for discharge on POD 4 or 5, once the patient tolerates diet with return of bowel function and ambulating with adequate pain control.

Patients should be encouraged to continue lifestyle modification, since alcohol and smoking cessation is associated with decreased risk of disease progression and morbidity. Patients need regular follow-up for exocrine and endocrine insufficiency, as they may require pancreatic enzyme supplementation or insulin.

Alternative Management

- Malnourished patients need nasojejunal feeding for enteral nutrition for 2–4 weeks preoperatively to promote an anabolic state. A feeding jejunostomy tube should be placed intraoperatively.
- Bile duct strictures should receive a preoperative biliary stent to assist duct identification prior to intra-pancreatic biliary sphincteroplasty following partial pancreatic head resection, to allow biliary drainage into the pancreaticojejunostomy,

Global Pearls

- Utilize lifestyle modification, when feasible, pre- and postoperatively
- Assess exocrine and endocrine function along with nutritional status for optimization
- Ensure adequate exposure of the pancreatic duct for complete debris removal
- Early initiation of enteral nutrition is a key postoperatively

References

1. Etemad B, Whitcomb DC. Chronic pancreatitis: diagnosis, classification, and new genetic developments. Gastroenterology. 2001;120(3):682–707.
2. Homma T, Harada H, Koizumi M. Diagnostic criteria for chronic pancreatitis by the Japan Pancreas Society. Pancreas. 1997;15(1):14–5.
3. Kloppel G, Maillet B. Pseudocysts in chronic pancreatitis: a morphological analysis of 57 resection specimens and 9 autopsy pancreata. Pancreas. 1991;6(3):266–74.
4. Kloppel G, Maillet B. Pathology of acute and chronic pancreatitis. Pancreas. 1993;8(6):659–70.
5. Whitcomb DC, Frulloni L, Garg P, Greer JB, Schneider A, Yadav D, et al. Chronic pancreatitis: an international draft consensus proposal for a new mechanistic definition. Pancreatology. 2016;16(2):218–24.
6. Lin Y, Tamakoshi A, Hayakawa T, Ogawa M, Ohno Y. Cigarette smoking as a risk factor for chronic pancreatitis: a case-control study in Japan. Research Committee on Intractable Pancreatic Diseases. Pancreas. 2000;21(2):109–14.
7. Talamini G, Bassi C, Falconi M, Frulloni L, Di Francesco V, Vaona B, et al. Cigarette smoking: an independent risk factor in alcoholic pancreatitis. Pancreas. 1996;12(2):131–7.
8. Yadav D, Hawes RH, Brand RE, Anderson MA, Money ME, Banks PA, et al. Alcohol consumption, cigarette smoking, and the risk of recurrent acute and chronic pancreatitis. Arch Intern Med. 2009;169(11):1035–45.
9. Yadav D, Whitcomb DC. The role of alcohol and smoking in pancreatitis. Nat Rev Gastroenterol Hepatol. 2010;7(3):131–45.
10. Ramstedt M. Alcohol and pancreatitis mortality at the population level: experiences from 14 western countries. Addiction. 2004;99(10):1255–61.
11. Frulloni L, Falconi M, Gabbrielli A, Gaia E, Graziani R, Pezzilli R, et al. Italian consensus guidelines for chronic pancreatitis. Digest Liver Dis. 2010;42(Suppl 6):S381–406.
12. Guidelines for the diagnosis and treatment of chronic pancreatitis (Nanjing, 2005). Chin J Digest Dis. 2005;6(4):198–201.
13. Tandon RK, Sato N, Garg PK. Chronic pancreatitis: Asia-Pacific consensus report. J Gastroenterol Hepatol. 2002;17(4):508–18.
14. Warshaw AL, Banks PA, Fernandez-Del Castillo C. AGA technical review: treatment of pain in chronic pancreatitis. Gastroenterology. 1998;115(3):765–76.
15. DiMagno EP, Go VL, Summerskill WH. Relations between pancreatic enzyme ouputs and malabsorption in severe pancreatic insufficiency. N Engl J Med. 1973;288(16):813–5.
16. Mergener K, Baillie J. Chronic pancreatitis. Lancet. 1997;350(9088):1379–85.
17. Imoto M, DiMagno EP. Cigarette smoking increases the risk of pancreatic calcification in late-onset but not early-onset idiopathic chronic pancreatitis. Pancreas. 2000;21(2):115–9.
18. Maisonneuve P, Lowenfels AB, Mullhaupt B, Cavallini G, Lankisch PG, Andersen JR, et al. Cigarette smoking accelerates progression of alcoholic chronic pancreatitis. Gut. 2005;54 (4):510–4.

19. Talamini G, Bassi C, Falconi M, Sartori N, Vaona B, Bovo P, et al. Smoking cessation at the clinical onset of chronic pancreatitis and risk of pancreatic calcifications. Pancreas. 2007;35 (4):320–6.
20. Caliari S, Benini L, Sembenini C, Gregori B, Carnielli V, Vantini I. Medium-chain triglyceride absorption in patients with pancreatic insufficiency. Scand J Gastroenterol. 1996;31(1):90–4.
21. Dominguez-Munoz JE. Pancreatic enzyme therapy for pancreatic exocrine insufficiency. Gastroenterol Hepatol. 2011;7(6):401–3.
22. Dumasy V, Delhaye M, Cotton F, Deviere J. Fat malabsorption screening in chronic pancreatitis. Am J Gastroenterol. 2004;99(7):1350–4.
23. Amann ST, Josephson SA, Toskes PP. Acid steatocrit: a simple, rapid gravimetric method to determine steatorrhea. Am J Gastroenterol. 1997;92(12):2280–4.

Total Pancreatectomy with Islet Autotransplantation

32

William P. Lancaster and Katherine A. Morgan

Case Scenarios

Case 1: Diffuse Small Duct Disease

A 42-year-old-woman presents for evaluation of chronic pancreatitis. She reports a 4-year history of disease, marked by progressive epigastric and left-sided abdominal pain with periodic episodes of significant exacerbation, requiring hospitalization for intravenous opiates. Between episodes, she requires daily narcotic pain medication. She has nausea and pain with eating and has had significant weight loss of 20 lb over the past year. She has oily stools with fatty meals. Her quality of life is poor and has deteriorated to the point that she has had to quit working. She has a history of endoscopic retrograde cholangiopancreatography (ERCP) with endoscopic stent placement, which provided no relief. She also has history of celiac plexus block, which provided temporary relief of her symptoms, but proved non-durable. She has no other significant medical problems and does not take medications. Her surgical history is significant for a laparoscopic cholecystectomy. She denies alcohol use, but admits to smoking one-half pack per day. She denies family history of pancreatitis or pancreatic cancer. On physical exam she appears older than her stated age and is thin. Her laboratory work is significant for an albumin of 3.2 g/dL and a vitamin D level of 8 ng/mL (normal 20–50 ng/ml).

W.P. Lancaster
Department of Surgery, Indiana University, 545 Barnhill Drive, EH 545, Indianapolis, IN 46202, USA
e-mail: wplancas@iupui.edu

K.A. Morgan (✉)
Medical University of South Carolina, 114 Doughty Street, Suite 249, Charleston, SC 29425, USA
e-mail: morganka@musc.edu

T.M. Pawlik et al. (eds.), *Case-Based Lessons in the Management of Complex Hepato-Pancreato-Biliary Surgery*, DOI 10.1007/978-3-319-50868-9_32

Imaging findings are notable for a magnetic resonance cholangiopancreatography (MRCP) demonstrating diminished parenchymal enhancement on T1 weighted imaging and, on T2 weighted images an irregular main pancreatic duct 3 mm in diameter along with multiple dilated side branches consistent, with chronic pancreatitis. Endoscopic retrograde cholangiopancreatography (ERCP) shows a similarly abnormal topography of the pancreatic duct, consistent with Cambridge classification type III, and endoscopic ultrasound (EUS) is high probability of chronic pancreatitis, revealing six criteria of chronic pancreatitis.

Case 2: Hereditary Pancreatitis

A 12-year-old-male presents with a history of pancreatitis since the age of 6. He reports episodes of pancreatitis marked by epigastric abdominal pain and intolerance of oral intake, which have become progressively more frequent and more severe over the past two years. He is well between episodes, but has had four episodes this past year, and has missed a significant amount of school. He has undergone multiple ERCPs with stent placement, which have resulted in transient symptom improvement. A celiac plexus block was not helpful. Most recent axial imaging shows diffuse calcifications throughout the gland, with associated atrophy. The pancreatic duct is 7 mm in maximal diameter on MRCP. He takes oral pancreatic enzyme supplementation with meals. He is not diabetic. Genetic testing is significant for a mutation at the PRSS1 gene. His father had chronic pancreatitis and died at age 42 from pancreatic cancer. His sister has pancreatitis as well.

Case 3: Salvage Pancreatectomy

A 48-year-old-female presents with a 6-year history of idiopathic chronic pancreatitis. She underwent a Frey procedure (local pancreatic head resection with a lateral pancreaticojejunostomy) 3 years ago for debilitating pain. She did well, with resolution of pain for approximately 2 years after surgery, but has had recurrence of her abdominal pain over the past year. She has developed diabetes requiring insulin over the past 3 months. Her past medical history and surgical history are otherwise unremarkable. She takes daily narcotic medication and oral pancreatic enzyme supplementation. She went back to school after her Frey and completed her degree, but is now unable to work. Her exam is benign and her labwork unremarkable. She underwent MRCP, which shows significant calcific disease and fibrosis in the remnant pancreas.

Case 4: Recurrent Acute Pancreatitis

A 37-year-old-female presents with recurrent episodes of acute pancreatitis. She reports her first episode was 3 years ago, and has since had progressively more frequent and severe bouts of acute pancreatitis. Her episodes are marked by severe epigastric abdominal pain with nausea, emesis, and intolerance of oral diet. These bouts are associated with elevated serum lipase and require hospitalization for intravenous hydration, antiemetics, and narcotics. The episodes last days to weeks, and she had four such episodes last year. She is well, without pain, between bouts. Her past medical history is unremarkable. Her surgical history is significant for a cholecystectomy. A CT scan during an episode reveals peripancreatic fat stranding and fluid. An MRI with MRCP done between episodes shows no evidence of chronic pancreatitis. EUS is low probability for chronic pancreatitis.

Preoperative Evaluation

The goals of the preoperative evaluation for total pancreatectomy with islet autotransplantation (TPIAT) are to establish the diagnosis of chronic pancreatitis or recurrent acute pancreatitis, to assess whether disease severity warrants intervention, to consider whether lesser interventions may be successful, to evaluate the physiologic fitness of the patient for surgery, and to consider the psychological preparedness of the patient [1].

Patients with diffuse small duct pancreatitis, those with genetic pancreatitis [2], patients who have failed lesser surgeries [3], and patients with recurrent acute pancreatitis may benefit from TPIAT.

History

The clinical hallmark of chronic pancreatitis is progressive, severe, debilitating abdominal pain. High healthcare utilization is common, and chronic narcotic use is frequently present. Patients report a severely diminished quality of life. Patients often have attendant nutritional failure due to PO intolerance, as well as to exocrine pancreatic insufficiency. Diabetes due to islet cell loss during parenchymal replacement with fibrosis occurs in late stages.

During the initial evaluation, risk factors for chronic pancreatitis should be sought. Alcohol use has traditionally been implicated in many cases with chronic pancreatitis, although direct causation is not evident, and susceptibility to alcohol-induced pancreatitis has been linked to genetic variation on the X chromosome. Alcohol is less commonly implicated in the morphologic patterns of pancreatitis that present as appropriate for TPIAT (diffuse small duct disease), and patients with alcoholic pancreatitis have been shown to have inferior outcomes after TPIAT [4]. Tobacco use has been found to be a significant factor for promoting fibrosis and for enhancing susceptibility to pancreatitis development, and has been found to correlate with lower islet yields and function after islet autotransplantation. Proper counseling should be undertaken with consideration of smoking cessation as a requirement for surgery [5].

Genetic Testing

Several genetic mutations have been identified that predispose to the development of chronic pancreatitis, including PRSS1, SPINK1, and CFTR. Genetic testing is an important component of preoperative evaluation, particularly in the setting of early-onset disease, as the natural history of hereditary pancreatitis may differ from pancreatitis of other etiologies. Patients with hereditary pancreatitis typically have progressive disease with subsequent development of endocrine and exocrine dysfunction, and often have disease refractory to conventional medical and surgical therapies. In addition, the lifetime risk of pancreatic cancer may be increased compared to the general population. Thus, these patients are often well suited to TPIAT [2]. Of the genetic mutations associated with pancreatitis, the best understood is PRSS1. The PRSS1 gene is located on the long arm of chromosome 7 and encodes cationic trypsinogen. It is inherited in an autosomal dominant fashion with an estimated penetrance of 80%. Disease onset is early, usually manifesting as pancreatic pain. Patients progress to endocrine and exocrine insufficiency by the third decade. The cumulative risk of pancreatic adenocarcinoma is approximately 50% at 75 years of age [6].

Recurrent Acute Pancreatitis

A subset of patients will have recurrent acute pancreatitis that is significantly debilitating, without evidence of chronic pancreatitis. These patients may benefit from TPIAT if disease progresses despite removal of aggravating environmental factors and despite endoscopic interventions. Pancreatitis should be definitively demonstrated to be causative of pain episodes by associated elevation in serum lipase during events to three times normal, and/or evidence of peripancreatic inflammation on axial imaging.

Imaging

Radiographic imaging is essential to the evaluation of patients for TPIAT. First, confirming diagnosis of chronic pancreatitis in patients with longstanding abdominal pain is fundamental, as abdominal pain can be multifactorial. Second, understanding the anatomy of the pancreatic duct and parenchymal disease distribution can help guide appropriateness of total pancreatectomy versus lesser intervention, such as a drainage procedure for dilated duct pancreatitis, or partial resection for focal pancreatitis. The pancreas is well evaluated with several different modalities. Computed tomography (CT) scan can demonstrate pancreatic inflammation as well as glandular atrophy and pancreatic calcifications commonly seen with chronic pancreatitis, though the overall sensitivity is low, particularly in early-stage disease and in the absence of calcifications or overt ductal changes (Fig. 32.1) Magnetic resonance cholangiopancreatography (MRCP), particularly with secretin administration, allows

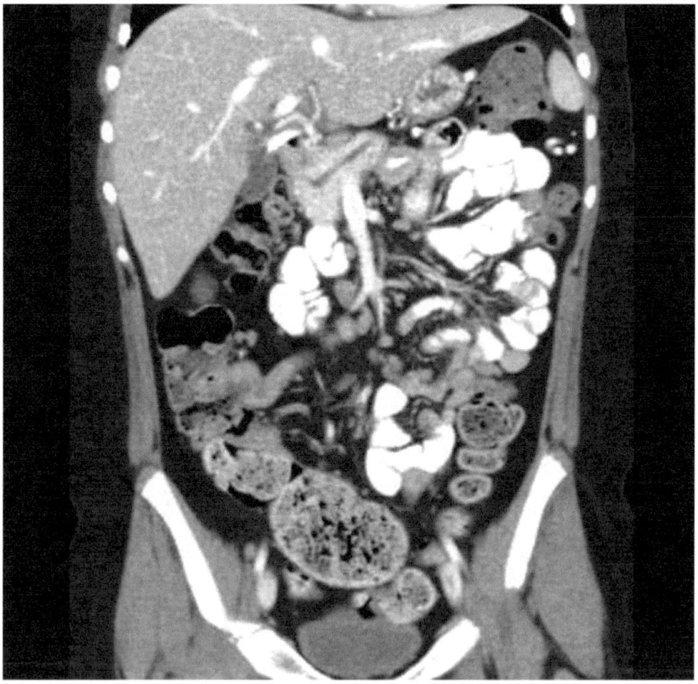

Fig. 32.1 Diffuse small duct pancreatitis is demonstrated in this CT scan of a patient with idiopathic chronic pancreatitis who underwent total pancreatectomy with islet autotransplantation. Noted are a prominent, mildly dilated main pancreatic duct, parenchymal fibrosis, and punctate calcifications

for reasonable ability to evaluate the pancreatic parenchyma as well as the pancreatic ductal anatomy. ERCP is rarely used purely for diagnosis in the modern era of MRCP, and is reserved for therapeutic use. The Cambridge classification system of pancreatic abnormalities seen on ERCP is used to define features of chronic pancreatitis, and has also been applied to MRCP. A sensitive assessment of the pancreas, although subject to interobserver variability, is with EUS. EUS assesses for abnormal parenchymal features as well as ductal abnormalities, and at least five features of pancreatitis should be present in order for the test to be considered high probability for chronic pancreatitis. Imaging features must be considered within the clinical context of these often complex patients with chronic abdominal pain.

Diabetes

Patients with chronic pancreatitis may develop pancreatic endocrine failure due to islet cell loss (type 3c diabetes). Patients with diabetes may still benefit from islet autotransplantation, as endogenous c-peptide production can ameliorate the severity of resultant surgical diabetes after pancreatectomy [7]. Patients with diabetes on evaluation for TPIAT should be evaluated for their level of islet function, however, to help weigh whether the potential benefits of islet autotransplantation warrant the risks inherent. Stimulated c-peptide response should be assessed, often with a mixed-meal tolerance test.

Nutritional Assessment

Patients with chronic pancreatitis are at risk for nutritional failure due to poor PO intake and from pancreatic exocrine insufficiency. A full nutritional evaluation and efforts to optimize nutritional status preoperatively are important for best outcomes. Pancreatic enzyme replacement therapy is best instituted preoperatively. Evaluation for malnutrition with assessment of serum albumin and pre-albumin levels are requisite. Preoperative oral supplementation or enteral feeds may be required in the severely affected. Deficiencies in the fat-soluble vitamins should be addressed.

Physiologic Assessment

As with other major elective abdominal operations, attendant comorbidities, including cardiac, pulmonary, and renal disease should be evaluated when considering patient candidacy for surgery. In particular, a history of hepatic disease is important, as the islet infusion is an embolic event, which may be a significant stressor to a previously compromised liver, increasing morbidity.

Behavioral Medicine Evaluation

Patients evaluated for TPIAT should undergo comprehensive psychological assessment to evaluate relative preparedness for surgery [8]. Evaluation assesses multiple psychological domains, including global cognitive functioning, quality of life, and coping. The patient's knowledge and expectations of the procedure are assessed, as well as the support system available. A complete psychiatric evaluation is performed to diagnose previously untreated psychiatric disorders, e.g. depression, anxiety. The patient's health behaviors and compliance are also assessed to screen for narcotic dependence/abuse and ability to manage complex medication regimens, e.g., pancreatic enzyme therapy, insulin.

Preoperative Counseling

In consideration of this radical, elective procedure, patient education is paramount. Patients should demonstrate understanding of proper expectations. The goals of the procedure are pain relief and improvements in quality of life. These expected outcomes come at the cost of lifelong (ameliorated) surgical diabetes and exocrine insufficiency.

Patient Selection Criteria for Total Pancreatectomy with Islet Autotransplantation for Chronic Pancreatitis

1. Chronic pancreatitis

Evidenced by: CT, MRCP, EUS (5 criteria, high probability), or prior surgical pathology

OR

Recurrent acute pancreatitis

Evidenced by: at least two documented episodes with lipase >3 time normal

2. Debilitating pain

Defined by daily narcotic use and/or inability to work, attend school, or engage in normal societal roles

3. Not amenable to lesser interventions

Includes medical, endoscopic, and lesser surgical options

4. Physiologically fit

No prohibitive cardiopulmonary conditions, no significant hepatic disease

5. Psychologically fit

Requires behavioral medicine evaluation

Surgical Technique

The patient is positioned supine under general anesthesia. A triple lumen central venous catheter is placed for durable intravenous access, primarily in anticipation of the continuous infusions required during the initial postoperative period. Additional large-bore peripheral intravenous access is also established because there is the potential for rapid fluid shifts. An arterial line is placed and continuous hemodynamic monitoring is used to allow for goal-directed fluid management.

An upper midline laparotomy incision extending from the xiphisternum to above the umbilicus is typically used. A wound protector is utilized. The gastrocolic ligament is divided and the lesser sac is entered. The greater omentum and short gastric vessels are taken down along the greater curvature of the stomach. The hepatic flexure is mobilized and retracted inferomedially. A full Kocher maneuver is performed, mobilizing the duodenum to the level of the aorta medially. The right gastroepiploic vein and middle colic vein are identified and followed toward the superior mesenteric vein. The right gastroepiploic vein is divided, taking care to preserve the middle colic vein. The inferior margin of pancreatic neck is identified over the superior mesenteric vein, and the plane between the portal vein and the pancreatic neck is developed. The gastroduodenal artery is ligated, confirming continued perfusion of the hepatic artery. If the gallbladder is present, it is removed.

The common bile duct is dissected circumferentially and is divided. The stomach is divided proximal to the pylorus with a surgical stapler. Just distal to the ligament of Treitz, the proximal jejunum is divided and the jejunal mesentery as well as the ligament of Treitz are taken down with an energy device. The proximal jejunum and the fourth portion of the duodenum are then rotated under the superior mesenteric vessels.

The pancreatic neck is divided over the portal vein, and the pancreatic head is rotated laterally and dissected from the portal vein. The periarterial vascular and lymphatic tissue between the uncinate process and the superior mesenteric artery is divided, and the head of pancreas and duodenum are removed from the abdomen and immediately placed in cold balanced-electrolyte preservative solution.

On the back table, the pancreatic head specimen is immediately prepared by flushing the gastroduodenal artery stump with cold preservative solution. The duodenum is removed and the pancreatic duct is cannulated with a 5 French pediatric feeding tube (Fig. 32.2a).

Next, attention is turned to removing the body and tail of the pancreas. The splenic artery is dissected and tagged but not yet ligated near its origin, the superior margin of the pancreatic body. Similarly, the splenic vein is tagged, taking care to preserve the coronary vein. Once the pancreas is dissected free from the surrounding structures, the splenic vessels are ligated and the distal pancreas and spleen are removed from the abdomen and placed in cold preservative solution.

On the back table, the spleen is removed sharply. The splenic vein is opened along its length to exsanguinate the specimen, and the splenic artery is flushed with cold preservation solution. The pancreatic duct is cannulated with a 5 French pediatric feeding tube, which is sutured in place (Fig. 32.2b, c). The pancreatic body and tail are packaged with the head, and the pancreas is then taken on ice to the islet cell laboratory for processing.

A 5 French KMP catheter to be used for islet infusion is threaded into the portal vein to the bifurcation via a tributary of the middle colic vein. The catheter is sutured to the transverse mesocolon. Reconstruction is undertaken with a retrocolic end-to-side choledochojejunostomy. Gastrointestinal continuity is restored with an antecolic Roux-en-Y gastrojejunostomy. The abdomen is closed with interrupted fascial sutures, allowing an opening for the KMP catheter to exit at the inferior aspect of the incision. The fascial sutures where the catheter emerges are placed, but not tied.

Islet Cell Preparation

The prepared pancreas is transferred to the cGMP cell processing facility. A modified Ricordi method is utilized for islet harvest [9]. Islets are released from the exocrine and connective tissues of the gland via enzymatic and mechanical digestion. Collagenase (Liberase MTF, Roche, Indianapolis, IN USA) is infused

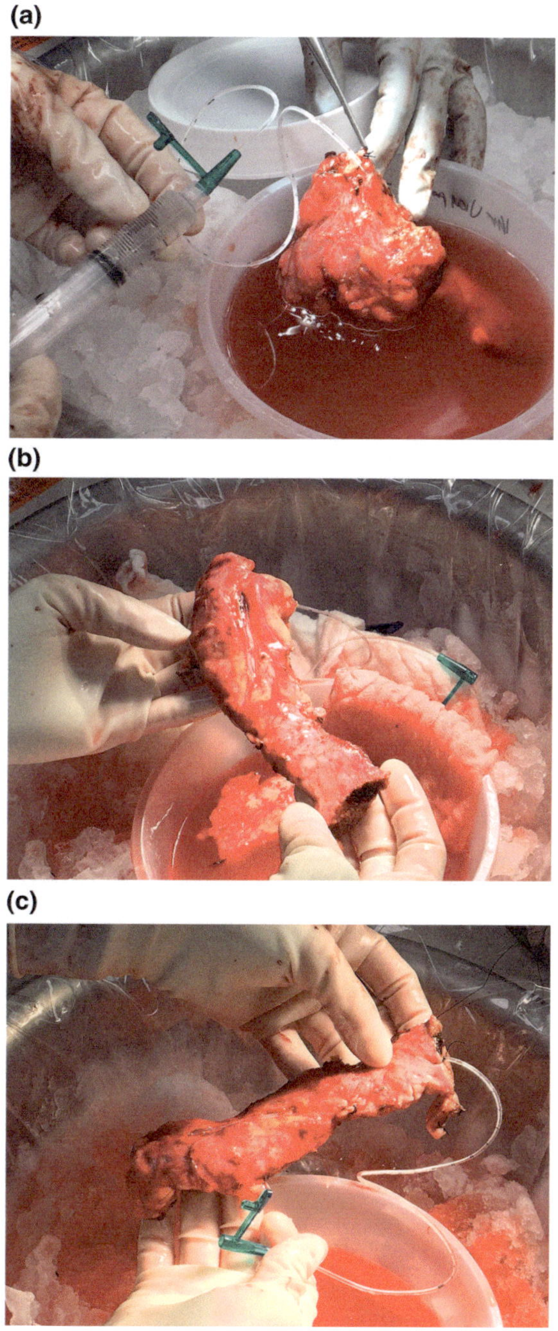

Fig. 32.2 **a** The head of the pancreas is prepared on the back table in cold preservation solution immediately upon extraction. The gastroduodenal artery is flushed to exsanguinate the organ. **b** Similarly, the body and tail of the pancreas are prepared. The splenic vein is opened and the splenic artery is flushed. **c** The main pancreatic duct of the prepared left pancreas is cannulated with a 5 French pediatric feeding tube, to be used in the cell processing lab for infusion of digestive protease

intraductally and/or injected directly into the pancreas for distension. The solution is perfused through a closed heated circuit to optimize enzymatic effect, and aliquots are examined periodically to determine timing of optimal islet separation. The islets are then separated by centrifugation. Islet yield, viability, function, and sterility are assessed. The isolated islets are then resuspended in 5% albumin solution with prophylactic antibiotic (cephazolin) and with heparin (70 U/kg body weight).

Islet Transplantation

The patient is admitted to the intensive care unit intubated and sedated following surgery. Once islet preparation is complete, the patient is transported to the interventional radiology suite, where catheter placement at the portal venous bifurcation is confirmed under fluoroscopy and the islets are infused by gravity through the catheter. Portal venous pressures are measured before, during, and after transplantation, as the portal system is a noncompliant system, and volume infusion can significantly raise portal venous pressure. Large increases in pressure and pressures greater than 30 mmHg have been shown to correlate with an increased incidence of portal vein thrombosis. Therefore, pressures greater than 25 mmHg prompts a delay in the infusion for 5 to 15 min. If the pressure does not come down in that time, the remaining islets can be infused into the peritoneal cavity. A completion portal venogram is performed (Fig. 32.3). The catheter is removed after transplant, and the venous branch clipped in the wound. The previously placed fascial sutures are tied and the skin closed.

Other centers perform intraoperative islet infusion, keeping the patient under anesthesia in the operating room during the islet harvest and autotransplanting the islets into the portal vein under direct visualization.

Technical Pearls for Total Pancreatectomy with Islet Autotransplantation

- Perfusion of the pancreas should be maintained during surgery to minimize warm ischemic time by ligating the vascular supply only when the organ is ready to be removed.
- Careful attention should be taken to preserve the left gastric (coronary) vein to maintain gastric vascular outflow and to minimize the incidence of postoperative delayed gastric emptying.
- A pylorus ablating procedure can be utilized to reduce the incidence of postoperative delayed gastric emptying.
- A Roux-en-Y alimentary reconstruction may improve postoperative gastric emptying and reduce risk of marginal ulceration when utilizing the pylorus ablating procedure with antrum intact.

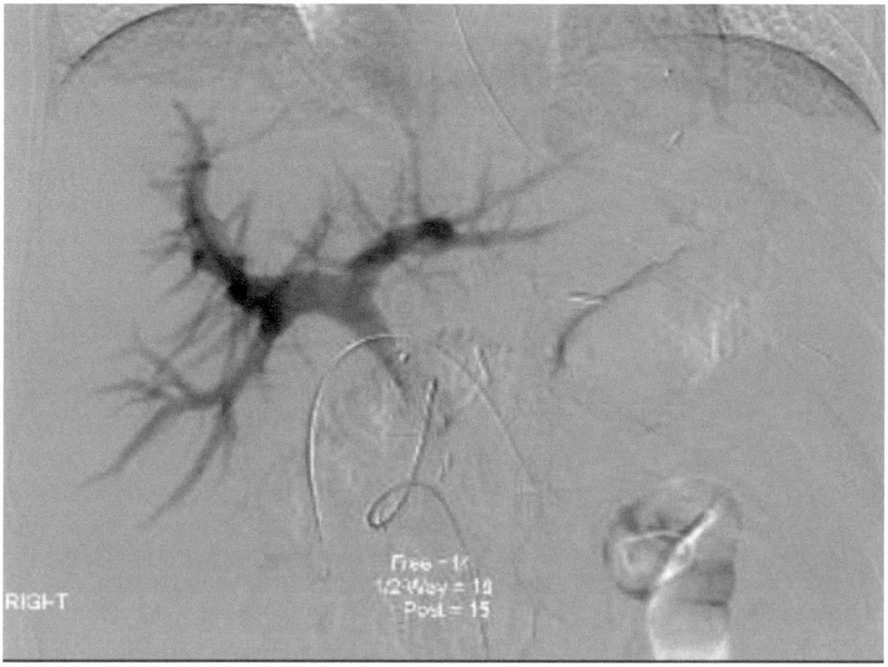

Fig. 32.3 Portal venogram after completion of islet infusion. Catheter enters through a portal venous tributary and the catheter tip is below the bifurcation

Postoperative Care

The patient is then transported back to the intensive care unit and extubated. Blood glucose levels are checked every 30 min for 2 h and then hourly thereafter. An insulin infusion is used to maintain blood glucose levels between 70–110 mg/dL. This is discontinued on postoperative day 3 and transitioned to low-dose long-acting insulin and sliding scale short-acting insulin, as needed. All patients are maintained on some dose of long-acting insulin except those with significant concerns for hypoglycemia, in order to rest the islets during engraftment.

A low-dose heparin infusion (250 U/h) is begun on the morning of postoperative day 1 if the hemoglobin has been stable. This is continued for 3 days, and the patient is transitioned to oral aspirin 81 mg.

A duplex ultrasound of the portal venous system is performed on the first postoperative day and again prior to discharge, to evaluate for portal vein thrombosis, which can be otherwise unrecognized and is well treated with therapeutic anticoagulation.

The islet preparation is sent for culture, and if gram stain or the final culture is positive, the patient is given prophylactic antibiotics to cover the offending organism for 3 days. The positive islet cultures do not seem to translate into meaningful clinical infections [10].

Postoperative pain control is achieved with a combination of epidural anesthesia, ketamine infusion, and intravenous narcotics. Non-narcotic adjuncts are maximally utilized. The ketamine infusion is tapered in 24 h, and the epidural is removed on the third day after surgery. Intravenous narcotics are slowly tapered with the addition of oral narcotics, as the patient is able to tolerate PO intake.

The nasogastric tube is removed on the first postoperative day and full liquids are begun, including oral nutritional supplements. Patients are advanced to full diabetic diet on the second day after surgery, as tolerated. Oral pancreatic enzymes are administered with diet. Early ambulation is supported [11].

Potential Complications

Complications associated with TPIAT are those seen with other major pancreatic surgeries, with the notable exception of postoperative pancreatic fistula.

Complications specific to islet autotransplantation include hemorrhage (from the anticoagulation given at infusion), portal vein thrombosis, and systemic inflammatory response. Acinar mantle cells surround the islets to keep them stable and intact. These cells, however, are a source of tissue thromboplastin, which is thrombogenic. Anticoagulation is administered with the islets during infusion to prevent portal vein thrombosis. Tissue thromboplastin as well as other factors associated with exocrine pancreatic tissue can incite systemic inflammatory response.

Long-Term Outcomes

After TPIAT, patients can expect pain relief and improvements in quality of life. On the Short Form Quality of Life questionnaire, significant improvements in all domains as early as 6 months postoperatively have been demonstrated by multiple centers. Narcotic weaning may be challenging, depending on patient history, support system, coping skills, and physician management. Thirty percent of patients will be insulin-free long-term (25% of adults, 55% of children) and 90% will have some demonstrable function of autotransplanted islets (serum c-peptide levels > 0.6 ng/ml) long-term [13] 1214]. Exocrine pancreatic insufficiency requires lifelong oral pancreatic enzyme supplementation and monitoring of nutritional health [15].

References

1. Bellin MD, Gelrud A, Arreaza-Rubin G, Dunn TB, Humar A, Morgan KA, et al. Total pancreatectomy with islet autotransplantation: summary of an NIDDK workshop. Ann Surg. 2015;261(1):21–9.
2. Chinnakotla S, Radosevich DM, Dunn TB, Bellin MD, Freeman ML, Schwarzenberg SJ, et al. Long-term outcomes of total pancreatectomy and islet autotransplantation for hereditary/genetic pancreatitis. J Am Coll Surg. 2014;218(4):530–43.
3. Morgan KA, Theruvath T, Owczarski S, Adams DB. Total pancreatectomy with islet autotransplantation for chronic pancreatitis: do patients with prior surgery have different outcomes? Am Surg. 2012;78(8):893–6.
4. Dunderdale J, McAuliffe JC, McNeal SF, Bryant SM, Yancey BD, Flowers G, Christein JD. Should pancreatectomy with islet cell autotransplantation in chronic alcoholic pancreatitis be abandoned? J Am Coll Surg. 2013;216(4):591–6.
5. Cote GA, Yadav D, Slivka A, Hawes RH, Anderson MA, Burton FR, et al. Alcohol and smoking as risk factors in an epidemiology study of patients with chronic pancreatitis. Clin Gastroenterol Hepatol. 2001;9(3):266–73.
6. Whitcomb DC, Gorry MC, Preston RA, Furey W, Sossenheimer MJ, Ulrich CD, et al. Hereditary pancreatitis is caused by a mutation in the cationic trypsinogen gene. Nat Genet. 1996;14(2):141–5.
7. Dorlon M, Owczarski SM, Wang H, Adams D, Morgan K. Increase in postoperative insulin requirements does not lead to decreased quality of life after total pancreatectomy with islet cell autotransplantation for chronic pancreatitis. Am Surg. 2013;79(7):676–80.
8. Morgan KA, Borckardt J, Balliet W, Owczarski SM, Adams DB. How are chronic pancreatitis patient selected for total pancreatectomy with islet autotransplantation? Are there psychometric predictors? J Am Coll Surg. 2015;220(4):693–8.
9. Ricordi C, Lacy PE, Finke EH, Olack BJ, Scharp DW. Automated method for isolation of human pancreatic islets. Diabetes. 1988;37(4):413–20.
10. Johnson CN, Morgan KA, Owczarski SM, Wang H, Fried J, Adams DB. Autotransplantation of culture positive islet product: is dirty always bad? HPB (Oxford). 2014;16(7):665–9.
11. Morgan KA, Lancaster WP, Walters ML, Owczarski SM, Clark CA, McSwain JR, et al. Enhanced recovery after surgery protocols are valuable in pancreas surgery patients. J Am Coll Surg. 2016;222(4):658–64.
12. Morgan K, Owczarski SM, Borckardt J, Madan A, Nishimura M, Adams DB. Pain control and quality of life after pancreatectomy with islet autotransplantation for chronic pancreatitis. J Gastrointest Surg. 2012;16(1):129–33.
13. Sutherland DE, Radosevich DM, Bellin MD, Hering BJ, Beilman GJ, Dunn TB, et al. Total pancreatectomy and islet autotransplantation for chronic pancreatitis. J Am Coll Surg. 2012;214(4):409–24.
14. Chinnakotla S, Beilman GJ, Dunn TB, Bellin MD, Freeman ML, Radosevich DM, et al. Factors predicting outcomes after a total pancreatectomy and islet autotransplantation lessons learned from over 500 cases. Ann Surg. 2015;262(4):610–22.
15. Crosby J, Bellin MD, Radosevich DM, Chinnakotla S, Dunn TB, Pruett TL, et al. Gastrointestinal symptoms before and after total pancreatectomy with islet autotransplantation: the role of pancreatic enzyme dosing and adherence. Pancreas. 2015;44(3):453–8.

Necrotizing Pancreatitis: Best Approaches

33

Attila Nakeeb and Nicholas J. Zyromski

Introduction

In the United States approximately 290,000 patients develop acute pancreatitis annually. More than 80% of cases of acute pancreatitis are due to either alcohol consumption or gallstone disease. More uncommon causes include metabolic disorders, trauma, tumors, and iatrogenic injuries (ERCP, surgery). The severity of acute pancreatitis ranges from edema to necrosis of the gland. The edematous form of the disease (mild acute pancreatitis) occurs in about 80–85% of patients and is self-limited, with recovery in a few days. In the 15–20% of patients with the most severe form of pancreatitis, hospitalization is prolonged, and commonly associated with the systemic inflammatory response syndrome (SIRS), multi-organ failure, and infection of the pancreatic necrosis. In these patients, mortality can be as high as 20% [1, 2].

Case Presentation

A 68-year-old-male with a history of coronary artery disease, atrial fibrillation, and diabetes mellitus, is transferred to a tertiary referral center 2 weeks into a course of severe necrotizing pancreatitis due to hypertriglyceridemia. On presentation, the

A. Nakeeb (✉) · N.J. Zyromski
Indiana University School of Medicine, 545 Barnhill Drive, Emerson Hall 539, Indianapolis, IN 46202, USA
e-mail: anakeeb@iupui.edu

N.J. Zyromski
e-mail: nzyromsk@iupui.edu

T.M. Pawlik et al. (eds.), *Case-Based Lessons in the Management of Complex Hepato-Pancreato-Biliary Surgery*, DOI 10.1007/978-3-319-50868-9_33

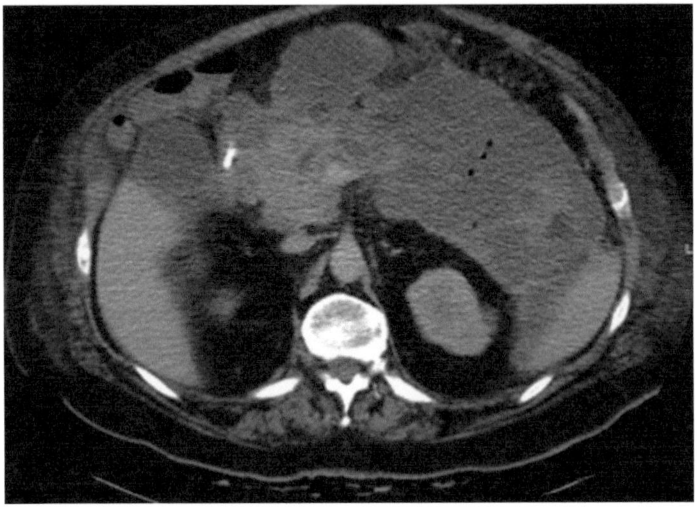

Fig. 33.1 IV contrast-enhanced CT scan showing pancreatic and peripancreatic necrosis and small gas bubbles, suggesting infected necrosis

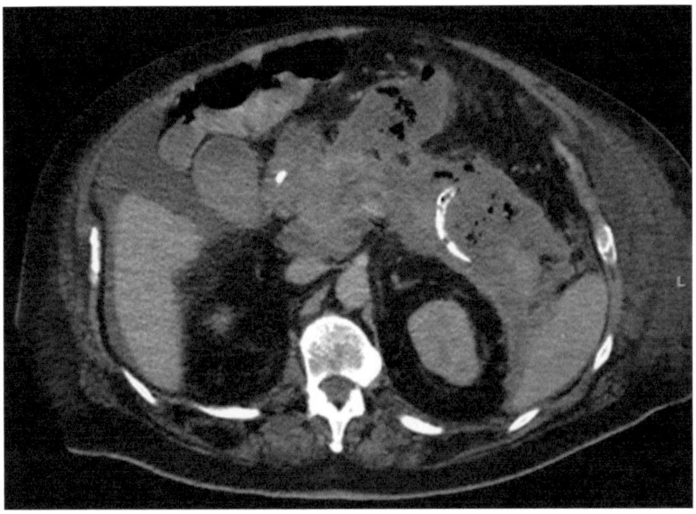

Fig. 33.2 CT scan showing percutaneous drain placed in a necrotic collection

patient was febrile to 39.5 °C and required norepinephrine to maintain a systolic blood pressure > 90 mmHg. He required mechanical ventilation for hypoxemia and required continuous veno-venous hemodialysis for an acute kidney injury. Contrast-enhanced computed tomography (CT) scan (Fig. 33.1) revealed necrotizing pancreatitis with evidence of infected pancreatic and peripancreatic necrosis

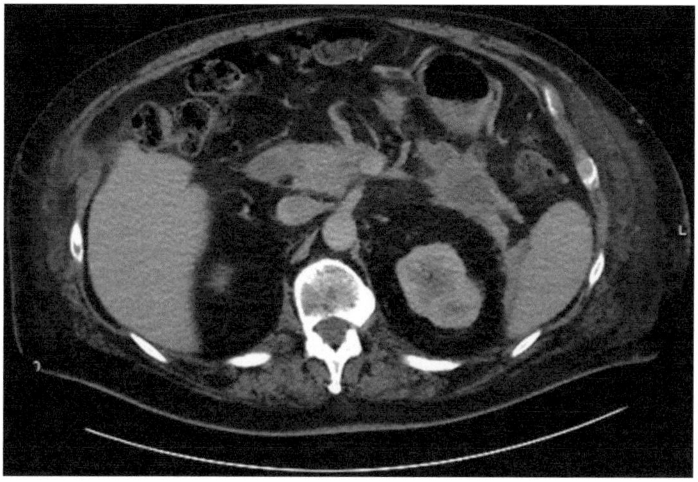

Fig. 33.3 Four-week post video-assisted retroperitoneal debridement CT scan demonstrating near complete resolution of the peripancreatic necrosis

in the lesser sac and tracking into the left pericolic gutter. He was started on broad-spectrum antibiotics and taken to interventional radiology for placement of a percutaneous drain into the infected fluid collection (Fig. 33.2). After percutaneous drainage his clinic course stabilized, and at four weeks he was taken to the operating room for a video-assisted retroperitoneal pancreatic debridement (VARD). Postoperatively he was able to be extubated, and his renal function recovered. Follow-up CT 1-month post debridement showed near complete resolution of his peripancreatic and pancreatic necrosis (Fig. 33.3).

Pathophysiology and Determination of Severity

Acute pancreatitis is a consequence of the intra-acinar cell cleavage of trypsinogen to trypsin, with subsequent activation of other enzymes. The local inflammatory response in the pancreas is associated with the liberation of oxygen-derived free radicals and cytokines, including interleukin (IL)-1, IL-6, IL-8, tumor necrosis factor alpha (TNFα), and platelet-activating factor (PAF) [3]; these mediators play an important role in the transformation of a local inflammatory response to systemic illness. The revised Atlanta classification of acute pancreatitis [4] stratifies patients with acute pancreatitis into mild, moderately severe, or severe categories based on the presence of organ failure and the presence of local or systemic complications. Organ failure is assessed by the modified Marshall scoring system (Table 33.1). Organ failure is defined by a score of two or more for the respiratory, cardiovascular, or renal systems. Local complications include acute peripancreatic fluid collections, pancreatic pseudocysts, acute necrotic collections (sterile or infected),

Table 33.1 Modified Marshall scoring system for organ dysfunction

Organ system	Score[a]				
	0	1	2	3	4
Respiratory (PaO_2/FiO_2)	>400	301–400	201–300	101–200	<101
Renal (serum Cr, mg/dl)	<1.4	1.4–1.8	1.9–3.6	3.6–4.9	>4.9
Cardiovascular (systolic BP, mm Hg)	>90	<90 fluid responsive	<90 not fluid responsive	<90 pH < 7.3	<90 pH < 7.2

[a]A score of 2 or greater defines organ failure

and walled of pancreatic necrosis (sterile or infected). Patients with mild pancreatitis have no evidence of organ failure or local or systemic complications. Moderately severe acute pancreatitis is defined by transient organ failure (resolves within 48 h) and/or local or systemic complications without persistent organ failure. Severe acute pancreatitis is characterized by persistent organ failure of one or multiple systems.

Medical Therapy

Initial therapy for patients with pancreatitis is mostly supportive. Severe acute pancreatitis is divided into two clinical phases; an early vasoactive and a late septic phase. The vasoactive phase typically occurs during the first 2 weeks and is dominated by the consequences of SIRS. Severe pancreatitis is associated with a marked increase in microvascular permeability, leading to large volume losses of intravascular fluid into the tissues, thereby decreasing perfusion of the lungs, kidneys, and other organs. The single most important element in preventing multiple organ failure is vigorous fluid resuscitation with electrolyte solutions in order to optimize cardiac output and to maintain hemodynamic stability. The management of the first phase of severe pancreatitis is summarized here:

Management of the First Phase of Severe Pancreatitis

- Fluid resuscitation
- Respiratory support
- Cardiovascular support
- Relief of pain
- Limitation of systemic complications
- Treatment of metabolic complications
- Nutritional support
- Prevention of infection

Table 33.2 Randomized controlled trials of enteral versus parenteral nutrition in severe pancreatitis

Author	Year	Country	Enteral	TPN	Rate of pancreatic infection
Kalfarentzos	1997	Greece	18	20	Decreased with enteral
Gupta	2003	UK	8	9	Decreased with enteral
Louie	2005	Canada	10	18	Decreased with enteral
Eckerwall	2006	Sweeden	23	25	Equal TPN and enteral
Petrov	2006	Russia	35	34	Decreased with enteral
Casas	2007	Spain	11	11	Decreased with enteral
Doley	2009	India	25	25	Equal TPN and enteral
Wu	2010	China	53	54	Decreased with enteral

The second phase of the disease is characterized by infection of pancreatic necrosis and subsequent sepsis. Both phases can result in multi-organ failure and death. Patients with mild pancreatitis usually experience resolution of their pain within 24–48 h after a regimen of no oral intake, narcotics for pain relief, and intravenous fluids.

Nutrition

Increasing evidence has suggested that enteral nutrition may be feasible, safe, and even desirable in severe pancreatitis (Table 33.2). Several randomized trials have documented that enteral nutrition, when tolerated, has the advantage of avoiding the high cost of total parenteral nutrition (TPN), as well as catheter-related complications, particularly line sepsis. Furthermore, the use of enteral nutrition, usually through a nasojejunal tube, may support intestinal mucosal integrity and avoid the alterations to intestinal barrier function and altered intestinal permeability associated with TPN. Enteral nutrition should be used if tolerated.

Prophylactic Antibiotics

Pancreatic infection is common with pancreatic necrosis, and the incidence of this infection increases with time, although it rarely occurs before the second week. Aerobic and anaerobic gastrointestinal flora are the primary organisms involved, and infections may be monomicrobial or polymicrobial. An association between pancreatic infection and mortality has been the rationale behind the widespread use of prophylactic systemic antibiotics in patients with pancreatic necrosis. Multiple prospective, randomized trials have compared prophylactic antibiotic treatment versus no treatment to prevent infection in patients with pancreatic necrosis (Table 33.3). Each trial has limitations; however, none have conclusively proved prophylactic antibiotic treatment decreases infectious complications, the rate of

Table 33.3 Randomized controlled trials of IV antibiotics for prophylaxsis for acute pancreatitis

Author	Year	Country	Abx	Treat group	Control group	Result
Howes	1975	US	Amp	48	47	No difference
Craig	1975	US	Amp	23	23	No difference
Finch	1976	US	Amp	31	27	No difference
Pederzoli	1993	Italy	Imipen	41	33	Decreased pancreatic infection
Sainio	1995	Finland	Cefurox	30	30	Decreased mortality
Delcenserie	1996	France	Ceftaz + Amik + Met	11	12	No difference
Schwarz	1997	Germany	Oflox + Met	13	13	No difference
Spicak	2003	Czech	Meropen	20	21	No difference
Isenmann	2004	Germany	Cipro + Met	58	56	No difference
Dellinger	2007	NA + Europe	Meropen	50	50	No difference
Rokke	2007	Norway	Imipen	36	37	Decreased pancreatic infection
Xue	2009	China	Imipen	29	27	No difference
Garcia-Barrasa	2009	Spain	Cipro	22	19	No difference

Amp Ampicillin, *Cefurox* Cefuroxime, *Ceftaz* Ceftazadine, *Amik* Amikacin, *Met* Metronidazole, *Cipro* Ciprofloxacin

need for surgical intervention, or mortality. The use of broad-spectrum antibiotics for this purpose is known to change the bacterial flora of pancreatic infection, and has been demonstrated to encourage the development of antibiotic-resistant bacterial and fungal infections [5]. The risk of superinfection is thought to be related to the length of treatment with prophylactic antibiotics. Currently, most authorities advocate against prophylactic antibiotic administration in necrotizing pancreatitis.

Management of Pancreatic Necrosis

Between 5 and 10% of patients with acute pancreatitis will develop necrosis of the pancreas and/or peripancreatic tissue. Intravenous contrast-enhanced CT scanning is the preferred imaging test for identifying pancreatic necrosis, as seen in Fig. 33.1. The impairment of pancreatic perfusion and subsequent pancreatic necrosis usually evolves over several days from the acute injury, and therefore early CT scanning may underestimate the degree of pancreatic necrosis. The sensitivity for identifying pancreatic necrosis using contrast-enhanced CT scan approaches 100% after four days from presentation. It is therefore reasonable to recommend an abdominal CT scan with intravenous contrast in patients with clinical and biochemical features of acute pancreatitis who do not improve after several days of conservative management. The extent of pancreatic and peripancreatic necrosis estimated on early contrast-enhanced helical CT is a specific predictor of morbidity and mortality.

Pancreatic and peripancreatic necrosis may be sterile or infected. There appears to be no correlation between the extent of necrosis and the development of infection. Infected pancreatic and peripancreatic necrosis is usually diagnosed by the demonstration of extra luminal gas on a contrast-enhanced CT scan, shown in Fig. 33.2, or by a positive gram stain or culture on image-guided fine-needle aspiration.

Sterile necrosis is best managed medically during the first 3–4 weeks. After this interval, if abdominal pain persists and prevents oral intake, debridement should be considered. This may be accomplished surgically, but percutaneous or endoscopic debridement is a reasonable choice in selected circumstances, if appropriate expertise is available. Delaying operative intervention for 4 weeks allows for consolidation of the peripancreatic necrosis, and allows for a safer debridement.

In the setting of infected pancreatic and peripancreatic necrosis the goal of intervention is to debride all necrotic infected tissue, drain infected fluid collections, minimize the risk of technical complications (including bleeding and enteric fistula), and ensure abdominal wall integrity. These goals can be accomplished either operatively, endoscopically, percutaneously, or by a combination of all approaches. Operative intervention should be delayed for at least 4 weeks after the original presentation due to the excessive mortality and morbidity from early operative debridement. Percutaneous drainage may be employed earlier if clinically indicated for control of sepsis.

Operative approaches can be categorized as either open (performed through a laparotomy incision) or minimally invasive, in which the retroperitoneum is reached endoscopically, laparoscopically, or through a small flank incision. The choice of approach depends on the specific anatomic locations of the areas to be drained or debrided and the severity of critical illness, which determines the rate at which source control needs to be achieved. Our approach is summarized in Fig. 33.4. In patients with necrosis limited to the lesser sac, we would recommend either an endoscopic or a laparoscopic transgastric necrosectomy. If the necrosis is limited to the lesser sac and tracks down the right or left pericolic gutter, we would favor a video-assisted retroperitoneal debridement (VARD) after establishing percutaneous drainage of the necrosis cavity. An open pancreatic debridement is preferred for patients with extensive necrosis that tracks into both pericolic gutters, or centrally down the root of the small bowel mesentery.

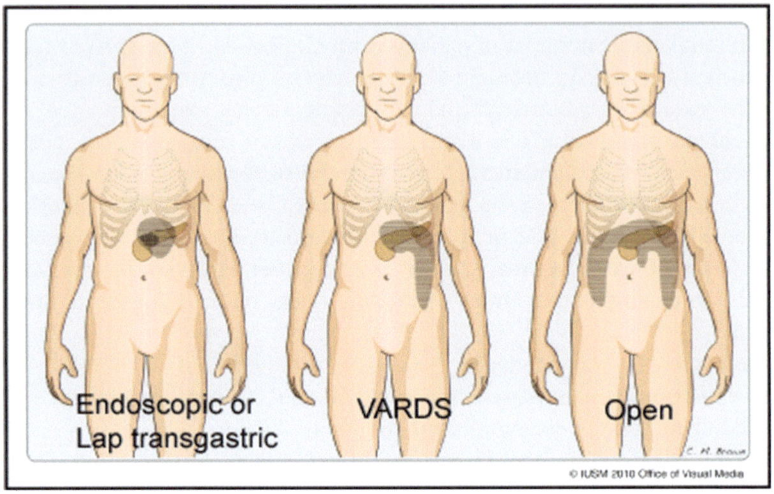

Fig. 33.4 Patterns of pancreatic necrosis and preferred debridement technique. Reprinted from Journal of Gastrointestinal Surgery. 2016; 20(2):445–9. Transgastric pancreatic necrosectomy: how I do it. Zyromski NJ, Nakeeb A, House MG, Jester AL. With permission of Springer

Management of Pancreatic Necrosis

- Supportive care during early phase of severe acute pancreatitis
- Avoid prophylactic antibiotic therapy
- Early enteral nutrition
- Percutaneous drainage of infected necrosis
- Delay pancreatic debridement for minimum of 4 weeks
- Individualize debridement technique to pattern of necrosis.

Endoscopic Necrosectomy

Endoscopic necrosectomy can be accomplished from either the stomach or the duodenum. Puncture of the fluid collection can be made either directly by visualizing a bulge or with endoscopic ultrasound (EUS) guidance. The collection is punctured with a 19-gauze needle and a guide-wire is advanced under fluoroscopic guidance. The tract is balloon dilated up to 8 mm and either two double pigtail plastic stents or a lumen-opposing metal stent is placed. The cavity is irrigated with 1 L of normal saline per 24 h via a nasogastric tube placed into the collection. Necrotic tissue is evacuated with a basket, a net, or a polypectomy snare [6, 7]. The endoscopic approach often requires multiple procedures to adequately remove all necrotic material. Lumen-opposing stents should be removed once the necrosectomy is completed. Several authors recommend leaving double pigtail stents in permanently, though long-term follow-up of this strategy is lacking.

Laparoscopic Transgastric Necrosectomy

An alternative approach to an endoscopic necrosectomy is the laparoscopic transgastric necrosectomy [8]. Advantages of this approach are the ability to accomplish debridement in a single procedure, the creation of a large cystogastrostomy to drain residual collections, and the ability to perform cholecystectomy for patients with gallstone pancreatitis. This approach can also be used in patients with gastric varices from sinistral portal hypertension, making endoscopic transgastric drainage too dangerous. The procedure is shown in Fig. 33.5. A gastrotomy is created in the anterior wall of the stomach between stay sutures, and a laparoscopic aspirating needle is placed thru the posterior wall of the stomach into the necrosis cavity to localize the collection. Alternatively, intraoperative ultrasound can be used to identify the point of contact between the posterior stomach and the necrosis cavity. A posterior stay suture is placed into the posterior gastric wall and used as a traction suture to facilitate a posterior gastrotomy made with an ultrasonic scalpel. The posterior gastrotomy is extended, and a running 2–0 monofilament suture or endovascular stapler can be used to secure the stomach to the cyst cavity wall. Laparoscopic instruments and suction irrigation are then used to debride all loose necrosis from the retroperitoneum and placed in an endocatch bag for extraction. The anterior gastrotomy is then closed with a linear stapler or suture. This transgastric approach is also feasible through a short (open) upper midline incision.

Video-Assisted Retroperitoneal Debridement (VARD)

The initial step to performing VARD procedure is to have the interventional radiologists place a 14 French percutaneous drain into the peripancreatic collection through a retroperitoneal flank approach. This drain may be serially upsized, and may provide definitive treatment for the necrosis in up to one-third of patients [9]. If percutaneous drainage does not lead to clinical improvement, VARD may be undertaken (Fig. 33.6). The patient is placed in supine position with the left side elevated 30°–40° A 5-cm incision is made close to the exit point of the percutaneous drain. The drain is then used as a guide to carefully dissect into the retroperitoneum, and the cavity entered. Irrigation and debridement of the superficial necrosis are carried out under direct vision. A 0° laparoscope or a videoendoscope can be placed into the cavity and further debridement can be accomplished using ring forceps or laparoscopic graspers and suction irrigators [10]. The debridement should be performed cautiously, removing only loose nonadherent necrosis, to avoid injury to any underlying blood vessels. Bleeding can be controlled with electrocautery or laparoscopic clips. In the rare case of extensive

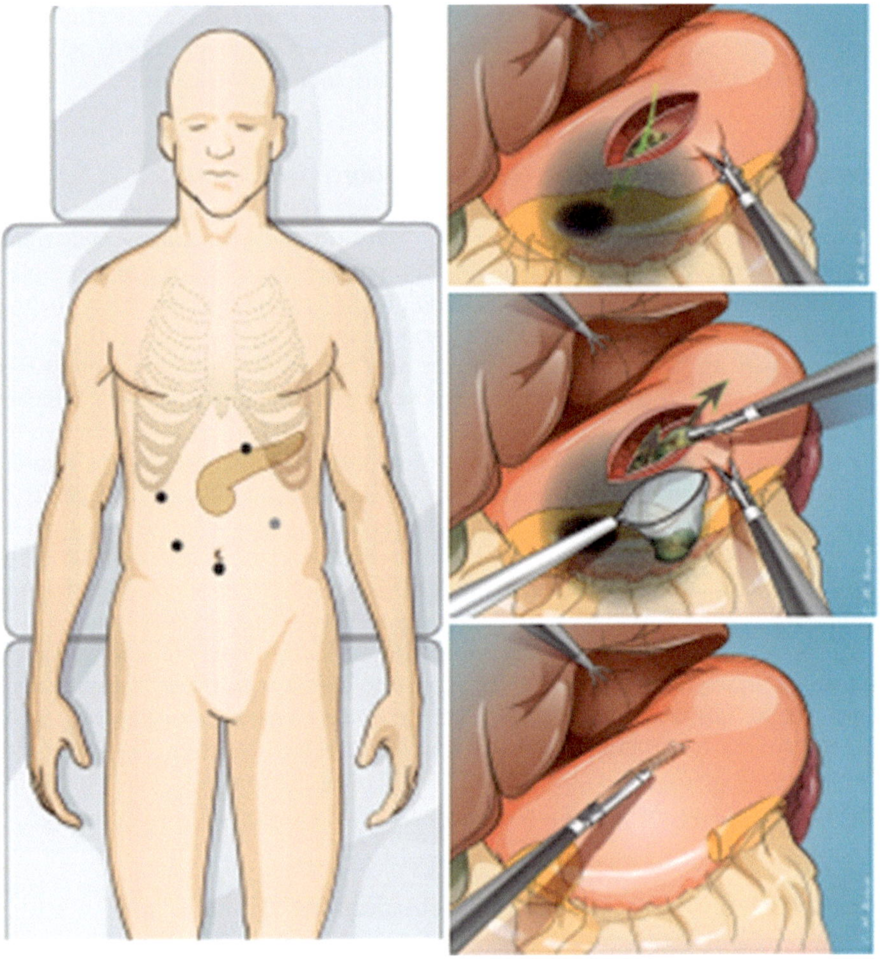

Fig. 33.5 Technique of laparoscopic transgastric debridement. Reprinted from Journal of Gastrointestinal Surgery. 2016; 20(2):445–9. Transgastric pancreatic necrosectomy: how I do it. Zyromski NJ, Nakeeb A, House MG, Jester AL; with permission of Springer

hemorrhage, packing of the retroperitoneal cavity can be performed and the procedure converted to a laparotomy, or the patient can be taken to radiology for angiographic embolization. After the debridement is completed, the percutaneous drain is exchanged for two drains that are brought out through the incision, and the fascia is closed. Continuous lavage is performed through the drains, with either normal saline or dialysis fluid, until the effluent is clear.

This step-up approach to the management of pancreatic necrosis was compared to traditional open debridement in a multicenter, randomized, prospective trial completed in the Netherlands [9]. The authors found that of the patients assigned to the step-up approach, 35% were treated with percutaneous drainage only.

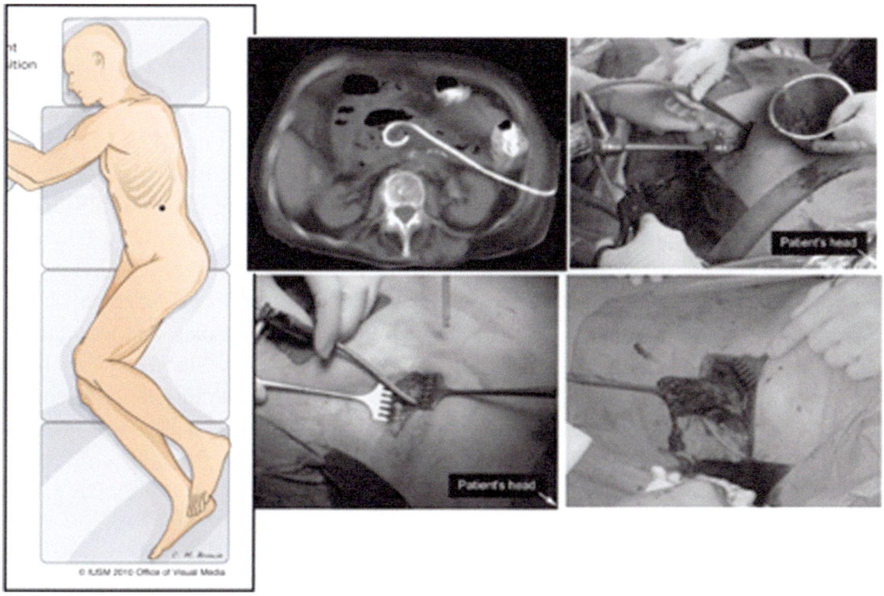

Fig. 33.6 Technique of video-assisted retroperitoneal debridement. Reprinted from HPB (Oxford) 2007;9:156–59. van Santvoort HC, Besselink MG, Horvath KD, Sinanan MN, Bollen TL, van Ramshorst B, et al. Videoscopic assisted retroperitoneal debridement in infected necrotizing pancreatitis; with permission from Elsevier

New-onset multiple organ failure occurred less often in patients assigned to the step-up approach than in those assigned to open necrosectomy (12% vs. 40%, $P = 0.002$). Mortality did not differ significantly between groups (19% vs. 16%). Additionally, patients assigned to the step-up approach had a statistically significant lower rate of incisional hernias (7% vs. 24%) and new-onset diabetes (16% vs. 38%) than patients treated with open debridement.

Open Pancreatic Debridement

Open pancreatic debridement remains a viable option for patients with infected pancreatic and peripancreatic necrosis that are not amenable to, or have failed, minimally invasive techniques. The goals of open pancreatic debridement are to control infection, to evacuate all peripancreatic fluid and necrotic debris, to externally drain any pancreatic fistulae, and to establish enteral access for postoperative nutrition. Surgical intervention should be delayed for a minimum of 4 weeks if possible. The extent of debridement should be based on careful interpretation of preoperative CT imaging to ensure all necrotic collections are addressed.

Open pancreatic debridement can be accomplished through a midline or bilateral subcostal incision. The pancreatic and peripancreatic necrosis can be accessed either through the transverse mesocolon or directly through the gastrocolic ligament. If a transverse mesocolon approach is chosen, the transverse colon and omentum are elevated anteriorly and an opening is made in the avascular plane to the left of the middle colic vessels to enter the lesser sac. Care must be taken to dissect any adherent small bowel away from the mesocolon. If a gastrocolic approach is chosen, the gastrocolic omentum should be divided inferior to the gastroepiploic vessels to enter the lesser sac. Oftentimes this plane is difficult to enter, due to significant inflammation in the lesser sac, and care should be taken not to injure the colon or its mesentery. Once the lesser sac is entered, all the peripancreatic fluid and necrosis can be gently debrided using a combination of ring forceps and suction/irrigation. Again, only nonadherent necrosis and devitalized tissue are removed, and care should be taken not to avulse any blood vessels. If the necrosis tracks down the pericolic gutters, the colon should be mobilized medially to facilitate debridement. Large-caliber drains should be placed into the necrosis cavity to control any potential pancreatic fistulae and to facilitate postoperative lavage. Our preference is to place a gastrojejunostomy tube for postoperative gastric decompression and enteral feeding.

Approaches to Pancreatic Debridement

- Percutaneous drainage
- Endoscopic transgastric
- Laparoscopic transgastric
- Video-assisted retroperitoneal debridement (VARDS)
- Open debridement (laparotomy).

Complications

The main complications associated with pancreatic necrosectomy include perioperative hemorrhage; pancreatic fistula and disconnected left pancreatic remnant; enteric fistulas (colon, duodenum, stomach); intestinal/gallbladder ischemia; and pancreatic endocrine and exocrine insufficiency.

Hemorrhage in acute pancreatitis may be venous or arterial, and may occur prior to or following intervention. Pre-intervention hemorrhage is reliably diagnosed by the presence of high attenuation (30 Hounsfield Units) material in peripancreatic collections visualized by contrast-enhanced computed tomography (CT). After intervention (either operation or percutaneous drainage of pancreatic necrosis), the presence of blood in surgical or radiologically placed drains is the most common manifestation of this complication. Though relatively minor venous bleeding (perhaps from irritation by the drains) is fairly common, potentially life-threatening bleeding from visceral arterial pseudoaneurysm (PSA) must be considered and ruled out. Currently, dedicated CT angiogram is the exam of choice to diagnose PSA; in addition to offering a high-contrast evaluation of the entire visceral arterial tree with a single contrast bolus, this test also provides cross-sectional abdominal images of residual peripancreatic collections. Angiographic embolization provides definitive therapy for PSA in nearly all cases [11].

Pancreatic fistula by definition involves disruption of the pancreatic ductal system, and may manifest as an external fistula (following intervention), or as pancreatic ascites or pleural effusion with amylase rich fluid in patients who have not been instrumented. Defining the pancreatic ductal anatomy is central to planning treatment; this work-up generally requires endoscopic retrograde cholangiopancreatography (ERCP)—which may be therapeutic as well as diagnostic. It is worthy of note that magnetic resonance cholangiopancreatography (MRCP) is less helpful in the setting of ascites or peripancreatic fluid collections, which obscure ductal anatomic features. Fistulae from smaller side branches are typically lower volume, on the order of 50 mL daily. These side branch fistulae generally "dry up" spontaneously, and may be managed by sequential "cracking" and withdrawal of drains. Fluoroscopic sinogram in these situations often provides valuable information. Major pancreatic fistulae result from "disconnection" of the main pancreatic duct, where a viable body/tail loses ductal continuity with the pancreatic head and duodenum. The viable, disconnected left pancreatic remnant generally requires operative intervention, with the patient's anatomy dictating ideal operation—pancreaticojejunostomy versus left pancreatectomy/splenectomy [12]. In the setting of disconnected left pancreatic remnant, transgastric debridement with "cyst-gastrostomy" draining the pancreatic tail at the time of initial debridement is an attractive solution for select patients.

Intestinal or colonic ischemia probably occurs with much greater frequency than is commonly recognized in patients with necrotizing pancreatitis; clinicians caring for these patients must keep a high degree of suspicion for this problem, especially in patients who suddenly turn for the worse after a period of relative stability. The only way to assuredly rule out (or rule in) ischemic bowel is by laparotomy and direct inspection of the abdominal contents. The price of a "nontherapeutic" laparotomy is small compared to that of missing the diagnosis and potential to treat ischemic bowel before perforation occurs.

Awareness of the abdominal compartment syndrome is important in patients with severe acute pancreatitis. Patients with findings of intra-abdominal compartment syndrome require decompressive laparotomy if they fail to respond to non-operative measures.

Conclusion

Management of patients with severe pancreatitis and pancreatic necrosis require a multi-disciplinary team. Surgeons, critical care physicians, gastroenterologists, and interventional radiologists must be involved in caring for these complex patients.

Over the past decade, better critical care, the introduction of early enteral nutrition, the appropriate use of antibiotics, delaying intervention for a minimum of 4 weeks, and the application of minimally invasive techniques have all led to lower morbidity and mortality in patients with pancreatic necrosis.

References

1. Fagenholz PJ, Fernandez-del Castillo C, Harris NS, Pelletier AJ, Camargo Jr CA. Direct medical costs of acute pancreatitis hospitalizations in the United States. Pancreas. 2007;35 (4):302–7.
2. Freeman ML, Werner J, van Santvoort HC, Baron TH, Besselink MG, Windsor JA, et al. Interventions for necrotizing pancreatitis: summary of a multidisciplinary consensus conference. Pancreas. 2012;41(8):1176–94.
3. Frossard JL, Steer ML, Pastor CM. Acute pancreatitis. Lancet. 2008;371(9607):143–52.
4. Banks PA, Bollen TL, Dervenis C, Gooszen HG, Johnson CD, Sarr MG, et al. Classification of acute pancreatitis–2012: revision of the Atlanta classification and definitions by international consensus. Gut. 2013;62(1):102–11.
5. Howard TJ, Tempel MB. Prophylactic antibiotics alter the bacteriology of pancreatic necrosis in severe acute pancreatitis. J Am Coll Surg. 2002;195(6):759–76.
6. Bakker OJ, van Santvoort HC, van Brunschot S, Geskus RB, Besselink MG, Bollen TL, et al. Endoscopic transgastric vs surgical necrosectomy for infected necrotizing pancreatitis: a randomized trial. JAMA. 2012;307(10):1053–61.
7. Haghshenasskashani A, Laurence JM, Kwan V, Johnston E, Hollands MJ, Richardson AJ, et al. Endoscopic necrosectomy of pancreatic necrosis: a systematic review. Surg Endosc. 2011;25(12):3724–30.
8. Zyromski NJ, Nakeeb A, House MG, Jester AL. Transgastric pancreatic necrosectomy: how I do it. J Gastrointest Surg. 2016;20(2):445–9.
9. van Santvoort HC, Besselink MG, Bakker OJ, Hofker HS, Boermeester MA, Dejong CH, et al. A step-up approach or open necrosectomy for necrotizing pancreatitis. N Engl J Med. 2010;362(16):1491–502.
10. van Santvoort HC, Besselink MG, Horvath KD, Sinanan MN, Bollen TL, van Ramshorst B, et al. Videoscopic assisted retroperitoneal debridement in infected necrotizing pancreatitis. HPB (Oxford). 2007;9(2):156–9.
11. Zyromski NJ, Vieira C, Stecker M, Nakeeb A, Pitt HA, Lillemoe KD, et al. Improved outcomes in postoperative and pancreatitis-related visceral pseudoaneurysms. J Gastrointest Surg. 2007;11(1):50–5.
12. Murage KP, Ball CG, Zyromski NJ, Nakeeb A, Ocampo C, Sandrasegaran K, et al. Clinical framework to guide operative decision making in disconnected left pancreatic remnant (DLPR) following acute or chronic pancreatitis. Surgery. 2010;148(4):847–56; discussion 856–7.

Pancreatic Pseudocyst: Operative Versus Endoscopic Approach

34

Benjamin D. Ferguson and Jeffrey B. Matthews

Introduction

A pancreatic pseudocyst is classically defined as a collection of peripancreatic fluid bordered by a non-epithelialized capsule that develops as a consequence of pancreatic parenchymal/ductal disruption. The clinical presentation varies. Symptoms may include persistent abdominal or back pain, nausea and vomiting, jaundice, and intolerance of oral intake in the weeks and months after an episode of pancreatitis or pancreatic trauma. Symptoms are often attributable to compression and distortion of local structures, leading to obstruction. Some patients are asymptomatic. The natural history is also highly variable. While pancreatic pseudocysts may resolve spontaneously, many persist and continue to cause chronic morbidity that is difficult to control without definitive management. Rarely, erosion into an adjacent vascular structure may lead to hemorrhage within the pseudocyst cavity; progressive enlargement of a pseudocyst may lead to arterial pseudoaneurysm, rupture of which may be fatal. For this reason, therapeutic intervention is generally indicated for even mildly symptomatic or enlarging pseudocysts. Options for pseudocyst management include surgical and endoscopic approaches. Historically, open surgical techniques have been the mainstay of treatment for symptomatic pseudocyst disease. More recently, laparoscopic and endoscopic approaches have become increasingly commonly employed.

B.D. Ferguson
Department of Surgery, University of Chicago, 5841 S. Maryland, MC6040, Chicago, IL 60637, USA
e-mail: benjamin.ferguson@uchospitals.edu

J.B. Matthews (✉)
The University of Chicago, 5891S, Maryland Avenue, MC 5029, Chicago, IL 60134, USA
e-mail: jmatthews@uchicago.edu

T.M. Pawlik et al. (eds.), *Case-Based Lessons in the Management of Complex Hepato-Pancreato-Biliary Surgery*, DOI 10.1007/978-3-319-50868-9_34

Pancreatic pseudocyst should be distinguished from walled-off pancreatic necrosis (WOPN), as these may require different management strategies. By consensus definition [1], WOPN evolves over several weeks from acute necrotic collections in the context of necrotizing pancreatitis, and represents solid and variably liquefied pancreatic parenchyma and surrounding retroperitoneal adipose and connective tissue surrounded by a fibrous non-epithelialized capsule. In contrast, a pseudocyst evolves from acute fluid collections that follow an attack of acute interstitial pancreatitis, and contains primarily thin, amylase-rich fluid with relatively little solid debris within a similarly encapsulated structure. Pancreatic pseudocyst and WOPN are not infrequently confused on CT and, indeed, in reality there is a continuum of peripancreatic fluid/debris collections within the spectrum of complicated acute pancreatitis. MRI or ultrasound may be particularly helpful to distinguish solid from liquid content within a walled-off collection.

Symptomatic pseudocysts are primarily managed by decompression and internal drainage, whereas WOPN usually requires drainage and often some degree of debridement to remove the solid debris from the necroma cavity, not infrequently requiring multiple staged procedures, particularly in the patient with infected necrosis. In practice, there is considerable overlap in the decision-making for treatment of symptomatic pseudocyst and WOPN.

Here, we present and discuss three cases that illustrate various aspects of planning, multidisciplinary treatment approaches, and associated technical challenges with respect to pancreatic pseudocyst and WOPN. For the purposes of this chapter, discussion is limited to the management of symptomatic, persistent, predominantly fluid-filled peripancreatic collections that can occur after either severe acute interstitial or necrotizing pancreatitis. For simplicity, the term “pseudocyst” is used throughout. The related topic of the treatment of suspected infected pseudocyst or WOPN in the acute and subacute setting is omitted.

Case 1

A 57-year-old man with a history of acute idiopathic necrotizing pancreatitis 2 months earlier developed left upper quadrant fullness and early satiety within 6 weeks following resolution of his pancreatitis. CT demonstrated a 10 × 8.5 × 5.8 cm cystic mass involving the majority of the pancreatic body and tail, with mass effect on the posterior wall of the stomach. Repeat CT subsequently demonstrated interval enlargement of the mass to 11 × 9.5 × 6.2 cm. A CT-guided percutaneous drainage catheter was placed into the cystic collection by interventional radiology. This procedure relieved the majority of his symptoms, but the percutaneous catheter continued to drain more than 250 cc daily for several weeks. During this time, he reported a decrease in weight from 200 to 147 lb. His care was transferred to our institution for ongoing management, and he was initially evaluated for roughly 10 weeks after resolution of his pancreatitis with ongoing left upper quadrant discomfort. Repeat CT again demonstrated a pancreatic pseudocyst that now measured

6.9 × 5.1 cm, with an indwelling percutaneous catheter (Fig. 34.1a). There was no clinical evidence of infection, but the persistent cyst cavity suggested incomplete drainage of what was likely to be superinfected fluid with or without infected solid necrosis.

Because the residual cystic cavity appeared be easily accessible through the posterior wall of the stomach and continued to demonstrate compression of the gastric wall, he was determined to be an excellent candidate for endoscopic drainage. Upper endoscopy revealed extrinsic compression of the posterior gastric body. Endoscopic ultrasound identified a 6.8 × 5.0 cm fluid collection in this region containing fluid and only a small amount of solid debris. Thus, while the cystic collection (which followed an episode of necrotizing pancreatitis) might more properly be termed WOPN, its predominantly fluid-filled nature more closely resembled a pseudocyst for practical purposes. There was no obvious evidence of communication with the main pancreatic duct, but the persistent high-output fistulous drainage suggested that this was likely the case. Using color Doppler imaging to identify any interposed vessels between the walls of the stomach and pseudocyst, the cyst was punctured under endosonographic guidance and a wire was inserted under fluoroscopic guidance. Thin fluid and thicker purulent material drained from the cyst (Fig. 34.1b); the fluid was sent for amylase level which later proved to be greater than 20,000 U/L. A larger cystotomy was made with an over-the-wire cautery-enhanced lumen-apposing self-expandable metal stent. The cystotomy was dilated to 12 mm using a balloon dilator, and a 10-French double-pigtail plastic stent was placed across the metal stent to prevent intermitted occlusion by necrotic debris. While in the recovery area following the procedure, he briefly developed a fever to 38.7 °C and was started on broad-spectrum antibiotics while awaiting culture results from the pancreatic fluid. This eventually grew *Streptococcus constellatus* and coagulase-negative *Staphylococcus*, and he was transitioned to oral ciprofloxacin and clindamycin for a total of 7 days.

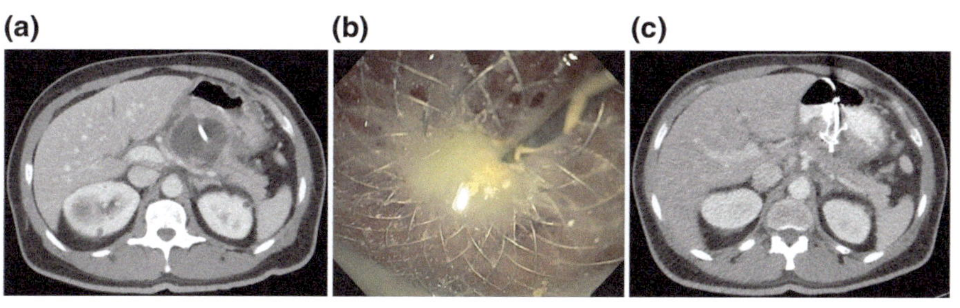

Fig. 34.1 **a** A residual pseudocyst is evident on repeat CT with indwelling percutaneous drain in place. Note compression of the posterior wall of the stomach. **b** Drainage of thin fluid and pus from the pseudocyst cavity upon placement of the self-expanding metal stent prior to balloon dilation and placement of an additional double-pigtail plastic stent. **c** Near-resolution of the pseudocyst, with the dumbbell-shaped metal stent in good position and plastic stent traversing through it

He tolerated sips of water on the day of the procedure and was advanced to a general diet within 2 days. His symptoms of left upper quadrant pain and early satiety resolved, his percutaneous drain was clamped, at its output had decreased dramatically, and he was discharged home on post-procedure day three. At that time, repeat CT showed that his pancreatic fluid collection had nearly resolved, with only a 1.5 × 1.2 cm residual collection remaining (Fig. 34.1c). He passed the plastic stent with a bowel movement at 2 weeks following the procedure, with no subsequent development of abdominal complaints. Surveillance MRI/MRCP at 5 weeks post-procedure demonstrated resolution of the collection. He continues to be free of symptoms from the pseudocyst at 2 months of follow-up; he has gained 10 lb, and his metal stent and percutaneous drain were removed at 3 months.

Case 2

A 52-year-old man with ulcerative colitis initially presented to pancreatology clinic after being referred for refractory back pain following an episode of severe acute necrotizing pancreatitis 11 months earlier that had been attributed to alcohol abuse. He did well after his initial 3-week admission, but 8 months later developed constant pressure-like back pain that was accompanied by abdominal cramping and occasional nausea with vomiting. His pain was poorly controlled despite multiple pain-control regimens. He also reported weight loss and steatorrhea consistent with exocrine insufficiency that improved with pancreatic enzyme replacement. His type 3c diabetes was relatively well controlled with long- and short-acting insulin supplementation. His lipase, triglyceride, and IgG4 levels were within the normal ranges. MRI/MRCP obtained prior to his presentation revealed a 13.5 × 5.8 cm well-encapsulated fluid collection nearly completely replacing the pancreatic parenchyma, associated with narrowing of the common bile duct and the confluence of the superior mesenteric and splenic veins (Fig. 34.2a). Subsequent pancreas-protocol CT confirmed the appearance of a large pancreatic pseudocyst with similar measurements and findings consistent with compression of adjacent structures (Fig. 34.2b).

The gastric body and splenic vein were noted to be displaced somewhat superiorly, the gastric antrum and transverse colon were veiled over the anterior aspect of the pseudocyst, and the lateral and posterior borders of the pseudocyst were closely associated with the spleen, left kidney, and loops of mid-jejunum. Because of these anatomic relationships, endoscopic and percutaneous approaches for drainage were felt to be unsafe. He was therefore evaluated in our pancreatic surgery clinic and underwent operation the following week. Diagnostic laparoscopy confirmed only limited apposition of the posterior gastric wall to the pseudocyst, a finding that was felt to preclude safe laparoscopic transgastric decompression. Instead, the procedure was converted to laparotomy and, after localization and aspiration of murky fluid from the pseudocyst, a 3-cm hand-sewn cystgastrostomy was created with a double-armed running locked Connell suture using absorbable monofilament. The pseudocyst cavity was almost entirely fluid-filled and contained

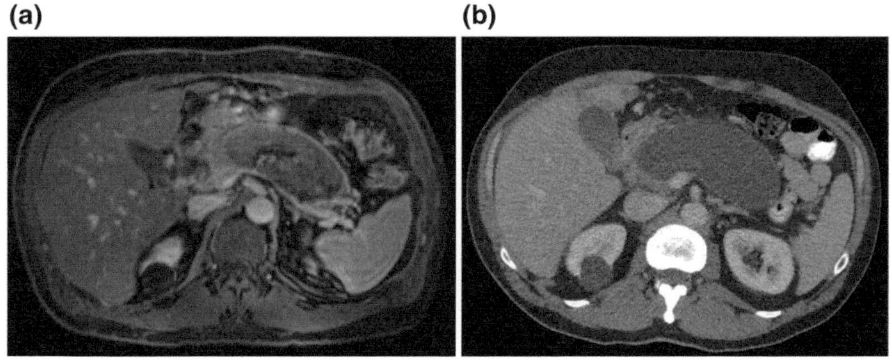

Fig. 34.2 **a** MRI with evidence of pancreatic parenchyma replacement by the pseudocyst, and essentially complete obliteration of the SMV-splenic vein confluence. **b** Pancreas-protocol CT with evidence of compression of adjacent structures, and poor apposition with the stomach and distal portions of the duodenum. Also note abutment of the splenic vein posteriorly, and several loops of jejunum and colon surrounding the lateral and anterior borders of the pseudocyst

only minimal solid necrotic debris. The patient tolerated a diabetic diet by post-operative day two and was discharged the following day on oral narcotic pain medication. He continued to have full symptomatic resolution over nearly 3 years of follow-up.

Case 3

A 54-year-old man who was initially diagnosed with recurrent pancreatitis of unknown etiology 16 months earlier presented to gastroenterology clinic with persistent vague upper abdominal pain associated with weight loss and decreased appetite. At presentation, lipase, triglyceride, and IgG4 levels were normal, and genetic panel testing that had been performed at an outside facility was negative for autoimmune or genetic/hereditary causes of pancreatitis. Abdominal ultrasound obtained at an outside center revealed a cystic mass in the left upper quadrant that was incompletely visualized. Subsequent MRI/MRCP demonstrated a 14.3 × 8.1 cm cystic mass in the distal pancreas with total replacement of the pancreatic body and tail that was felt to represent a pseudocyst, although a cystic neoplasm could not be excluded (Fig. 34.3a). The portal confluence was severely compressed with splenic thrombosis and associated collateral vessels. Endoscopic ultrasound was performed for further characterization, and again identified a septated, thin-walled cystic mass within the distal pancreas (Fig. 34.3b) as well as prominent adjacent vessels consistent with gastric varices. Because there was limited contact between the posterior gastric and cyst walls, and because neoplasm could not be excluded, fine-needle aspiration was performed for laboratory analysis, which revealed thin fluid with an amylase level of 9830 U/L, low CEA, and

(a) (b)

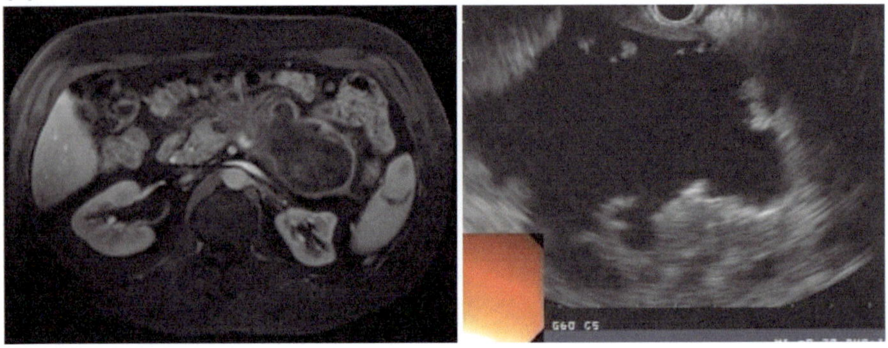

Fig. 34.3 **a** MRI with evidence of a large, thin-walled, septated cystic pancreatic mass. Note loops of jejunum and colon draped over the anterior surface of the pseudocyst, with no close apposition to the stomach, which precluded safe endoscopic management. **b** Endosonographic appearance of the septated cystic mass without direct apposition between the stomach and cyst wall

non-malignant cells on cytologic evaluation. Following this procedure, he developed mild recurrent pancreatitis with persistent fever that was treated with oral antibiotics and allowed to resolve prior to further invasive therapy.

Surgical rather than endoscopic internal drainage of the pseudocyst was chosen on the basis of limited abutment of the pseudocyst on the stomach as well as concern for gastric varices and extensive venous collateralization. A laparoscopic approach was undertaken. Varices were predominantly contained within the omentum and could be avoided during exposure of the posterior gastric wall, which was able to be drawn over toward the pseudocyst capsule without tension. A laparoscopic 2.5-cm hand-sewn cystgastrostomy with running nonabsorbable suture was performed in Connell fashion. The patient tolerated a low-fat diet by postoperative day two and was discharged the same day on oral narcotic pain medications. He continued to be asymptomatic over 6 months of observation.

Discussion

Optimal management of pancreatic pseudocyst requires multidisciplinary planning and nuanced clinical judgment. Adequate pre-intervention imaging is particularly important. MRCP can non-invasively distinguish the relative amount of liquid versus solid debris contained within peripancreatic collection, indicating the extent of debridement that may be necessary in addition to establishing internal drainage. MRCP also non-invasively outlines the pancreatic duct system, which also may be useful in determining whether a given patient might also benefit from pancreatic duct stenting to dilate ductal strictures or bridge areas of ductal disruption. Various technical "tricks of the trade" are summarized here

Clinical Pearls

- Transgastric internal drainage (cystgastrostomy) can be established by open or laparoscopic surgery, or endoscopically.
- A Roux-en-y enteric conduit is a versatile solution to pseudocysts that are otherwise not easily amenable to the transgastric route.
- The relative amount of solid debris contained within the cystic collection as defined by pre-intervention imaging indicates the likely extent of debridement that may be necessary.
- Cystgastrostomy suture line hemostasis should be achieved through the use of appropriate laparoendoscopic staple height or a running suture method.

Symptomatic or enlarging pancreatic pseudocysts should ideally undergo a decompressive procedure that achieves internal drainage. Percutaneous external catheter drainage has a higher failure rate due to incomplete decompression and persistent external pancreatic fistula. Because most pseudocysts form in the lesser sac, a transgastric route for drainage is most commonly chosen. Historically, open drainage with cystgastrostomy was the mainstay of therapy. The procedure consists of anterior gastrostomy, followed by identification of the pseudocyst by palpation or visualization of a bulging of the posterior wall of the stomach. Localization is confirmed by needle aspiration of typically dark, murky pseudocyst fluid (sometimes described as crankcase oil in consistency). Aspiration of frankly bloody fluid should raise suspicion for the presence of pseudoaneurysm, which should be treated by angiographic embolization. After needle localization, the common wall between the pseudocyst and stomach is widely opened using electrocautery. The cavity is digitally explored, and then solid and liquid debris are aspirated completely. Definitive marsupialization of the pseudocyst is achieved by a continuous suture technique that also ensures hemostasis. The anterior gastrotomy is then closed in single- or two-layer fashion.

More recently, as minimally invasive procedures have become more widely adopted, endoscopic and laparoscopic approaches have repeatedly been shown to be safe and effective and have largely supplanted open surgical approaches as the preferred approach (see box below). The principles of laparoscopic cystgastrostomy are essentially the same as the open approach: anterior gastrotomy is performed (usually with an energy device such as the harmonic scalpel), followed by localization of the bulge of the pseudocyst into the posterior gastric wall. A posterior cystgastrostomy may be created using laparoendoscopic stapler (with appropriate staple height to ensure hemostasis) or by a hand-sewn technique.

Endoscopic approaches rely on favorable anatomic relationships between the pseudocyst and an adjacent gastrointestinal lumen in order to achieve a reliably safe result. Most commonly, the posterior wall bulge of the pseudocyst is readily visible at endoscopy, allowing localization and confirmation of the target. Often, visualization is supplemented by endoscopic ultrasound to confirm the presence of fluid within the cystic collection, as well as the absence of interposed vascular or other critical structures that may be damaged with inadvertent puncture or disruption. Broad apposition between the gastric wall and the pseudocyst capsule is also important. Lesions that do not meet these criteria are much riskier for endoscopic management, and these patients are often best suited to surgical management. Pseudocysts that abut the duodenum rather than stomach may sometimes be approachable for endoscopic cyst-duodenostomy, although this may be technically more challenging and riskier. Roux-en-Y cyst-jejunostomy, performed by open or laparoscopic technique, is a versatile and generally straightforward surgical option for internal drainage of pseudocysts that are not amenable to cystgastrostomy.

Alternative Approaches and Controversies

- Overall treatment options for pancreatic pseudocyst include operative, endoscopic, and percutaneous approaches.
- There is a substantial lack of evidence to suggest superiority of any of these approaches over alternative approaches.

There is a substantial lack of high-quality clinical evidence comparing the effectiveness of endoscopic versus surgical approaches, and the available literature to date mostly consists of case series and retrospective reviews. The single such randomized prospective trial found that surgical and endoscopic management of pancreatic pseudocyst were essentially equal in their treatment efficacy and recurrence rates, although endoscopic management tended to be associated with shorter hospital length of stay, lower overall cost of treatment, and higher postprocedural health-related quality of life compared to open surgical management [2]. However, this study was limited by low patient enrollment at a single institution and was ultimately underpowered to detect meaningful differences in outcomes between the two groups. The largest retrospective case series of patients managed endoscopically identified a treatment success rate of 75%, complication rate of 10%, and recurrence rate of 5.6%; 14% of patients required subsequent surgical management [3]. Another large case series reviewing patients managed endoscopically noted a treatment success rate of 93.5% and recurrence rate of 5%, with 13% requiring subsequent surgical management [4]. One case series of 106 patients undergoing laparoscopic management of pancreatic pseudocysts found a treatment success rate of 100%, with a recurrence rate of only 0.9% and complication rate of 6.6% [5]. In general, minimally invasive techniques are felt to confer less postprocedural pain, fewer complications, non-inferior technical success, shorter length of stay, and lower cost than open surgical approaches.

There is unfortunately a considerable paucity of randomized trials that compare these techniques head-to-head, and therefore most of the available literature comprises retrospective case series and reviews. The single prospective randomized trial to date compared patients who underwent open surgical or endoscopic management but did not enroll patients treated laparoscopically. While rates of treatment success, complications, and need for further intervention were not significantly different between groups, endoscopic therapy was associated with shorter hospital length of stay (2 vs. 6 days) and lower overall treatment cost ($7011 vs. $15,052) [6]. One retrospective review of patients undergoing endoscopic, laparoscopic, or open cystgastrostomy found no significant differences in treatment success rates or complication rates across the three treatment approaches, though a significantly higher rate of crossover from initial endoscopic therapy to any surgical therapy was noted, as compared to the rate of crossover from any initial surgical therapy to endoscopic therapy [7].

Notably, endoscopic techniques have improved substantially in recent years with the advent of devices more adept at stenting cystenterostomies with larger and more durable communications. In particular, lumen-opposing expandable stents have gained more frequent use, as the dumbbell configuration limits stent migration, and its self-expanding nature creates a larger cystenterostomy diameter to promote prolonged drainage, avoid stent occlusion by necrotic debris, and facilitate endoscopic debridement [8, 9].

Conclusion

Debate continues about the relative merits of surgical versus endoscopic approaches. However, most experienced practitioners agree that patients with pancreatic pseudocysts are best served by the least invasive approach possible, and that, ultimately, an individualized treatment approach based on the characteristics of the pseudocyst and its relationship to adjacent structures should be undertaken. The relationship of the pseudocyst to the wall of the stomach, duodenum, or jejunum is paramount in determining the feasibility and safety of endoscopic therapy; patients with pseudocysts that are not well apposed to adjacent enteral structures or that have critical structures interposed, such as solid organs, major vessels, or other uninvolved viscera, are generally felt to be less suitable candidates for safe endoscopic therapy and therefore are likely better served by initial laparoscopic or open surgical management.

Overall Management Pearls

- Internal drainage by surgical or endoscopic means is generally far preferable than external percutaneous drainage.
- Endoscopic management of pancreatic pseudocysts should be pursued when safe and technically feasible.
- In cases of pancreatic pseudocyst suitable for surgical management, a laparoscopic approach to cystgastrostomy or cystenterostomy may be indicated depending on availability of appropriate instrumentation and assistance, and the degree of surgeon experience/expertise.

- In general, the treatment approach for the patient with symptomatic pancreatic pseudocyst should progress from less invasive options (endoscopic/laparoscopic) to more invasive options (open operation), as less invasive approaches tend to be associated with equivalent success rates, less pain, shorter hospital length of stay, and fewer complications.
- Appropriate management must be tailored to individual patients taking into consideration the situation of the pseudocyst in relation to other structures, including stomach and bowel, major vessels, and dilated venous collaterals that may preclude safe undertaking of one approach over another.

References

1. Banks PA, Bollen TL, Dervenis C, Gooszen HG, Johnson CD, Sarr MG, et al. Classification of acute pancreatitis–2012: revision of the Atlanta classification and definitions by international consensus. Gut. 2013;62(1):102–11.
2. Varadarajulu S, Bang JY, Sutton BS, Trevino JM, Christein JD, Wilcox CM. Equal efficacy of endoscopic and surgical cystogastrostomy for pancreatic pseudocyst drainage in a randomized trial. Gastroenterology. 2013;145(3):583–90.
3. Weckman L, Kylänpää M-L, Puolakkainen P, Halttunen J. Endoscopic treatment of pancreatic pseudocysts. Surg Endosc. 2006;20(4):603–7.
4. Varadarajulu S, Bang JY, Phadnis MA, Christein JD, Wilcox CM. Endoscopic transmural drainage of peripancreatic fluid collections: outcomes and predictors of treatment success in 211 consecutive patients. J Gastrointest Surg. 2011;15(11):2080–8.
5. Palanivelu C, Senthilkumar K, Madhankumar MV, Rajan PS, Shetty AR, Jani K, et al. Management of pancreatic pseudocyst in the era of laparoscopic surgery–experience from a tertiary centre. Surg Endosc. 2007;21(12):2262–7.
6. Varadarajulu S, Bang JY, Sutton BS, Trevino JM, Christein JD, Wilcox CM. Equal efficacy of endoscopic and surgical cystogastrostomy for pancreatic pseudocyst drainage in a randomized trial. Gastroenterology. 2013;145(3):583–90.
7. Melman L, Azar R, Beddow K, Brunt LM, Halpin VJ, Eagon JC, et al. Primary and overall success rates for clinical outcomes after laparoscopic, endoscopic, and open pancreatic cystgastrostomy for pancreatic pseudocysts. Surg Endosc. 2009;23(2):267–71.
8. Shah RJ, Shah JN, Waxman I, Kowalski TE, Sanchez-Yague A, Nieto J, et al. Safety and efficacy of endoscopic ultrasound-guided drainage of pancreatic fluid collections with lumen-apposing covered self-expanding metal stents. Clin Gastroenterol Hepatol. 2015;13(4):747–52.
9. Patil R, Ona MA, Papafragkakis C, Anand S, Duddempudi S. Endoscopic ultrasound-guided placement of AXIOS stent for drainage of pancreatic fluid collections. Ann Gastroenterol. 2016;29(2):168–73.

Index

Note: Page numbers followed by *f and* t indicate figures and tables respectively

T.M. Pawlik et al. (eds.), *Case-Based Lessons in the Management of Complex Hepato-Pancreato-Biliary Surgery*, DOI 10.1007/978-3-319-50868-9

MIX
Papier aus verantwortungsvollen Quellen
Paper from responsible sources
FSC® C105338

If you have any concerns about our products,
you can contact us on
ProductSafety@springernature.com

In case Publisher is established outside the EU,
the EU authorized representative is:
Springer Nature Customer Service Center GmbH
Europaplatz 3, 69115 Heidelberg, Germany

Printed by Libri Plureos GmbH
in Hamburg, Germany